3⁷ ⁰⁰

X - RAY ANATOMY OF THE VASCULAR SYSTEM

X-ray Anatomy of the Vascular System

G. Luzsa, M. D.

Chief Physician of the Radiological Department
City Hospital, Mosonmagyaróvár (Hungary)

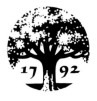

J. B. Lippincott Company

PHILADELPHIA AND TORONTO

Translated

by

A. DEÁK

Library of Congress Catalog Card Number: 73−8047

ISBN −0−397−58088−6

Published 1974 jointly by

J. B. LIPPINCOTT COMPANY, PHILADELPHIA AND TORONTO

BUTTERWORTH & CO. (PUBLISHERS) LTD., LONDON

and

AKADÉMIAI KIADÓ, BUDAPEST

To the memory of my father

PREFACE

Of the morphological branches of medicine it is perhaps in roentgenology that the necessity to approach problems from a functional point of view is greatest. In vivo visualization of the vascular system by means of radio-opaque matter reveals a phase in the actual functioning of a given segment, while postmortem angiography presents all possible varieties in which blood vessels are filled with contrast medium. Postmortem angiography is, therefore, anatomically superior and functionally inferior to intravital radiography, a fact that lends importance to the study of postmortem angiograms. Knowledge of anatomical details enables the roentgenologist to achieve correct evaluation of clinical manifestations. The aim of the present work on postmortem angiography is to serve as a handbook for a correct interpretation of vasograms made in vivo. It was intended to offer anatomical information for clinical application.

It seemed necessary to make these remarks in order to justify the postmortem radiographic representation of vascular anatomy. Though perhaps unusual, this procedure has made it possible to present a comparatively large area of the vascular system. The almost unlimited increase in literature has prevented the author from making this work as complete as he would have wished it to be. Nevertheless, he hopes to have succeeded in presenting to the reader all essential details in an adequately proportioned arrangement.

As regards the fundamentals of theoretical anatomy, indispensable for the writing of this book, I was trained at the Anatomical Institute, Semmelweis Medical University, Budapest, then under the leadership of the late Professor F. Kiss. It was at the side of J. Halmi, chief radiologist of the hospital at Győr, that I became conversant with the various aspects of roentgenology. I shall always cherish the memory of these two scientists. My gratitude is due to Professor J. Szentágothai, presently director of the Anatomical Institute, Semmelweis Medical University, Budapest, whose assistance and encouragement meant so much to me when writing this work. I wish to express my thanks for his valuable advice, and I am indebted to him as also to M. Erdélyi, Professor of Roentgenology at the Postgraduate Medical School of Budapest, for the supervision of the present work. I am glad to express my gratitude for the zealous and untiring help rendered by my collaborators Miss E. Gincsay, Mrs. T. Schwendtner, Mr. S. Meszlényi, Mrs. E. Vagyon, Miss K. Nagy and Mr. Z. Tatár in connection with the dissections, taking of X-ray pictures, the preparation of drawings and the typing. I must not omit to mention Mr. and Mrs. M. Seregdy, both of them engineers, to whom credit is due for the precise and true drawings in India ink. Also Mr. M. Borsa, technical assistant, is entitled to thanks in this respect. I am obliged to Dr. I. Gorácz and Dr. S. Szücs for the permission to use roentgenograms. Credit is due to the Publishing House of the Hungarian Academy of Sciences for the publication and excellent layout of my book.

GYÖRGY LUZSA

CONTENTS

9

INTRODUCTION

By reason of the special conditions of radiology, X-ray anatomy of the vascular system is a morphological science based on functional considerations. Although blood vessels were visualized in cadaveric organs in the very year of the discovery of X-rays (Haschek and Lindenthal 1896, Addison 1896, cit. by Sutton 1962) technical difficulties prevented their employment in vivo for a long time. It required lengthy studies of postmortem angiography (Jamin and Merkel 1907, Crainicianu 1922, Laubry et al. 1939, Czmór and Urbányi 1939) before the technique of contrast material injection into the living blood vessels, i.e. angiography, was elaborated (Moniz and Lima 1927, Sicard and Forestier 1923, Berberich and Hirsch 1923, Dos Santos 1935, Castellanos et al. 1937, Robb and Steinberg 1940). Angiography as a method has been introduced in clinical practice in the past twenty years.

Progress in surgical procedures and clinical therapy has considerably increased the importance of the recognition of vascular diseases. While the anatomy of the vascular system was restricted to mere morphology at the beginning of the 20th century, the routine application of angiography has made it possible to study the "morphological picture" from a functional angle. Though a young branch of science, roentgenology has been enjoying a renaissance since the introduction of angiography. Accurate knowledge of anatomy is a *conditio sine qua non* for correct diagnosis. Textbooks on anatomy and topographical anatomy describe the course and regional distribution of blood vessels in several dimensions. There are, however, certain areas which cannot be studied without angiography, e.g., anastomoses, organic angioarchitecture, relationships to bones, regions hardly explorable by dissection, further projection anatomy. Knowledge about the polymorphism of the vascular system has made vast progress since the injection of vessels with contrast material has become a routine procedure. While, previously the anatomical variations were only of theoretical interest, now their knowledge is indispensable in the daily practice of the angiologist.

The anatomy of blood vessels and their variants has been studied on anatomical preparations by numerous investigators. Although many authors have carefully evaluated thousands of cases, most of the works on angiography deal with normal morphology only to the extent that is necessary for the interpretation of the pathological phenomena occurring within the sphere of their special interest. Thus, the necessity arose to collect the available data into a synthesis. Accordingly, the present work has a twofold aim: (*i*) to provide clinicians and roentgenologist, engaged in angiography, with precise x-ray anatomical details which cover the entire vascular system and include normal variants; (*ii*) to acquaint medical students concerned with anatomy and specialists with the true relationship of vessels to the adjacent organs and with their distribution in the organs in areas that cannot be explored by any other technique.

The present work is thus a roentgenological presentation of vascular anatomy which shows the typical vessel courses by way of two- or three-dimensional radiography. By filling in situ even the smallest vessels that can be found in the anatomical nomenclature, by isolating certain organs or groups of organs, the vessels can be visualized regionally without the disturbing shadows of bones and soft tissues. Besides the description of the typical vessels it seemed necessary to illustrate the variations in origin, distribution and division with line drawings. The present work follows the Paris Nomina Anatomica (1955).

The application of the terms *variation* and *anomaly* in the literature is rather inconsistent. The present work discusses the variations that exist under normal haemodynamic conditions. Thus, anomalies causing pathological circulation are not dealt with. Distinction in this respect is often difficult because certain vascular variations may persist throughout life without causing trouble, while they cease to ensure the required blood supply if circulatory insufficiency supervenes. A good example in this respect is offered by faulty development of the circle of Willis which cannot be correctly diagnosed without angiography. Such questions must, of course, be dealt with by treating the variants in extent. Opening of the pulmonary veins into the left atrium with a common trunk is a variant, whereas their course into the portal vein is regarded as anomaly. It was intended to present the variants, as extensively as possible and within the limit of their clinical significance. Description of the collateral circulation of the various organs and parts of the body as a supplement to clinical anatomy, should enable the clinician to judge anatomical variations reliably when faced with a specific pathological picture. Chapters dealing with contrast filling refer briefly to in vivo application, while the description of postmortem angiography should facilitate the correct interpretation of the radiograph.

It should be noted that postmortem angiography is not sufficient for a correct interpretation of angiograms made in vivo, since the two pictures are not identical. This question is discussed in detail in this book. The illustrations and the text give the morphology of the vascular system that forms the basis for the evaluation of in vivo angiograms.

METHODS

The usefulness of postmortem angiography depends on the correct injection and preparation techniques.

Contrast media must be easily injectable, uniformly spreading and strongly radio-opaque substances. The currently used *pure barium sulphate*, after the addition of some viscosity-promoting colloid, fills the vessels up to 0·5 to 1 mm. We did not attempt to visualize smaller structures since our aim was postmortem reconstruction of the intravital angiograph. Contrast material was injected on the roentgen table, and the pictures were taken immediately after injection so that the application of 5 to 10 per cent formalin, currently used, was often unnecessary. *Novobarium oralis*, a Hungarian water-soluble preparation, diluted to cream thickness, proved to be the most suitable. Although increase in contrast can be obtained by higher concentrations, higher viscosity of the medium requires increased pressure of the injections which, exceeding certain limit, results in the supersaturation of the central vessels at the expense of the periphery. If the dilution of the contrast medium by blood is to be expected, as in the case of the major veins, this method is applicable to decrease the intensity of shadows. Contrast material of excessive density should therefore never be employed for filling the arteries because more air bubbles will develop in this dense mixture which disturb the evaluation of the pictures.

Technique of injection. Uniform filling of the peripheral vessels is best obtained by rhythmic administration at medium pressure through an easily moving syringe. The filling is accomplished when no more contrast material can be injected without increased pressure. The piston of the syringe is pushed backward on account of overpressure. Injection with the aid of an apparatus replacing normal blood pressure (Tucker and Krementz 1957) is not necessary, since postmortem filling depends on the nature of the contrast material and the physical properties of the vessel walls; intravital haemodynamic conditions need not be regarded (Schoenmackers 1960). Correct filling requires skill.

Preparation preceding injection is made by a blunt exposure with the slightest possible damage to the tissues. When a particular vascular segment is free, a ligature is applied proximally and distally from the point of the intended filling. The proximal segment must be tied up, while the distal segment lies in a loose loop. The next step is to make an aperture on the vessel that should be somewhat narrower than the cannula into which a properly fitting glass tube, filled with radio-opaque matter, is then inserted. The cannula must be fixed at once, particularly in case of arteries, because it slips back very easily. The end of the tube distal to the body is connected by a rubber pipe with the syringe. Before the actual injection the piston of the syringe must be pulled back in order to remove the air from the vessel. While finely emulsified air does not disturb the shadow of the greater vessels, air bubbles may render the analysis of the minute vasculature difficult.

Contrast filling of the *entire arterial system* can be achieved via the subclavian artery with the use of about 170 to 220 ml of radio-opaque material. In this case initial pressure should be higher in order to obtain a closure of the aortic valves. When filling the *veins* (1,000 to 1,500 ml) the pulmonary vessels can also be visualized. About 100 to 150 ml of the contrast medium is needed for the visualization of the *portal system*, and 100 to 200 ml for that of the *branches of the pulmonary trunk*. We often filled up isolated regions of the body: the necessary amount of contrast material varied according to the individual case which determined also the site and the manner of injection.

To demonstrate the *arteries of the extremities* it is necessary to perform anterograde filling through the subclavian artery and the distal portion of the abdominal aorta, respectively. This way also the vessels of the shoulder girdle and the pelvis are uniformly visualized. In order to demonstrate the *arteries of the head*, first the aorta around the isthmus must be ligated and then the radio-opaque substance injected into the ascending aorta. Such injection fills simultaneously both the carotid and the subclavian arteries. Separate ligature of the external or internal carotid artery ensures individual visualization of the vessels of the brain or the skeleton of the face. The lateral picture of the external carotid artery is best obtained by unilateral filling in order to avoid a superposition of the bilateral shadows. This method cannot be used in the case of the internal carotid artery because of the numerous connections of the two sides. Moniz (1940) attempted to obtain isolated filling of one hemisphere by taking postmortem angiograms immediately after having simultaneously injected water into one side and contrast material into the other. We filled the brain completely through all the four arteries, a procedure which yields pictures notably different from those seen in vivo. Analysis of such pictures facilitates, however, the study of the superimposed details of the internal carotid artery and the vertebral artery. In this case we can present an in vivo angiogram as well which supplements the postmortem pictures with the demonstration of normal haemodynamic conditions (radiographs by Gorácz). The *thoracic arteries* can be filled either through the abdominal aorta or the subclavian artery. The aorta must be ligated at the height of the diaphragm. Thus the coronary arteries are filled, too. Although their initial segment is confluent with the shadow of the bulb of aorta, topographical conditions are still better demonstrable in this way than by their separate filling following exposure (Schoenmackers and Vieten 1954). Arteriographic visualization of the *abdominal viscera* can be obtained by anterograde injection of the thoracic aorta or by synchronous retrograde filling through the two femoral arteries. For the demonstration of the vessels of the individual abdominal organs (e.g., kidney, liver, spleen, intestines) it is advisable to dissect them after complete filling, freed from the neighbouring tissues. Of the organs with filled vascular system the x-ray pictures are taken extra-abdominaly. This way we may avoid the otherwise frequent occurrence of the accessory vessels remaining uninjected. Arteries filled with white contrast medium are well distinguishable at dissection.

In order to demonstrate the *veins of the extremities* it is necessary to prepare a minor vessel in the distal portion of the limbs. Centripetal injection will fill the veins lying proximally to the site of injection. The veins of the fingers and the toes cannot be demonstrated by this method on account of the presence of valves. Filling through the capillaries by means of the arterial circulation can be performed in vivo only, and the contrast shadow so obtained is pale. The *veins of the head* are best demonstrated through the superior vena cava. With the isolated filling of the internal jugular vein, the injected material usually escapes through the collaterals without filling the veins of the brain appreciably. Superposition of the shadows of the great veins and venous plexus renders differentiation in the roentgenograms of the cervical region difficult. The *thoracic veins* can be best filled through a tube inserted in the right auricle. The contrast medium does not pass into the lesser circulation if the pulmonary trunk is ligated. The intercostal veins are demonstrated by filling them with an intraspongiosal procedure (radiograph by Szücs). Demonstration of the *abdominal veins* is carried out by retrograde filling through the thoracic segment of the inferior vena cava or anterogradely through the femoral vein. Since the hepatic veins are highly vulnerable, the injection should be given at a moderate pressure, and repeated roentgenograms should be taken to check the degree of filling.

Precapillary angiography of the *lesser circulation* can be carried out with simultaneous phlebography of the thoracic veins via the filling of the right heart or the isolated preparation of the pulmonary trunk. Care must be taken in this case not to injure the pleura because vessels collapsed owing to the resulting pneumothorax will no longer represent intravital conditions. Postcapillaries of the pulmonary vessels are filled retrogradely through the left auricle or the aorta. In the latter case the cannula should be passed into the left ventricle through the aortic valve. Pressure required for the demonstration of the peripheral minor branches may abnormally dilate the left atrium. Enlargement of the atrial contours seen in roentgenograms becomes still more pronounced by the overlapping projections of the terminal segments of the pulmonary veins.

The *portal system* can be visualized through a mesenteric vein. Provided the width of the portal vessels is normal, the contrast medium, more viscous than blood, can pass into the caval system only through rectal anastomoses and never through the collaterals. This is also confirmed by the fact that, after the portal apparatus has been filled and all rectal communications tied up, the entire complex of abdominal organs can be lifted out without a drop of the contrast material in the caval system being lost, even though the vessels are cut in many places.

The arterial system of the *newborn* together with the arteries of the lesser circulation can be demonstrated best through the aorta or the umbilical artery; the veins, through the right auricle. In the latter case also the pulmonary and portal veins are filled. The aorta and the initial portion of the pulmonary trunk must be ligated for such manipulation. Veins of the extremities lying distal to the proximal valves are not demonstrable due to retrograde filling.

Contrast filling, performed by the described methods, may be supplemented by the radiograms of *isolated organ preparations* which must be carried out in every case, following injection in situ and secondary preparation of the organ. Pictures obtained in this way illustrate the angioarchitecture of the vessels of the various organs—brain, heart, lungs, liver, spleen, stomach, intestines, kidneys, genital organs—with sharper contrast. In case of the liver, the combined demonstration of the hepatic artery and the portal vein or of the bile ducts gives a better view of interrelations, just as it is the case with the simultaneous filling of the hepatic veins and the portal vein. If, after the filling of the arterial or portal part of the abdominal vessels, the abdominal viscera are removed in toto, the x-ray pictures of the organs will be without the disturbing shadows of the soft tissues of the abdominal wall and of the bones. Combined in situ illustration of the arteries of the pulmonary circulation and the thoracic veins, as well as of the pulmonary veins and the aorta facilitates a correct view of their dimensional arrangement. For the same reason the combined filling of the inferior vena cava and the portal system demonstrates conditions of projection in and around the liver. Since the isolated organ complexes are not preserved preparations, they do not retain their shape after removal. Accordingly, radiographs taken in such cases do not aim at topographical orientation but are to demonstrate the distribution and division of vessels.

The applied **x-ray technique** demonstrates the vascular regions in question in the typical manner, just as it is done for in vivo examinations. Dimensional arrangements are thus not demonstrated by stereoscopic pictures (Jamin and Merkel 1907, Vastesaeger et al.1955, Heinz 1968) but by pictures taken from two directions. These pictures, offering in most cases considerably more projected representations than angiographic procedures in vivo, should afterwards facilitate a better understanding of conditions in vivo. The three-plane pictures of the neck and the skull mean a further improvement of this technique. The adjustment of two- or three-plane roentgenograms is hard and time-consuming owing to the characteristics of the dead body, e.g., rigor mortis. In some instances, as in the case of the lateral view of the neck, in vivo roentgenological conditions cannot be reproduced. We used for our *roentgenograms* a four-valve x-ray apparatus of the type Auto-Heliophos 500, further Ferrania, Supervidox and Forte films. The typical pictures were made on films in light-tight paper containers provided with an intensifying screen. Foil-free films were employed for isolated organ preparations in order to increase image contrast. Examinations in such cases were repeatedly performed with the aid of a one-tank Siemens ball (10 mA). It should be noted that the exposure factors of typical radiograms is 15 to 20 per cent less than of pictures of the same regions made in vivo. Considering that radiographic examinations were usually performed 2 to 6 hours after death, it was merely the sinking of blood following death that meant a difference as compared to in vivo conditions. This, however, does not influence the radiological characteristics. Further observations, measurements and phantom experiments are required to clarify the problem.

DIFFERENCE BETWEEN IN VIVO AND POSTMORTEM ANGIOGRAPHY

Filling of blood vessels in vivo and postmortem differ from each other in certain aspects. Postmortem filling is determined by the width of the vessels, the physical properties of the contrast material and the applied pressure. Blood pressure drops to zero after death. Owing to the increasing number of smooth muscles, the lumina of peripheral arteries appear to be wider than that of the central vessels, more abundantly provided with elastic fibres. Postmortem roentgenograms present a "more abundantly vascularized" pattern than those made during life. Structural differences between the walls of major and minor veins are negligible so that discrepancies of this nature need not be considered (Schoenmackers and Vieten 1954).

Conditions of filling the vessels in vivo depend on the tone of the muscles, the direct action of substances regulating physiologic circulation, temperature and vascular innervation. This manifests itself in the filling of vessels that provide the circulation of the organ. Extensive collaterals connecting two vascular areas may thus remain invisible. Incomplete filling under these conditions is therefore not to be attributed to the underdevelopment or pathologic alteration of the vessels, but to the necessary humoral and neurogenic regulation of circulation. At rest relatively few vessels participate in the circulation under normal conditions, while the collaterals are filled at increased exertion (Ránky 1962). Deficient vascular pattern under postmortem conditions is due either to congenital or acquired anatomical anomalies or to some error in the filling. Another difference is that the contrast substance, diluted by blood in the living organism flows in the midline of the vessels where the rate of flow is the fastest so that their marginal zone remains more radiolucent. Frik and Persch (1969) found that water insoluble contrast substances that caused emboli in the blood make the lumina of the vessels larger than do water soluble materials that mix with blood. In cadavers the entire cross-section of vessels gives a homogenous shadow. The most striking example in this respect is the superior sagittal sinus, which appears as a narrow band in x-ray pictures made in vivo, but shows the true anatomical form if filled after death. Under these circumstances, it is natural that postmortem angiograms facilitate only morphological orientation, and no conclusions can be drawn concerning physiological functions. The speed of the rate of flow cannot be ascertained; the angiographic "capillary phase" is also lacking since vessels with diameters less than 0.5 to 1.0 mm cannot be filled from either side. Application of a contrast medium able to fill still narrower vessels produces pictures that cannot be evaluated because of the superposition and confluence of shadows. The situation is different in microradiography.

The interpretation of both in vivo and postmortem angiograms is influenced by physical properties of the x-ray pictures. Instead of taking stereoscopic roentgenograms when trying to represent dimensional arrangements on flat sheets, up-to-date radiology prefers pictures taken from two directions. On this occasion many difficulties arise in contrast filling in vivo which do not present themselves in postmortem filling when studying the pathological-anatomical alterations of vessels. It is indispensable to study the precise course of the vessels in order to obtain a correct anatomical view. Appreciation of the intersections and ramifications of vessels is facilitated by the simultaneous visualization of two pictures taken from opposite directions. The actual and not the projected length and the cross section of vessels can be estimated much better this way. Based on the studies by Frik and Persch (1969) it can be stated that the measurement of vessels obtained by postmortem angiography indicates in vivo conditions only in case of the larger vessels. Ramification of larger into smaller vessels and the angle of their division can be better observed if viewed from two directions. Examinations of isolated organ complexes facilitates a better understanding of in vivo observations. Angioarchitecture remains unchanged in postmortem angiograms and only the didactic value of postmortem angiograms is higher. Though, corrosion and other anatomical procedures serve the same purpose, those engaged in the analysis of roentgenograms will nevertheless find postmortem angiograms more useful in preliminary studies for the everyday clinical practice.

BLOOD VESSELS OF THE THORAX

THE HEART

Topography and projection anatomy

The heart is situated in the mediastinum with two thirds to the left and one third to the right of the median line. The entire organ is between the two layers of the pericardium. Through the major vessels and through the pericardium it is in close connection with its surroundings. The three sides and the base of the pyramidally shaped organ stands out as a well-definable surface among the neighbouring structures. The heart is attached to the respiratory system and the major vessels by the aorta saddling the left principal bronchus, as well as by the superior vena cava, which, via the azygos vein, is closely connected with the right principal bronchus. Connection with the diaphragm and the liver is through the inferior vena cava. The pulmonary arteries and veins together with the bronchi, ensure the anatomical unity of the heart and the respiratory system.

Projection topography of the surfaces and orifices. The *sternocostal, the anterior surface of the heart* lies against the anterior wall of the thorax, partly directly and partly slightly covered by the two lungs. The left membrane of the pleura turns laterally behind the fourth sternocostal joint, while the right membrane continues its downward course. Thus, the pericardium lies free in an approximately triangular area, the size of which varies according to the position of the heart. It extends, as a rule to the anterior angle of the 4th to 8th ribs. The free area is in contact with the sternum and the ribs. The distance between the pericardium and sternum amounts to 1 to 5 cm. The distance increases upwards (Testut and Jacob 1921). The retrosternal space increases on deep inspiration (Zdansky 1962). One third of the heart is to the right of the median line in the projection of the chest's anterior surface. It includes the right atrium—excepting the apex of the auricle—the interatrial septum, half of the left atrium, a small portion of the right ventricle as well as the contact surface of the aorta and the pulmonary trunk (Joessel 1889). Half of the left atrium with the left auricle, the apex of the right auricle, the major part of the right ventricle, the left ven-

tricle and the interventricular septum are to the left of the median line.

Projected on the anterior wall of the thorax, the heart shows an approximately quadrangular picture (Fig. 1). Its *upper border* lies transversely across the upper part of the body of the sternum at a distance of 1 to 1·5 cm from the edge of the manubrium sterni (Paturet 1958). The *right border*, running at a distance of 1 cm from the sternum, passes steeply downward from the upper edge of the 2nd intercostal space or the 3rd rib to the 5th sternocostal joint. This line is constituted by the superior vena cava and the margin of the right atrium. Its upper part extends beyond and its lower part coincides with the projection of the right border of the vertebral column. The *left border* begins 2 cm from the margin of the sternum in the 2nd intercostal space or at the upper edge of the 3rd rib and

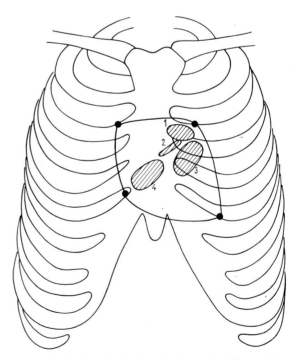

Fig. 1. Projection of the boundaries and orifices of the heart on the anterior thoracic wall. (*1*) Orifice of the pulmonary trunk; (*2*) orifice of the aorta; (*3*) left atrioventricular orifice; (*4*) right atrioventricular orifice.

runs obliquely downward to the apex of the heart. The latter is in the 5th intercostal space in the medioclavicular line, at a distance of 8 to 10 cm from the midline. The apex of the heart is in the 4th intercostal space in children, and in the 6th in old age (Knese 1963). The projection of the left border lies along a straight line formed by the left auricle and the left ventricle. Above, it is joined by the projection of the pulmonary trunk and the aortic arch. The *lower border* runs from right to left from the 6th sternocostal joint to the apex of the heart. This line corresponds to the right margin resting on the diaphragm, while its end on the right coincides with the lower end of the right atrium.

If a line is drawn from the right lower to the left upper corner of this tetragon, it will approximately run along the projection of the coronary sulcus. The superjacent triangle corresponds to the atria, while the subjacent triangle to the ventricles (Knese 1963).

Projections of the various cardiac orifices on the thoracic wall can be summed up as follows.

The longitudinal axis of the *right atrioventricular orifice* (Figs 1/4, 10/1, 37/4, 38/4, 39/4, 40/2) may be characterized by a line which connects the anterior end of the right 6th rib with the sternal end of the 3rd rib. The right border of the orifice is at the sternal end of the height of the 5th or 6th rib (Joessel 1889). The centre of the ostium is at the intersection of the above line with the perpendicular line at the height of the 5th rib. The line is 40 to 42 mm long (Debierre 1908).

The *left atrioventricular orifice* (Figs 1/3, 10/3, 37/13, 38/12, 39/13, 40/5) is projected on the sternal end of the left 4th rib and the parasternal parts of the 3rd and 4th intercostal spaces. The centre of the orifice is approximately behind the border of the sternum. Its length is generally 38 to 44 mm (Debierre 1908).

The *pulmonary orifice* (Figs 1/1, 10/2, 37/5, 38/5, 39/5, 40/3) has a diameter of 20 to 22 mm (Debierre 1908) and can be found in or somewhat to the left of the projection of the sternal end of the left 3rd rib (Sick 1885). Its centre is at a distance of 28 mm from the median plane (Virchow 1913).

The *aortic orifice* (Figs 1/2, 10/4, 37/14, 38/13, 39/14, 40/6) shows a line which runs from the sternal end of the 3rd left rib obliquely to the 4th right intercostal space. Its right border reaches the median plane, while its middle part is at the sternal end of the 4th left rib at a distance of 16 mm from the midline (Virchow 1913).

The *lower surface* of the heart rests on the diaphragm. This area is occupied by the left and right ventricles and by the inferior vena cava entering into the right atrium. The plane of the diaphragm is slightly arched in the frontal view and oblique in the sagittal view. Separated from the pericardium and the diaphragm lies the left lobe of the liver and to its left the fundus of the stomach is situated below the heart.

Since the size of the left hepatic lobe is variable, the mutual arrangement of these organs shows individual differences according to the dimensions of the air bubble ("Magenblase"). In case of an empty stomach the left flexure of the colon is seen next to the heart's lower surface between the left hepatic lobe and the spleen.

The *surfaces facing the mediastinum* are in contact with the adjacent pulmonary lobes. To the right, the right atrium together with a small part of the ventricle impress the upper and middle lobes, while to the left the upper and lower lobes are impressed by the left ventricle and auricle (cardiac impression). On the two sides of the pericardium the pericardiacophrenic vessels and the phrenic nerve run towards the diaphragm.

The projection of the *posterior surface* of the heart appears at the height of the 4th to 8th thoracic vertebrae (Testut and Jacob 1921). The surface contacting with the neighbouring organs is formed here by a small portion of the right atrium, by the left atrium and by the left ventricle. The left atrium is situated anterior to and somewhat downward from the hilus of the lung. Above it, behind the right atrium, runs the right pulmonary artery, the backside of which contacts with the bifurcation of the trachea. The left principal bronchus lies against the pulmonary veins, whereas the right principal bronchus in front of and above the right inferior pulmonary vein adheres to the right upper border of the left atrium. The left atrium is separated from the esophagus by the pericardium only. The contact surface is 2 to 4 cm long (Gäbert 1924). The descending aorta is behind and to the left of the gullet, and the azygos vein runs behind and to the right of the esophagus.

Comparative projections of the chambers of the heart. The projections of the heart chambers in their correlative arrangements can be studied by means of serial sections (Pernkopf 1937, Töndury 1959), chamber casts (Pernkopf 1937, Sprer 1959) and angiocardiograms (Thurn 1958, Zdansky 1962, etc.). Serial sections serve just as a basis for the three-dimensional view, while casts cannot be prepared in situ. Postmortem filling facilitates the interpretation of angiocardiograms made during life because a simultaneous filling of the vessels belonging to both the pulmonary and the systemic circulation allows the visualization of a much larger vascular area. Comparative study of the projections is much easier this way. Based on the data of the above-

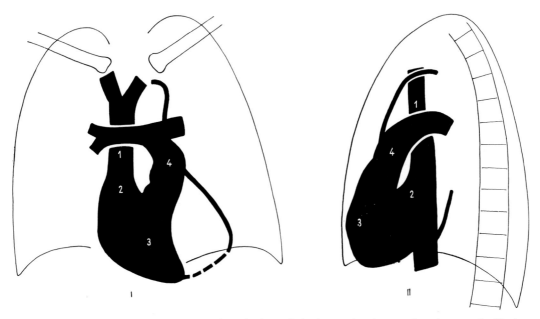

FIG. 2. Roentgenanatomical conditions of projection of the heart chambers and major vessels (dextro-cardiogram) I, anteroposterior view; II, lateral view. (1) Superior vena cava; (2) right atrium; (3) right ventricle; (4) pulmonary trunk.

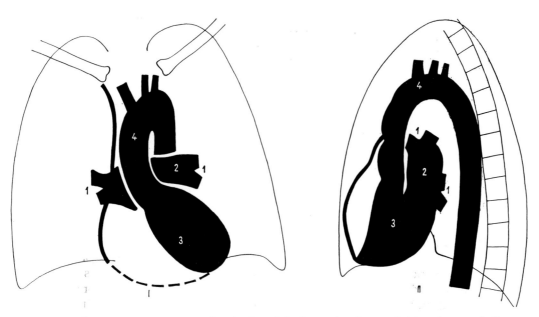

FIG. 3. Roentgenanatomical conditions of projection of the heart chambers and the major vessels (laevo-cardiogram). I, anteroposterior view; II, lateral view. (1) Pulmonary veins; (2) left atrium; (3) left ventricle; (4) aorta.

mentioned authors and our own studies, the summary of the projections of the heart and the major vessels is as follows (Figs 2, 3, 4).

The *right atrium* (Figs 2/2, 4/3, 36/1, 43/1, 47/7, 48/5, 52/3, 55/5) lies to the right of and dorsal to the right ventricle. Situated in the area between the lower sternal edge of the right 4th rib and the middle of the 3rd right costal cartilage on the right partly behind the right ventricle it occupies the right side of the heart. The auricle is projected in front of the aorta. The right inferior pulmonary vein passes in a transverse direction behind the upper end of the atrium, while the right superior pulmonary vein appears behind the superior vena cava. The *right ventricle*

21

(Figs 2/3, 4/4, 36/3, 43/3, 47/25, 52/4, 55/6, 56/7) is in anterior position, and its right margin marks the lower border of the heart shadow. It covers the inferior-medial part of the right atrium and more than two thirds of the left ventricle. Viewed laterally, the posterior half of the right ventricle overlaps three quarters of the left ventricle, while its anterior half together with the entire conus arteriosus are freely visible. In the anteroposterior view the conus

Radiological anatomy

Analysis of the x-ray anatomy of the heart may be carried out in four standard views: posteroanterior, first and second oblique, and right to left (Fig. 5).

The shadows of the heart and the great vessels appear between the radiolucent lungs as a part of the so-called *middle shadow* on the **sagittal** (postero-

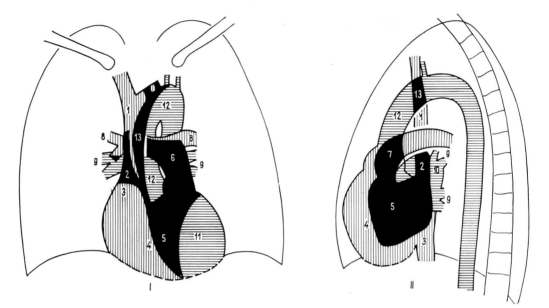

FIG. 4. Roentgenanatomical arrangements of the projection of the heart chambers and major vessels (superposition of laevo- and dextrocardiograms). I, anteroposterior view; II, lateral view. (*1*) Superior vena cava; (*2*) right and left atria; (*3*) right atrium; (*4*) right ventricle; (*5*) right and left ventricles; (*6*) pulmonary trunk and left atrium; (*7*) pulmonary trunk and aorta; (*8*) right and left pulmonary arteries; (*9*) pulmonary veins; (*10*) left atrium; (*11*) left ventricle; (*12*) aorta; (*13*) aorta and superior vena cava.

overshadows the left half of the left atrium as well as the aortic orifice. The *left atrium* (Figs 3/2, 4/10, 36/2, 43/2, 59/14), the most posterior part of the heart, extends downward somewhat below and behind the infundibulum. Its left half is covered by the right ventricle, its inferior third by both ventricles, its middle part by the aorta, and its right edge by the right auricle. Viewed laterally, its larger part is free and constitutes the posterior contour of the heart. The left ventricle is projected on its antero-inferior border, the inferior vena cava and the right atrium are projected on its anterior margin. The *left ventricle* (Figs 3/3, 4/11, 36/4, 43/4, 52/5, 59/5, 60/6, 61/3) is obscured by more than two thirds of the right ventricle. In the lateral view, three quarters of its shadow coalesces with the right ventricle, and behind, a minor part overlaps with both atria.

anterior, Fig. 37) **thoracic roentgenograms**. This mainly homogenous shadow passes without sharp contours into the surroundings below the sternal end of the clavicles and in the projection of the diaphragm. After hard exposure of the film, the sharper outline of the vertebral column may show in the midline. The air stripe of the trachea (Fig. 37/21) is visible in or slightly to the right of the median. It may be followed to the bifurcation in thin persons. It is especially in children that the orthodiagraphic projection of a part of the azygos vein, its proximal section opening into the superior vena cava, can be seen in the right tracheobronchial angle (Th. 5—6). With a pale contour the middle shadow continues laterally and upward-sideways forming a laterally concave curve and disappears in the projection of the clavicle. This area is the initial section of the right brachiocephalic vein (Fig. 37/1). Two curved parts of approximately equal lengths are traceable on the *right contour* of the middle shadow between the origin of the brachiocephalic vein and the diaphragm. The *upper flatter arch* corresponds to the right margin of the superior vena cava (Fig. 37/2). Depending on constitutional factors, the ascending aorta (Fig. 37/15), the margin of which is scarcely in the shadow of the superior vena cava, may extend beyond the border of this vein. The upper arch

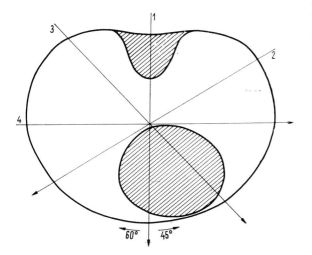

FIG. 5. Standard views for the examination of the heart. (*1*) Posteroanterior; (*2*) first oblique; (*3*) second oblique; (*4*) lateral view.

turns with a slight angle into the convex lower arch, which is formed by the right atrium. The right ventricle begins to the left of the boundary between the atrium and diaphragm. In the low position of the diaphragm in asthenic types, it may form a border. A pale shadow can sometimes be traced that fills the angle formed at the *transition of the lower arch and the diaphragm*. This corresponds to the adipose tissue or the supradiaphragmatic orifice of the right hepatic vein (Fig. 37/3). A slightly concave area, the so-called cardiac sinus, at the *left border* of the middle shadow is situated between two marked arches. Starting below the clavicle, the *upper arch* projects strongly forward. This regional projection of the isthmus of the aorta is called the *aortic knob* (Fig. 37/16). The laterally concave curve extending from the upper edge of the aortic knob to the clavicle represents the shadow of the left subclavian artery (Fig. 37/20). The depth of the cardiac sinus below the aortic knob is variable. Its two curved parts, the pulmonary arch and the left auricle, are more pronounced in young persons than in adults. The *pulmonary arch* (Fig. 37/6) represents the initial portion of the pulmonary trunk. The division of this vessel is not visible. The extent to which the *arch of the left auricle* protrudes be-

tween the pulmonary arch and the left inferior arch of the heart varies from individual to individual. It is in most cases confluent with the lower arch. The *lower left arch*, which is the longest and most pronounced, is formed by the border of the left ventricle with the *apex of the heart* at its lower end. The extent to which the left ventricle forms the left margin of the heart shadow depends on the position of the diaphragm and the respiratory phase. It is easier to determine the projection of the apex of the heart in children and thin adults. Often there is a small amount of adipose tissue in this area. It usually forms a concave boundary laterally, and the apex of the heart can be better seen therein during deep inspiration. The *lower border of the heart* is lost in the diaphragm without any distinguishable contour. However, this can be determined with fair accuracy by drawing a convex, slightly curved downward line from the apex of the heart to the right angle formed by the heart and the diaphragm.

First oblique view (right oblique view, fencing position, Fig. 38). When rotating the chest 60° to the left, the edge in front and at the back is formed by the right ventricle and the left atrium, respectively. The vertebral column and the heart are clearly distinguishable in this projection: the former is seen behind the latter. The more radiolucent area between them is Holzknecht's space; it includes the mediastinal and pulmonary configurations. Its upper part has a retrovascular, its lower part a retrocardiac position. The *right border* of the heart shadow is formed by the left atrium which making a slightly convex backward turn recedes from the vertebral column when approaching the diaphragm. The heart shadow forms here an angle with the diaphragm which is filled with the pale shadow of the inferior vena cava (Fig. 38/3). The translucent strip of the trachea (Fig. 38/20) and the right principal bronchus, covering the shadow of the superior vena cava, run above the heart shadow behind the posterior wall of the ascending aorta. The left bronchus is lost in the projection of the heart shadow. In the uppermost part of Holzknecht's space, the left angle of the scapula is projected on the posterior aspect of the aortic arch, while the descending aorta (Fig. 38/16) can be followed in front of the spine to the diaphragm. On account of the mediastinal structures it is the retrocardiac space that can best be studied during deep inspiration or during esophageal passage. Roentgenograms made in this view show above the ascending aorta (Fig. 38/14) and the anterior contour of the left brachiocephalic vein (Fig. 38/1) on the *left border* of the heart shadow. The shadow of the brachiocephalic vein is lost in the projection of the clavicle. The initial segment of the

23

pulmonary trunk (Fig. 38/6) casts a slightly curved shadow below the inferior margin of the ascending aorta. Its extent is variable. The arch formed by the pulmonary trunk passes without sharp boundary into the contour of the right ventricle or into the lower third of the contour of the left ventricle. It is impossible to draw the line between the two ventricles. The size of the area, forming the marginal contour, depends on the angle of rotation as also on the constitutional configuration of the heart.

Second oblique view (left oblique view, boxing position, Fig. 39). Projections made following a 45° rotation of the chest to the right offer a good view of the ventricles, atria and thoracic aorta. The heart appears in this projection in front of the spine shadow. Uppermost the arch of the left ventricle may cast a shadow on the edge of the latter. The *left margin of the heart* is formed by the left atrium above and the left ventricle below. The boundary between the two arches is marked by a slight retraction. The left border of the heart is much more convex than the right one. With the diaphragm in a low position, it is in this projection that the heart shadow can be best distinguished from the homogenous mass of the abdominal viscera. At the lower end of the ventricular arch, the shadow of the inferior vena cava (Fig. 39/3) passes steeply into the contour of the diaphragm. In case of the low position of the diaphragm, the heart shows an oval shape, whereas it appears round in case of the high position of the diaphragm. The shadow of the superior vena cava extends above the heart shadow and is projected largely on the ascending aorta. The origin of the brachiocephalic veins (Fig. 39/1) is situated above the aortic arch. Their shadow is lost upwards in the projection of the clavicle. The entire thoracic section of the aorta can be best visualized in this oblique view (Figs 39/15, 16, 17). The air stripe of the trachea (Fig. 39/21) crosses the aortic arch transversely, while the left principal bronchus is projected behind the heart and the right bronchus (Fig. 39/22) on the heart shadow. The pulmonary trunk (Fig. 39/6) is not visible, whereas the upper edge of the right pulmonary artery (Fig. 39/7) can be visualized in the projection of the right hilum. The left pulmonary artery is projected on the aortic window. On the *right margin of the heart* two arches are visualized. The *upper arch* is the anterior contour of the ascending aorta (Fig. 39/15) which passes with a slight curve into the *lower arch*, i.e., into the border of the shadow of the right ventricle. The latter is less curved than the projection of the border of the left ventricle. The contour passes with sharp border into the shadow of the diaphragm.

Lateral view (dextrosinistral view; Fig. 40). Radiographs taken in this view show the *retrosternal space* between the sternum and the heart. Becoming narrower in its downward course it terminates approximately at the height of the sternal end of the 4th ribs. From here downwards the anterior margin of the heart is in contact with the thoracic wall. This space dilates during deep inspiration and constricts during expiration. The *anterior border* of the heart shadow is formed in this view by the almost perpendicularly rising ascending aorta (Fig. 40/7) which, in its upper course, passes into the shadow of the brachiocephalic trunk with an indistinct margin (Fig. 40/10). The confluent, somewhat protruding border of the pulmonary trunk and the conus pulmonalis (Fig. 40/4) is visible below the aorta. The conus pulmonalis passes without sharp border into the shadow of the right ventricle which extends to the diaphragm. On the *posterior margin*, the coalescent boundary of the left atrium and of the left ventricle cannot be separated. The major part of the shadow is provided by the atrium. The ventricular section is usually obscured by the pale edge of the inferior vena cava (Fig. 40/1). In the *retrocardiac space*, the anterior margin of the descending aorta (Fig. 40/9) is often visible in its entire length in front of the vertebral column.

Determination of the normal size of the heart by x-rays

The irregular elliptic shape of the heart renders it difficult to determine by x-ray the size of the heart and the morphological and magnitudinal deviations of its components. Whatever method is used, the results are decisively influenced by the physiological variability of factors concerning size and morphology. Size and shape may be studied by means of linear diameters, by the determination of surfaces and of the heart volume.

Linear diameters of the heart. *Sagittal view* (Fig. 6): *Median line* is running in the median sagittal plane (M). *Right* and *left median diameters* are the maximum distances between the right and left cardiac margins, respectively, measured from the median line (Md and Ms). The left is longer than the right diameter. The results are influenced by the position of the diaphragm. The ratio of the right and left diameters is $1 > 2$ in case of the high, and $1 < 2$ in case of the low position of the diaphragm. *Transverse diameter* (Tr) is the sum of the right and left median diameters ($Md + Ms$). It does not give the true length of the heart because it occupies an oblique position in the chest. The value of this diameter increases in the higher position of the diaphragm and decreases in the lower position. *Longitudinal diameter* (L) is the line linking together the

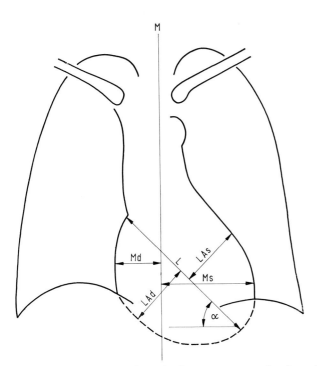

FIG. 6. Linear diameters in sagittal roentgenograms for the determination of the size of the heart. *Md:* right median diagonal; *Ms:* left median diagonal; *Md + ms: Tr* (transverse diameter); *M:* median line; *L:* longitudinal diameter; *α:* angle of the heart's inclination; *LAd:* right diameter in width; *LAs:* left diameter in width.

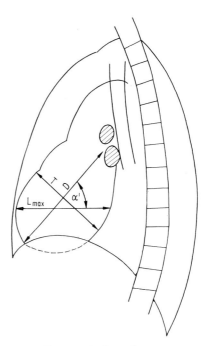

FIG. 7. Linear diameters in frontal roentgenograms for the determination of the size of the heart (after Zdansky, E.: *Röntgendiagnostik des Herzens und der großen Gefäße.* 3rd ed. Springer, Wien, 1962). *L_max:* transverse depth diameter; *D:* longitudinal depth diameter; *T:* depth diameter in width; *α':* angle of inclination.

junction of the curves of the right cardiac margin with the apex of the heart. Its determination is often uncertain owing to the difficulty in judging the place of the apex of the heart. *Angle of inclination of the heart* is the angle formed by the transverse and longitudinal diameters (α). It gives the most reliable indication for determining the heart's position. The mean value of the angle is 45°. We speak of transverse position if its degree is less, and of vertical position of the heart if its degree is higher. *Broad diameter (LAd + LAs)* is the amount of the maximum distance of the right lower cardiac point and of the left upper cardiac point measured from the longitudinal diameter. The left upper point is the junction of the pulmonary and the auricular arches. The determination of the right lower point is frequently just guessed, since it lies in the projection of the diaphragm.

Frontal view (Fig. 7): *Transverse depth diameter* (L_{max}) is the line connecting the extreme anterior with the extreme posterior point of the heart. Its value is strongly influenced by the position of the diaphragm (Rohrer 1916). *Longitudinal depth diameter* (D) is the line lying in the longitudinal axis of the heart; its upper point is at the junction of the pulmonary arteries and the anterior border of the left principal bronchus, while its lower point is the apex of the heart (Assmann 1934). *Broad depth diam-*

eter (T) forms a right angle with the longitudinal diameter and connects the extreme anterior and the extreme posterior points. The *angle of inclination* in

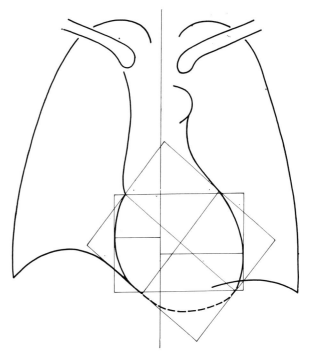

FIG. 8. Auxiliary lines for the determination of the cardiac surface.

the frontal view (α') is the angle formed by the longitudinal and transverse depth diameters. Its mean value is 45°.

Determination of the cardiac surface (Fig. 8). The surface of the heart in roentgenograms taken in the sagittal view can be measured by means of a planimeter or graph paper (Kirsch 1929, Moritz 1931, 1932, 1934).

Determination of the cardiac volume would seem the ideal object of radiographic measurements. The three-dimensional measurements involve a wide margin of error, therefore their values are questionable (Rohrer 1929).

All former radiographic methods for the measurement of the heart have been replaced by angiocardiography.

Physiological changes of radiological morphology

Under physiological conditions, a dynamic equilibrium exists between the activity of the heart and the work it has to perform. Factors influencing its shape and size are summed up in the following.

Pulsation. The size and shape of the heart change with the phases of cardiac function. During ventricular systole, contraction of the left ventricle coincides with a pronounced dilatation of the aorta and the pulmonary trunk. Quick medial expansion (systole) is followed by a slow lateral one (diastole). Stumpf (1928) writes of pulsation type I or II according to whether the amplitude is wider at the apex or at the base of the heart. Its value varies from 2·5 to 6 mm at rest. Besides the ventricular amplitude simultaneously with the systole a left-to-right pendulation, the elevation and the rounding of the apex of the heart can be visualized. The movement of the left auricle is partly its own pulsation and partly taken over from the ventricle and aorta. This is of a lesser degree (1 to 2·6 mm). Movements at the right margin of the heart are of an atrial character on the upper part of the atrial arch, and more of a ventricular character on the lower part. Changes in pulsatory movements can be studied by kymography.

Age. The size and shape of the heart change according to age (Fig. 9). Laënnec (cit. by Rauber and Kopsch 1951) proportioned the size of the heart with the fist of the individual. With the diaphragm situated lower in *older age* in general, the heart becomes paradoxically larger, chiefly due to the preponderance of its left half (Fig. 9/IV). The heart of a *newborn* is relatively large (Fig. 9/I). The borders of the heart shadow are less jagged, the shadow of the major vessels is broader, and the aortic knob is

mostly missing. This configuration is due to the high position of the diaphragm and the broad chest. Owing to the thymic involution, the upper part of the cardiac shadow becomes narrower from birth to *school age*. The shape of the chest changes; its long axis becomes elongated, its transverse diameter becomes shorter. The configuration of the heart develops towards the adult type. Marked protrusion of the pulmonary arch (puerile type of heart) is frequent at this age, which disappears often only after puberty.

Sex. In accordance with the constitution and body weight of females, their hearts are smaller than those of males (Fig. 9/II—III). Owing to the comparatively higher diaphragm, the transverse position of the heart is more common in women (Holzmann 1952). Comparing males and females of identical stature, Ludwig (1941) found the hearts of women to be 20 per cent smaller.

Constitution. It is commonly known that constitutional factors influence the size of the heart and its morphological variations. The transversely situated heart of the *pyknic* type seems to be larger not only on account of the body weight but also because of the higher position of the diaphragm (Fig. 9/VI). Cardiac hypertrophy found in *athletes* is the result of biological adaptation to more work being thrown upon the heart. The drop heart (cor pendulum) in *asthenic* individuals is well-known (Fig. 9/V). Cardiac configuration should be regarded as hypoplasia only if the size of the heart is smaller than normal even in recumbent position (Dietlen 1909). Within constitutional factors, the size of the heart depends on stature, body weight, circumference of the chest and body surface.

Increase in *stature* affects the longitudinal rather than the transverse diameter of the heart. With unchanged body weight but increased body height the longitudinal axis increases, while the transverse diameter becomes markedly diminished. The volume of the heart grows in proportion with its size but becomes relatively smaller if the individual's stature increases but his weight remains stationary (Ludwig 1939).

The effect of *body weight* on the size of the heart depends not on the increase of volume but on the development of the musculature. Changes in the transverse and longitudinal measurements of the heart are directly proportional to body weight.

The *circumference of the chest* varies directly with cardiac size. It is influenced by the simultaneous increase in body weight. According to the measurements performed by Rautmann (1951), the transverse diameter of the heart does not increase, but the longitudinal diameter reduces if the circumference of the chest becomes larger while the body weight and stature remain unchanged.

There exists a linear relationship between the *body surface* and the volume of the heart (Lilje-strand et al. 1939).

Position of the diaphragm. The influencing effect of the position of the diaphragm on the morphological more pronounced, and the distance between the ascending and descending aorta increases. Configuration of this kind was called the *adult type* by Zdansky (1962), whereas the pattern resulting from the high diaphragm in young children and pregnant women was termed by him the *infantile type*. Owing to the repletion of the cardiac sinus, the shape of

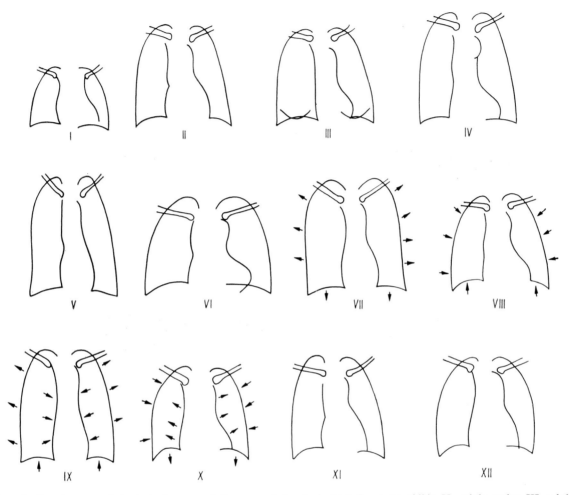

FIG. 9. Roentgenmorphological changes of the normal heart shadow. I, young child; II, adult male; III, adult female; IV, old person; V, asthenic person; VI, pyknic person; VII, maximum inspiration; VIII, maximum expiration; IX, Valsalva's manoeuver; X, Müller's manoeuver; XI, standing position; XII, recumbent position.

and dimensional variations of the heart is realized through the factors of age, sex and body build. Considering the mean value between expiration and inspiration depending on the high or low position of the diaphragm the heart undergoes changes.

The angle formed by the axis of the heart and the transverse diameter of the thorax is reduced if the diaphragm is in *high position*. Since the central tendon is relatively fixed, the cupolae of the diaphragm are elevated (Klaften and Palugyay 1927). The heart makes a left twist around its axis. The roentgenogram shows a transverse turn, the cardiac sinus becomes deeper, the arch of the aorta becomes the heart is rather similar to a mitral configuration in the latter type.

With the diaphragm in *low position*, the angle closed by the cardiac axis and the transverse diameter increases, i.e., more than 45°. The heart occupies a deeper position, and its long axis declines to the right. In roentgenograms, the left border of the heart is to a greater extent made up of the left ventricle, while the right ventricle forms the right border of the cardiac shadow (Dietlen 1923). The left border of the heart appears to be more completely filled owing to the diminution of the transverse diameter.

Apart from constitutional factors, the position of the diaphragm determines the shape of the heart depending on changes in intraabdominal and intrathoracic pressure, and on the phase of respiration. The latter factors are in close correlation with the extent to which the heart is filled with blood. Increased *intraabdominal pressure* elevates the diaphragm. Increase in *intrathoracic pressure* depresses and flattens the diaphragm, whereas decreased pressure produces a contrary effect. Valsalva's experiment, viz. expiratory effort with closed glottis after maximum inspiration, is based on this phenomenon (Fig. 9/IX). Return of blood to the heart is reduced and the heart becomes smaller owing to increased intrathoracic pressure. In Mueller's experiment, during a forced inspiratory effort with closed glottis after maximum expiration (Fig.9/X) the thoracic pressure decreases and the cardiac shadow becomes larger (Teschendorf 1952).

Respiration affects the heart both through changes in the position of the diaphragm and through the fluctuations of intrathoracic pressure. On maximum expiration, the heart's long diameter shortens, the organ broadens and the diaphragm moves upward (Fig. 9/VIII). On maximum inspiration the long diameter becomes still longer, and the heart becomes narrower owing to the downward movement of the diaphragm (Fig. 9/VII; Dietlen 1910); all arches of the heart are more clearly visible than in the expiratory phase.

Position of the body. Size, shape and position of the heart change according to bodily position. In standing position (Fig. 9/XI) the heart is 25 per cent smaller than in recumbent position (Fig. 9/XII). König and Bichmann (1967) have demonstrated that regarding heart volume, changes in the horizontal position like prone or dorsal position make no difference. The force of gravity affects the shape of the heart in lateral position. In right lateral position the heart sinks to the right, the cardiac sinus flattens, the right border of the heart protrudes markedly. In left lateral position the apex of the heart sinks to the left and rotates, and the cardiac sinus becomes deeper. The shape of the right border of the heart remains essentially unchanged (Zdansky 1962). Discrepancies of the cardiac configuration, as observed in the erect and the recumbent positions, show great individual differences (Dietlen 1909).

Variations in the position of the heart

The organs of the thorax and the abdomen develop in close correlation during embryonic life. Any change of this correlation in the course of develop-

ment may result in severe cardiac and vascular anomalies. Changes that do not involve abnormal haemodynamic conditions are regarded as anatomical variations (Bauer 1944). Anatomical variations in the position of the heart may be due to the inverted position of the thoracic and abdominal organs: thoracic or abdominal inversion, abnormal rotation of the heart or its inversion and rotation (Bopp 1947). In *dextrocardia*, the major part of the heart is on the right side. The abdominal organs may be in inversion or normal position. In *laevocardia*, the heart is situated on the left side, while the abdominal viscera are in inverted position.

Situs inversus viscerum is the complete inversion of the thoracic and abdominal viscera. Heart and circulation are normal. Variations in the origin of the branches of the aortic arch may also occur (Sanders and Poorman 1968). It is often a familiar phenomenon. We observed such inversion in five of 70,000 thoracic fluoroscopics. Four of the observed five cases belonged to the same family.

Dextrocardia with normal abdominal position is due to the isolated inversion of the heart. It may be associated with other congenital anomalies (Christiaens et al. 1964). The venous half of the heart together with the tricuspid valve occupy a sinistro-anterior, the arterial half together with the mitral valve, a dextroposterior position.

Dextrocardia is present if the *heart is dextrorotated* (Paltauf 1901). This conditions is usually accompanied by other congenital malformations (Ayres and Steinberg 1963). Van Praagh and his associates (1964) found normal haemodynamic conditions in 18 per cent of 51 cases of dextrocardia examined.

Two types of *laevocardia* are known. In the first form, situs inversus abdominalis with normally placed heart with normal configuration remains on the left side. In the second form, in the situs inversus totalis *laevotorsion* develops. Anatomical conditions are normal in the first, other anomalies occur in the second case (Campbell and Forgács 1953). Laevocardia is considerably less frequent than dextrocardia.

Angiocardiography

Anatomy of the heart and the great vessels has for long been a central problem in research. Owing to the close correlation between morphology and function, first the in vivo examinations completed our knowledge in this respect. The most suitable here was the in vivo examination of the chambers of the heart by means of angiocardiography.

Forssmann's self- and animal experiments (1931) were milestones concerning the filling of the heart with contrast media. Castellanos et al. (1937) successfully filled the heart and the vessels of the lungs, and were the first to demonstrate congenital defects by angiocardiography. Robb and Steinberg (1938) determined the time of circulation. Postmortem filling of the heart and great vessels facilitated the study of topographic conditions (Laubry et al. 1935a, b, c, 1936). Janker (1936, 1950) elaborated numerous methods for the examination of the heart by filling with contrast media. Serial angiograms (Wegelius and Lind 1950), further the method of cineangiocardiography (Janker 1950) considerably promoted the study of the dynamics of circulation.

According to Zdansky (1951) the *in vivo filling with contrast substance* first of the right, then of the left half of the heart (*dextrocardiogram—laevocardiogram*) takes place the following way: During systole, both ventricles get into a state of maximum contraction. The right ventricle is notably smaller than the left ventricle, the atria are dilated. Between the right atrium and ventricle a ridge, the supraventricular crest can be seen. The conus pulmonalis is displaced slightly to the left. During diastole the ventricles are dilated and show smooth contours, while the atria are constricted with regard to the systole. The supraventricular crest is invisible, and the conus pulmonalis is pushed to the right. The movement of the right outflow portion is pronounced owing to the heart's systolic rotation (Fig. 10). The apex of the heart moves forward from left below during systole, at the same time the conus approaches it. The elevation and dilation of the pulmonary root is followed by descent during diastole. While expansion of the ventricles is fast during diastole, systolic evacuation is slower. With angiography first the superior vena cava is filled, then the right atrium in 1 to 2 sec, the right ventricle after 1·5 to 2·5 sec, the left atrium after 5 to 7 sec, and the left ventricle after 8 to 10 sec (Zsebők 1969).

In *postmortem angiograms* the *shadow of the right atrium and ventricle* are confluent, while the supraventricular crest remains distinguishable. In **anteroposterior pictures** (Fig. 47), also the retrogradely filled coronary veins (Fig. 47/27) are visible in the projection of the ventricle's trabecular left border. In **lateral view** (Fig. 48), the *right atrium* (Fig. 48/5), arching backward between the superior and inferior venae cavae, further the great cardiac vein that runs in the coronary sulcus, and sometimes also the coronary sinus (Fig. 48/16) can be distinguished from one another. The anterior border of the *right ventricle* (Fig. 48/15) fills with a blurred

contour. The thickness of the anterior wall of the ventricle can be estimated in soft pictures. The shadow of the pulmonary trunk (Fig. 48/17), turning backward and upward after its origin, falls in the lateral view behind the projection of the superior vena cava.

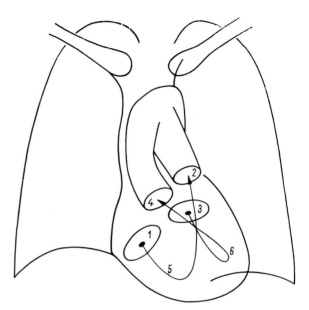

FIG. 10. The paths of blood flow in the heart chambers (after Zdansky, E.: *Röntgendiagnostik des Herzens und der großen Gefäße*. 3rd ed. Springer, Wien, 1962). (*1*) Right atrioventricular orifice; (*2*) orifice of pulmonary trunk; (*3*) left atrioventricular orifice; (*4*) orifice of aorta; (*5*) right path of flow; (*6*) left path of flow.

When *filling the left half of the heart*, the shadow of the *atrium* (Fig. 59/14) appears larger than in reality because—**anteroposteriorly** (Fig. 59)—the roots of the pulmonary veins (Figs 59/15, 29, 38, 54) are superimposed from both directions. The atrium and the left border of the auricle run approximately parallel with the spine, while the right border runs obliquely downward in front of the spine. The atrioventricular boundary appears in both views as a curved depression. The inside of the *left ventricle* seems to be oval in the **anteroposterior view** (Fig. 59/5), but appears to be pointed downward and shows an approximately triangular shape if viewed **laterally** (Fig. 60/6). On the marginal contours fringes caused by the papillary muscles are observable. The coronary vessels are filled. The origin of the ascending aorta can be distinguished from the atrium in the lateral view (Fig. 60/7), but their projections are superimposed in sagittal pictures (Fig. 59/8).

Coronary arteries

The coronary vessels, ensuring the blood supply of the heart, are in communication (Spalteholz 1924). Their physiological significance is indicated by the fact that they utilize 10 per cent of the blood flowing through the aorta.

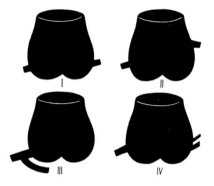

FIG. 11. Variations in origin of the coronary arteries in the systemic circulation. I, normal type; II, high origin on the left side; III, solitary right coronary artery; IV, multiple coronary arteries.

The right coronary artery arises from the right, the left coronary artery from the left sinus of aorta. Their origin is completely or partially obscured from view by the cusps of the aortic valve (Fig. 11/I).

Variation in origin may be due to abnormal origin from the systemic circulation or ectopic origin from the pulmonary circulation.

1. Within the systemic variation the coronaries may arise from the aorta immediately above the valvules (Fig. 11/II), first observed by Brücke (1885), in 4 per cent of the examined cases. Occasionally the coronaries may start off 1 or 2 cm above the valvules (Adachi 1928, Doerr 1955). In case of origin within the sinus, its depth may vary. Sometimes both arteries originate from the same sinus, in which case their further course deviates from the normal, too (Wilson 1965, Benson and Lack 1968, Ogden 1970). Origin from the posterior sinus is also possible (White and Edwards 1948). Further cases have been described in which the coronaries arose from the subclavian artery, the common carotid artery (Evans 1933) or the internal thoracic artery (Robicsek et al. 1967).

Variations may also be due to the number of the arising arteries. Single coronary artery (Fig. 11/III) is extremely rare, only 70 cases had been published until 1961 (Longenecker et al. 1961). Smith (1950) classified anatomical variations of the single coronary artery in three groups: (*1*) The artery runs like the right or the left coronary artery (Davis and Compton 1962, Vestermark 1965, Hillestad and Eie 1971). (*2*) After a short course, the single artery divides into two normal coronaries (Luschka 1858, Hallman et al. 1966). (*3*) Atypical course. In this case the irregular coronary or its branch may even form a fistula with one of the ventricles (Murray 1963).

Supernumerary coronary arteries consist mostly of accessory minor vessels (Fig. 11/IV, Symmers and Clair 1907, Gross 1921, Adachi 1928). The supernumerary vessels are sometimes equally strong (Schlesinger et al. 1949). This variant occurs more frequently than the single coronary (Castellanos et al. 1953). Meckel (cit. by Rauber and Kopsch 1951) described a case of quadruple coronary. Double origin of the right coronary artery is comparatively the most frequent anomaly (Doerr 1955). Triple origin of one coronary is rare (Mason and Hunter 1937).

Irregular origin of the coronaries from the systemic circulation is a normal variation. Patients may reach a great age. However, abnormal connections with the chambers of the heart give rise to the same pathological conditions as origin from the lesser circulation (Edwards 1958, Neil and Mounsey 1958, Neufeld et al. 1961).

2. Ectopic origin from the lesser circulation may arise from the pulmonary trunk (Brooks 1886). The left coronary artery originates from the lesser circulation more frequently than the right coronary artery (Bland et al. 1933, Sabiston et al. 1960, Jameson et al. 1963, Wilder and Perlman 1964, Stein et al. 1965). Sometimes, however, the left coronary artery may arise from the right pulmonary artery (Dutra 1950). The right coronary artery arises considerably less frequently from the lesser circulation (Bland et al. 1933, Pribble 1961, Ranninger et al. 1967). Only sporadic cases are known in which both coronaries arose from the pulmonary trunk (Soloff 1942, Szederkényi and Steczik 1964, Feldt et al. 1965, Ogden and Stansel 1971). There exist a few reports on the ectopic origin of the accessory coronary artery (Hackensellner 1955a).

Origin of the coronaries from the lesser circulation gives rise to greater or lesser circulatory disorders. In addition to variations concerning origin other anomalies of the angioarchitecture may likewise occur: intimal pads or communicating blind pouches may develop which are sometimes in contact with the cavity of the heart (Rubli 1933/34).

Right coronary artery (Figs 12/2, 41 and 42/2, 44/10, 45/8, 46/11, 58/7, 61/4). After its origin, it passes between the pulmonary trunk and the right auricle, and runs then backward in the coronary sulcus. At its root the vessel has a lumen of 3 to

4 mm. After passing around the right border of the heart it reaches the diaphragmatic surface and ramifies into terminal branches on the posterior surface of the right ventricle. The average diameter of the right coronary artery is 4 mm (1·5 to 5·5 mm; Paulin 1964). It supplies the right atrium and

Posterior interventricular branch (Figs 12/6, 41 and 42/6, 44/11, 45/10, 46/12). A terminal branch of the right coronary artery, which runs toward the apex of the heart in the similarly named groove. Its course is variable; it sends off numerous side branches to the posterior part of the ventricular septum.

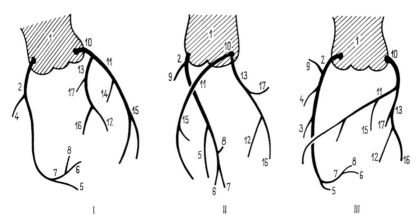

FIG. 12. X-ray anatomy of the coronary arteries in various projections. I, anteroposterior; II, lateral; III, left oblique. (*1*) Aorta; (*2*) right coronary artery; (*3*) anterior right ventricular branch; (*4*) anterior right atrial branch; (*5*) right marginal branch; (*6*) posterior interventricular branch; (*7*) posterior left ventricular branch; (*8*) posterior right atrial branch; (*9*) ramus coni pulmonalis dexter; (*10*) left coronary artery; (*11*) anterior interventricular branch; (*12*) branch of the obtuse margin; (*13*) circumflex branch; (*14*) ramus coni pulmonalis sinister; (*15*) anterior left ventricular branch; (*16*) posterior left auricular branch; (*17*) anterior left auricular branch.

ventricle, the posterior third of the septum, and a part of the infundibulum. It has the following *branches:*

Right anterior atrial branch (Figs 12/4, 41 and 42/3). After origin this branch passes on the right auricle supplying its anterior surface and the left side of its posterior surface. It forms anastomoses with the branches of the left coronary artery in the area of the sinoatrial node (Hayek 1958). Besides, it sends off a branch to the smaller part of the atrial septum.

Right anterior ventricular branch (Figs 12/3, 41 and 42/4). It begins opposite the auricular artery and ramifies downwards on the anterior surface of the right ventricle. It sends off a small side branch to the infundibulum (*ramus coni pulmonalis dexter*; Fig. 12/9), which often arises directly from the aorta (Bianchi, cit. Hayek 1958). The terminal branches may run as far as the anterior part of the ventricular septum (Paturet 1958).

Right marginal branch (Figs 12/5, 41 and 42/5). This branch follows the right border of the heart and runs toward the apex of the heart. It is the largest collateral vessel of the right coronary artery. Before reaching the apex of the heart, it divides into an anterior and a posterior branch.

Right posterior ventricular branch arises from the posterior surface of the atrioventricular groove. It is a minor vessel, which is often absent.

Right posterior atrial branch (Figs 12/8, 41 and 42/7) usually bifurcates on the posterior surface of the right auricle, but sometimes extends to the area between the two caval veins (Paturet 1958).

Left posterior ventricular branch (Figs 12/7, 41 and 42/8, 44/12, 45/9, 46/13). This is the other terminal branch of the main trunk; it runs to the left in the coronary sinus; at the same time it gives off a side branch to the diaphragmatic surface of the left ventricle.

Left coronary artery (Figs 12/10, 41 and 42/9, 44/13, 45/11, 46/14, 61/5). After its origin the left coronary artery, passing between the pulmonary trunk and the left auricle, reaches the sternocostal surface of the heart where it divides into branches. The initial section is dilated, elsewhere it has a diameter of 2 to 7 mm (Paulin 1964). The length of the main trunk amounts to 0·5 to 2 cm (Paturet 1958). Hellwing (1967) found its length to exceed 1 cm only in 45 per cent of the cases. The vessel supplies the left ventricle, left atrium, the larger anterior part of the ventricular septum and the larger posterior part of the atrial septum. It has the following *branches*:

The *anterior interventricular branch* (Figs 12/11, 41 and 42/10, 44/14, 45/12, 46/15, 57/6) bifurcates after a short course. The shorter branch runs towards the left side of the conus pulmonalis (*ramus coni pulmonalis sinister*; Figs 12/14, 41 and 42/11);

31

the longer, towards the apex of the heart in the anterior interventricular groove, and inclines there to the posterior side. If well developed, this branch supplies two thirds of the backside.

Circumflex branch (Figs 12/13, 41 and 42/13, 44/15, 45/13, 46/16, 57/5, 58/6) is the other, the larger branch; it turns to the posterior side of the heart below the left auricle in the coronary sulcus and takes there a downward course. Also, it may spring off independently from the aorta or from the right coronary artery (Hackensellner 1955b). The vessel has three minor branches at its origin, but these may arise from the main trunk as well. The *ramus septi sinister anterior* (Figs 41 and 42/14) runs to the septum between the aorta and the left atrium. The *left anterior atrial branch* (Figs 41 and 42/15) runs upward to the anterior surface of the left atrium and meets there the corresponding branch of the right coronary. This branch supplies blood to the sinoatrial node. The *left anterior ventricular branch* (Figs 12/15, 41 and 42/16) ramifies on the left obtuse margin of the left ventricle. The origin of the further branches is more constant but their area of supply is rather varied. The *left posterior auricular branch* (Figs 12/16, 41 and 42/17) is a larger branch which runs to the atrium between the auricle and the left superior pulmonary vein. It emits a side branch towards the superior vena cava (Belou 1934). Anastomoses are formed between the bilateral auricular arteries. The *left posterior atrial branch* (Figs 41 and 42/19) runs to the left atrium, the *left posterior ventricular branch* (Figs 12/7, 41, 42/18, 45/14) to the posterior surface of the left ventricle. The latter passes downwards parallel to the interventricular groove without reaching the apex of the heart. It supplies the upper two thirds of the wall of the ventricle.

Branch of the obtuse margin (*ramus diagonalis*; Figs 12/12, 41 and 42/12, 44/16, 45/15) passes downwards behind the obtuse margin of the left ventricle. It is either a branch of the circumflex branch or springs off directly from the left coronary artery in which case one speaks of a trifurcation of this coronary artery. Crainicianu (1922) observed this variation in 60, Di Guglielmo and Guttadauro (1954) in 9·4 per cent of the examined cases.

Area supplied by the coronary arteries. The above anatomical description of the coronary arteries with respect to the area they supply holds true only when they are more or less equally large. Various deviations may occur if one coronary artery is larger than the other.

The relative development of the coronary arteries may be studied by intravital coronarography, and by comparison three types can be distinguished (Di Guglielmo and Guttadauro 1954, Düx et al. 1961,

1964, Thurn et al. 1963, Schaede 1963, Hettler 1966).

Normal type. The posterior interventricular branch springs off from the right coronary artery and extends to the upper three quarters of the posterior wall. Passing around the apex of the heart, the anterior interventricular branch of the left coronary artery supplies one fourth to one third of the posterior wall. The circumflex branch is well developed.

Left-supply type. The well-developed circumflex branch has a longer course in the posterior interventricular groove. The proportion between the anterior and posterior interventricular branches is shifted in favour of the first.

Right-supply type. The determination of this type is much more difficult. The posterior interventricular branch of right coronary artery is well developed and extends to the apex of the heart, while the anterior interventricular branch of left coronary artery is short.

Hettler (1966) encountered the normal type in 79, left-supply type in 17, and right-supply type in 4 per cent of the examined cases. Paulin (1964) determined the degree of supply by the development of the calibre. He found equal development in 26, left-sided preponderance in 66, and right-sided preponderance in 8 per cent.

The *angioarchitecture* of the coronary arteries (Figs 41, 42) varies in the different parts of the heart. The *ventricles* are abundantly provided with blood vessels originating from the primary side branches of approximately equal diameter. These side branches have a superficial position as compared to the main trunk. They run a tortuous course in the epicardial adipose tissue. The secondary branches enter the myocardium at right angles, the tertiary branches divide at acute angles. The latter extend to the endocardium. This arrangement ensures undisturbed blood supply during ventricular systole (Wiggers 1952, Thurn et al. 1963, Kádár 1963). Types of division are similar in the ventricular septum. Numerous capillary anastomoses between the two coronary arteries may maintain a good collateral circulation (Nagy 1949, James 1970). Estes et al. (1966) distinguish two types of vessels in the ventricular wall, one which ramifies immediately after its origin while the other runs as far as the endocardium. There are several anastomoses between the branches of the latter.

The blood supply of the *atria* is much poorer. Dividing at acute angles, the side branches plunge downward in a uniform manner. The branches of the two coronaries form an arch around the fossa ovalis in the atrial septum.

The *papillary muscles* are penetrated by vessels which are corkscrew-like in the muscular segment and run a straight course along the chordae tendineae, an arrangement which ensures good blood supply during contraction and elongation. The arteries of the *valvules* enter the valves from the base of the cusps and from the chordae tendineae. Intimal pads in the precapillaries serve to multiply the normal size of lumina in cases of increased stress.

Collateral circulation, The following anastomoses connect the coronary arteries with each other and their surroundings for the maintenance of the collateral circulation.

(1) Arterio-arterial communications can develop between the coronary arteries and their branches, according to James (1970), between two segments of the same artery (intracoronary anastomosis), between two branches (intercoronary anastomosis), transatrially, transseptally, in the epicardium of the ventricular muscles, subendocardially, and finally, through specific arteries (r. coni pulmonalis dexter, artery of the sinoatrial node, artery of the atrioventricular node). Such intercoronary communications can be perhaps demonstrated in case of an intact heart also in vivo (Cheng 1972).

2. Arterio-arterial extracoronary anastomoses ensure communication mainly with the bronchial arteries (Voss 1856, Robertson 1930). The anastomoses have sometimes a diameter of 2 mm. With arteriography, Björk (1966) demonstrated their existence in 48 per cent of the examined cases. These anastomoses can be visualized also in healthy heart (Smith et al. 1972). With postmortem angiography Moberg (1967) could demonstrate anastomoses on the precapillary level. Well developed side branches of the bronchial arteries may maintain a good circulation in the atrial muscles (arteria atrialis bronchialis; Petelenz 1965, Debiec 1967). Anastomosis can occur also with the system of the pulmonary trunk (Gobel et al. 1970).

3. Regional circulation may be established with the vasa vasorum of the veins and great arteries as well as with the pericardial vessels (Halpern 1954).

4. By their opening, arteriovenous anastomoses in the myocardium may accelerate the rate of circulation (Correia 1939). Their regulatory role is similar to that of the obstructing arteries; their clinical occurrence is rare.

Coronarography. Roentgenological study of the coronary arteries was preceded by postmortem observations (Czmór and Urbányi 1939, Schoenmackers and Vieten 1954). Radner (1945) and later Jönsson (1948) could first achieve intravital visualization of the coronary arteries. Anatomical and physiological observations have benn adjusted to clinical practice (Di Guglielmo and Guttadauro 1954, Düx et al. 1961, Nordenström et al. 1962a,

Thurn et al. 1963, Paulin 1964, Hettler 1965, Düx 1967).

Examinations can best be carried out in the left oblique view and in the left lateral position. Anteroposterior pictures show less complete filling than those taken in a lateral position. Sones and Shirey (1962) recommend the right and left lateral view and in some cases posteroanterior projection. Intravital and postmortem coronarograms are discrepant owing to changes in the position of the heart (Düx 1967).

Anteroposterior radiographs (Figs 12/I, 44) may be used as supplements. The coronary arteries show a backward curving course at the right and the left borders of the heart. The shadows of the branches of the *left coronary artery* (Figs 12/10, 44/13) are often superimposed. The position of the *anterior interventricular branch* (Figs 12/11, 44/14) regarding the *circumflex branch* (Figs 12/13, 44/15) depends on the shape and position of the heart.

From the **lateral view** (Figs 12/II, 45), the *right coronary artery* (Figs 12/2, 45/8) shows a downward and then a backward course. It is crossed by the *anterior interventricular branch* (Figs 12/11, 45/12) which is more curved and is running downward and forward. The origin of the *left coronary artery* (Figs 12/10, 45/11) is projected on the bulb of the aorta. The *circumflex branch* (Figs 12/13, 45/13) passes downward at the posterior border of the heart.

The **left oblique view** (Figs 12/III, 46) is the most suitable also for the postmortem visualization of the *right coronary artery* (Figs 12/2, 46/11) and its branches. The *left main trunk* (Figs 12/10, 46/14) and the the *anterior interventricular branch* (Figs 12/11, 46/15) and the proximal segment of the *circumflex branch* (Figs 12/13, 46/16) are likewise clearly visible in this view. The right coronary artery is projected on the anterior, the left coronary artery on the posterior aspect of the heart. The anterior interventricular branch crosses the cardiac shadow from behind forward and obliquely downward (Gensini et al. 1967).

Veins of the heart

The veins of the heart open partly into the right atrium through the coronary sinus and several minor vessels, partly into all four chambers through the venae cordis minimae (Laux and Marchal 1948). Covered by the visceral pericardium, the great veins of the heart run parallel with but more superficially than the arteries (Kádár 1956). They contain three rudimentary valves. The principal veins are anastomosing. Part of the adventitia of the coronary sinus is formed by the muscle fibres which are carried over from the atrium so that there is a close connection between the sinal adventitia and the atrial musculature (Bucciante 1940, cit. by Hayek 1958). Drainage of the heart's venous blood is in harmony with the volume of blood that is rhythmically expelled by the myocardium (Di Giorgi and Gensini 1965).

The *coronary sinus* (Figs 13/1, 43/5, 48/16), situated in the coronary sulcus, collects the blood of the great cardiac veins. Together with the oblique vein of the left atrium, it develops from the sub-

The *great cardiac vein* (Figs 13/2, 43/6, 52/8) begins at the apex of the heart and ascends in the anterior interventricular groove to reach the coronary sulcus. It then curves to the left in this groove, and, reaching the back of the heart, opens into the left extremity of the coronary sinus. Its root at the apex of the heart never curves round to the dorsal side. The great cardiac vein collects the blood of the ventricles on the anterior surface of the heart, generally from four trunks. Its diameter is 4 to 5 mm.

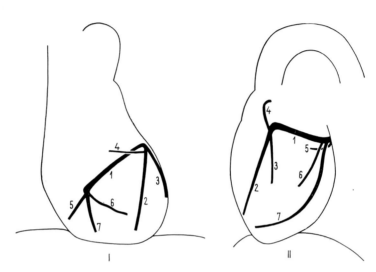

FIG. 13. X-ray anatomy of the cardiac veins. Anteroposterior and lateral views (after Gensini, G. et al.: Anatomy of the coronary circulation in living man. *Circulation* 31, 1965, 778). I, anteroposterior view; II, lateral view. (*1*) Coronary sinus; (*2*) great cardiac vein; (*3*) diagonal vein; (*4*) oblique vein of left atrium; (*5*) small cardiac vein; (*6*) posterior vein of left ventricle; (*7*) middle cardiac vein.

sequently disappearing left superior vena cava (Cuvier's duct). It runs from left to right and has a funnel-shaped opening into the right atrium. It is continuous with the great cardiac vein and frequently shows widenings. It has a semilunar valve at the orifice (valve of the coronary sinus or Thebesius' valve) which is often rudimentary and therefore incompetent (Mochizuki 1933). Sarrazin (1965) observed its presence in 71 per cent. The transition of the sinus into the great cardiac vein is at the opening of the oblique vein of the left atrium. The sinus is provided there with an underdeveloped valve (Vieussens' valve) which is, however, often missing. The sinus measures 5 cm (3 to 7 cm) in length and 0·8 to 1 cm in its maximum width (Cordier and Heffez 1952). The coronary sinus may be absent if the left superior vena cava is persistent in which case the cardiac veins open separately into the atria (Raghib et al. 1965). It can also happen that the coronary sinus is in connection also with the right atrium (Ceballos 1970).

The *middle cardiac vein* (Figs 13/7, 43/9) ascends in the posterior interventricular groove and opens into the great cardiac vein or into the coronary sinus. It does not, as a rule, open directly into the right atrium. Usually it has a valve at the proximal end (valvula of the middle cardiac vein); the initial segment often inclines to the anterior side where an anastomosis with the great cardiac vein is frequently formed (Mochizuki 1933). The largest diameter of the middle cardiac vein is 5 mm.

The *small cardiac vein* (Fig. 13/5), originating on the anterior aspect of the right ventricle, passes to the right around the coronary sulcus and opens into the coronary sinus. The vein is fairly variable and, according to Paturet (1958), it is absent in 40 per cent of the cases. Very rarely, it empties directly into the right atrium (Parsonnet 1952).

The *oblique vein of the left atrium (Marschall's vein)* (Figs 13/4, 43/8), a small vessel, 2 mm wide, descends on the back of the left atrium and opens into the major veins at the boundary between the coronary sinus and the great cardiac vein.

The *posterior vein of the left ventricle* (Figs 13/6, 43/7) is formed on the posterior surface of the left ventricle and opens into the coronary sinus or may end in the great cardiac vein. It is often a multiple vessel.

The *anterior cardiac veins* (Fig. 43/10), comprising 1 to 6 small vessels, collect blood from the front of the right ventricle and from the right atrium, bridge the coronary sulcus and empty into the right atrium.

The *venae cordis minimae* (*Thebesian veins*) comprise a number of minute vessels which lie in the muscular wall of the heart and open directly into all its four cavities. Their inlets are mostly on the septa. The blood may flow retrogradely in them if the coronaries are incompetent (Nagy 1962).

Venography. The venous circulation of the heart can be directly visualized in vivo by increasing the intrabronchial tension (Boerema and Blickman 1955). By means of this method, the contrast medium, accumulating in the myocardium, becomes visible (myocardiography) and also the larger coronary veins are filled (Nordenström et al. 1962b). Tori (1952) filled the coronary veins by retrograde catheterization of the coronary sinus.

For roentgenograms *in vivo* the right oblique view is best suited for examination (Gensini et al. 1963). As regards anatomical configuration, deviations are considerably less than in the case of arteries.

As described by Gensini et al. (1965), the larger coronary veins occupy two approximately triangular areas in the **anteroposterior picture** (Fig. 13/I). The *coronary sinus* (Fig. 13/1) passes upward from the left border of the projection of the vertebral column, while its continuation, the *great cardiac vein* (Fig. 13/2), runs steeply downward and can be followed as far as the apex of the heart. The *middle cardiac vein* (Fig. 13/7) lies beneath and medially to it. The *posterior vein of the left ventricle* (Fig. 13/6) runs along the descending part of the great cardiac vein. The *small cardiac vein* (Fig. 13/5) runs to the coronary sinus from the right, and the *oblique vein of the left atrium* (Fig. 13/4) opens into the upper extremity of this sinus. The smaller veins are not easy to distinguish.

In the **lateral view** (Fig. 13/II), the *great cardiac vein* (Fig. 13/2), opening into the anterior extremity of the *coronary sinus* (Fig. 13/1), usually communicates at the apex of the heart with the *middle cardiac vein* (Fig. 13/7) which passes upward along the posterior border of the heart. The veins of the ventricles are situated between these three vessels. The projection of the atrial veins appears above the coronary sinus.

Orientation is more difficult in *postmortem angiography* (Fig. 43 (because of the simultaneous filling of the cardiac cavities: only certain details of the venous system can be seen. The cadaveric position of the diaphragm causes a slight modification of the projection.

THORACIC ARTERIES
(ARTERIES OF THE GREATER CIRCULATION)
THE THORACIC AORTA AND ITS BRANCHES

The aorta arises from the left ventricle at the aortic orifice. It is the beginning of the greater circulation. Its physiological significance is due to its elasticity which ensures the transport of the blood during the phase of diastole. In accordance with its topographical situation, the aorta is described in several portions, viz., the ascending aorta, the arch of the aorta and the descending aorta (thoracic aorta + abdominal aorta).

Ascending aorta

At the height of its beginning, the ascending aorta (Figs 37/15, 38/14, 39/15, 40/7, 44/7, 45/5, 46/8, 57/7, 58/8, 59/6, 60/7) is dilated (bulb of the aorta);

this dilatation is formed by three pouchlike sinuse (right, left and posterior sinuses). With reference to the anterior wall of the thorax, the projection of the ascending aorta falls on the 3rd left sternocostal joint. Arising, the ascending aorta passes obliquely upward, forward and to the right as high as the upper border of the 2nd right sternocostal joint where it passes into the arch of the aorta. The pulmonary trunk is situated before its origin, the right auricle lies to the right, while the left atrium is behind and to the left of it. The superior vena cava runs along the further course of the ascending aorta. The pulmonary trunk passes to the left side of the ascending aorta. Behind it lies the right pulmonary artery, in front of it is the sternum, the latter being separated from the lower part of the ascending aorta by the pleura and from its upper part by the thymus. The entire ascending aorta lies within the pericardium. Its upper extremity is somewhat wider in adults. The length of the ascending aorta varies from 5 to 6 cm; its diameter, from 3 to 3·5 cm (Paturet 1958). The right coronary artery springs off from the right, the left coronary artery from the left aortic sinus.

Arch of the aorta

The aortic arch (Figs 37/16, 38/15, 39/16, 40/8, 44/8, 45/6, 46/9, 57/8, 58/9, 59/7, 60/8) is a continuation of the ascending aorta. It begins behind the 2nd right sternocostal joint at the bend of the pericardium. Its whole course shows the shape of an upward convex arch. First it runs upward, backward and to the left; it is then directed downward on the left, and finally it is continuous with the descending aorta. The highest point of the arch lies behind the manubrium of the sternum, 2·5 cm below the incisura sterni. Rarely it reaches above the upper margin of the sternum (Deffrenne and Verney 1968). Its initial part is covered anteriorly by the right lung and the corresponding portion of the pleura. In its later course, it is crossed by the left brachiocephalic vein. The posterior surface is in front of and impresses the trachea. The right pulmonary artery runs caudally from it to the right of the midline. The left principal bronchus runs toward the hilum below the aortic arch to the left of the midline. The vagus nerve is placed in front of the arch, while the left recurrent laryngeal branch of the left vagus hooks around below the vessel. Besides the trachea, also the esophagus and the thoracic duct are found on the left side behind its posterior surface. The accessory hemiazygos vein and the left phrenic nerve nestle against the left side of the aortic arch. It is at this point where it contacts the aortic sulcus of the left lung. The remnant of the embryonic ductus arteriosus (ligamentum arteriosum) which forms a connection to the left pulmonary artery, is found on the anterior aspect of the aortic arch, 1 to 1·5 cm distal to the origin of the left subclavian artery. This segment is somewhat narrower after birth (isthmus of the aorta) but becomes like the rest in later life. The aortic arch is attached to the neck and the upper mediastinum by the descending aorta, the major vessels emerge from there, and by the endothoracic fascia, which fixes it to the spinal column (Hayek 1958). Its initial part is projected on the 2nd to 3rd, its distal part on the 3rd to 4th thoracic vertebrae. The length of the aortic arch is 5 to 6 cm; its diameter 2·1 to 3·0

cm at the origin, 1·7 to 2·5 cm at the extremity (Adachi 1928, Nagy 1962).

Branches. The brachiocephalic trunk is the first, and the left common carotid artery the second to emerge from the convexity of the aortic arch above the border of the pericardium. Arising from the midpoint of the arch, the carotid lies nearer the brachiocephalic trunk than to the subclavian artery, the third and last branch of the aortic arch. The subclavian artery originates from the posterior border of the arch; its distance from the left common carotid amounts to 1·0 to 1·5 cm.

Brachiocephalic trunk (Figs 37/18, 38/17, 39/18, 40/10, 44/17, 45/16, 46/17, 57/10, 58/11, 59/9, 60/10). This is the first, most ventral and thickest branch of the aortic arch. It arises about 1 to 1·5 cm above the bend of the pericardium. The origin of the left common carotid lies a few mm distally. The brachiocephalic trunk passes obliquely upward and to the right at the level of the upper border of the right sternoclavicular joint and divides into the right subclavian and the right common carotid arteries. Its initial segment is traversed by the left brachiocephalic vein; the left common carotid artery runs to its left, the right brachiocephalic vein to its right. The trachea runs downward behind and to the left of the trunk. The brachiocephalic trunk measures 3 to 5 cm in length and 1 to 1·3 cm in width (Adachi 1928, Paturet 1958).

The brachiocephalic trunk usually has no branches, but if present, usually the arteria thyroidea ima arises from it.

On *native radiographs* it is in the **first oblique** (Fig. 38/17) and in the **lateral views** (Fig. 40/10) that the anterior border of the brachiocephalic trunk is distinguishable. In the **2nd oblique view** (Fig. 39/18) the most anterior vessel, i.e., the brachiocephalic trunk is transversely crossed by the left brachiocephalic vein in the projection of the sternum. The right brachiocephalic vein is situated before the anterior border of and runs approximately parallel with the brachiocephalic trunk. After being *filled with radio-opaque substance*, the **anteroposterior picture** (Fig. 44/17) shows the vessel running upward from left to right, in front of the right side of the 3rd and 4th thoracic vertebrae. In the first oblique view, its projection coalesces with the other two major vessels, whereas all the three can be differentiated in the **second oblique view** (Fig. 46/17). In the **lateral view** (Fig. 45/16), the shadows of the first two vessels are summated so that only the left subclavian artery remains separately visible.

Arteria thyroidea ima. The presence of this supernumerary vessel was observed in 10 per cent by some authors (Adachi 1928, Rauber and Kopsch 1951) and in 0·6 to 1·0 per cent by others (Liechty et al. 1957, Pontes 1963). It may arise from the aortic arch, the brachiocephalic trunk, the right common carotid, the internal thoracic, right subclavian and inferior thyroid arteries or the thyrocervical trunk. It originates most frequently from the brachiocephalic trunk or the aortic arch. Having examined 500 cases, Pontes (1963) found the vessel to be single in 0·6, multiple in 0·4 per cent. It runs along the vena thyroidea ima to the inferior

Variations of the aortic arch. 1. Normal type (Fig. 14/I): The branchial arches are formed between the second and sixth weeks of intrauterine life and develop together with the heart. The artery of the fourth left branchial arch persists and gives rise to the left aortic arch with the typical vascular pattern. This has been found to take place in 83 to 85 per cent of the cases (Adachi 1928, Pontes 1963).

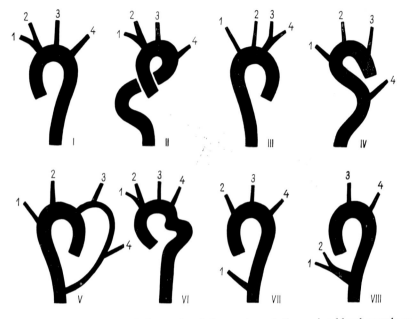

FIG. 14. Frequent variations of the arch of the aorta and the major blood vessels originating outside its convexity. I, normal type; II, left circumflex arch of aorta; III, right arch of aorta (situs inversus aortae); IV, right circumflex arch of aorta; V, double aortic arch; VI, pseudocoarctation of the aorta; VII, arteria lusoria dextra; VIII, right brachiocephalic trunk on the left side. *(1)* Right subclavian artery; *(2)* right common carotid artery; *(3)* left common carotid artery; *(4)* left subclavian artery.

pole of the thyroid gland. The presence of the vessel may be associated with the total or partial absence of the inferior thyroid arteries.

Variations of the aortic arch and its branches. The aortic arch and its larger branches may form numerous variations. Such irregularities, caused by some disturbance in the intricate development of the aorta, may be variations which give rise to no clinical complaints but may be anomalies accompanied by pathological changes. Their differentiation is difficult. It is not proposed here to expatiate upon anomalies in connection with the transposed origin of the aorta, nor upon its communications with the lesser circulation. Atypical possibilities without number arise from the combinations of the various irregularities. Whereas variations of the arch may be associated with the anomalous origin of the branches, variations of the branches may arise even if the arch is normal.

2. Left circumflex arch of the aorta (Fig. 14/II): The aortic arch is normal, but the descending aorta runs downward on the right side. It gets to the right behind the gullet (Edwards 1948, Grob 1949). The primordial aortic roots unite paramediastinally. The aortic knob is normal, but the border of the descending aorta appears on the right side on the roentgenogram. The gullet is impressed from behind at its intersection with the aorta; this impression can be visualized when the radio-opaque substance is ingested (Franke 1950). The turn to the right may be at the height of the arcus or deeper, behind the bifurcation of the trachea. In spite of the right turn of the descending aorta, the main branches of the arch may have normal origins. The right subclavian artery or the right brachiocephalic trunk occasionally arises from the origin of the descending aorta as the last branch of the aorta.

3. Two forms of the right arch of the aorta are known. *a. Situs inversus aortae* (Fig. 14/III): If the fourth right arch persists, the aortic arch is placed on the right side. The mirror image of the normal pattern is seen if it is in the right half of the thorax that the descending aorta runs downward. In such case the origin of the branches may be normal or the order of their origin may change (Fray 1936, Thurner 1951, Murray and Baron 1971). Owing to its retroesophageal position, the vessel which crosses the esophagus slightly to the left (the left brachiocephalic trunk or the left subclavian artery = arteria lusoria sinistra) encompasses with the ascending aorta the trachea and the gullet in both cases. This may cause symptoms of impression (Grollman et al. 1968). Diverticulumlike dilatation may occur at the origin of the vessels (Keats and Martt 1962, Zdansky 1962) or at the root of the ligamentum arteriosum (Wheeler and Keats 1963). The ligamentum arteriosum connects the left pulmonary artery with the left subclavian artery. The roentgenogram shows a constriction of the left side of the esophagus in cases of inverted aortic site. The individual branches of the aortic arch can be identified only by angiography.

b. Right circumflex arch of the aorta (Fig. 14/IV): If, in case of right-sided aortic arch, the descending aorta turns to the left, it hooks over between the spine and the gullet. It may do so also between the gullet and the trachea (Grob 1949, Álmos and Lónyay 1962). The aorta shows a complicated triple curvature: the first curve is the aortic arch, the second is the descending aorta; the third curvature inclines slightly towards the midline (Bedford and Parkinson 1936, Franke 1950). In this case the arch may extend considerably above the jugular notch (Bender et al. 1964). The order in which the main branches arise may show several variations in this case. On roentgenograms the aortic knob is visible on the right side, and the descending aorta on the left side. The esophagus is impressed on its posterior aspect. If the descending aorta inclines to the left, it can be clearly seen in the right oblique view. The downward coursing tortuous shadow of the aorta, seen below the left clavicle, curves back toward the midline at the level of the bifurcation (Zdansky 1962).

4. Double aortic arch (Fig. 14/V): Both aortic arches persist if the development of the aortic ring is unrestrained. This double arch surrounds the windpipe and the gullet, less frequently the former only. This variation is rare and usually not associated with other anomalies (Snelling and Erb 1933, Exalto et al. 1950, Kis-Várday 1963). It occurs occasionally that the two arches form a uniformly developed vascular ring (Neuhauser 1946) but more often one of the arches (mainly the right arch) is better developed and the other rudimentary (Arkin 1936, Hevitt and Brewer 1970). Provided the double aortic arch is symmetrically developed, with roentgenography the double aortic knob, the trachea and the stricture of the esophagus can be visualized. If the two arches are unevenly developed, the descending aorta may run downwards on either side (Zdansky 1962).

5. Absence of the aortic arch: The ascending aorta originates from the left ventricle, the descending limb is continuous with the ductus arteriosus so that no arch can be formed (Adachi 1928) which means a partial transposition of the large vessel.

6. Coarctation of the aorta: Partial constriction of the aorta in the region of the isthmus gives rise to pathological circulation and is regarded as anomaly.

7. Pseudocoarctation of the aorta (kinking; Fig. 14/VI). The descending aorta, curving back at the height of the isthmus, forms a second arch which passes with a bend into the lower segment of the descending part. If not accompanied by stricture it represents an anatomical variation. The backward arched segment below the aortic knob can be distinguished on well exposed x-ray pictures or on aortograms. This variation is very rare (Sonders et al. 1951, Steinberg 1962, Simay et al. 1967).

Variations in origin of the main branches of the aortic arch. Under normal conditions, the three principal branches may arise outside the convexity or from the arch.

I. Major vessels originating outside the convexity of the aorta. 1. Right subclavian artery arising on the left side (arteria lusoria dextra; Fig. 14/VII): The right subclavian artery arises at the boundary between the arch and the descending aorta. Its initial segment often shows a diverticulum-like dilatation. The artery sometimes runs upward from left to right between the esophagus and the trachea (Schmidt 1957). This configuration has long been known (Bayford 1789) and occurs in 0·5 to 2·0 per cent of the cases (Adachi 1928, Hayek 1958). While as a rule, it does not give rise to complaints, it is occasionally accompanied by disturbed deglutition (dysphagia lusoria; Holzapfel 1899). Beside the protruding aortic arch, an impression of the esophagus can be seen in the esophagogram below the aortic knob.

2. Brachiocephalic trunk arising on the left side (Fig. 14/VIII): If the right brachiocephalic trunk arises as the last branch of the aortic arch it can be recognized only via angiography (Grosse-Brockhoff et al. 1954). The impression of the esophagus is in such cases at the point where a similar irregularity is caused by the left principal bronchus under normal conditions (Zdansky 1962).

II. Major vessels originating from the convexity of the aortic arch. 1. Normal type (Fig. 15/I): Three large vessels, namely the brachiocephalic trunk, the left common carotid and the left subclavian arteries, spring off (in this order) from the convexity of the aortic arch. This variation is found in 83 to 85 per cent of the cases (Adachi 1928, Pontes 1963). Deviations from the normal may consist of a decrease in the number of vessels, their

5. Bicarotid trunk (Fig. 15/V): While the two common carotids have a common origin in the midline, the two subclavian arteries arise separately on the two sides.

6. Separate origin of all four branches (Fig. 15/VI): The brachiocephalic trunk is absent (Aleksandrowicz 1967).

7. Origin of the left vertebral artery from the aorta (Fig. 15/VII): The left vertebral artery arises

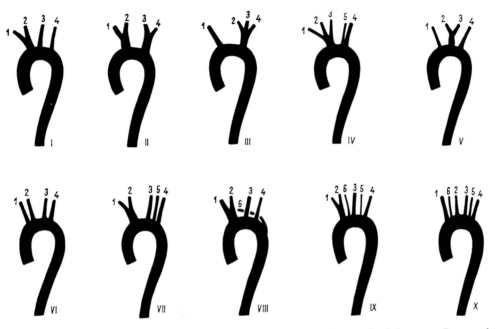

FIG. 15. Variations of the major blood vessels arising from the convexity of the arch of the aorta. I, normal type; II, double brachiocephalic trunks; III, left bicaroticosubclavian trunk; IV, right bicaroticosubclavian trunk; V, bicarotid trunk; VI, separate origin of the four vessels; VII, left vertebral artery springing off from the aorta; VIII, right vertebral artery arising from the aorta; IX, both vertebral arteries arising from the aorta; X, six vessels arising from aorta. (1) Right subclavian artery; (2) right common carotid artery; (3) left common carotid artery; (4) left subclavian artery; (5) left vertebral artery; (6) right vertebral artery.

fusion or an increase in their number. Also other vessels may arise from the aorta. Two to six variations and their combinations are possible (Liechty et al. 1957, Jungblut 1966).

2. Double brachiocephalic trunk (Fig. 15/II): The four principal vessels spring from two symmetrically placed brachiocephalic trunks.

3. Left bicaroticosubclavian trunk (Fig. 15/III): The right subclavian artery emerges alone, the other vessels arise jointly.

4. Right bicaroticosubclavian trunk (Fig. 15/IV): The brachiocephalic trunk and the left common carotid artery have a common origin, and the left vertebral artery forms an independent branch between the jointly emerging vessels and the left subclavian artery. This is the most frequently observed variation, occurring in 10 per cent of the cases (Adachi 1928).

between the left common carotid and the left subclavian artery. Four vessels emerge from the arch. The frequency of this variation is 4·3 per cent (Adachi 1928). Seldom the left vertebral artery may also arise as a separate side branch of the aortic arch behind the left subclavian artery.

8. Origin of the right vertebral artery from the aorta (Fig. 15/VIII): Situated behind the left subclavian artery, the right vertebral artery, the last branch of the aorta, runs obliquely to the opposite side (Krause 1880, cit. Adachi 1928).

9. Origin of both vertebral arteries from the aorta (Fig. 15/IX): The left common carotid arises in the midline, and the vertebral arteries are on its two sides.

10. Origin of six vessels from the aorta (Fig. 15/X): The brachiocephalic trunk is absent and the vertebral arteries arise independently.

11. Supernumerary vessels: The arteria thyroidea ima (0·6 per cent), the internal thoracic artery (0·2 per cent), the thymic artery (0·2 per cent) and muscular arteries (Pontes 1963) may arise from the aorta as supernumerary vessels.

Descending (thoracic) aorta

The thoracic portion of the descending aorta (Figs 37/17, 38/16, 39/17, 40/9, 44/9, 45/7, 46/10, 57/9, 58/10, 59/8, 60/9) begins at the left border of the 4th thoracic vertebra where it is continuous with the aortic arch. It courses downward, somewhat obliquely toward the midline. The upper extremity of the vessel is 2 to 2·5 cm laterally to the median plane, while its supradiaphragmatic part lies in the midline (Paturet 1958). Its entire course runs in the posterior mediastinum behind, or in its upper segment to the left of the esophagus. Passing through the aortic opening of the diaphragm in the midline, at the height of the 12th thoracic vertebra, it continues as the abdominal aorta.

It is by means of the endothoracic fascia that the aorta is attached to the vertebral column that runs behind it. The branches of the hemiazygos vein are between the aorta and the spine. In front of its origin is the left principal bronchus, above which the thoracic aorta is crossed by the left pulmonary artery, while the left inferior pulmonary vein crosses it under the bronchus. The middle segment of the aorta is separated from the left ventricle and the left atrium by the pericardium. The aortic groove of the left lung is placed to the left of the thoracic aorta, while, to its right, we find the gullet above, and the azygos vein imbedded in loose connective tissue below. Running first to the right and in front, the esophagus crosses the thoracic aorta from its anterior aspect. The diaphragm is then pierced by the esophagus on the left side and in front of the aorta. The vessel is surrounded in its entire course by the aortic plexus. Its length is 30 cm, its diameter 2·5 cm (Paturet 1958). The thoracic aorta has the following *branches*:

Because of its close correlation with the lesser circulation, the *bronchial branches* will be discussed in context with the lesser circulation.

The *esophageal branches* (Figs 16/6, 44/31, 45/28) arise in variable numbers from the front of the aorta. Shapiro and Robillard (1950) distinguish short and long arteries which, after a course of 3 to 5 cm, pass obliquely downward to the posterior wall of the esophagus where they divide into ascending and descending parts. One of the long arteries arises at the height of the 7th, the other at that of the 9th thoracic vertebra (Anson 1951). The vessels,

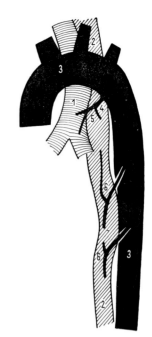

Fig. 16. Arteries of the thoracic segment of the esophagus. Second oblique view: (*1*) trachea; (*2*) esophagus; (*3*) aorta; (*4*) left bronchial branch; (*5*) esophageal branch (from the left bronchial branch); (*6*) esophageal branches.

ensuring the segmental supply of the esophagus (ascending pharyngeal, inferior thyroid, left gastric and splenic arteries), are closely interconnected by a submucosal arterial plexus (Póka and Nagy 1952). Also, the left bronchial artery supplies blood to the esophagus. The abundant arterial supply suffices for the maintenance of collateral circulation, but blood supply becomes insufficient if several larger trunks are incompetent (Nagy 1962). Angiograms, made in both oblique views, are necessary to demonstrate the vessels of the thoracic portion of the esophagus. Major trunks fill usually at the height of the 7th to 9th thoracic vertebrae.

The *pericardial branches* consist of a few small vessels which, distributed to the posterior surface of the pericardium, can hardly be visualized by angiography.

The *posterior intercostal arteries* (Figs 17/2, 44/32, 45/29, 46/28) arise in pairs from the back of the ascending thoracic aorta and are distributed to the 3rd to 11th intercostal spaces. The *subcostal artery* below the 12th rib is similarly situated. The arteries run forward between the veins and nerves in the costal grooves along the costal arches between the outer and inner intercostal muscles. Those on the right side are somewhat longer because they have to reach their intercostal space by passing in front of the vertebral column. Doing so, they run behind the esophagus, the thoracic duct, the azygos vein and the sympathetic trunk. Those of the left side

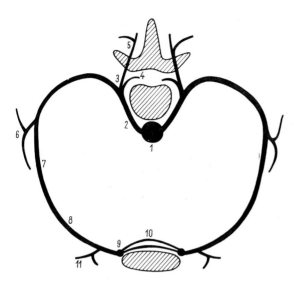

FIG. 17. Circle of intercostal arteries in the middle third of the thorax. (1) Aorta; (2) posterior intercostal artery; (3) dorsal branch; (4) spinal branch; (5) medial and lateral cutaneous branches; (6) lateral cutaneous branch; (7) collateral branch; (8) anterior intercostal branch; (9) internal thoracic arterior; (10) sternal branches; (11) perforating branches.

run behind the azygos vein. The terminal branches, anastomosing with the internal thoracic artery, form an arterial circle which provides good collateral circulation (Fig. 17). The diameter of the posterior intercostal arteries averages 2 mm. Variations occur chiefly in the longitudinal anastomoses in the upper part of the thorax (Ennabli 1967). It is in 80 per cent that the right fourth vessel sends off a branch to the right bronchial artery (Paturet 1958). Two intercostal vessels may emerge with a common trunk.

Branches of the intercostal arteries: The *dorsal branch* (Figs 17/3, 44/33, 45/30, 46/29) curves backward along the vertebral bodies and bifurcates after a short course. The *spinal branch* (Fig. 17/4), entering the vertebral canal across the corresponding vertebral foramen, communicates there with the spinal arteries. The *medial* and *lateral cutaneous branches* (Figs 17/5, 17/6, 44/34, 46/30) terminate in the muscles and the skin. The lateral branch supplies part of the blood to the breast. Arching forward, its terminal branches (*rami collaterales*; Figs 17/7, 44/35, 45/31, 46/31) communicate with the anterior intercostal branches. Also the corresponding branch of the highest intercostal artery forms a part of this arch-shaped connection. The three lowest vessels communicate with the superior epigastric and musculophrenic arteries in the abdominal wall.

Roentgenograms in the **anteroposterior** view (Fig. 44) are eminently suited for the visualization of the

principal trunks. The relation between the vessels and the ribs, further the posterior aspect of the collaterals as well as the lateral cutaneous branches can be conveniently examined in this view, whereas—owing to its almost sagittal course—the dorsal branch is hardly distinguishable. In the **lateral view** (Fig. 45) also the posterior branches become visible beside the arched course of the main trunks, although their summated shadows make examination difficult. We found radiographs taken in both **oblique views** (Fig. 46) to be best suited for the visualization of the posterior branches; the branches running to the spine are well outlined in such pictures.

The *superior phrenic arteries*, consisting of two (sometimes three) trunks, arise from the lowest part of the descending thoracic aorta and are distributed to the upper surface of the diaphragm. They can be better examined in the anteroposterior than in the lateral view.

Radiological anatomy of the thoracic aorta

Radiological conditions are examined in the following in the posteroanterior and the first and second oblique views.

Posteroanterior roentgenograms (Fig. 37) show only the left half of the aortic arch and the beginning of the descending aorta which form the first arch of the middle shadow known as the *aortic knob* (Fig. 37/16). It is visible in the area of the isthmus, between the shadow of the medial end of the left clavicle and that of the pulmonary trunk. With a straight border, the *descending aorta* (Fig. 37/17) runs downward from the aortic knob and is slightly directed toward the spinal column. It is sometimes possible to see the left subclavian artery which, running upward, forms a laterally concave border along the mediastinum. The *ascending aorta* (Fig. 37/15) cannot be distinguished in this projection. Under special constitutional conditions its right border may extend beyond the border of the superior vena cava, which forms the right upper arch.

Radiographs taken in the **first oblique view** (Fig. 38) show the anterior border of the *ascending aorta* (Fig. 38/14) running above the pulmonary trunk in an upward and backward direction. Its upper extremity is lost in the shadow of the left brachiocephalic vein. The posterior border of the ascending aorta coalesces with the adjacent tissues. The anterior border of the *descending aorta* (Fig. 38/16) is outlined before the vertebral column.

In the **second oblique view** (Fig. 39), the *ascending aorta* (Fig. 39/15) forms a sharp border which extends upward from the upper end of the cardiac

41

shadow. Its shadow is cast on the projection of the superior vena cava and that of the right pulmonary artery, but becomes visible before them on stronger rotation. Its right border curves into the arch of the aorta, while the left border is sharply outlined against the trachea and the right principal bronchus. The inferior border cannot be distinguished from the right pulmonary artery and the right pulmonary veins. The width of the upper section of the ascending aorta is reliably appreciable if the posterior

anterior border is less frequently outlined. Thus the entire course of the thoracic aorta is visible in this view.

Measurement of the aorta

Projections revealing the aortic wall in its width make it possible to make a *direct* measurement of the aorta. With the *indirect* method we compare

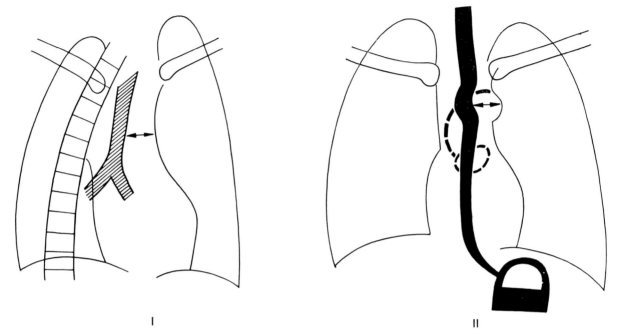

FIG. 18. Methods for the measurement of the aorta. I, in the first oblique view (after Assmann); II, in the postero-anterior view (after Kreuzfuchs).

border of the ascending aorta touches the anterior border of the trachea. Owing to the brachiocephalic trunk emitted by it and the soft tissues situated behind, the initial portion of the *arch of the aorta* (Fig. 39/16) cannot be distinguished. In its subsequent course, the arch becomes distinguishable again owing to the translucent band of the trachea. The upper border of the posterior part of the arch is outlined particularly well. This area corresponds to that segment of the left subclavian artery which lies immediately after its origin. Though projected on the trachea, sometimes also the shadow of the left common carotid artery is visible. The surrounding soft tissues prevent the inferior border from being visualized in the posterior two thirds of the arch. The shadow of the posterior border of the *descending aorta* (Fig. 39/17), thrown upon the projection of the anterior border of the spine, can be followed over a stretch the length of which depends on the constitution and age of the individual. The

a well distinguishable segment to some other fixed line. Assmann (1934) carried out determinations in both oblique views. In the first oblique view (Fig. 18/I), he determined the distance between the outer border of the aorta and the trachea at the junction of the arch and the ascending portion. Using the posteroanterior projection, Vaquez and Bordet (1928) determined the distance from the midline to the border of the ascending aorta as well as the aortic knob. Kreuzfuchs (1936), after filling the esophagus with radio-opaque material, determined the distance from the lateral edge of the aortic knob to the point of the esophageal impression (Fig. 18/II). He found it to amount to 2 to 2·5 cm in adults between 20 and 50 years; to 1 cm in children of 5 years, and to 1·3 cm at the age of 10. Fleischner (1926) and Zdansky (1932) modified Kreuzfuchs' method. They recommend the patient's rotation to the left until the segment they want to examine comes to lie in the path of the ray.

The modified measurement is carried out in this position.

The limitation of all these methods is that they can be employed only in certain variations of the aortic arch. Aortography eliminates this difficulty. Its employment enables to study the thoracic aorta in its entire course. Owing to its simplicity, the modified method of Kreuzfuchs can still be used to advantage.

Physiological changes in radiological morphology

Physiological conditions with respect to the radiological anatomy of the aorta are influenced by pulsation, the width of the aorta, the position of the diaphragm as also by differences in age and sex.

Pulsation, as perceptible on the aortic knob, consists of vigorous dilatation during systole and of slow contraction during diastole. The aortic knob is displaced upwards and to the left in systole. The amplitude of deviations is influenced by the position of the diaphragm and the entire elongation of the aorta.

Among the factors on which the *width of the aorta* depends, are, according to Zdansky (1962), the volume of blood flowing through it, the intraaortic tension, mural elasticity and muscular tonicity. Hypoplastic aorta (aorta angusta) is a congenital anomaly. The whole aorta is thin. Abnormally reduced aorta is present only if its width is less than normal in a recumbent position (Reuterwall 1922, Zdansky 1962). A diffusely wide aorta is not an anatomical variation but the result of some disease.

Diaphragm in *high position* elevates the entire aorta so that its arch is displaced upwards, while its ascending and descending limbs are shifted laterally. Hence, the ascending aorta forms a border on the right side, while on the left the descending aorta widens the upper border of the cardiac shadow over a longer stretch. The distal third of the arch turns somewhat transversely, so that the aorta looks wider on the roentgenogram. In the second oblique view, the aorta which generally looks like a "shepherd's crook", here assumes the approximate form of a semicircular arch. Both the ascending and the descending aorta become elongated along the axis of the body if the diaphragm occupies a low position. The aorta becomes more vertical in this case. When examined in the posteroanterior view, the aorta appears to be narrower, and at the same time the border of the aortic knob becomes less conspicuous.

Age. The position of the diaphragm becomes lower with advancing age, while paradoxically, the aorta, instead of appearing to be narrower, seems to be wider. Therefore, posteroanterior roentgenograms of older persons often show the border of the ascending aorta to extend beyond the shadow of the superior vena cava (Holzmann 1952).

Sex. The fact that the diaphragm is relatively higher in females makes their aortic configuration slightly wider in contrast to males.

Aortography

In connection with angiocardiography, Castellanos and his associates (1937) were the first to examine the aorta via radio-opaque filling. Aortography, i.e., the selective filling of the thoracic aorta and its branches, was first performed by Jönsson and his coworkers (1951), and it was Janker (1955) who elaborated the method and outlined its applicability.

With *postmortem angiography* in **anteroposterior view** (Figs 44, 57, 59), the *bulb of the aorta* (Figs 44/6, 57/4) is placed to the right of, and half a costal space lower than the origin of the pulmonary trunk. The *ascending aorta* (Figs 44/7, 57/7, 59/6) tends to the right and upwards and is continuous with the arch of the aorta behind the sternal end of the right 2nd rib. Owing to its anatomical position, in this view it seems to be somewhat shorter than in reality. Owing to the almost sagittal position of the *arch of the aorta* (Figs 44/8, 57/8, 59/7), the three major vessels, originating in three different planes, show side by side in the projection. The first, i.e., the *brachiocephalic trunk* (Figs 44/17, 57/10, 59/9), runs upward and to the right. The *left common carotid artery* next to it (Figs 44/18, 57/11, 59/13), is projected on the left side of the trachea and climbs steeply upwards. The last of the three is the *left subclavian artery* (Figs 44/19, 57/12, 59/11). The two latter vessels run a parallel course over a length of a few centimetres. The arch of the aorta extends from the sternal end of the second right ripple to the left border of the 4th thoracic vertebra. Its last portion forms part of the aortic knob visible in plain radiographs. The *descending aorta* (Figs 44/9, 57/9, 59/8) runs from the left border of the 4th thoracic vertebra towards the diaphragm in a right-downward course.

In the **lateral view** (Figs 45, 58, 60), the arched shape of the *bulb* (Figs 45/4, 58/5) is determined by the arrangement of the semilunar valves. The *ascending aorta* (Figs 45/5, 58/8, 60/7) runs steeply upward and bends slightly backward. The *arch of the aorta* (Figs 45/6, 58/9, 60/8) is shortened in this projection also, for both its right and its left turn are projected on the same plane. The *brachiocephalic* trunk (Figs 45/16, 58/11, 60/10) cannot be distinguished from the *left common carotid artery* (Figs 45/18, 58/11, 60/10), while the projection of the *left subclavian artery* appears behind them (Figs 45/19, 58/14, 60/11). The arch of the aorta approaches the spine, and the *descending aorta* (Figs 45/7, 58/10, 60/9) passes downward and obliquely slightly forward from the inferior border of the 4th thoracic vertebra along the anterior border of the vertebral column. The area between the aorta and the spine at the diaphragm is about 1·5 cm wider than the upper segment.

In the **second oblique view** (Fig. 46) the projection of the entire thoracic aorta lies in a plane parallel to that of the x-ray film so that the whole characteristic shape resembling a shepherd's crook is outlined. The *ascending aorta* (Fig. 46/8) runs slightly upward and forward from the *bulb of the aorta* (Fig. 46/7). The three large vessels emitted by the *arch* (Fig. 46/9) are distinguishable. The *descending aorta* (Fig. 46/10) passes downward and slightly forward in the projection of the right border of the spinal column. The narrow segment formed by the isthmus of the aorta on the border of the arch of the aorta and the descending aorta can be well visualized most of the time.

THORACIC VEINS
(VEINS OF THE GREATER CIRCULATION)
SYSTEM OF THE SUPERIOR VENA CAVA AND THE AZYGOS VEIN

Superior vena cava

The **superior vena cava** (Figs 37/2, 38/2, 39/2, 47/10, 48/8, 55/10, 56/10) is formed by the union of the brachiocephalic veins; it collects blood from the veins of the upper half of the body and opens into the right atrium. It is situated in the anterior part of the superior mediastinum. The upper half of the vein is covered anteriorly with connective tissue, its lower half is in the pericardial sac. To the right of its origin it forms a slightly convex arch and runs toward the heart. The ascending aorta and the initial segment of the arch of the aorta are to its left, the right upper lobe of the lung to its right, behind it the right pulmonary artery occupies a higher, and the right superior pulmonary vein a lower position. The lower half of its anterior portion is covered by the pericardium and within the latter by the right auricle, while the higher half is covered by the mediastinal connective tissue. The azygos vein opens into its posterior side above the border of the pericardium. The superior vena cava is devoid of valves. The length of the superior vena cava is 6 to 8 cm; its diameter 1·5 to 2·2 cm (Paturet 1958). The projection of the superior vena cava on the anterior thoracic wall extends parasternally from the sternal end of the 1st right rib to the sternal end of the 3rd rib (Hayek 1958).

Variations. Persistent left superior vena cava (Figs 19, 221/7). Two superior venae cavae are present if the left duct of Cuvier and the initial segment of the left superior cardinal vein persist. This is the most frequent variation of the venous system, and its occurrence is estimated to occur in 1 to 3 per cent (Drewes and Seling 1966). The vessel of the size of a little finger's breadth forms the continuation of the left brachiocephalic vein and passes in front of the arch of the aorta and the hilum of the lung to reach the pericardium. Its orifice is variable. A communication may persist between the two caval veins (transverse jugular vein). The right vena cava may be absent (Grosse-Brockhoff et al. 1960). Other congenital cardiac anomalies may be concomitant, such as defect of the atrial septum (Winter 1954), transposition of a pulmonary vein (Gensini et al. 1959), bilateral persistence of the azygos veins (Glasgow 1963), simultaneous existence of variations of the inferior vena cava (Derra et al. 1965), doubling of the subclavian vein (Drewes and Seling 1966). The occurrence of the persistent left superior vena cava is estimated at 40 per cent in the cases of dextrocardia (Campbell and Deuchar 1954).

Grouping according to the opening of the persistent left superior vena cava shows the following comparatively frequent possibilities (Doerr 1955):

1. It opens into the left auricle (Fig. 19/I), a phenomenon often accompanied by some other anomaly (Friedrich et al. 1950). Normal circulatory conditions are present only if the supernumerary vein is extremely thin.

2. Opening into the coronary sinus (Fig. 19/II) is the most frequent variation which, provided haemodynamic conditions are normal, is not pathologic (Beuren 1966). Opening into the right atrium has also been described (Zágreanu et al. 1964).

44

3. The persistent vein, opening into the occluded coronary sinus (Fig. 19/III), is emptied by the right vena cava via the simultaneously existing transverse jugular vein (Reed 1938).

4. It may open into the inferior vena cava (Fig. 19/IV) under normal circulatory conditions (Hagedorn 1954).

Branches of the superior vena cava. Minor veins, such as the *pericardial* and *mediastinal veins* and sometimes also the *right internal thoracic vein* open into the superior vena cava. The most significant branch is the constant *azygos vein* through which communication is maintained between the superior vena cava and the inferior vena cava.

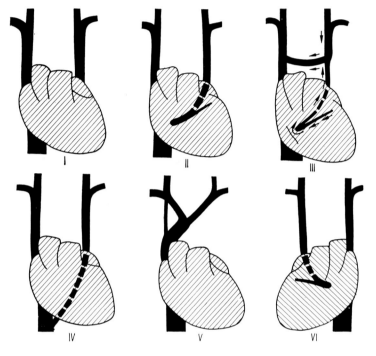

FIG. 19. Variable openings of the persistent left superior vena cava. I, left auricle; II, coronary sinus; III, occluded coronary sinus (circulation via the anastomosis); IV, inferior vena cava; V, right atrium (occlusion of the superior vena cava); VI, situs inversus (the left vena cava is normal, the right is supernumerary).

5. Instead of the typical superior vena cava, it opens alone into the right atrium (Knappe et al. 1968; Fig. 19/V). Normal circulation between them is possible only with adequate anastomosis (Goerttler 1958). Only an occluded bundle can be found in such cases in the lower part of the right superior vena cava.

6. In cases of situs inversus (Fig. 19/VI), the left vena cava is normal, while the right vena cava is the variation (Halpert and Coman 1930). In laevocardia, the persistent vein may empty into the left atrium (Beuren 1966).

7. Association with other irregularities brings about numerous possibilities which are conjoined with congenital cardiac anomalies. Also opening into the pulmonary veins (Gardner and Oram 1953) and into the portal vein (Chlyvitch 1932) have been described.

Radiological anatomy. Seen in the **anteroposterior view** (Fig. 37), the *superior vena cava* (Fig. 37/2) constitutes the right upper arch of the middle shadow. Its right edge may be obscured by a wider aorta. It continues in the right brachiocephalic vein, the right border of which is always visible. In cases of persisting left superior vena cava, provided the vessel is thick enough, it is possible to study the widening left border of the mediastinum as well as the venous pulsation (Holzmann 1952). Roentgenograms made in the **first oblique view** (Fig. 38) show the lower third of the vena cava superior between the ascending and the descending aorta, its middle third in front of, and its upper third above the arch of the aorta. In the **2nd oblique view** (Fig. 39), it is to a great extent obscured by the ascending aorta, and only a small segment below the orifice of the brachiocephalic veins can be seen covered by the

45

manubrium sterni. In **lateral view** (Fig. 40), the superior vena cava, covered by the ascending aorta, cannot be distinguished in the soft tissues. The orifice of the brachiocephalic veins is occasionally visible.

Pulsation observable on the superior vena cava is of both venous and also of arterial type. No pulsation is perceptible if it is covered by the ascending aorta.

System of the azygos and hemiazygos veins

These veins arise as *ascending lumbar veins* from the abdominal cavity on the two sides of the spine. They are connected by the transversely running

The **hemiazygos vein** (Figs 20/2, 49/5) runs on the left side of the spine upward behind the aorta, then turns to the right at the level of the 6th to 9th thoracic vertebrae and opens into the azygos vein. Sometimes, it arches to the right side before the aorta. The *accessory hemiazygos vein* (Fig. 20/3), which may have a variable course, collects blood from the upper left quadrant of the chest. One or more anastomoses connect the azygos and hemiazygos veins.

Variations of the azygos system. In case of irregular course, the azygos vein cuts through the right upper lobe of the lung to the superior vena cava (Wrisberg 1778, cit. Szücs 1964). Schinz et al. (1952) estimate the incidence of the so-called "azygos lobe" at 0·5 per cent. The vein may be redoubled in

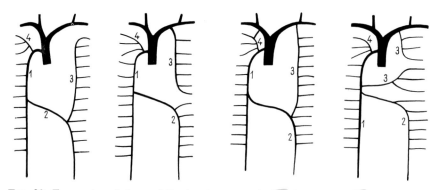

FIG. 20. Frequent variations of the hemiazygos vein. (*1*) Azygos vein; (*2*) hemiazygos vein; (*3*) accessory hemiazygos vein; (*4*) right superior intercostal vein.

lumbar veins. The ascending lumbar veins enter the thorax between the crura of the diaphragm; the vein on the right-hand side is called then azygos, that of the left-hand side the hemiazygos vein. There are several anastomoses with the inferior vena cava in the abdominal cavity.

The **azygos vein** (Figs 20/1, 47/13, 48/9, 49/4, 55/13, 56/13) ascends in the posterior mediastinum in front of the right border of the spinal column. With azygography, Szücs (1964) found its course to be on the right in 50, in the middle in 36, and on the left in 14 per cent. The azygos vein intersects the posterior intercostal arteries anteriorly. The thoracic duct and the aorta are to the left, and the sympathetic trunk to the right of the azygos vein. At the height of the 4th or 5th thoracic vertebra, it curves mildly to the right, then arching forward at right angles, it passes above the right principal bronchus to open into the superior vena cava, just before that vessel pierces the pericardium. In two-third of the cases 1 to 4 valves can be found in it (Zrivets 1970). The azygos vein measures 20 to 25 cm in length and 0·4 to 1·0 cm in diameter (Paturet 1958).

case of persistent left superior vena cava (Saxena 1965), or typical vena cava superior (Düx et al. 1967). Nagy (1962) described the following more important variations of the accessory hemiazygos vein (Fig. 20/3): it may open into the hemiazygos vein (40 per cent; Fig. 20/I), into the brachiocephalic vein (30 per cent; Fig. 20/II), into the azygos vein (5 per cent), or it enters a connecting arch between the hemiazygos and brachiocephalic veins (15 per cent; Fig. 20/III). It is sometimes doubled (10 per cent; Fig. 20/IV) in which case the upper part terminates in the brachiocephalic, the lower in the hemiazygos or azygos vein.

Branches of the azygos system. *Posterior intercostal veins* (Figs 48/10, 49/6). These vessels drain the thoracic wall and the spinal column (*dorsal and spinal branches*). The latter are in communication with the other venous plexuses through the external and internal vertebral plexuses. The branches running in the thoracic wall drain the intercostal spaces. The azygos vein receives, on the right side, the three veins with a tributary, the *right superior intercostal vein* (Fig. 48/11), while all other veins empty directly into the main trunk. The upper 4 to 6 veins of the left side open into the accessory hemiazygos, the lower ones into the hemiazygos vein. The middle veins open directly into the azygos vein by means of transverse communications. The lowest intercostal veins of both sides are known as *subcostal veins*. Like the arteries, the intercostal veins form a venous ring with the branches of the internal thoracic vein (Fig. 49/8). They communicate with the lateral thoracic vein in the middle axillary line. There are valves 2 to 3 cm before the orifice of the intercostal veins.

The *superior phrenic veins* extend from the posterosuperior part of the diaphragm.

The *esophageal veins* (Fig. 47/15), begin with the submucosal plexus of the gullet. They maintain communication between the various longitudinal veins supplying the gullet, viz., the inferior thyroid, the azygos, hemiazygos, superior phrenic and left gastric veins (Nakayama and Kitagawa 1965). The collateral anastomoses between the superior vena cava and the portal vein are of clinical significance.

The *bronchial veins*, being closely correlated with the lesser circulation, will be discussed in connection with the pulmonary circulation.

The numerous plexiform *pericardiac* and *mediastinal veins* (Fig. 47/14) empty into the azygos system.

Radiological anatomy. Plain roentgenograms show only the pre-orificial segment before the orifice of the azygos vein. It is especially in childhood that this vein can be seen in the right tracheobronchial angle on sagittal radiographs. Wishart (1972) when studying the thoracic roentgenograms of children found the diameter of the azygos vein between 0 to 6 months to be 3.5 mm, between 6 months and 2 years 4.1 mm, between 2 and 7 years 4.8 mm and between 7 and 14 years 5.1 mm in normal cases. The vein appears to be smaller in standing than in recumbent position (Zdansky 1962). It decreases during Valsalva's experiment (Swart 1959). The azygos vein can be much better visualized by tomography (Erdélyi 1944, Bozsó 1966). In frontal tomograms (at an approximate depth of 8 cm), the vein can be identified in the angle of the trachea and the right principal bronchus in the form of a tear-drop. In sagittal tomograms (at an approximate depth of 10 cm, in a right-side position), the vein segment can be seen as an arch extending from the point where it inclines forward from the spine, right to its orifice, mainly in pneumomediastinum. The width of the vein can thus be reliably determined. The "azygos lobe" can be identified on sagittal roentgenograms by means of the orthodiagraphic shadow cast by the interlobar space (Wessler, cit. Szücs et al. 1960).

Brachiocephalic veins

The brachiocephalic veins (Figs 37/1, 38/1, 39/1, 47/11 and 12, 48/12, 55/11, 56/11 and 12, 110/5 and 6) are large trunks, formed by the union of the internal jugular and subclavian veins (venous angle), which open into the superior vena cava. They collect blood from the head, neck and the upper extremities.

Originating behind the left sternoclavicular joint, the *left brachiocephalic vein* runs obliquely downward to the superior vena cava in front of the internal thoracic artery, the phrenic nerve, the subclavian artery, the vagus nerve, the left common carotid artery, the trachea and the brachiocephalic trunk. The aortic arch lies caudal to the vessel. The initial segment of the vein runs in front of the costal pleura, and its termination is overlapped by the bend of the pleura. The *right brachiocephalic vein* passes steeply from behind the right sternoclavicular joint downward to the superior vena cava. Posteriorly and to its left are the vagus nerve and the brachiocephalic trunk; to the right the phrenic nerve and the internal thoracic artery run almost parallel with it. Its course is covered by the sternoclavicular articulation and, lower, by the manubrium of the sternum as well as by the 1st rib and the sternal muscles. The angle formed by the union of the bilateral veins is more than 90° in the newborn, 90° in the adult and acute angle in old age (Adachi 1933). The brachiocephalic veins are devoid of valves.

The projection of the left brachiocephalic vein on the anterior chest wall corresponds to the line between the left sternoclavicular and the right first sternocostal joints. The right brachiocephalic vein runs almost vertically downward from the right sternoclavicular joint. The left vein has a length of 6 to 8 cm (5·1 to 8·5 cm); the right is 3 to 3·5 cm long (2·6 to 5·5 cm; Paturet 1958). The diameter of both veins averages 1·3 to 1·6 cm (Paturet 1958).

Variations. In cases of persistent left superior vena cava, the left vein runs steeply downward and passes into the superior vena cava without interruption. A rare variation is when the left vein passes in front of the aortic arch, then turns right and unites with its counterpart (Jakubczik 1963). This vein may sometimes reach the superior vena cava through the substance of the thymus (Krause 1876, cit. Adachi 1933).

Radiological anatomy. **Posteroanterior view** (Fig. 37): the slightly laterally curving right border of the *right brachiocephalic vein* (Fig. 37/1) in continuation of the superior vena cava disappears in the shadow of the inferior border of the sternoclavicular joint. **First oblique view** (Fig. 38): the shadow of the *left* *vein* (Fig. 38/1), running in a posteroanterior direction, can only be guessed in the projection of the posterior border of the manubrium sterni. The *right vein* projects mostly on the air band of the trachea (Fig. 38/1). **Second oblique view** (Fig. 39): the anterior border of the *right vein* is projected on the shadow of the manubrium sterni. The *left vein* cannot be distinguished from the mediastinal structures (Fig. 39/1). Neither vein can be visualized in the **lateral view.**

The *branches* of the brachiocephalic veins spring off from the neck and the thorax. Part of the cervical branches carry blood from the thyroid (*inferior thyroid vein*) and the larynx (*inferior laryngeal vein*). The thyroid plexus (*thyroid impar venous plexus;* Fig. 47/16), originating from the thyroid isthmus is in front of the trachea, in anastomotic communication with the inferior thyroid and laryngeal veins. One or more branches (*vena thyroidea ima*) empty into the left brachiocephalic vein. The inferior laryngeal vein empties most frequently into the right vein. Several branches of the inferior thyroid vein open into the internal jugular vein (Rauber and Kopsch 1951). Extensive collateral circulation may be maintained via the superior-inferior-posterior-median plexuses of the thyroid between the brachiocephalic and the jugular veins (Chevrel et al. 1965).

Another venous plexus, originating from the neck, collects the blood of the spine and the occiput (*vertebral vein,* Figs 110/14, 112/18, 115/26; *anterior vertebral vein, accessory vertebral vein, suboccipital venous plexus,* Figs 112/17, 115/25; *deep cervical vein,* Figs 47/21, 112/20). These veins unite in 2 to 3 trunks and open posteriorly into the brachiocephalic veins.

The visceral parts of the thoracic branches arise from the mediastinal organs after which they are named (*thymic, pericardiac, pericardiacophrenic, mediastinal, bronchial, tracheal, esophageal veins;* Figs 47/14 and 15). Among them, particularly the bronchial and esophageal veins are of clinical significance.

The parietal branches originate from the chest wall, the anterior part of the diaphragm and the supero-anterior part of the abdominal wall. The *internal thoracic veins* (Fig. 49/8), two veins accompanying the artery of the same name, extend from the abdominal wall into the thorax (*superior epigastric veins*) establishing in this way communication between the system of the portal vein and the inferior vena cava. The anterior and thoracic branches running from the diaphragm (*musculophrenic* and *anterior intercostal veins*) form a venous ring with the azygos system. The supreme intercostal veins behave differently. The *supreme intercostal vein* receives blood from the two right superoanterior intercostal veins and opens into the right brachiocephalic vein, sometimes into the superior vena cava. The size of the *left superior intercostal vein* depends on the size of the hemiazygos vein. Usually it carries the blood of the upper 3 to 4 intercostal segments to the left brachiocephalic vein. It returns blood from the left bronchial veins and communicates with the azygos veins as well (Rauber and Kopsch 1951).

The thoracic duct opens into the left venous angle and the right lymphatic duct into the right venous angle.

Subclavian vein

The subclavian veins (Figs 47/19, 48/13, 55/12, 110/7) open into the brachiocephalic veins behind the sternoclavicular joint. They drain the arms, the shoulder girdles and a part of the anterior thoracic wall. They follow the course of the corresponding arteries from which they are separated by the scalenus anterior muscle. They run along and are attached to the inner surface of the clavicle. The left subclavian artery is situated more medially than its contralateral partner (Land 1972). They are usually provided with valves. The terminal valve is in the venous angle or sometimes slightly below it (Drewes 1963). Its function is influenced by the intrathoracic pressure (Rominger 1958).

Variations. Drewes and Seling (1966) observed reduplication in one per cent of the examined cases. Sometimes an accessory subclavian vein can be found between the clavicle and the subclavius muscle. Islet formation has occasionally been observed around the tendon of the scalenus anterior muscle (Drewes 1963).

Branches. The subclavian vein is the continuation of the *axillary vein.* Its main branches are the *thoracoacromial, transverse cervical,* and *transverse scapular veins.* The latter two vessels frequently empty with a common orifice into the subclavian vein.

Collaterals between the major thoracic and abdominal veins

Performed communications may ensure extensive collateral circulation between the system of the superior and inferior vena cava (Fig. 21; Carlson 1934, Abrams 1957, Steinberg 1962, Markhashow 1970). Anatomical structures offer basis for the following connections: 1. with the azygos system via the ascending lumbar veins (Fig. 21/5 and 6);

2. with the internal thoracic vein via the superior and inferior epigastric and also through the external iliac veins (Figs 21/11, 15 and 19); 3. with the thoracoepigastric vein via the subclavian and the external iliac veins (Figs 21/20 and 15). 4. The vertebral veins maintain communication between the superior and inferior venae cavae via the brachiocephalic, intercostal, lumbar and sacral veins (Figs 21/23, 3, 10 and 16).

Collaterals between the systems of the superior caval and the portal veins will be dealt with in chapter of the portal system.

Contrast-filling of the thoracic veins

"Superior" cavography. Sicard and Forestier (1922), further Dünner and Calm (1923) were the first to fill the major thoracic veins intravitally with radio-opaque substance. Sgalitzer and his associates (1931) studied the valves and the conditions of blood flow in their work on phlebography. Drewes' communication (1963), based on 500 examinations, presents a detailed study of the possible anatomical variations.

In *postmortem angiography* the large thoracic veins can best be studied in **anteroposterior pictures** (Figs 47, 55). The *subclavian vein* (Figs 47/19, 55/12), the continuation of the axillary vein, shows a slightly curved course above the projection of the 1st rib. Sometimes impressions due to the pressure of soft tissues can be observed on the vein. Drewes (1963) regarded this as nonpathologic, so-called "pelott's effect". Occasional collaterals with the jugular and cephalic veins can be observed. Only a few of the tributaries of the *brachiocephalic veins* (Figs 47/11 and 12, 55/11) can be visualized if the latter are filled *in vivo*. The *vena thyroidea ima* can be demonstrated with relative frequency. Süsse and Aurig (1954) demonstrated the bilateral *internal thoracic veins* by injecting contrast material into the sternum. In *postmortem* examination the *impar thyroid plexus* and the *mediastinal veins* cannot easily be distinguished on account of their simultaneous filling (Figs 47/14 and 16). The vertebral plexus is also frequently projected on this area. Variously wide, the *superior vena cava* (Fig. 47/10) borders with a sharp outline the upper arch of the right margin of the heart. Mediastinal veins form a plexus on the medial aspect of the vessel. The *azygos vein* (Fig. 47/13), entering from behind, is distinguishable only in the lateral view since it is usually obscured by the shadow of the superior vena cava in anteroposterior pictures. Its orthodiagraphic shadow may sometimes be observed on the medial side of the superior vena cava also in sagittal

pictures. In **lateral view** (Figs 48, 56), anatomical conditions cannot be visualized so well because of superposition of shadows The *azygos vein* (Fig. 48/9) is here in its entire thoracic course distinctly visible.

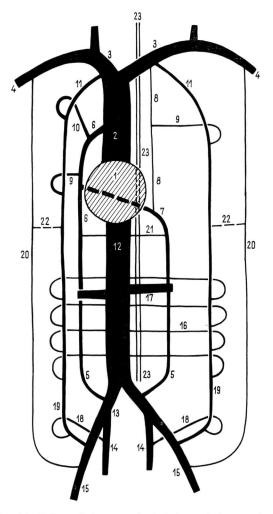

FIG. 21. Collaterals between the inferior and the superior vena cava. (*1*) Right atrium; (*2*) superior vena cava; (*3*) brachiocephalic veins; (*4*) axillary vein; (*5*) ascending lumbar veins; (*6*) azygos vein; (*7*) hemiazygos vein; (*8*) accessory hemiazygos vein; (*9*) posterior intercostal veins; (*10*) right superior intercostal vein; (*11*) internal thoracic vein; (*12*) inferior vena cava; (*13*) common iliac vein; (*14*) internal iliac vein; (*15*) external iliac vein; (*16*) lumbar veins; (*17*) renal vein; (*18*) iliolumbar vein; (*19*) inferior epigastric vein; (*20*) thoracoepigastric vein; (*21*) inferior and superior phrenic veins; (*22*) anastomosis between thoracoepigastric and internal thoracic veins; (*23*) vertebral venous plexus.

Azygography (Fig. 49). Osteomedullary venography of the ribs, i.e., azygography, employed first by Tori (1954) and Süsse and Aurig (1954), is the suitable method for the radiological demonstration of the azygos vein in vivo. Schobinger (1960) reviewed a large number of anatomical variations.

Szücs (1964) studied anatomical and physiological conditions in 400 cases. Düx and his co-workers (1967) introduced the retrograde method of direct azygography in order to fill the entire thoracic segment of the azygos vein in vivo.

Postmortem phlebography. After the filling of the inferior vena cava, the *azygos vein* (Fig. 48/9) in the **lateral view** (Fig. 48) is projected along its entire course on the anterior border of the vertebral column. The *right superior intercostal vein* (Fig. 48/11) and, beneath, the *posterior intercostal veins* (Fig. 48/10) — which latter segmentally cross the projection of the vertebrae in an oblique direction, — fill at the upper, backward convex bend of the last segment of the azygos vein which forms here an angle of 90°. Through them the external and internal vertebral plexuses are sharply outlined in their entire length. The further course of the *intercostal veins* cannot be visualized with this method on account of the valves they contain. The *esophageal veins* can be injected through the portal vein (Jonnesco 1914).

With *in vivo intraosseal azygography* the best filling can be achieved following injection into the lower ribs which can be observed in the roentgenograms taken in anteroposterior or lateral but particularly in the **second oblique view** (Fig. 49). The course and the shepherd's crook-like upper end of the *azygos vein* (Fig. 49/4) become visible when the *posterior intercostal veins* have been filled. Usually also the *internal thoracic vein* (Fig. 49/8) fills through the collaterals.

With **meningorachidography** the veins of the spinal cord can be studied *in vivo* by means of direct filling through the intercostal veins (Tarkiainen 1967).

BLOOD VESSELS OF THE LUNG

Pulmonary circulation secures the exchange of oxygen and carbon dioxide so basic for the maintenance of the body. The lesser circulation carries blood from the right ventricle to the left atrium through the pumonary trunk and its branches then through the capillaries and the pulmonary veins. These pulmonary vessels are called vasa publica, whereas the pulmonary tissues themselves are supplied by the so-called vasa privata, namely, the bronchial arteries and veins. The two vascular systems communicate at several levels.

In contrast to the greater circulation, the main characteristic of the lesser circulation is low blood pressure, which can be attributed to the short afferent and efferent vascular segments between the two halves of the heart and also to the arterioles of low resistance. The precapillaries and the postcapillaries have thin walls, and a few smooth muscles are present only in the former. Their diameters vary between 125 and 150 mμ. Without the smooth muscles, the postcapillaries of the lung can be disregarded as far as constriction is concerned. Only veins over 150 mμ have been found to contain muscular elements (Sielaff 1964). Concerning regulation of the lesser circulation, Fishman (1961) considers the following conditions decisive: Constriction and dilatation via the smooth muscles. During constriction increased tension can be measured in the small vessels provided with smooth muscles; they maintain the pressure. Vessels of larger diameter are more likely to produce construction than passive dilatation.

Apart from supplying the parenchyma, the role of the vasa privata is to compensate differences of pressure between the arterial and the venous circulation. This is made possible via the collaterals connecting the two systems. The importance of these communications does not arise under physiological but under pathological conditions. Nevertheless, they must be known under normal conditions too.

VASA PUBLICA

The pulmonary trunk and its branches

The arrangement of the pulmonary arteries is influenced by intraarterial pressure and the pulsatory movements. They are longer than the straight line between the heart and their area of distribution. This is particularly significant in case of increasing internal pressure. Arteries connected with the position of the bronchi have an arched course which makes their elongation, when necessary, possible. The close connection applies to segmental and minor branches alike (Felix 1928). The position of the arteries in relation to the bronchi alternates in various parts of the lung. The ascending arteries of the upper lobe run mediodorsally, the horizontal arteries craniodorsally, and the basal ones laterodorsally with reference to the corresponding bronchi. There are differences, not only in relation to the bronchi but also in relation to each other, in the course and ramification of the bilateral upper lobar branches. The left pulmonary artery crosses the bronchus in a cranial, the right pulmonary artery in a ventrocaudal direction. The branches running to the upper lobes ramify differently on the two

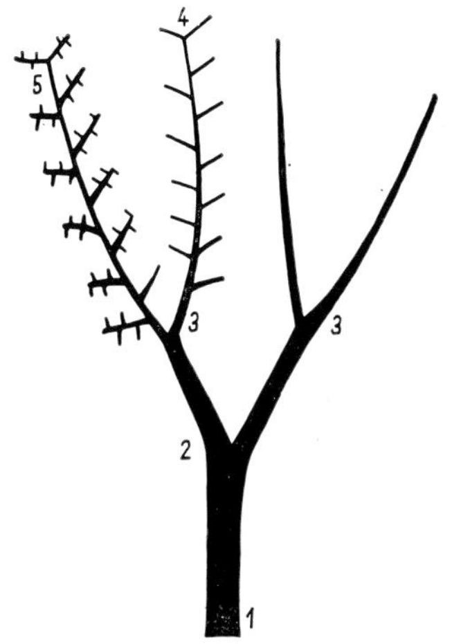

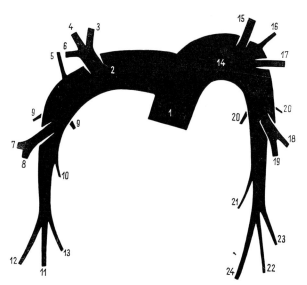

FIG. 22. Division of the pulmonary segmental arteries. (*1*) Segmental artery; (*2*) subsegmental artery; (*3*) prelobular artery; (*4*) lobular artery; (*5*) terminal artery.

sides. The bronchus is not always eparterial above the right pulmonary artery (Narath 1901). Eparterial bronchus on the left side is extremely rare (Herrnheiser and Kubat 1951). Anomalous bronchus of a tracheal origin is not always accompanied by an accessory artery (Kubik and Müntener 1971).

The *segmental arteries* emit small side branches toward the periphery with steadily increasing angles. The lumen diminishes continuously, and the vessel shows a curvature. Segmental arteries are able to dilate at a high degree, their volume depending on intrathoracic pressure (Brown et al. 1939). The extent to which pulmonary arteries can be filled depends also on posture and respiratory function (Karpati 1957). The vascular structure is affected by the size and shape of the thorax, the volume of air, and the conditions of pressure. The angles at which vessels divide is closely connected with the volume of air. Angles of ramification diminish simultaneously with decreasing volume of air, while they grow with increasing volume of air. Hornykiewytsch (cit. Sielaff 1964) distinguished different types of ramification of the pulmonary artery. If the trunk of the pulmonary artery can be followed in its entire length after the emission of the larger branches, he speaks of magistral division. We speak of scattered type if the pulmonary artery divides into segmental branches immediately after entering the lung. The mixed type of division is a transition between the two extreme types. The magistral type accounts for 20, the scattered type for 60 and the mixed type for 20 per cent of the cases (Melnikow 1924).

The segmental arteries divide into the subsegmental arteries and these bifurcate at acute angles into two arteries which supply an area 2 to 5 cm long, 2 to 4 cm wide with a diameter of 1·2 to 1·8 cm (Junghans 1958; Fig. 22). Junghans called the latter *prelobular arteries* because they form six to ten *lobular arteries* after repeated divisions. The diameter of the latters varies from 0·4 to 0·8 mm. The more terminal the vessels, the more their angle of division approaches the right angle. The area supplied by the lobular arteries measures 0·8 to 2·8 cm in length and 0·6 to 1·5 cm in width. *Terminal arteries* with diameters of 0·2 to 0·3 mm spring off at right angles from the lobular arteries; they ramify after a course of 1 to 2 mm. This area corresponds to the subdivision of terminal bronchiole into respiratory bronchioles.

The pulmonary arteries have a great number of variations. The left upper lobe offers the widest possibilities for variable origins and courses. Therefore, identification of the segmental arteries in this lobe is not always possible (Cory and Valentini 1959).

The **pulmonary trunk** (Figs 23/1, 37/6, 38/6, 39/6, 40/4, 47/26, 48/17, 52/9, 55/14, 56/15) originates from the conus pulmonalis of the right ventricle, and runs to the left, upward and backward. The origin of the pulmonary trunk is situated about 1·5 cm higher than the aorta to the left and before it (Paturet 1958). Its first portion is situated in front

FIG. 23. Branches of the pulmonary trunk. (*1*) Pulmonary trunk; (*2*) right pulmonary artery; (*3*) A_1; (*4*) A_2; (*5*) A_{2a}; (*6*) A_3; (*7*) A_4; (*8*) A_5; (*9*) A_6; (*10*) A_7; (*11*) A_8; (*12*) A_9; (*13*) A_{10}; (*14*) left pulmonary artery; (*15*) A_1; (*16*) A_2; (*17*) A_3; (*18*) A_4; (*19*) A_5; (*20*) A_6; (*21*) A_7; (*22*) A_8; (*23*) A_9; (*24*) A_{10}.

of the aortic bulb. The left coronary artery is here behind the pulmonary trunk and curves then left and forward. The right coronary artery arises from behind to the right and passes then to the right side of the trunk. In its further course, the pulmonary trunk lies closely against the left anterior surface of the aorta. Having reached the concave surface of the aortic arch, it bifurcates (Fig. 23). Seldom in case of normal origin, the trunk turns right and not left. In this case the left pulmonary artery reaches the hilum above the left bronchus (Castellanos and Garcia 1951). The division of the pulmonary trunk forms an upward open angle of 130° to 150° (Paturet 1958). Its initial part is covered by the pericardium, which turns backward before the division of the trunk. Thus, anatomically it may be divided into intrapericardial and extrapericardial segments. The left auricle is placed to the left, the right auricle to the right, the ascending aorta to the right and behind the intrapericardial segment. On the left, the extrapericardial segment is in contact with the mediastinal surface of the left lung, the phrenic nerve and the pericardiacophrenic artery, while the left border of the ascending aorta and the concavity of the aortic arch are on its right side. The pulmonary trunk measures 3 to 6 cm in length (Brown et al. 1939) and 3·2 cm (2·2 to 3·5 cm) in diameter (Dotter and Steinberg 1949).

In relation to the anterior chest wall, the projection of the pulmonary trunk falls on the second intercostal space to the left of the sternum. Its left border extends 1·5 to 1·8 cm beyond the border of the sternum (Paturet 1958). Conditions of projection are decisively influenced by constitutional factors (Delmas 1954). In extreme cases the upper border of the vessel's projection reaches the inferior border of the first rib. This "high position" occurs more frequently in females. In case of "deep position" of the diaphragm, the projection may fall on the foremost part of the 4th rib. Age and shape of the heart are likewise influencing factors. Division takes place at the height of the 4th vertebra at the sternal end of the 2nd rib (Töndury 1959).

Blood circulation is more or less seriously affected by the *variations* of the pulmonary trunk. Common origin, communication with the vessels of the greater circulation are regarded as anomaly. The left coronary artery arises fairly often, the right coronary artery or both coronary arteries arise very rarely from the pulmonary trunk (Brooks 1886, Bland et al. 1933, Sabiston et al. 1960, Jameson et al. 1963, Szederkényi and Steczik 1964, Stein et al. 1965). Ectopic origin of branches of the pulmonary artery may occur from the subclavian, common carotid, celiac, superior mesenteric arteries, from the abdominal (Manhoff and Howe 1949), the

ascending (Weintraub 1966, Waldhausen et al. 1968), or the descending aorta (Bruwer et al. 1950), and from the brachiocephalic trunk (Kassai and Kurotaki 1967). The left pulmonary artery may arise from the right pulmonary artery (Tan et al. 1968). Also, the left pulmonary artery (Jovanovic et al. 1967) or the right pulmonary artery (Fonó 1968) may be missing. All these variations in origin disturb the circulation more or less and are therefore considered anomalous.

The **right pulmonary artery** (Figs 23/2, 37/7, 38/7, 39/7, 50/4, 51/7, 52/10, 53/2, 55/15, 56/16, 57/15, 58/15) turns transversely to the right and runs below the arch of the aorta after its origin, between the inner and outer sheets of the pericardium toward the right hilum. From the pericardium, fibres of connective tissue extend to the adventitia of the artery which at the same time have a fixing effect (Hayek 1953). The ascending aorta, the phrenic nerve and the superior vena cava are in front of the pulmonary artery which crosses these structures transversely from behind. Behind its initial portion is the space below the bifurcation of trachea. It has, thus, a deeper position than the left pulmonary artery. It crosses the right bronchus from below upward and passes to its anterior aspect and arrives in front of the bronchus intermedius. Its course is very rarely above the bronchus of the right upper lobe (Narath 1901, Richter and Böck 1967). The right superior pulmonary vein runs almost *parallel* below and slightly before the artery. Immediately before its division anteriorly, lies the superior vena cava; posteriorly, the right principal bronchus; infero-anteriorly, the superior right pulmonary vein; and above it the azygos vein. The superior vena cava crosses it transversely from above downward, and the azygos vein passes sagittally across it. The length of the right pulmonary artery is 5 to 6 cm according to Paturet (1958) and 3·5 to 5·5 cm according to Hayek (1958). Its diameter measures 2 to 2·3 cm (Paturet 1958, Hayek 1958) or, with angiography, 2·34 cm (1·7 to 3·0 cm; Robb and Steinberg 1938).

The artery is projected on the fourth or on the upper border of the fifth thoracic vertebra. Compared to the anterior costal arches, the projection falls on the line connecting the second costal spaces of the two sides. It extends beyond the border of the sternum on the right side and ramifies at the lateral edge of the superior vena cava.

1. *Arteries of the right upper lobe* (Fig. 24). The right upper lobe is mainly supplied by the upper branch (truncus superior) of the right pulmonary artery. This is the only artery which runs caudally from the corresponding lobar bronchus. In few cases the entire lobe is supplied by this branch

alone. Generally three arteries supply the entire right upper lobe: the apical branch, A_1; the posterior branch, A_2; and the anterior branch, A_3. According to the site of their origin they can be distinguished as recurrent vessels that spring off from that part of the right pulmonary artery which faces the interlobar space and ascendant branches that arise from the mediastinal side (Felix 1928, Appleton 1945). Boyden (1955) encountered arteries of exclusively mediastinal origin in 8 per cent, and

$(A_{1a,b})$ to S_1. It supplies this segment independently only in one fifth of the cases. Often it gives off minor branches to the adjacent segments. It lies medially to the bronchus, and its subsegmental branches have a dorsomedial position (Hayek 1953). The main trunk passes toward the apex of the lung in an upward-backward and lateral direction. It supplies the apex of the upper lobe (Löhr et al. 1959).

Posterior branch, A_2 (Figs 23/4, 24/2, 25/2, 26/1, 50/8, 51/9, 52/12, 53/4, 55/17, 56/17, 57/19, 58/16).

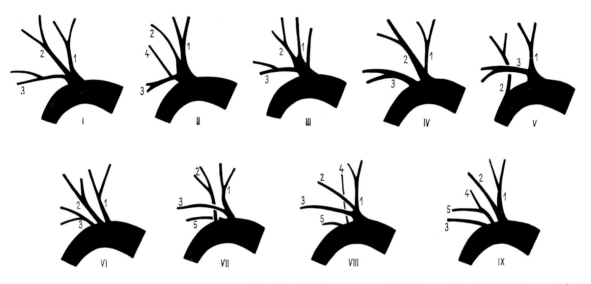

FIG. 24. Variations of the arteries of the right superior lobe. I–III, one artery; IV–V, two arteries; VI–IX, three arteries; (*1*) A_1; (*2*) A_2; (*3*) A_3; (*4*) A_{2x}; (*5*) A_{3x}.

arteries of mediastinal and interlobar origin in 92 per cent. Kassai (1950) found the upper lobe to be supplied by one artery in 20, by two arteries in 50, and by three in 30 per cent of the examined cases. If there is one artery to supply the upper lobe (Figs 24/I to III) it reaches the segments in three branches (A_1, A_2, A_3). It may occur in these cases that before the trifurcation a separate fourth branch runs to a subsegment of S_1. More seldom, one of the three branches supplies the S_3, the others supply the S_1 and S_2. The artery A_3 may emit a subsegmental branch to S_2 in such cases. Two alternatives are possible if two arteries supply the upper lobe (Figs 24/IV, V): arteries A_1 and A_2 arise together and A_3 arises separately or, A_1 and A_3 have a common, and A_2 has a separate origin (Sanish and Gessner 1958). Numerous variations are possible if there are three arteries (Fig. 24/VI to IX). Most frequently A_1, A_2 and A_3 origin separately. Further alternatives are offered by variations of the subsegmental branches of A_2 and A_3.

Apical branch, A_1 (Figs 23/3, 24/1, 25/1, 50/5, 51/8, 52/11, 53/3, 55/16, 56/17, 57/16, 58/16) gives off most frequently two subsegmental branches

Its origin and course are variable. It occurs only in 30 per cent as a separate branch (Zenker et al. 1954, Löhr et al. 1959). In about half of the cases it arises from the interlobar part and reaches the segment from a posteroinferior direction. This pulmonary segment is supplied by several arteries in 70 per cent of the cases. The posterolateral portion is supplied caudally (*ramus posterior ascendens*, A_{2a}), the medial upper portion is supplied from the front (*ramus posterior descendens*, A_{2b}). It happens occasionally that the *recurrent branch*, A_{2x} (Fig. 24/4) arising from the A_6 supplies one of the subsegments (Hayek 1953, Kováts and Zsebők 1961). A_2, forming a curve, runs upward, backward and slightly laterally and supplies the posterior basal and the subapical upper lobar segment.

The *anterior branch*, A_3 (Figs 23/6, 24/3, 25/3, 50/11, 51/10, 52/13, 53/5 and 6, 55/18, 57/22, 58/17) originates, according to Boyden (1955), from the anterior aspect of the right pulmonary artery in 58 per cent, while, in the remaining 42 per cent, vessels from both sides may lead here (*ramus anterior ascendens*, A_{3a}; *ramus anterior descendens*, A_{3b}). Only a small portion of the lobe is reached by recur-

53

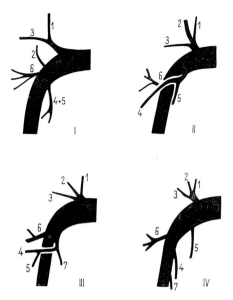

FIG. 25. Variations of the arteries of the right middle lobe. I, A_{4+5} in the distal part of the pars interlobaris; II, A_{4+5} in the proximal part of the pars interlobaris; III, A_{4+5+7} springing off together; IV, A_4 and A_5 springing off separately. (1) A_1; (2) A_2; (3) A_3; (4) A_4; (5) A_5; (6) A_6; (7) A_7.

rent branches. These ascending vessels with a backward running course usually originate from the interlobar trunk, near, or together with the artery of the middle lobe (Felix 1928). Numerous variations of the subsegmental arteries may be present. The artery A_3 supplies the lateroinferior part of the upper lobe (Löhr et al. 1964).

2. *Arteries of the right middle lobe* (Fig. 25). In 50 per cent of the cases, one artery (*ramus lobi medii*; Figs 51/12, 52/14, 56/18) and in another 50 per cent two arteries lead to the right middle lobe (Appleton 1944, Lindskog 1949, Kassai 1950, Oliveros 1951, Boyden 1955). They originate from the interlobar trunk. The origin is usually on the anterior surface, above, laterally to the middle lobar bronchus. It may further arise from the distal (Fig. 25/I) or the proximal part (Fig. 25/II) of the interlobar trunk, from the artery A_7 (Fig. 25/III) or from the common trunk of the arteries A_7 and A_8 (Boyden 1955). If there are two arteries, the proximal vessel arises from above the artery A_6, the distal one 0·5 to 1·0 cm below it (Fig. 25/IV). The origin is frequently adjacent to that of the artery A_{2x} or A_{3x} which recurs to the upper lobe. If blood is supplied by one trunk, it bifurcates (or rarely trifurcates) after a short course (Zenker et al. 1954). One of these side branches divides in the posterolateral (*ramus lateralis*, A_4; Figs 25/4, 26/2, 50/15, 51/12, 52/14, 53/10, 55/19, 57/26), the other in the middle or anterior part of the lobe (*ramus medialis*, A_5; Figs 25/5, 26/3, 50/18, 51/12, 52/14, 53/9, 55/20, 57/29). The distribution of the arteries is not quite identical

with that of the bronchi. The artery A_5 extends sometimes to part of the segment S_4. Both segments may be supplied by both trunks.

3. *Arteries of the right lower lobe* (Fig. 26). This lobe is supplied by the downward curving portion of the right pulmonary artery. It passes round the bronchus intermedius from before laterally and running beside the bronchus of the middle lobe, arrives at its outer side where it sends the ramus lobi medii to the middle lobe. In its further course, the vessel passes behind the inferior lobar bronchus and divides into branches which go to the basal segments (pars basalis). The branch of the right pulmonary artery which runs to S_6 arises at or above the level of the middle lobar artery from the right pulmonary artery (Kováts and Zsebők 1961).

The *apical (superior) branch to the inferior lobe*, A_6 (Figs 25/6, 26/4, 50/22, 23 and 24, 51/13, 52/15, 53/8, 55/21, 56/20, 57/33, 34 and 35, 58/18) is generally of higher origin than the artery of the middle lobe. It springs off from the posteromedial side of the right pulmonary artery. It is solitary in 80 per cent (Boyden 1955). It bifurcates after a short course into its subsegmental branches (*ramus mediosuperior*, A_{6a} and *ramus lateralis*, A_{6b}; Fig. 26/III). Sometimes there are three arteries. Its course follows the corresponding bronchus only in half of the cases. The vessel supplies the apical portion of the inferior lobe.

Basal part (Figs 50/25, 51/15, 52/16, 53/7, 55/22, 56/21, 57/36, 58/19). Hornykiewytsch and Stender (1954) distinguish three types of its division: Magistral type: the artery A_{10} or sometimes A_9 is stronger and is so to speak a continuation of the right pulmonary artery (Figs 26/I—III). Bifurcation: division in respect of A_9 and A_{10} is of equal degree (Figs. 26/V—VI). Trifurcation: A_7 and A_8 form a branch each, and a third branch is formed by A_{9+10} (Figs. 26/IV, VII, VIII).

The *medial basal (cardiac) branch*, A_7 (Figs 25/7, 26/6, 50/26, 52/17, 53/11, 55/23, 56/22, 57/37), the first branch of the basal part, has frequently a common origin with A_8 (Fig. 26/IV). From the front it goes around and crosses the bronchus of the inferior lobe and joins it at the point where the basal medial bronchus bifurcates. In case of two arteries (Fig. 26/V), one passes round the bronchus of the inferior lobe from the front, the other one from behind. It is rarely missing (4 per cent); but if so, it is replaced by the other basal branches (Kassai 1950).

The *anterior basal branch*, A_8 (Figs 26/7, 50/27, 51/18, 52/18, 53/12, 55/24, 56/22, 57/38) supplies its own segment independently in 50 per cent of the cases. It begins below the artery A_7 on the anterior part of the medial side. It may have two arteries, i.e., it may have a common origine with A_7 (Fig. 26/IV) or with A_9 (Fig. 26/VI; Boyden 1955).

The *lateral basal branch*, A_9 (Figs 26/8, 50/28, 51/17, 52/19, 53/13, 55/25, 56/23, 57/39) is one of the terminal branches of the right pulmonary artery. This vessel may be paired (Fig. 26/VII) and give off branches to the adjacent vascular areas A_8 and A_{10}.

The *posterior basal branch*, A_{10} (Figs 26/9, 50/29, 51/16, 52/20, 53/14, 55/26, 56/23, 57/40), the other terminal branch, is situated posterolaterally to its

where it ramifies. The left pulmonary artery runs upward at a steeper angle and thus occupies a higher position than its counterpart. After its beginning it is situated downward and laterally along a 2 cm long portion from the concave border of the arch of the aorta. Its course is parallel to the corresponding section of the aorta. As on the right side, from the pericardium thick bundles extend to it which can be followed as far as the emission of the first branches (Hayek 1953). The recurrent branch

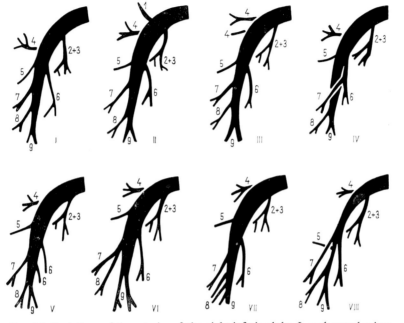

FIG. 26. Variations of the arteries of the right inferior lobe. I, each vessel arises separately; II, ascending origin of A_2; III, A_6 double; IV, A_{7+8} together; V, A_7 double; VI, A_{8+9} together; VII, A_9 double; VIII, A_x from A_{10}. (*1*) A_2; (*2*) A_4; (*3*) A_5; (*4*) A_6; (*5*) A_x; (*6*) A_7; (*7*) A_8; (*8*) A_9; (*9*) A_{10}.

own bronchus. It frequently sends off subsegmental branches to S_9 (Zenker et al. 1954).

The *subapical (subsuperior) branch*, A_x (Figs 26/5, 53/15) supplies the subapical segment of the inferior lobe. It shows many variations and may originate from the artery of any adjoining basal segment (Fig. 26/VIII; Ferry and Boyden 1951).

The **left pulmonary artery** (Figs 23/14, 37/9, 38/9, 50/30, 51/6, 52/21, 54/2, 55/27, 56/16, 57/41, 58/15) differs from its contralateral artery in length, course and topographical position. After its origin, it takes a course obliquely to the left, upward and backward, then in front of the left bronchus it crosses the principal bronchus of the upper lobe transversely and arrives then above this. Making a backward and downward curve, it runs deep into the interlobar fissure. From here it passes to the lateral side of the principal bronchus of the inferior lobe

of the vagus nerve can be found between the aorta and this artery (n. recurrens). In the hilum of the lung, the arch of the aorta is situated above, and the left superior pulmonary vein above and in front of the artery. In this region the left principal bronchus is below, the descending aorta behind the artery. In its further course it goes around the posterior surface of the left principal bronchus and gives off branches to the superior lobe. This segment (arcus arteriae pulmonalis sinistrae) gives off branches both from its anterior and interlobar surface. In contrast to the slightly backward and downward course of thet lef principal bronchus, the course of the left pulmonary artery between its arch and its division into basal segments was found to be almost vertical by Kováts and Zsebők (1961). Since the various lobes of the lung are not supplied here by separate trunks, there is a wide range of variations in this area (Zenker et al. 1954, Herrnheiser and Kubat 1936, Boyden 1955, Hayek 1958, Kováts and Zsebők 1961). The artery has a length of 3 cm (Paturet 1958, Hayek 1958) and a diameter of 1·8 to 2·1 cm.

The projection of the vessel falls on the left border of the 4th thoracic vertebra, and extends beyond

Seldom, eparterial origin of the bronchus of S_1 may be on the left side too. It is most convenient to study the various arterial trunks according to the site of their origin (Zenker et al. 1954).

Segmental arteries originating from the anterior aspect (Figs 27/I to IV, VIII to XII): *apical*

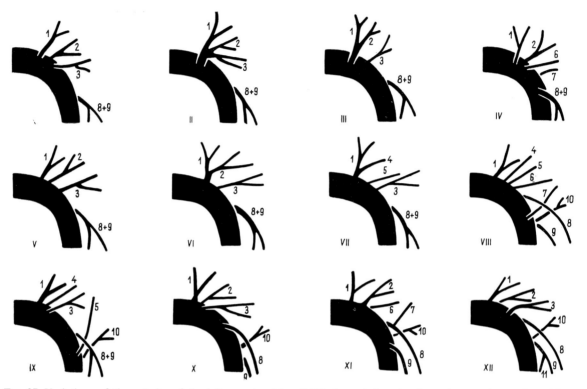

Fig. 27. Variations of the arteries of the left superior lobe. I–IV, A_1 and A_3 arise from the anterior surface; V–VII, A_1, A_2 and A_3 arise from the upper surface; VIII–XII, variations of A_4 and A_5. (1) A_1; (2) A_2; (3) A_3; (4) A_{2a}; (5) A_{2b}; (6) A_{3a}; (7) A_{3b}; (8) A_4; (9) A_5; (10) A_6; (11) A_7.

the border of the sternum at or slightly above the level of the sternal edge of the 2nd rib.

1. Arteries of the left upper lobe (Fig. 27). Arteries supplying the left upper lobe may spring off from the superior or from the anterior and interlobar surface of the arch of the left pulmonary artery. Therefore, many variations are possible. The number of arteries varies from 4 to 8. According to Boyden (1955) the number of arteries may be four (18 per cent), five (40 per cent), six (28 per cent) seven (12 per cent) and eight (2 per cent). The great variability is due to three anatomical factors. Segments S_3, S_4 and S_5 may be supplied by vessels arising both from the mediastinal and the interlobar surface. Besides, segments S_1 and S_2 may be provided with divided arteries. Finally, there may exist supernumerary vessels according to the number of bronchi. The anterior branch leading to S_3 arises and runs before, the other segment arteries originate and run usually behind the segmental bronchus.

branch, A_1 (Figs 50/31, 52/22, 57/42, 58/16), *anterior branch*, A_3 (Figs 50/37, 51/10, 52/24, 57/48, 58/17); variations: A_2, A_4, A_5 (Figs 50/40, 57/51).

In 80 per cent of the cases arteries belonging to A_1 and A_3 arise separately from the anterior surface of the left pulmonary artery (Hayek 1958). In case of a common origin, this vessel supplies segments S_1, S_2 and S_3 (truncus superior) or only the first two segments (truncus anterior). This common trunk is at the same time the first branch of the left pulmonary artery, and it may give off branches to S_4 and S_5 as well. If only segment S_1 is supplied, the trunk passes to the posteromedial side of the bronchus, but it lies against the anterior side of the bronchus if it supplies S_3 as well; finally it runs along and ramifies on the anterior side of the bronchus if S_4 and S_5 too are supplied.

If the pulmonary vessel gives off two arteries, one supplies the anterior part of S_1 and the other supplies the posterior part of S_1 and a part of S_2. In

56

those cases (about 20 per cent), when S_4 and S_5, too, are supplied by this group of arteries, simultaneously it may get a branch from the interlobar side as well. The blood supply of these segments is extremely complicated in such cases (Boyden 1955).

Boyden 1955). A_4 and A_5 arise with a common trunk in one third of the cases. The height of origin is in this case facing A_6. Kent and Blades (1942) observed it in a lower position in exceptional cases. It is rather frequent that A_3, and less frequent that

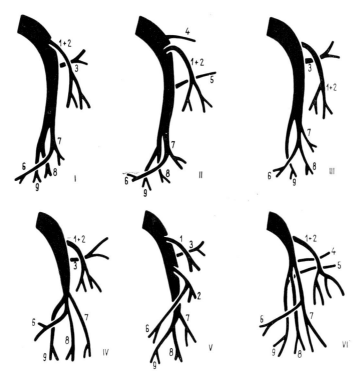

FIG. 28. Variations of the arteries of the left inferior lobe. I, A_{7+8} arise together and A_{9+10} arise together; II, A_6 double; III, A_{7+8+9} together; IV, A_{7+9} together, A_8 and A_9 separately; V, A_{5+7} and A_{9+10} together, A_8 separately; VI, A_{6b+10} and A_{7+8} together. (1) A_4; (2) A_5; (3) A_6; (4) A_{6a}; (5) A_{6b}; (6) A_7; (7) A_8; (8) A_9; (9) A_{10}.

Segmental arteries originating from the upper side (Figs 27/V to VII): *apical branch*, A_1 (Figs 54/3, 55/28, 56/17), *posterior branch*, A_2 (Figs 54/4, 55/29, 56/17), *anterior branch*, A_3 (Figs 54/5, 55/30). Arteries A_1 and A_2 arise frequently from the upper side of the left pulmonary artery. Origin with common trunk is rare (12 per cent according to Boyden, 1955). Arteries supplying the lingular segments have a separate origin even if they, too, arise from the same side as the aforesaid arteries. In 4 per cent of the cases aberrant trunks run to segment S_6 (A_{6x}). A_3 arises occasionally from the upper side.

Segmental arteries springing off from the posterior interlobar side (Figs 27/VIII to XII): *superior lingular branch*, A_4 (Figs 52/25, 54/6, 55/31, 56/18) and *inferior lingular branch*, A_5 (Figs 52/26, 54/7, 55/32, 56/18); variation: A_2, A_3.

The lingular segments may be supplied from the interlobar side (72 per cent), from the anterior side (8 per cent) and from both sides (20 per cent;

A_7 and A_8 have a common origin with these arteries. Sometimes, the subsegmental artery of A_2 and the main trunk of A_6 have a common origin.

2. *Arteries of the left inferior lobe* (Fig. 28). After the left pulmonary artery has given off the branches supplying the upper lobe, it continues as interlobar part. Below the origin of A_6 the trunk is called basal part. It divides after a short course into the mediobasal part (A_7, A_8) and the laterobasal part (A_9, A_{10}). These branches give off the corresponding segmental arteries after repeated ramification.

Apical (superior) branch to the inferior lobe, A_6 (Figs 27/10, 28/3, 50/43, 51/13, 52/27, 54/8, 55/33, 56/19, 57/54, 58/18), is a solitary vessel in half of the cases originating opposite to the artery A_4 from the posterior side of the main trunk and supplying the apical area of the inferior lobe. It divides into two branches after a short course. If they have separate origins (Fig. 28/II), a separate branch may run to the lower basal segments (Fig. 28/VI; Hornykiewytsch and Stender 1955). An aberrant branch may reach this area from the A_2 trunk of the upper lobe. Contrasted with the right side, there are no ascending vessels here. The *subapical (subsuperior) branch*, A_x usually arises from the basal segments (Hayek 1958).

Basal part (Figs 50/47, 51/14, 52/29, 54/9, 55/34, 56/21, 57/58, 58/19). Hornykiewytsch and Stender (1955) classified the division of the basal part just as that of the right-hand side in three types. Magistral type: A_{7+9} originate together, A_{10} arises separately. The latter is a continuation of the main trunk (Fig. 28/IV). Bifurcation: A_{7+8} just as A_{9+10} arise as a common branch. This is the most frequent type of division, accounting for 42 per cent of the cases (Figs 28/I to III, V). Trifurcation (Fig. 28/VI): several variations are possible. A_{10} is an independent branch.

The *medial basal branch* A_7 (Figs 27/11, 28/6, 50/48, 52/30, 54/10, 56/22, 57/59) and *anterior basal branch* A_8 (Figs 28/7, 50/51, 51/18, 52/31, 54/11, 55/35, 56/22, 57/60) form a common trunk in 50 per cent of the cases, and are one of the terminal branches of the left pulmonary artery. After a short course it bifurcates. Boyden (1955) observed the common origin of A_7 and A_9 in 10 per cent. The variation A_{8+9} may be present too. The medial and anterior basal branches supply the medial anterior and segments of the base of the inferior lobe.

Lateral, A_9 (Figs 28/8, 50/50, 51/17, 52/32, 54/12, 55/36, 56/23, 57/61, 58/20) and *posterior*, A_{10} (Figs 28/9, 50/49, 51/16, 52/33, 54/13, 55/37, 56/23, 57/62, 58/21) *basal branches* constitute the other terminal branch. Separate origin is more frequent here and the variation is A_{7+9} or the A_{8+9}, respectively. A_{10} is always a solitary branch which sometimes gives off a subsegmental branch to A_6. The artery A_{10} may sometimes produce an independent terminal branch in which case the basal part divides into three parts (Hayek 1958). The area supplied by the basal lateral and posterior arteries is similar to that of the right side.

Radiological anatomy of the pulmonary arteries

Visualization of the pulmonary circulation contained in the air-filled lungs makes their radiological study possible. Schwartz (1910) did not only describe the expansive pulsation of the vessel contours but also the rhythmical changes in the intensity of the shadows. The shadow of the hilum and the configuration of the lungs are mainly visualized by way of the vessels (Assmann 1911). Fluoroscopy

enables the study of vascular changes during respiration due to the transparency of the air-filled lungs. In accordance with the changes in blood volume, transparency diminishes on deep expiration and increases during inspiration. While the volume of blood increases 50 per cent during inspiration, the volume of air increases two- to threefold (Csákány 1965). X-ray pictures combined with tomograms are suitable for detailed morphological study of the branches of the pulmonary vessels.

Owing to its upward and backward course, the *pulmonary trunk* appears shorter in **anteroposterior roentgenograms** than in reality (Fig. 37/6) and forms the second arch of the left heart contour. It is distinguishable only by kymography in native pictures. Dotter and Steinberg (1949) demonstrated by angiography that the conus pulmonalis does not reach the left border of the heart so that contrast filling is required for its visualization. Besides the trunk the pulmonary arch is composed of the left pulmonary artery as well (Robb and Steinberg 1938). The pulmonary arch is more pronounced in children. Its protrusion during adolescence can be observed also under physiological conditions, although tomograms reveal that it does not become wider in this period (Richter 1963). On **lateral radiographs** of the chest (dextrosinistral) the pulmonary trunk, joining the right ventricle, is usually difficult to identify (Fig. 40/4). A considerable part of the anterior contour of the heart is formed by the right ventricle on roentgenograms made in the **right oblique view** (Fig. 39/6). The conus pulmonaris and the pulmonary trunk form the border in the upper part of such pictures.

Frontal plane **tomograms** do not show the pulmonary trunk clearer than summation pictures taken in the same view. On *sagittal plane* tomograms the trunk can be visualized in its entire length. The anterior contour of the cardiac shadow is separated from the retrosternal space. The sharp anterior contour of the pulmonary trunk passes gradually into the shadow of the left pulmonary artery. The lower end of the trunk cannot be reliably distinguished from the cardiac shadow. Tomograms made in the *transverse* plane are more relevant under pathological than under physiological conditions (Gremmel 1962, Richter 1963). Tomography *combined with pneumo-mediastinography* is less suited for the exploration of normal anatomical correlation (Bogsch 1958).

Pulsation seen on the pulmonary trunk, as on the aorta, consists of rapid systolic dilatation and subsequent slow diastolic contraction. The amplitudes are considerably smaller than those of the aorta.

The *right pulmonary artery* does not produce a margin in native x-ray pictures and can be visualized only by contrast-filled examinations.

The *left pulmonary artery* is the principal constituent of the left hilum and is clearly visible in **anteroposterior pictures** (Fig. 37/9). Owing to its anatomical position, the projection of this artery lies higher than that of the right artery. It forms a part of the pulmonary arch (Robb and Steinberg 1938, Miller 1947). Its oblique upward, lateral and backward course shows considerable individual variations. In children the situation of the artery approaches the transverse line, while in adults it is rather ventrodorsal (Kreuzfuchs 1937). Therefore, the shadow of the artery is often visible below the knob of the aorta in children, while in adults, its projection falls on the pulmonary trunk so that only its branches form the arterial picture of the hilum. Seen in the **right oblique view** (Fig. 39/6), the vessel appears as an orthodiagraphic round shadow within the cardiac shadow in the projection of the origin of the aorta (Richter 1963). The epibronchial portion is clearly visible in *sagittal plane* **tomograms** and is thus suitable for the objective determination of the width. The diameter of the left pulmonary artery can be exactly measured by prolonging the radius of the left bronchus to the upper border of the left pulmonary artery. It is thus possible to distinguish the width of the main trunk from the overlapping projections of the arteries of the upper lobe (Richter 1963). In contradiction with the pulmonary trunk, the epibronchial portion of the left pulmonary artery is clearly outlined in *frontal plane* tomograms because here it is seen in its oblique section.

The *interlobar part* and *basal part* of the left pulmonary artery (Fig. 37/10) can be visualized on both summation radiographs and tomograms taken in the frontal and the sagittal views. They show an arched course.

Methods for measuring the diameter of the pulmonary vessels. Apart from the direct angiographic method there are several ways to determine the diameter of the pulmonary trunk and its branches.

Assmann (1911) measured the width of the right truncus intermedius in anteroposterior roentgenograms. The upper limit of the normal value is 1·6 cm for males and 1·5 cm for females (Chang 1965). Kreuzfuchs (1937) saw the diameter of the left pulmonary artery in underexposed chest radiographs as a round shadow in the projection of the upper end of the pulmonary trunk. He measured the portion above the principal bronchus of the left upper lobe in a similar manner and found the normal width to be 2·6 cm maximally. Moore and his associates (1959) determined the width of the pul-

monary trunk in posteroanterior chest radiographs by means of auxiliary lines. The correlation between the length of the line drawn from the intersection of the thoracic median line and the arch of the aorta to the intersection of the left inferior arch and the left diaphragm, and the length of the line running to the first line from the convexity of the pulmonary arch, as seen in posteroanterior pictures made during deep inspiration, is thought by Csákány (1965) to be suitable for determining the width of the pulmonary trunk. This method is based exclusively on the characteristics of the middle shadow and can be well applied for the differentiation between normal and pathologic conditions. Of course, it is much more reliable to determine the diameter directly by angiography.

The course of the branches of the pulmonary arteries. In their studies Hornykiewytsch and Stender (1953a, b, c, 1954a, b, c, d, e, 1955a, b, c) dealt in detail with the study of this field.

Pneumoangiography

Forssmann (1931) was the first to examine the arteries of the lung in vivo by filling them with contrast material. Examinations were initially restricted to the more central vessels (Dotter and Steinberg 1949). Subsequently, tomography enabled the study of more and more details (Hornykiewytsch and Stender 1953a, b, c, 1954a, b, c, d, e, 1955a, b, c, Kováts and Zsebők 1961, Richter 1963). The development of cineradiography meant a great step forward (Janker 1954). The selective filling enables the study of minor branches as well (Bolt et al. 1957, Bell et al. 1959).

In *postmortem* **anteroposterior** *pneumoangiograms* (Fig. 50) the *pulmonary trunk* with its two main arteries can be visualized as in the x-ray-anatomical description (Fig. 50/4 and 30). Its characteristic course starts from the right ventricle with an even transition. The trunk runs steeply upward and somewhat to the left, and gives off two main branches which appear fairly wide in comparison to the main trunk. While the left pulmonary artery can be visualized in summation roentgenograms and tomograms, the right pulmonary artery can only be seen by angiography. The vessel shows a somewhat oblique downward course to the right at the height of the 4th and 5th thoracic vertebrae. Comparisons with the contralateral vessel as to height, length and course are most convenient in this projection. In the **lateral view** (Fig. 51), due to overlapping, the contours of the two main branches of the pulmonary trunk (Fig. 51/6 and 7) are only partly separable.

By inserting a catheter into the *segmental arteries*, they can be separately demonstrated in vivo. It is thus possible to penetrate trunks of about 2·5 mm in diameter (Bolt et al. 1957, Bell et al. 1959). The diameter of the segmental arteries is 2 to 3 mm, of the subsegmental vessels 1·5 to 2 mm, of the pre-lobular vessels 1·2 to 1·5 mm, of the lobular branches 0·4 to 0·8 mm, and of the terminal vessels 0·2 to 0·3 mm (Löhr et al. 1964). Peripheral circulation and functional capillary network are best observable if the catheter, pushed forward, completely obliterates the vessel ("Wedge's arteriogram"). Circulatory condition of the parenchyma of the lung can be best studied with this method. Giese (1957), using tubes with fine focus, could demonstrate vessels of 20 to 40 μ by means of selective angiography.

For the study of segmental and minor vessels *postmortem angiograms* are more suitable than tomograms. Frequently, only details of A_6 (the most hidden artery) and its branches can be identified, mostly on the right side from the **anteroposterior view** (Fig. 50). Because the two sides cover each other the **lateral view** (Fig. 51) is not complete. Trunks A_1 and A_2 as well as the peripheral details of A_3 are relatively distinct. In this position, the trunks A_4, A_5 and A_6 run approximately parallel with the plane of the film and are in some respects easier to observe than in an anteroposterior position. It is possible to study the relative positions of A_8, A_9 and A_{10}. Being usually projected on the shadow of some other branch, A_7 cannot reliably be separated.

If postmortem pneumoangiography is combined with the *simultaneous filling of the right half of the heart and the great veins*, the *right pulmonary artery* (Fig. 55/15), running to the right behind the superior vena cava, is partly obscured in **anteroposterior view** (Fig. 55). Its bifurcation is usually behind the trunk of the superior vena cava. The projection of the right pulmonary artery is crossed from behind by the azygos vein. In **lateral view** (Fig. 56), the dividing *pulmonary trunk* (Fig. 56/15) and the anterior part of the *pulmonary arteries* (Fig. 56/16) are obscured by the superior vena cava. The further course of the main trunks behind the superior vena cava, they is covered by one another only. Of the segmental branches A_1 and A_2 intersect sagittally the azygos vein that runs forward above the convexity of the pulmonary arteries. The high contrast shadow covers the artery A_3 as far as the margin of the upper third of the superior vena cava and the pulmonary trunk. Only the origins of A_4, A_5 and A_8 are visible; their further course is lost in the projection of the right atrium. Branches of A_6 and A_{10} are crossed by the ascending azygos vein. The entire course of A_9 is visible.

By *simultaneous contrast filling of the pulmonary arteries and the aorta* the *right pulmonary artery* (Fig. 57/15), running below the arch of the aorta and turning behind the ascending aorta, is covered in **anteroposterior pictures** (Fig. 57). The *left pulmonary artery* (Fig. 57/41) crosses the descending aorta transversely from in front and runs to the left. Of the segmental branches the simultaneously filling left coronary artery crosses the projection of A_7 and A_8 at several points. The right coronary artery is more medially placed than the right pulmonary arteries. In **lateral view** (Fig. 58), the superimposed shadows of the *pulmonary arteries* (Fig. 58/15) appear below the arch of the aorta between the ascending and the descending aorta. Only the origin and the peripheral portions of A_1 and A_2 are visible; the middle portion is covered by the upper part of the descending aorta. Lost in the projection of the ascending aorta, arteries A_3, A_4 and A_5 are not separable. A_6 and A_{10} cross the descending aorta in transverse and oblique directions, respectively. The way of A_7, A_8 and A_9 is crossed by the arched course of the right coronary artery and its branches.

Making *isolated organ preparations* after the joint removal of the lungs and heart, in the **anteroposterior view** (Fig. 52), the vascular structure shows the relative position of the dividing vessel trunks flattened out as far as the terminal arteries. **Lateral roentgenograms** (Figs 53, 54) show the ramifications more precisely and the outlines of the smallest vessels more sharply.

The pulmonary veins and their branches

The course of the pulmonary veins is independent of the arteries. Owing to intravascular pressure and vigorous pulsation, the course of the arteries is somewhat curved, whereas, owing to subatmospheric tension, veins are almost taut and are seen as straight lines. The larger veins pass radially toward the hilum and the left atrium. The orifice of the veins is at a more obtuse angle than the ramification of the arteries. Both the smaller and the larger veins intersect one another as well as the arteries and the bronchi at several points. In contrast to the latter veins running in the septa between the segments, subsegments and lobules are fixed by loose connective tissue. One vein lies between two arteries (Kováts and Zsebők 1961). The larger veins converge from two segments. Junghans (1958) demonstrated by stereoscopic roentgenograms that veins run along the poorly vascularized interarterial paths. Two to four veins collect the blood of each artery. There is no anastomosis between the pulmonary veins. Orifice of the veins occurs always at a less acute angle than the division of the arteries.

The portion of the veins which runs between the segments (*infrasegmental part*) must be distinguished from the trunks situated deep in the parenchyma (*intrasegmental part*). The arrangement is not the same in all pulmonary regions. Veins respect the boundary of the lung segments between the upper lobe and the lingular segments as also between the apical and the basal parts of the inferior lobe, whereas venous blood flow deviates from the segments elsewhere. The veins of these segments carry the blood not only from the superjacent artery but from the arteries of the adjoining subsegments as well. Pulmonary veins lie more horizontally and open into the heart more caudally than the arteries. They are devoid of valves.

In general, two **pulmonary veins** enter the left atrium on each side. These veins originate in the hila from the confluence of pulmonary segmental vessels. Their course is longer on the right side than on the left.

The right superior pulmonary vein is in the hilum of the lung below and in front of the right pulmonary artery. It collects the blood from the upper and the middle lobes. The right inferior pulmonary vein can be found below the principal bronchus and behind the preceding vein and collects the blood from the right inferior lobe. Both veins run into the left atrium behind the superior vena cava and then behind the aorta and below the right pulmonary artery. They enter separately into the atrium, the superior vein somewhat higher and more anteriorly than the inferior. Their intrapericardial portion is shorter than that of the corresponding veins of the left side. The left superior pulmonary vein is placed below and in front of the left pulmonary artery, behind the ascending aorta, and in front of the left principal bronchus. It collects the veins of the left upper lobe. The left inferior pulmonary vein is before the thoracic aorta and below the left principal bronchus. It drains the blood of the left inferior lobe. Both left pulmonary veins pass through the pericardium below the left pulmonary artery and, running behind the artery, enter the left atrium in comparison with those of the right-hand side after a considerably longer course. The superior vein enters the atrium at the top, the inferior vein in the left posteroinferior corner (Nagy 1962).

The cardiac muscles from the left atrium spread over the pulmonary veins. Their length varies even on the anterior and the posterior side of the same vessel's wall (Adachi 1933). As a rule, the muscles strengthening the veins extend as far as the peri-

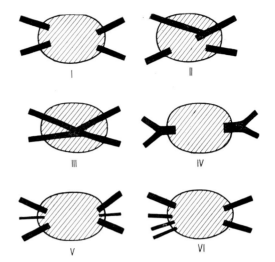

FIG. 29. Variations in the opening of the pulmonary veins. I, typical opening; II, partial crossing; III, complete crossing: common trunk; IV, bilateral common trunk; V, right and left medial pulmonary vein; VI, apical branch, the superior and inferior basal veins have separate openings.

cardium (Benninghoff 1930). They can sometimes be traced as far as the segmental veins (Franceschi 1927). In the absence of valves these muscle fibres regulate the volume of blood streaming into the atrium. Therefore their physiological importance is significant. In addition to the pulmonary branches, they collect the following veins: *hilar, pleural, mediastinal* and *bronchial* (Paturet 1958). Diameters of the pulmonary veins: right superior pulmonary vein: 1·6 cm; left superior pulmonary vein: 1·5 cm; right inferior pulmonary vein: 1·5 cm; left inferior pulmonary vein: 1·4 cm (Paturet 1958).

Numerous *variations* and anomalies of the pulmonary veins are known (Fig. 29). Doerr (1955) estimates their occurrence at 10 per cent. Variations are possible because, instead of four, more or less veins may open into the left atrium. We speak of right or left common pulmonary vein (Figs 29/II to IV) if the two pulmonary veins of the right or left side unite to form a common trunk before they empty into the left atrium. There are in such cases three instead of four pulmonary veins. The common trunk may be formed within or outside the pericardium (Adachi 1933). Intrapericardial trunk formation is relatively more frequent, and it occurs more often on the right side than on the left. In case of bilateral common pulmonary veins one may open into the contralateral one, in which case only one pulmonary vein is formed (Didion 1942). The occurrence of more pulmonary veins is mostly due to the separate openings of the veins of the middle lobe or the lingula (right or left middle pulmonary vein, Fig. 29/V; Brantigan 1952, Boyden 1955). Isolated openings of other segmental veins may oc-

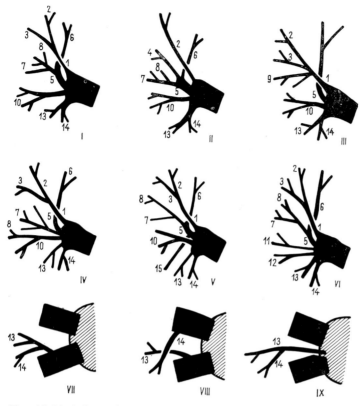

FIG. 30. Variations of the veins of the right superior and middle lobes. I, V_1, V_2, V_3 arise separately, V_{4+5} together; II, V_{2+1x} together; III, V_{1+2x} together; IV, V_{3+2c} together; V, V_{2+6x} together, V_4 and V_5 separately; V_{3a}, V_{3b}, V_4, V_5 separately; VII, V_{4+5} open into the right inferior pulmonary vein; VIII, V_4 opens into the right inferior, V_5 into the right superior pulmonary vein; IX, V_{4+5} into the right middle pulmonary vein. (1) V_1; (2) V_{1a}; (3) V_{1b}; (4) V_{1x}; (5) V_2; (6) V_{2c}; (7) V_{2b}; (8) V_{2c}; (9) V_{2x}; (10) V_3; (11) V_{3a}; (12) V_{3b}; (13) V_4; (14) V_5; (15) V_{6x}.

cur as well (Fig. 29/VI). Their number may vary from two to five on one side (Töndury and Weibel 1958).

Clinically it is more important if one or more veins open into the greater circulation (transposition of pulmonary veins) than if, though in anomalous number, they open into the left atrium. The transposition of pulmonary veins according to postmortem examination varies from 1·8 to 10·0 per cent (Romoda et al. 1963). With anomalous orifice of one or more veins, partial transposition with ectopic opening of all the veins complete transposition exists. Complete transposition makes life impossible unless accompanied by a defect of the atrial septum. Life is still possible if at least 50 per cent of the blood flows into the left atrium, and no clinical manifestations arise in case if 75 per cent blood flows there. (Doerr 1955). Transposition into the following veins may take place:

Right superior vena cava (complete: Swan et al. 1953; partial: Campbell and Deuchar 1954, Csákány and Varga 1966, Bhagvant et al. 1967); left superior vena cava (Abrams 1957, Csákány and

Varga 1966); left brachiocephalic vein (complete: Anderson et al. 1961; partial: Harley 1958); inferior vena cava (Fogel et al. 1959, Fiandra et al. 1962); hepatic veins (Downing 1953); azygos vein (Winter 1954, Diaz et al. 1959); right atrium (Blake et al. 1965, Csákány and Varga 1966); coronary sinus (Campbell and Deuchar 1954, Bhagvant et al. 1967); ductus venosus (Mehn and Hirsch 1947, cit. Doerr 1955); portal vein (Lüdin 1952); thoracic duct (Healey 1952).

The **right superior pulmonary vein** collects the veins of the right upper and middle lobes (Figs 30, 59/15, 60/12, 61/7, 62/2). The number of these veins is variable. They do not follow the segmental distribution. Viewed from the hilum, superficial (subpleural) and deep (central) veins are distinguishable. The preponderance of one vein may replace the other (Hayek 1953).

There arise generally three veins from the *upper lobe*, namely the apical (V_1), posterior (V_2) and anterior (V_3) branches.

The *apical branch*, V_1 (Figs 30/1, 59/16, 60/13, 61/8, 62/3) runs superficially below the visceral surface of the pleura behind the corresponding bronchus. In general, it unites two larger branches. It receives the veins of the septum between segments S_1 and S_3 (Fig. 30/I). Its variant branch may be a subsegmental vein of V_2 (Fig. 30/III).

The *posterior branch*, V_2 (Figs 30/5, 59/20, 60/13, 61/9, 62/4), is the largest vein of the upper lobe which goes round the anterior bronchus from below. As a rule, it collects the veins lying between segments S_1 and S_2 and between S_2 and S_3, furthermore the veins of the dorsal part of S_2 (Fig. 30/I). The vessel is called vena magna if the veins open posteriorly into it from the surrounding subsegments (Appleton 1944, Oliveros 1951). The superficial and central branches of V_2 sometimes open separately into the main trunk (Figs. 30/II to IV). It is claimed by Boyden (1955) that in 56 per cent of the cases the accessory vein of V_6 enters into the main trunk (Fig. 30/V).

The *anterior branch*, V_3 (Figs 30/10, 59/23, 60/14, 61/10, 62/6) runs below the corresponding bronchus in 50 per cent of the cases. It receives the veins of the subpleural part of segment S_3. The two branches of the vessel have separate orifices (Fig. 30/VI) in

30 per cent (Boyden 1955). In such cases, one of the branches may open into the veins of the middle lobe.

It is either with a common trunk that the veins of the *right middle lobe* (*ramus lobi medii*) open into the right superior pulmonary vein (Figs 30/I to III, 60/15, 61/11, 62/7) or, in some cases, they may have separate orifices (Figs. 30/IV to VI). They collect blood from two venous trunks: the *lateral part*, V_4 (Figs 30/13, 59/27, 62/8) drains the veins between S_4 and S_5, the *medial part*, V_5 (Figs 30/14, 59/28, 62/9) the superficial mediastinal vessels of S_5. The main trunk runs and ramifices below the bronchus of the middle lobe. As a variant, it may happen that the branch of the middle lobe or the vein V_4 gets into the inferior pulmonary vein (Figs. 30/VII and VIII; Boyden 1955). Occasionally the branch of the middle lobe reaches the left atrium as a direct branch (Fig. 30/IX; Brantigan 1952).

As a rule, the veins of the right inferior lobe open separately into the **right inferior pulmonary vein** (Figs 31, 59/29, 60/12, 61/12, 62/10). It happens but exceptionally that it receives an occasional branch from a segment of the upper or middle lobe. In the hilum it is usually formed by the union of three vessels (Fig. 31/II), viz. the apical (superior) branch V_6 unites the veins of the highest lying segments, the superior and inferior basal veins which drain the basal segments. If the latter two veins form a common trunk before they empty into the main trunk it is called common basal vein (Fig. 31/I).

The *apical (superior) branch* to the inferior lobe, V_6 (Figs 31/1, 59/30, 60/16, 61/13, 62/11) has usually three tributaries, two of which arise in 60 per cent of the cases from the segment S_6 (intrasegmental part) and one from the area between segments S_6 and S_{10} (infrasegmental part). These veins converge usually resembling a star in shape. There are many possible variations, so many that Boyden and Scannel (1946) were unable to classify them in 40 per cent of their cases. V_{6x} (Fig. 30/15) may sometimes end in the posterior branch of the upper lobe via a paravertebrally formed parenchymal bridge.

The *superior basal vein*, V_{8+9} (Figs 59/31, 60/17, 61/28, 62/13) opens, according to Boyden (1955), usually into the common basal vein. As a rule, it ascends obliquely from the lateral toward the hilum behind the medial bronchus. It lies in the intersegmental septum between S_7 and S_8 as well as S_9 and S_{10}, only its root is in the interlobar septum. The superior basal branch drains segments S_8 and S_9. Zenker and his associates (1954) distinguish two types to demonstrate its ramification. One is composed of the trunks V_{8+9} and V_8, the other of the vein uniting the branches of V_{8+9}, V_8, V_9 and V_{10}.

The *inferior basal vein*, V_{9+10} (Figs 59/35, 60/17, 61/18, 62/17) usually drains segments S_9 and S_{10}

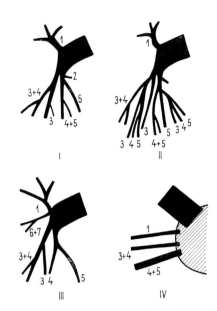

FIG. 31. Variations of the veins of the right inferior lobe. I, two trunks: V_6 and common basal vein; II, three trunks: V_6 and superior and inferior basal veins (diverging type); III, four trunks: V_6, V_{4+5}, superior and inferior basal veins, V_7 is not visualized; IV, three branches open into the left atrium: V_6, V_{8+9}, V_{9+10}. (*1*) V_6; (*2*) V_7; (*3*) V_8; (*4*) V_9; (*5*) V_{10}; (*6*) V_4; (*7*) V_5.

into the common basal vein. It may receive tributary from S_8. Also in this case Zenker et al. (1954) distinguish two types of confluence: the main trunk is formed by V_{10} and V_{9+10} in the first, by V_{9+10}, V_{10} and V_8, V_9, V_{10} in the second type.

V_7 is usually small (Figs 31/2, 62/14), and may open either into the superior or the inferior basal vein, and cannot always be visualized.

Variations in the confluence of the veins of the right inferior lobe are as follows (Boyden 1955): There are two veins (78 per cent): apical (superior) and common basal vein (Fig. 31/I). There are three veins: apical (superior) branch, superior and inferior basal veins (Fig. 31/II). There are four veins composed of the above three and an accessory vessel. The latter may be the branch of the middle lobe (10 per cent) or the descending branch of V_2 (4 per cent; Fig. 31/III). There is only a single vein formed by the confluence of the three main trunks (Healey and Gibbon, cit. Zenker et al. 1954). It occurs in 3 per cent. A rare variant is the direct opening of the inferior lobar veins into the right atrium (Brantigan 1952; Fig. 31/IV).

The veins of the left upper lobe open into the **left superior pulmonary vein** (Figs 32, 59/38, 60/12, 61/19, 63/2). In respect of the right side, the difference arises from the fact that they have a superficial orifice on the mediastinal side. The central and posterior veins open into the anterior venous trunks. Certain veins may drain several segments. Their

63

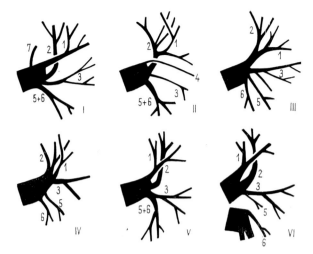

FIG. 32. Variations of the veins of the left superior lobe. I, V_{4+5} arise together, superior hilar vein; II, V_{1+2}, V_{4+5} together, V_3 and V_{3x} separately; III, V_{1+2} together, V_4 and V_5 separately; IV, V_{1+2+3} together, V_4 and V_5 separately; V, V_{3+4+5} together; VI, V_5 into the left inferior pulmonary vein. (1) V_1; (2) V_2; (3) V_3; (4) V_{3x}; (5) V_4; (6) V_5; (7) superior hilar vein.

course is fairly constant. There are usually three main branches: *apicoposterior branch* V_{1+2} (Figs 32/1 and 2, 59/39, 60/13 61/20, 63/3), *anterior branch* V_3 and *lingular branch* V_{4+5}. Boyden and Hartmann (1946) distinguish three types in which the veins returning blood from the three upper segments ramify: V_{1+2} arise together (Fig. 32/II) — the most frequent alternative (68 per cent); V_{1+2a+b} arise together as well as V_{2c+3c} (Fig. 32/III); V_{1+3a} arise together (Fig. 32/IV) and V_2 receives V_{3c}. Relations to the neighbouring bronchi and arteries vary according to the type of division.

The *anterior branch*, V_3 (Figs 32/3, 59/47, 60/14, 61/23, 63/6) receives the veins from S_3 and from the septum between S_3 and S_4. It has a separate

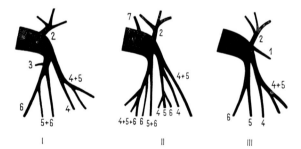

FIG. 33. Variations of the veins of the left inferior lobe. I, common basal vein, V_7 opening into the inferior basal vein, V_8, V_{8+9} into the superior basal vein; II, the superior and inferior basal veins open separately, the inferior hilar vein empties into the left inferior pulmonary vein, V_8, V_{8+9}, V_8, V_9, V_{10} open into the superior basal vein, V_{8+9+10}, V_{10} and V_{9+10} into the inferior basal vein; III, V_5 into the left inferior pulmonary vein. (1) V_5; (2) V_6; (3) V_7; (4) V_8; (5) V_9; (6) V_{10}; (7) inferior hilar vein.

opening between the two other veins. Trifurcation of the upper lobar veins results in case of independent orifice of V_3. If it has a common opening with the neighbouring veins bifurcation arises. V_3 consists of two (Figs. 32/I and IV), sometimes of one (Fig. 32/II), and in 10 per cent of three (Fig. 32/III) separate branches which course radially into the left superior pulmonary vein.

In half of the cases the *lingular branch*, V_{4+5} (Figs 32/5 and 6, 59/50, 60/15, 61/24, 63/7) enters the left superior pulmonary vein with separate *superior, part*, V_4 and *inferior part*, V_5 (Fig. 32/III and IV), in the other half with a common trunk (Figs. 32/I, II, V). V_5 opens into the left inferior pulmonary vein in 10 per cent of the cases (Figs 32/VI; Boyden 1955). Thus, this is the only vein of the upper lobe entering into the inferior pulmonary vein. Variations of the lobar veins, like those on the right side, have not been observed here. Both veins drain from the corresponding segments.

The **left inferior pulmonary vein** (Figs 33, 59/54, 60/12, 61/25, 63/10) drains the blood of the left inferior lobe, and the pattern of its ramification resembles that of the contralateral vessel. It is usually formed by the union of two branches (Fig. 33/I), namely the common basal vein and the apical (superior) branch, but may be formed also by three branches (Fig. 33/II), namely the superior and inferior basal veins, further the apical (superior) branch. The vein V_5 (Fig. 33/III) and a retrohilar vein (*inferior hilar vein*; Figs 33/II, 59/53), too, may open into this vessel. The *apical (superior) branch*, V_6 (Figs 33/2, 59/55, 60/16, 61/26, 63/11) is usually formed by three branches arising from S_6 and from the septum between S_6 and S_{10}. It is better developed than the corresponding vessel on the other side. The *common basal vein* (Figs 59/56, 60/17, 61/27, 63/12), consisting of two branches, runs to the hilum with a lateral-oblique course. It can usually be found in the angle of division between B_{9+10} or B_{7+8}. The branch coursing from S_6 is called *paramediastinal vein*. Further divisions of the main trunk are similar to the right side.

Radiological anatomy of the pulmonary veins

Steinbach and his associates (1955) tried to differentiate the pulmonary veins by means of summation roentgenograms. In the **anteroposterior view** (Fig. 37) particularly on the righ-hand side the great veins of the upper lobe can be distinguished. They can be more clearly visualized by means of tomography. In the **second oblique view** (Fig. 39), the veins of the middle and inferior lobes can be

64

demonstrated in the projection of the cardiac shadow by hard ray technique. Veins of the inferior lobes can be well followed from the periphery to the right atrium in **lateral x-ray pictures** (Fig. 40).

Only the upper veins are involved in the visualization of the hilar structures, whereas the inferior veins run independently of the hilum. They have a more horizontal position and a more caudal opening than the arteries. The right superior pulmonary vein appears at the height of the upper border of the seventh, the left at that of the lower border of the sixth, the right inferior pulmonary vein at that of the upper border of the eighth, the left at the height of the lower border of the seventh thoracic vertebra.

Concerning the detailed analysis of the radiological anatomy of the pulmonary veins reference has been made to the work by Hornykiewytsch and Stender (1954a, b, c, d, e, 1955a, b, c).

Pneumovenography

It is in the venous phase of pneumoangiography that the pulmonary veins can be studied in vivo. Dotter and his coworkers (1949) succeeded first in demonstrating the anomalies of the pulmonary venous trunks by filling them with radio-opaque matter. This method allows the identification of central branches only; peripheral details remain more or less obscure owing to the dilution of the contrast medium.

Even the most peripheral veins can be filled retrogradely in *postmortem pneumovenography* with adequate pressure. In **anteroposterior pictures** (Fig. 59), the radial convergence of the trunks in the hilum give a perfectly clear view of the various segmental and subsegmental veins and smaller branches. At or proximally to the hila the overlapping shadows of the four *pulmonary veins* are barely distinguishable (Figs 59/15, 29, 38, 54). Thus the opening into the left atrium cannot be reliably localized. If the left ventricle and the aorta are also filled a combination of the projective conditions is produced. The shadows of the left V_7 and V_8 and possibly also V_{10} are cast upon the projection of the left ventricle. The projection of about the 7th thoracic vertebra is crossed by the border of the left atrium which curves upward and slightly to the right. Three quarters of it lies to the left of the median line. The bulb of the aorta and the initial portion of the ascending aorta cover the atrium from the front. The descending aorta behind the left atrium is obscured from view at the height of the upper border of the atrium. In **lateral view** (Fig. 60), the origin of the *pulmonary veins* cannot be

distinguished in the oval projection of the left atrium (Fig. 60/12). The ascending branches of V_1 and V_2 after their division intersect the arch of the aorta. V_3, V_4 and V_5 run across the ascending aorta. The descending aorta is crossed obliquely, somewhat upward and horizontally by V_6, and obliquely downward by V_9 and V_{10}. V_7 is visible between the aorta and the left atrium. V_8 can be found in full usually in the overlapping of the atrium and ventricle.

In **anteroposterior pictures** (Fig. 61) following the joint removal of the lungs and heart in *isolated organ preparations* the ramifications of the flattened venous trunks can be traced from their origin to their orifice. Even minor details and also the relative position of the trunks entering at the hila can be observed in the **lateral view** (Figs 62, 63).

VASA PRIVATA

The bronchial vascular system secures the blood supply to the tissues of the lungs. With respect to the vasa publica, it is termed vasa privata. Already Ruysch (1696) was familiar with their existence. Their importance has considerably increased during the last decade, ever since their normal and pathological conditions can be registered by physiological and clinical methods.

The bronchial arteries of the newborn are relatively thicker than those of adults (Halmágyi 1957). Normal circulation is established with the first breath. While all the blood, entering the right ventricle, passes through the pulmonary system, only a slight fraction of the blood in the aorta gets into the bronchial vessels.

Bronchial arteries

The number of bronchial arteries is variable (Fig. 34). As a rule, one right and two left bronchial arteries can be found (Miller 1906a, b, 1925, 1947; Cauldwell et al. 1948). This typical variation in origin could be found only in about 40·6 per cent of the cases, whereas, according to Cauldwell et al. (1948), two to five bronchial arteries are in 59·4 per cent. The two left bronchial arteries arise from the ventral aspect of the descending aorta at the height of the fourth to sixth thoracic vertebrae (Latarjet and Juttin 1951). The origin of the right branches is more variable. The most common is the common origin with the first posterior intercostal artery, but it may arise directly from the wall of the aorta, from the subclavian artery (O'Rahilly et al. 1950), from the internal thoracic artery (Quain 1884),

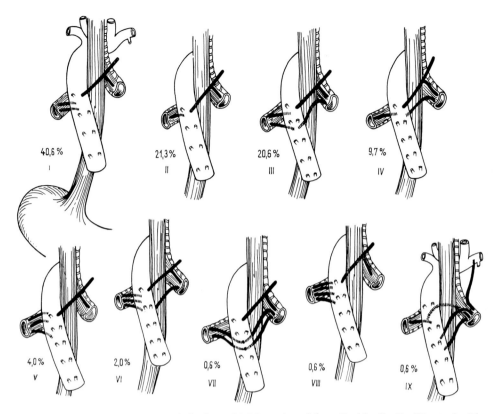

FIG. 34. Variations in the origin of the bronchial branches (after Cauldwell, E. W. et al.: The bronchial arteries. An anatomic study of 150 human cadavers. *Surg. Gynec. Obstet.*, 86, 1948, 395).

from the brachiocephalic trunk (Romankevitch 1931) as also from the arteria lusoria (Abesi 1966).

The *right bronchial artery* (Figs 45/27, 46/25) runs first behind the left bronchus and then behind the bronchopericardiac membrane. Reaching the right principal bronchus, it usually bifurcates. One branch runs to the anterior surface of the principal bronchus and joins the bronchus of the upper lobe (*superior branch*, Fig. 44/30), the other passes from the posterior surface of the bronchus intermedius to the posterior surface of the middle or lower lobar bronchus (*inferior branch*, Fig. 44/29).

The *left bronchial arteries* (*superior*, Figs 16/4, 46/27 and *inferior*) reach the lung running along the anterior surface of the corresponding bronchi (Hayek 1953).

After the origin, the bronchial branches pursue a spiral course in loose connective tissue around the bronchi. In front of the hila, they adhere persistently to the wall of the bronchi and follow their ramification. In their mediastinal course, they give off side branches to the pericardium, the lymph nodes, esophagus and pleura. They usually communicate with a branch of the pericardiacophrenic artery (*anterior bronchial branch*) and the tracheal vessels (Hayek 1953, Bikfalvi et al. 1967). Communication with the coronary arteries has likewise been de-

scribed (Delarue et al. 1960, Moberg 1967). The right and left branch are frequently anastomosing at the level of the bifurcation (Latarjet and Juttin 1951). Verloop (1948) could follow the terminal branches as far as the surface of the diaphragm. The repeatedly ramifying vessels can be observed in the lung as far as the terminal bronchiole where they form an arterial plexus (Miller 1925, Marchand et al. 1950). The capillaries of the alveolar wall are fed by the terminal branches of the pulmonary artery (Hayek 1958). These vessels represent the vasa vasorum of the branches of the pulmonary artery (Florance 1960).

Blood to the visceral pleura over the whole convex and diaphragmatic surface is supplied by small branches of the pulmonary artery coming from the parenchyma of the lung, while the mediastinal and interlobar parts are supplied by the bronchial arteries (Latarjet and Juttin 1951, Silver 1952).

Bronchial veins

Veins of the bronchial walls form plexuses and the small venules form a *peribronchial network* (Miller 1947, Schoenmackers 1960a). Veins arising here run along the bronchial walls towards the hila. Most of them end in the pulmonary veins, while some enter directly into the left atrium (Zuckerkandl 1882, Miller 1947, Aviado 1965). They are called *bronchopulmonary veins*.

Veins originating from the extrapulmonary bronchi, from the hilar structures and the pleuromediastinal surface are called *pleurohilar-bronchial veins*. Vessels from the anterior and posterior part of the latter group open into the vena azygos on the right side, while the posterior veins on the left side into the hemiazygos vein or the accessory hemiazygos vein or into the left brachiocephalic vein; the anterior veins of the left side open into the posterior bronchopulmonary veins (Zuckerkandl 1882). These veins are also in communication with the pulmonary veins (Schoenmackers, 1960a). There are valves in the larger pleurohilar veins.

The bronchial veins communicate in the mediastinum with the mediastinal, pericardiac, tracheal, esophageal and diaphragmatic veins chiefly through the branches of the internal thoracic and the intercostal veins (Zuckerkandl 1882, Schoenmackers 1960a). Collateral circulation, mediated by the esophageal veins, may also be formed with the system of the portal vein (Schoenmackers and Vieten 1953, 1954).

Bronchial angiography

Contrast filling of the bronchial arteries by means of selective angiography offers convenient orientation in respect of their anatomical pattern and their role in the pulmonary circulation (Schober 1964, Viamonte et al. 1965, Nordenström 1967). Pictures made by the subtraction technique present a still better view of the minor branches (Groen et al. 1966). Even minor branches can be visualized by selective filling (Botenga 1968).

While the origin of the small vessels arising from the anterior wall of the aorta is invisible in *postmortem* **anteroposterior angiograms** (Fig. 44), the *right branch*, running below the arch of the aorta upward from left to right, can be well seen. The origin is usually at the height of the fifth thoracic vertebra. Of the branches descending in the lung, the *right superior bronchial artery* passes toward the clavicle (Fig. 44/30) and the *right inferior bronchial artery* (Fig. 44/29) advances toward the diaphragm. Mostly they ramify in the hilum. The *left superior bronchial artery* (Fig. 46/27) passes first upward along the mediastinal border and runs then obliquely lateral. Its extrahilar segment is most often covered by projection of the descending aorta, which is intersected by the branch from in front. The further course in the lung of both the upper and lower

arteries is similar to the right side. In **lateral view** (Fig. 45), the origin of the *bronchial vessels* can often be observed on the anterior wall of the aorta (Fig. 45/27), but their further course remains hidden owing to their progressive tenuity.

Postmortem the bronchial veins can be filled with contrast material through the pulmonary veins (Schoenmackers 1960b).

COLLATERAL CIRCULATION OF THE PULMONARY VESSELS

The vasa publica and privata of the lung form an anatomical unit maintained by anastomoses existing between the two functionally different vascular systems. Ruysch (1696) was the first to recognize the bronchopulmonary anastomoses. By means of corrosion preparations Hayek (1940) demonstrated collaterals connecting the pulmonary artery with the peribronchial venous plexus; with the injection of radio-opaque matter Cudkowicz and Armstrong (1951) found numerous collaterals between the bronchopulmonary vessels. The significance of anastomoses between the various veins increases in pathological conditions (Viamonte 1967). The anatomical aspects of communications existing between the two arterial and venous systems and the vessels of the adjoining organs are described in the following.

1. Arterio-arterial anastomoses. Being terminal vessels, there is no communication between the branches of the pulmonary artery (Fig. 35/I; Cohnheim and Litten 1875). There are numerous anastomoses between the various parts of the bronchial arteries (Fig. 35/II; Miller 1947, Marchand et al. 1950). These arteries communicate with the surrounding vessels of the systemic circulation (Fig. 35/III), through the mediastinal, pleural, esophageal, tracheal and diaphragmatic branches through the branches of the coronary artery and through the vasa vasorum of the posterior intercostal artery and aorta (Hayek 1940, Verloop 1948, Delarue et al. 1960, Björk 1966, Rémy et al. 1972). Between the pulmonary and the bronchial artery (Fig. 35/IV), anastomoses, 0·08 mm in diameter, exist at the level of middle-sized and small bronchi. Morphologically, they correspond to the branch of the bronchial artery and are provided with circular and facultatively with longitudinal muscles (Töndury and Weibel 1956, 1958). They regard these muscles as the result of a functional change caused by the extension of the lung. The number of anastomoses at the precapillary level in the lung of normal individuals totals 200 to 300 (Weibel 1959). They can be visualized in vivo under patho-

logical conditions (Shedd et al. 1951, Massumi et al. 1965, Szabó and Simay 1972). There are spiral communications between the pulmonary and bronchial vascular systems on the pleural surface of the lung (Zuckerkandl 1882). Blood flows under normal conditions in a bronchopulmonary direction through the connecting precapillary branches. The average

that there are many anastomoses between the pleurohilar and the other veins of the greater circulation.

3. Arterio-venous anastomoses. Prinzmetal and his associates (1948) demonstrated pulmonary arteriovenous communications in physiological model experiments. No such anastomoses have so far been

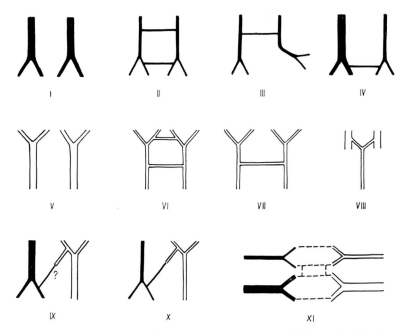

FIG. 35. Diagram of the bronchopulmonary anastomoses. I–IV, arterio-arterial; V–VIII, veno-venous; IX–X, arterio-venous; XI, intercapillary anastomoses. I, pulmonary arteries; II, bronchial arteries; III, bronchial—mediastinal arteries; IV, pulmonary—bronchial arteries; V, pulmonary veins; VI, bronchopulmonary—pleurohilar veins; VII, bronchopulmonary—pleurohilar veins; VIII, mediastinal—bronchial—pulmonary veins; IX, pulmonary arteries—veins; X, bronchial arteries—bronchial veins; XI, bronchial and pulmonary arteries—bronchial and pulmonary veins.

blood pressure before anastomosis in the pulmonary branches is 25 mm Hg and 30 mm Hg in the bronchial branches (Töndury and Weibel 1958).

2. Veno-venous anastomoses. No postcapillary anastomoses (Fig. 35/V) exist between the branches of the pulmonary vein (Weibel 1959). Branches of the bronchial veins communicate at various levels (Figs 35/VI and VII). There are anastomoses in the bronchopulmonary plexuses (Miller 1947, Schoenmackers 1960a), between the pleurohilar veins (Marchand et al. 1950, Weibel 1959), further between the two systems in the hilum (Marchand et al. 1950). The communications between the bronchial and the pulmonary veins are more significant (Fig. 35/8). Most of the blood of the bronchial veins but also some of the blood from the pleurohilar vessels gets into the pulmonary veins (Schoenmackers 1960a, Aviado 1965). It has already been mentioned

demonstrated anatomically (Fig. 35/IX; Weibel 1959). Anastomoses between the bronchial arteries and bronchial veins can be found also in normal lungs (Fig. 35/X; Watzka 1936). Their number in healthy lungs varies from 25 to 30 (Weibel 1959).

4. Intercapillary anastomoses. There are abundant capillary interconnections between the bronchial and the pulmonary vessels (Fig. 35/XI) around the terminal bronchioles (Miller 1925, Hayek 1953).

Significance of the bronchopulmonary collateral circulation (Fig. 36). Only a fraction of the cardiac output flows through the bronchial vessels under normal conditions. The clinical significance of the vasa privata is enhanced if the pulmonary terminal arteries become insufficient in which case the supply of the lung tissues is secured through the collaterals (Ellis et al. 1952). According to Kovács (1965), we

68

present here a brief anatomical description of the normal collateral circulation between the vasa privata and vasa publica.

1. Bronchopulmonary collateral circulation (Fig. 36/9). Pressure being higher in the bronchial than in the pulmonary vessels, circulation has a bronchopulmonary direction and takes place at three levels.

veins. Its volume depends on the width of the paths of communication.

3. Cavo-pulmonary collateral circulation (Fig. 36/21). The direction of blood flow through the anastomoses described above is reversed if intravenous pressure in the greater circulation exceeds that of the pulmonary veins. In this case revers-

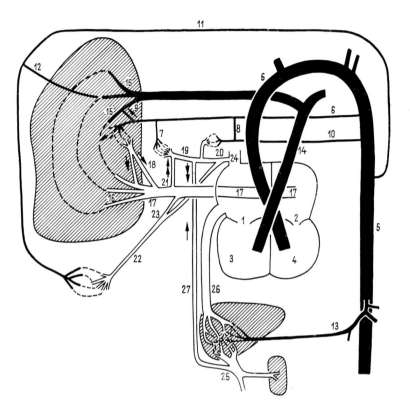

FIG. 36. Diagram of the bronchopulmonary circulation (after Kovács, G.: *A bronchopulmonalis kollateralis keringés vizsgálata* [Study of the bronchopulmonary collateral circulation]. Thesis. Szeged, 1965, modified). (*1*) Right atrium; (*2*) left atrium; (*3*) right ventricle; (*4*) left ventricle; (*5*) aorta; (*6*) bronchial branch; (*7*) bronchial branch—pleurohilar bronchial veins; (*8*) bronchial branch—mediastinal artery; (*9*) bronchial branch—pulmonary artery; (*10*) mediastinal artery; (*11*) posterior intercostal artery; (*12*) pleuropulmonary anastomosis, (*13*) hepatic artery; (*14*) pulmonary trunk; (*15*) branches of the right pulmonary artery; (*16*) branches of the right pulmonary vein; (*17*) pulmonary vein; (*18*) bronchopulmonary veins; (*19*) pleurohilar bronchial veins; (*20*) azygos vein; (*21*) pleurohilar bronchial veins—pulmonary veins; (*22*) pleural veins; (*23*) pleural—pulmonary veins; (*24*) superior vena cava; (*25*) portal vein; (*26*) inferior vena cava; (*27*) portal vein—mediastinal veins.

There is a precapillary circulation between the branches of the bronchial and pulmonary arteries, and an intercapillary communication between the capillaries of the two systems which accounts for 50 per cent of the regional circulation (Schoedel 1964). Furthermore, there are postcapillary anastomoses through the bronchopulmonary veins which open into the pulmonary veins.

2. Pulmobronchial collateral circulation (Fig. 36/21). Blood flowing from the pulmonary veins passes into the caval system via the pleurobronchial

ed flow is established through the system of anastomosis.

4. Portopulmonary collateral circulation (Fig. 36/27). If the normal portal pressure (8 to 12 mm Hg) is notably elevated, a portopulmonary flow may result by direct communications between the portal and the pleurohilar veins. No such phenomenon occurs under physiological conditions. Under normal condition bronchopulmonary blood flow being the most significant among the circulatory alternatives.

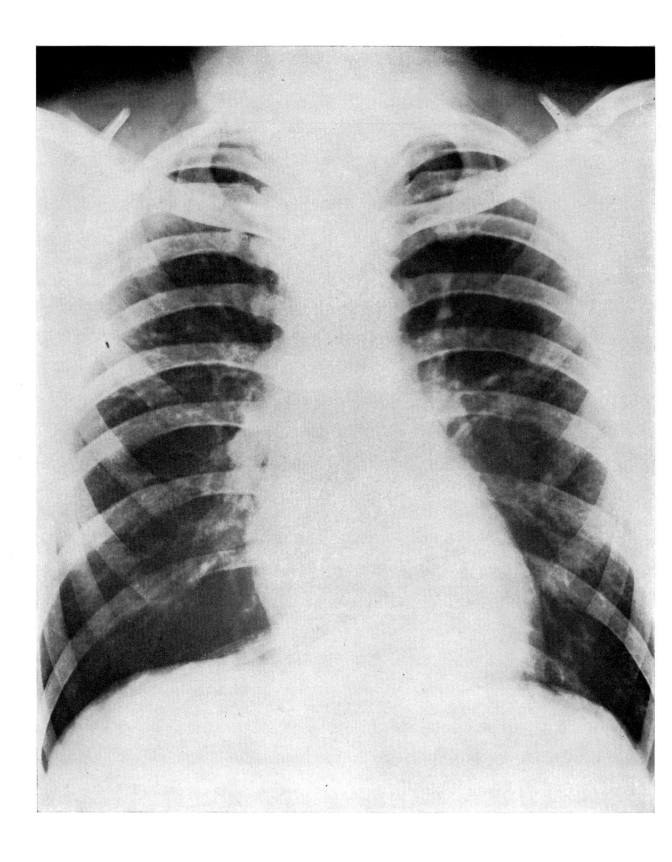

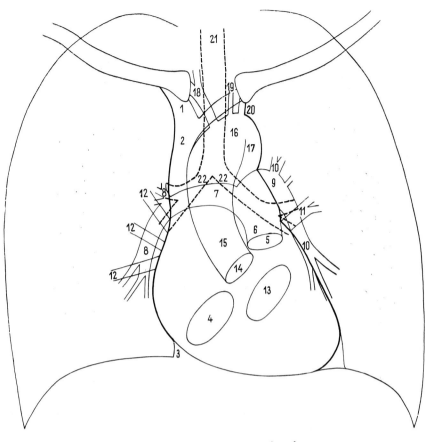

FIG. 37. The heart, I. Posteroanterior view.

1. Brachiocephalic veins
2. Superior vena cava
3. Inferior vena cava (right hepatic vein)
4. Right atrioventricular orifice
5. Orifice of pulmonary trunk
6. Pulmonary trunk
7. Right pulmonary artery
8. Branches of right pulmonary artery
9. Left pulmonary artery
10. Branches of left pulmonary artery
11. Left pulmonary veins
12. Right pulmonary veins
13. Left atrioventricular orifice
14. Orifice of aorta
15. Ascending aorta
16. Arch of the aorta
17. Descending aorta
18. Brachiocephalic trunk
19. Left common carotid artery
20. Left subclavian artery
21. Trachea
22. Right and left bronchus

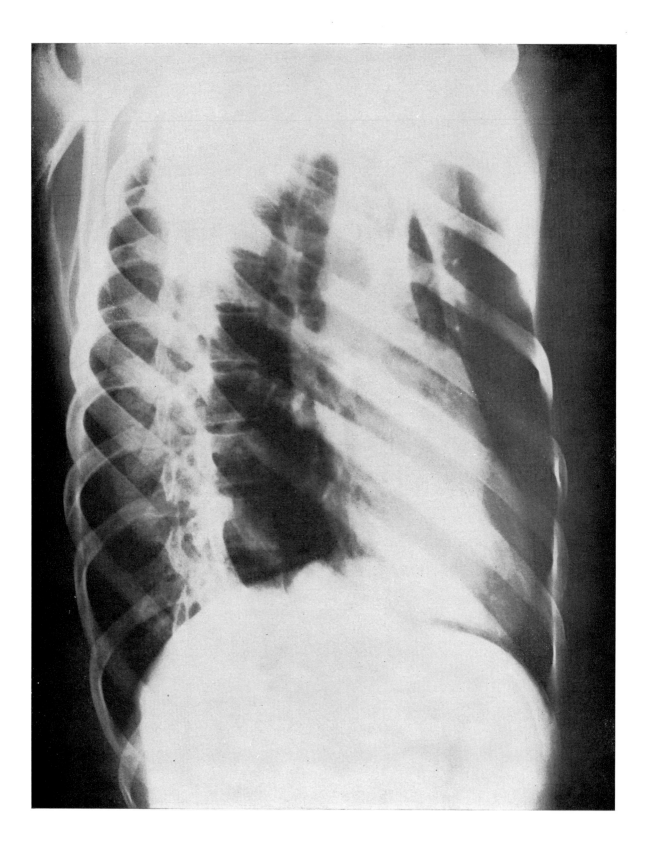

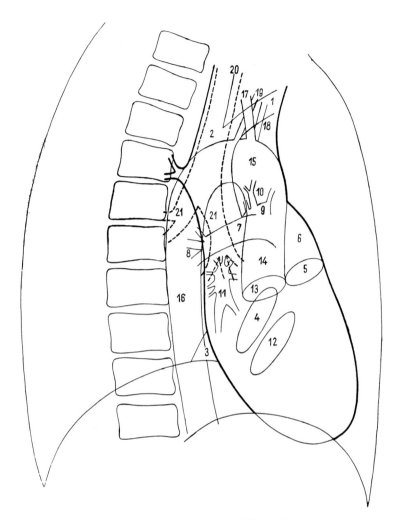

FIG. 38. The heart, II. First oblique view.

1. Brachiocephalic veins
2. Superior vena cava
3. Inferior vena cava
4. Right atrioventricular orifice
5. Orifice of pulmonary trunk
6. Pulmonary trunk
7. Right pulmonary artery
8. Branches of right pulmonary artery
9. Left pulmonary artery
10. Branches of left pulmonary artery
11. Left pulmonary veins
12. Left atrioventricular orifice
13. Orifice of aorta
14. Ascending aorta
15. Arch of the aorta
16. Descending aorta
17. Brachiocephalic trunk
18. Left common carotid artery
19. Left subclavian artery
20. Trachea
21. Right and left bronchus

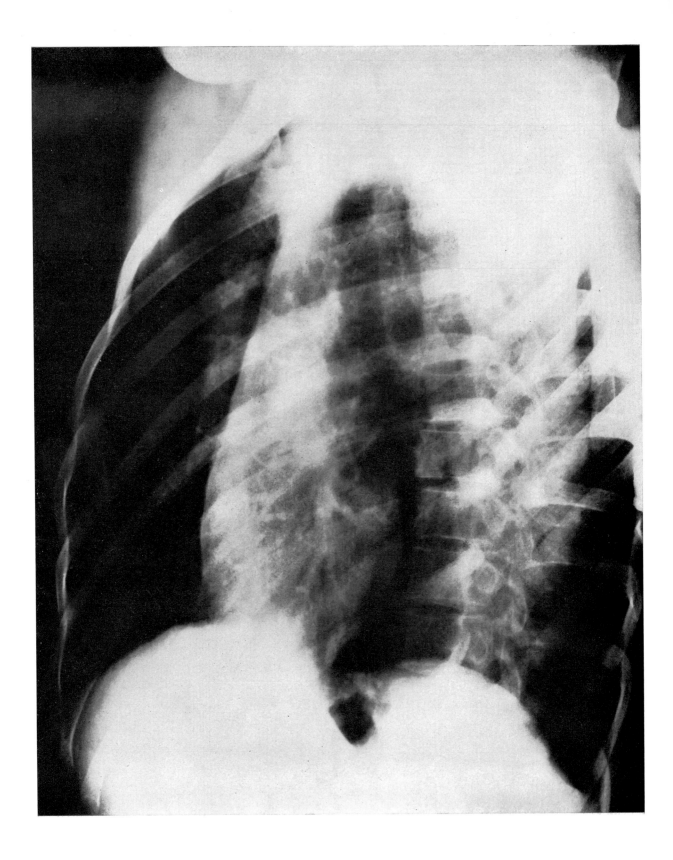

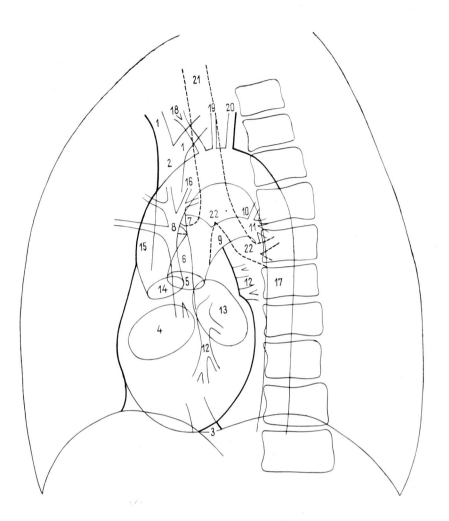

FIG. 39. The heart, III. Second oblique view.

1. Brachiocephalic veins
2. Superior vena cava
3. Inferior vena cava
4. Right atrioventricular orifice
5. Orifice of pulmonary trunk
6. Pulmonary trunk
7. Right pulmonary artery
8. Branches of right pulmonary artery
9. Left pulmonary artery
10. Ligamentum arteriosum
11. Branches of left pulmonary artery
12. Branches of left pulmonary veins
13. Left atrioventricular orifice
14. Orifice of aorta
15. Ascending aorta
16. Arch of aorta
17. Descending aorta
18. Brachiocephalic trunk
19. Left common carotid artery
20. Left subclavian artery
21. Trachea
22. Right and left bronchus

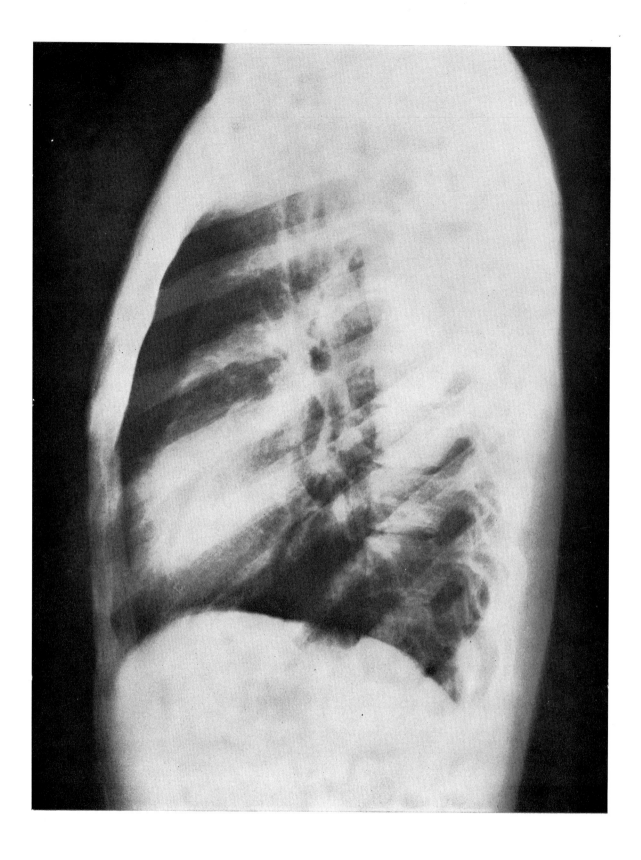

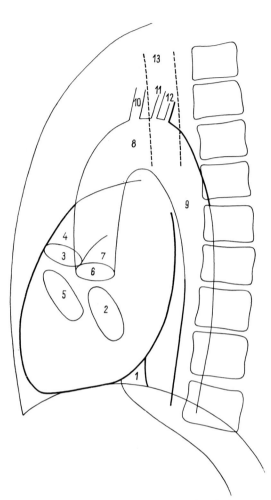

FIG. 40. The heart, IV. Dextrosinistral view.

1. Inferior vena cava
2. Right atrioventricular orifice
3. Orifice of the pulmonary trunk
4. Pulmonary trunk
5. Left atrioventricular orifice
6. Orifice of the aorta
7. Ascending aorta
8. Arch of the aorta
9. Descending aorta
10. Brachiocephalic trunk
11. Left common carotid artery
12. Left subclavian artery
13. Trachea

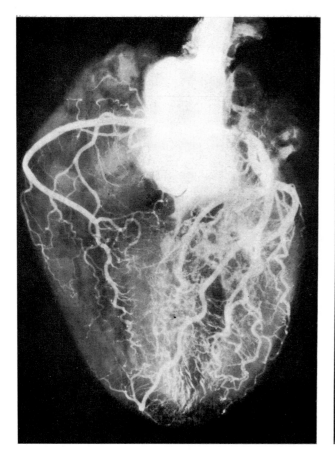
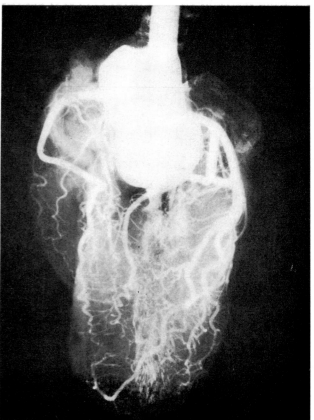
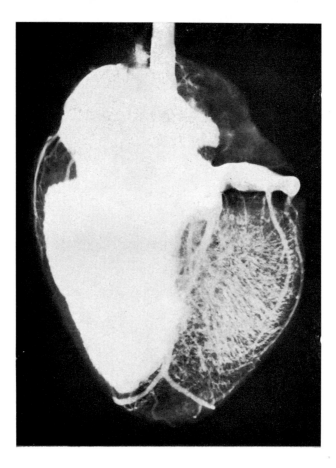

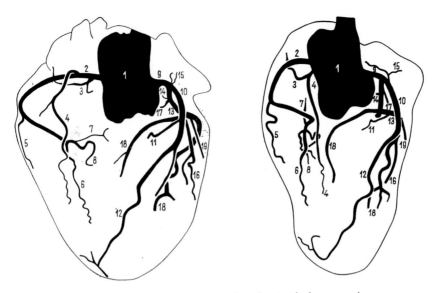

FIGS 41 and 42. The coronary arteries. Anatomical preparation.
Anteroposterior view (Fig. 41), dextrosinistral view (Fig. 42).

1. Bulb of aorta
2. Right coronary artery
3. Right anterior atrial branch
4. Right anterior ventricular branch
5. Right marginal branch
6. Posterior interventricular branch
7. Right posterior atrial branch

8. Left posterior ventricular branch
9. Left coronary artery
10. Anterior interventricular branch
11. Ramus coni pulmonalis sinister
12. Diagonal branch
13. Circumflex branch

14. Left anterior septal branch
15. Left anterior atrial branch
16. Left anterior ventricular branch
17. Left posterior auricular branch
18. Left posterior ventricular branch
19. Left posterior atrial branch

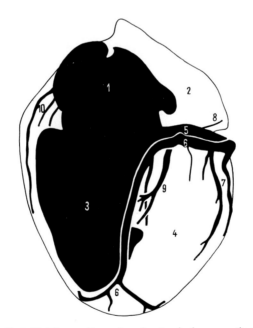

FIG. 43. The cardiac veins. Anatomical preparation.
Anteroposterior view.

1. Right atrium
2. Left atrium
3. Right ventricle
4. Left ventricle
5. Coronary sinus

6. Great cardiac vein
7. Posterior vein of left ventricle
8. Oblique vein of left atrium
9. Middle cardiac vein
10. Anterior cardiac veins

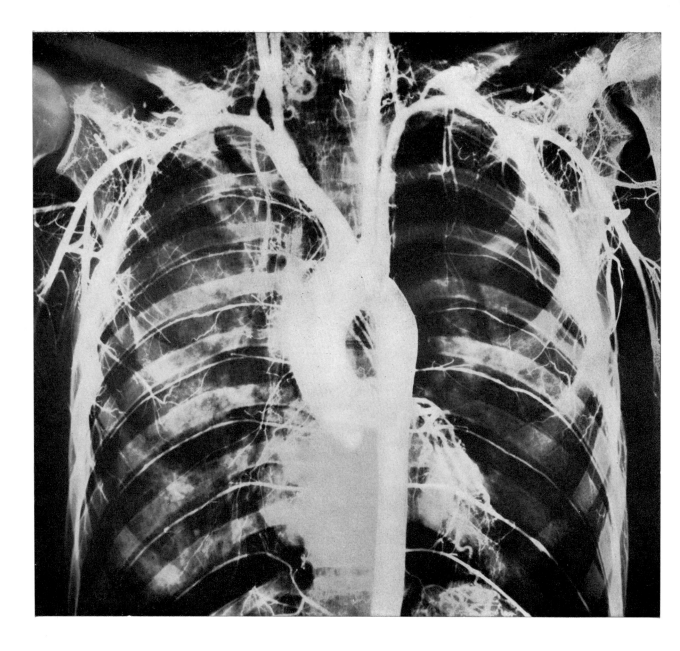

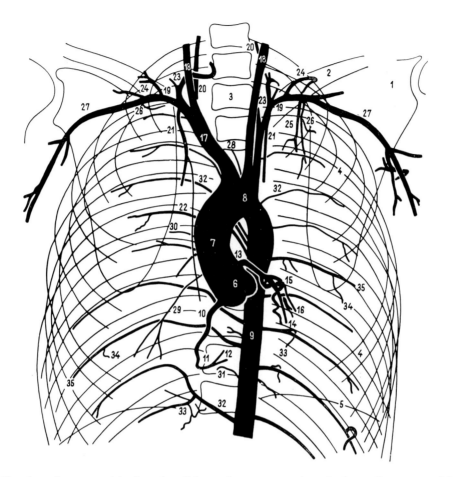

FIG. 44. The thoracic aorta and its branches, I (ascending aorta, aortic arch, descending aorta and branches). Anteroposterior view.

1. Scapula	*13.* Left coronary artery	*26.* Transverse cervical artery (deep branch)
2. Clavicle	*14.* Anterior interventricular branch	*27.* Axillary artery
3. Thoracic vertebrae	*15.* Circumflex branch	*28.* Mediastinal branch
4. Ribs	*16.* Ramus marginalis obtusus	*29.* Right (inferior) bronchial branch
5. Diaphragm	*17.* Brachiocephalic trunk	*30.* Right (superior) bronchial branch
6. Bulb of the aorta	*18.* Common carotid artery	
7. Ascending aorta	*19.* Subclavian artery	*31.* Esophageal branches
8. Arch of the aorta	*20.* Vertebral artery	*32.* Posterior intercostal arteries
9. Descending aorta	*21.* Internal thoracic artery	
10. Right coronary artery	*22.* Pericardiacophrenic artery	*33.* Dorsal branches
11. Posterior interventricular branch	*23.* Thyrocervical trunk	*34.* Lateral cutaneous branch
	24. Costocervical trunk	*35.* Collateral branch
12. Left posterior ventricular branch	*25.* Highest intercostal artery	

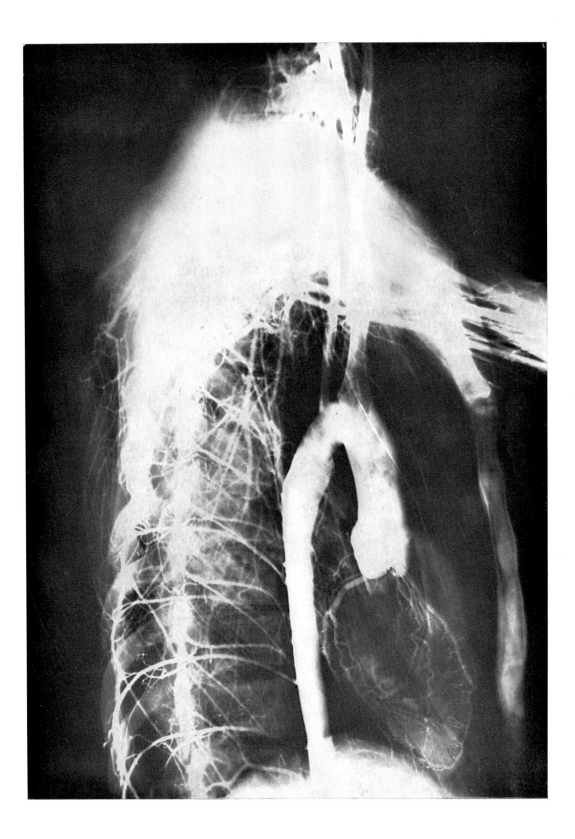

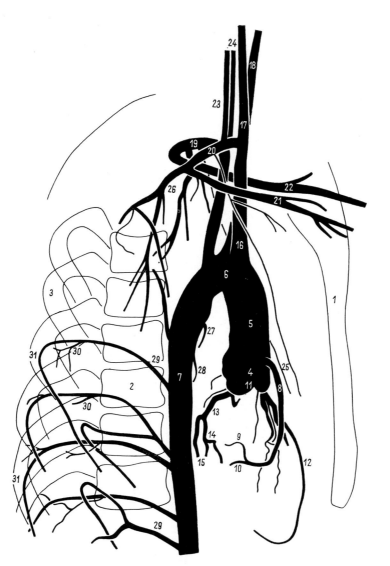

FIG. 45. The thoracic aorta and its branches, II (ascending aorta, aortic arch, descending aorta and branches). Dextrosinistral view.

1. Sternum
2. Thoracic vertebrae
3. Ribs
4. Bulb of the aorta
5. Ascending aorta
6. Arch of the aorta
7. Descending aorta
8. Right coronary artery
9. Left posterior ventricular branch
10. Posterior interventricular branch
11. Origin of left coronary artery
12. Anterior interventricular branch
13. Circumflex branch
14. Left posterior ventricular branch
15. Ramus marginalis obtusus
16. Brachiocephalic trunk
17. Right common carotid artery
18. Left common carotid artery
19. Left subclavian artery
20. Right subclavian artery
21. Right axillary artery
22. Left axillary artery
23. Right vertebral artery
24. Left vertebral artery
25. Pericardiacophrenic arteries
26. Transverse cervical artery (deep branch)
27. Bronchial branch
28. Esophageal branches
29. Posterior intercostal arteries
30. Dorsal branch
31. Collateral branch

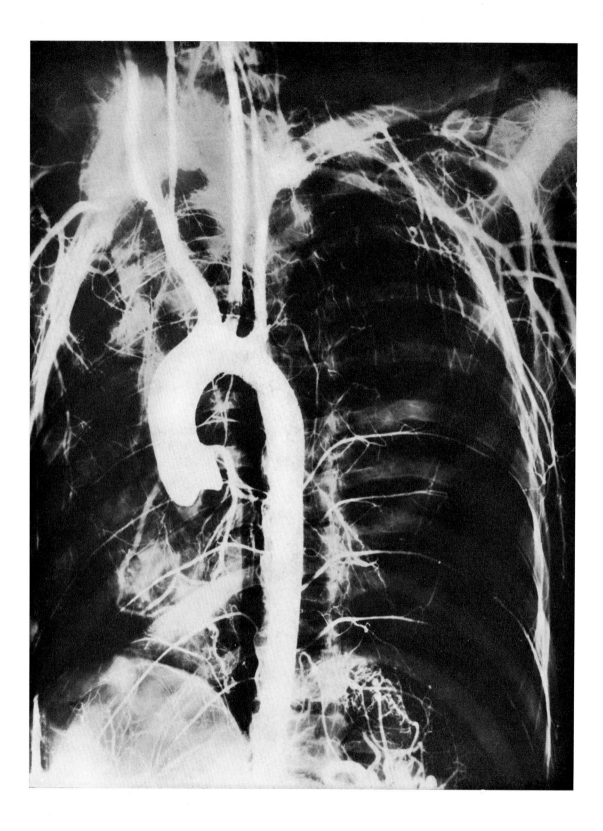

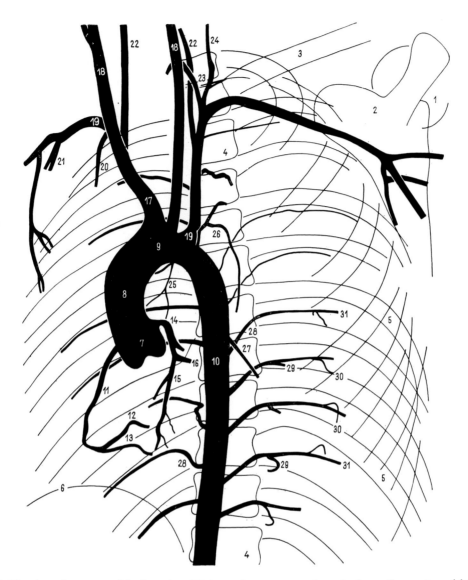

FIG. 46. The thoracic aorta and its branches, III (ascending aorta, aortic arch, descending aorta and branches). Second oblique view.

1. Humerus
2. Scapula
3. Clavicle
4. Thoracic vertebrae
5. Ribs
6. Diaphragm
7. Bulb of the aorta
8. Ascending aorta
9. Arch of the aorta
10. Descending aorta
11. Right coronary artery

12. Posterior interventricular branch
13. Left posterior ventricular branch
14. Left coronary artery
15. Anterior interventricular branch
16. Circumflex branch
17. Brachiocephalic trunk
18. Common carotid artery
19. Subclavian artery
20. Internal thoracic artery

21. Transverse cervical artery
22. Vertebral artery
23. Thyrocervical trunk
24. Ascending cervical artery
25. Right bronchial branch
26. Mediastinal branch
27. Left bronchial branch
28. Posterior intercostal arteries
29. Dorsal branch
30. Lateral cutaneous branch
31. Collateral branch

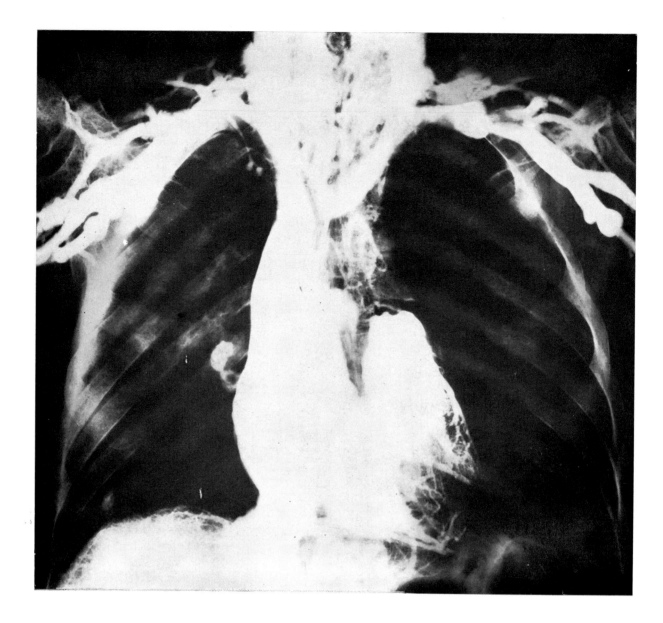

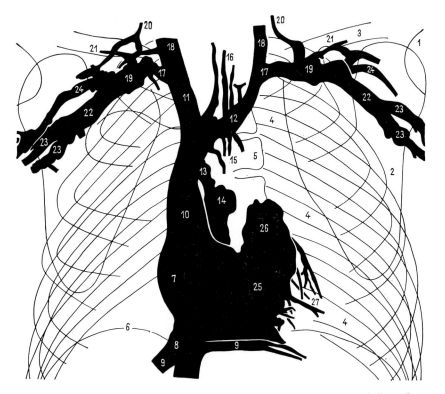

FIG. 47. The superior vena cava and its branches, I (pulmonary trunk ligated).
Anteroposterior view.

 1. Humerus
 2. Scapula
 3. Clavicle
 4. Ribs
 5. Thoracic vertebrae
 6. Diaphragm
 7. Right atrium
 8. Inferior vena cava
 9. Hepatic veins
10. Superior vena cava

11. Right brachiocephalic vein
12. Left brachiocephalic vein
13. Azygos vein
14. Mediastinal veins
15. Thymic, tracheal, esopha-
    geal veins
16. Thyroid impar and pha-
    ryngo-esophageal venous
    plexus
17. Venous angle

18. Internal jugular vein
19. Subclavian vein
20. External jugular vein
21. Deep cervical vein
22. Axillary vein
23. Brachial veins
24. Cephalic vein
25. Right ventricle
26. Pulmonary trunk
27. Cardiac veins

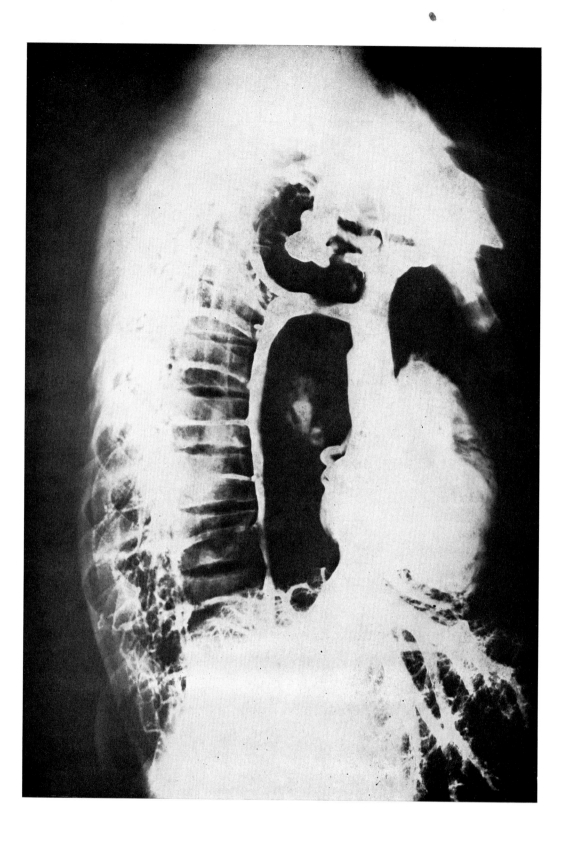

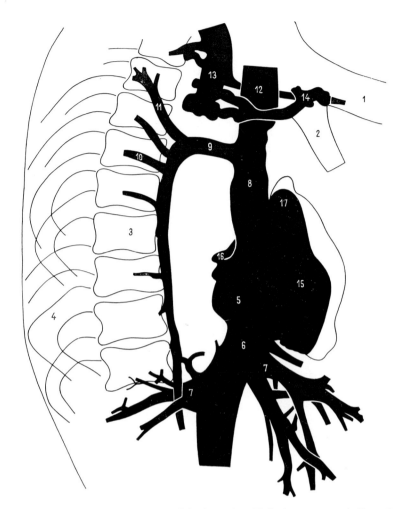

FIG. 48. The superior vena cava and its branches, II (pulmonary trunk ligated). Dextrosinistral view.

1. Humerus	*7.* Hepatic veins	*12.* Brachiocephalic veins
2. Sternum	*8.* Superior vena cava	*13.* Subclavian veins
3. Thoracic vertebrae	*9.* Azygos vein	*14.* Axillary veins
4. Costal angles	*10.* Posterior intercostal veins	*15.* Right ventricle
5. Right atrium	*11.* Right superior intercostal	*16.* Coronary sinus
6. Inferior vena cava	vein	*17.* Conus arteriosus

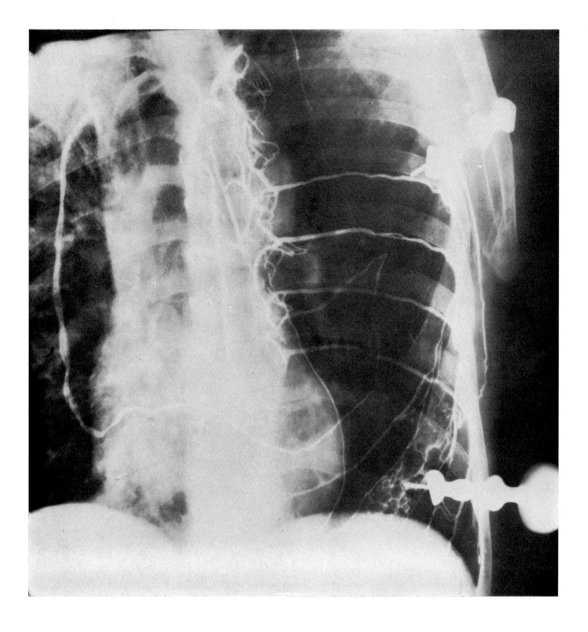

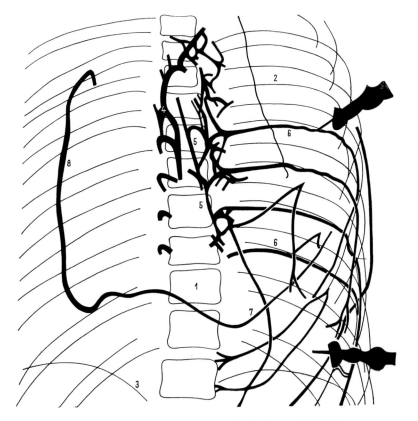

FIG. 49. The azygos system (azygography in vivo by S. Szücs).
Second oblique view.

1. Thoracic vertebrae
2. Ribs
3. Diaphragm
4. Azygos vein

5. Hemiazygos vein
6. Posterior intercostal veins
7. Collateral branch
8. Internal thoracic vein

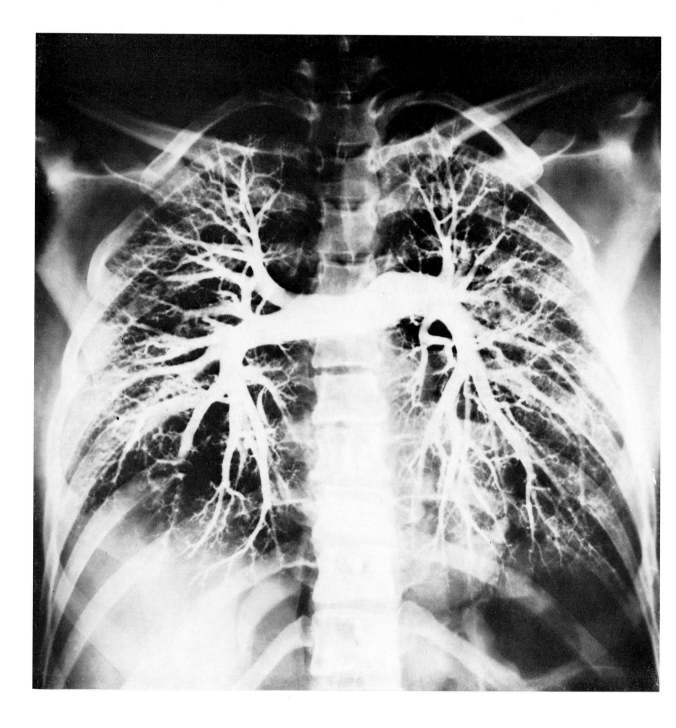

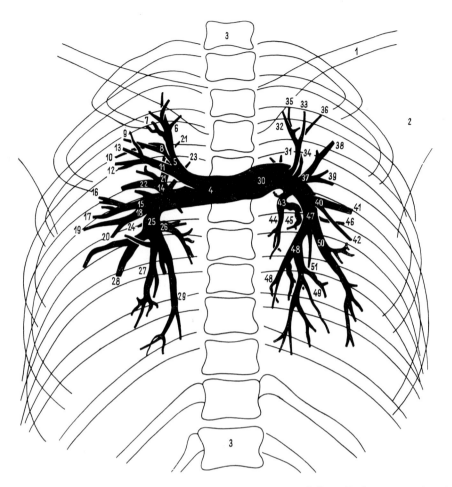

FIG. 50. The branches of the pulmonary trunk, I (pulmonary trunk ligated). Anteroposterior view.

1. Clavicle
2. Scapula
3. Thoracic vertebrae
4. Right pulmonary artery
5. Apical branch, A_1
6. A_{1a}
7. A_{1b}
8. Posterior branch, A_2
9. A_{2a}
10. A_{2b}
11. Anterior branch, A_3
12. A_{3a}
13. A_{3b}
14. Apical superior branch of inferior lobe, A_6
15. Lateral branch of middle lobe, A_4
16. A_{4a}
17. A_{4b}
18. Medial branch of middle lobe, A_5
19. A_{5a}
20. A_{5b}
21. A_{2x}
22. A_{6a}
23. A_{6b}
24. A_{6c}
25. Basal part
26. Medial basal branch, A_7
27. Anterior basal branch, A_8
28. Lateral basal branch, A_9
29. Posterior basal branch, A_{10}
30. Left pulmonary artery
31. Apical branch, A_1
32. A_{1a}
33. A_{1b}
34. Posterior branch, A_2
35. A_{2a}
36. A_{2b}
37. Anterior branch, A_3
38. A_{3a}
39. A_{3b}
40. Lingular branch, A_{4+5}
41. Superior lingular branch, A_4
42. Inferior lingular branch, A_5
43. Apical (superior) branch of inferior lobe, A_6
44. A_{7x}
45. A_{6a}
46. A_{6b}
47. Basal part
48. Medial basal branch, A_7
49. Posterior basal branch, A_{10}
50. Lateral basal branch, A_9
51. Anterior basal branch, A_8

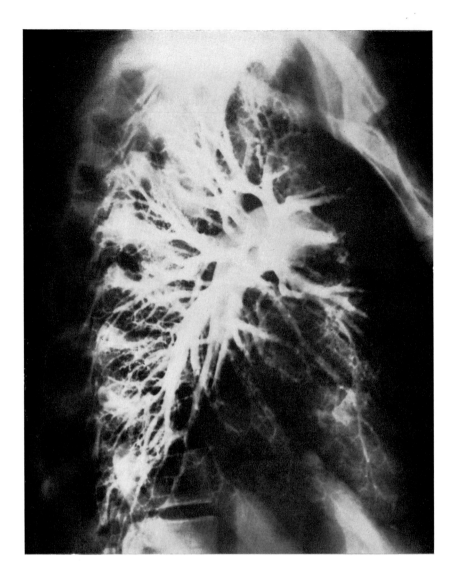

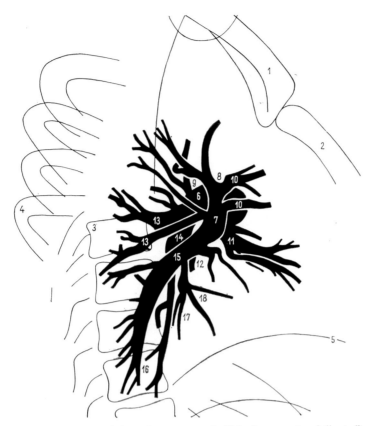

Fig. 51. The branches of the pulmonary trunk, II (pulmonary trunk ligated).
Dextrosinistral view.

1. Clavicle	*11.* Lingular branches, A_4, A_5
2. Sternum	*12.* Branches of the middle lobe,
3. Thoracic vertebrae	A_{4+5}
4. Costal angles	*13.* Apical (superior) branches
5. Diaphragm	of the inferior lobes, A_6
6. Left pulmonary artery	*14.* Left basal part
7. Right pulmonary artery	*15.* Right basal part
8. Right apical branch, A_1	*16.* Posterior basal branches, A_{10}
9. Right posterior branch, A_2	*17.* Lateral basal branches, A_9
10. Anterior branches, A_3	*18.* Anterior basal branches, A_8

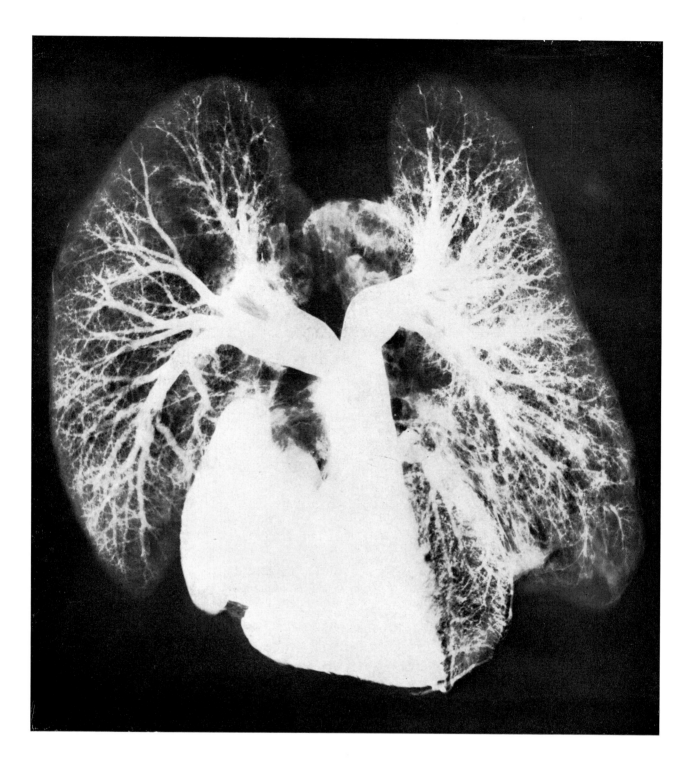

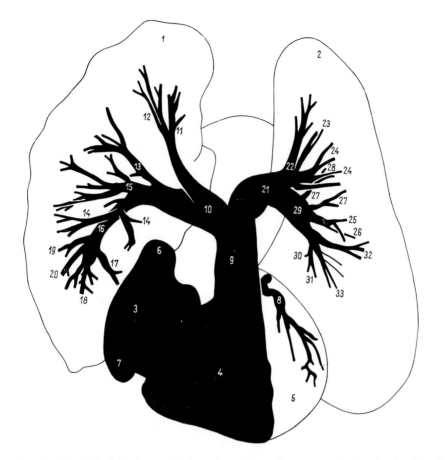

FIG. 52. The right half of the heart with branches of the pulmonary trunk (caval veins ligated).
Anatomical preparation. Anteroposterior view.

1. Right lung
2. Left lung
3. Right atrium
4. Right ventricle
5. Left ventricle
6. Superior vena cava
7. Inferior vena cava
8. Great cardiac vein
9. Pulmonary trunk
10. Right pulmonary artery
11. Apical branch, A_1
12. Posterior branch, A_2
13. Anterior branch, A_3
14. Branch of the middle lobe, $A_{4,5}$
15. Apical (superior) branch of inferior lobe, A_6
16. Basal part
17. Medial basal branch, A_7
18. Anterior basal branch, A_8
19. Lateral basal branch, A_9
20. Posterior basal branch, A_{10}
21. Left pulmonary artery
22. Apical branch, A_1
23. Posterior branch, A_2
24. Anterior branch, A_3
25. Superior lingular branch, A_4
26. Inferior lingular branch, A_5
27. Apical (superior) branch of inferior lobe, A_6
28. A_{3x}
29. Basal part
30. Medial basal branch, A_7
31. Anterior basal branch, A_8
32. Lateral basal branch, A_9
33. Posterior basal branch, A_{10}

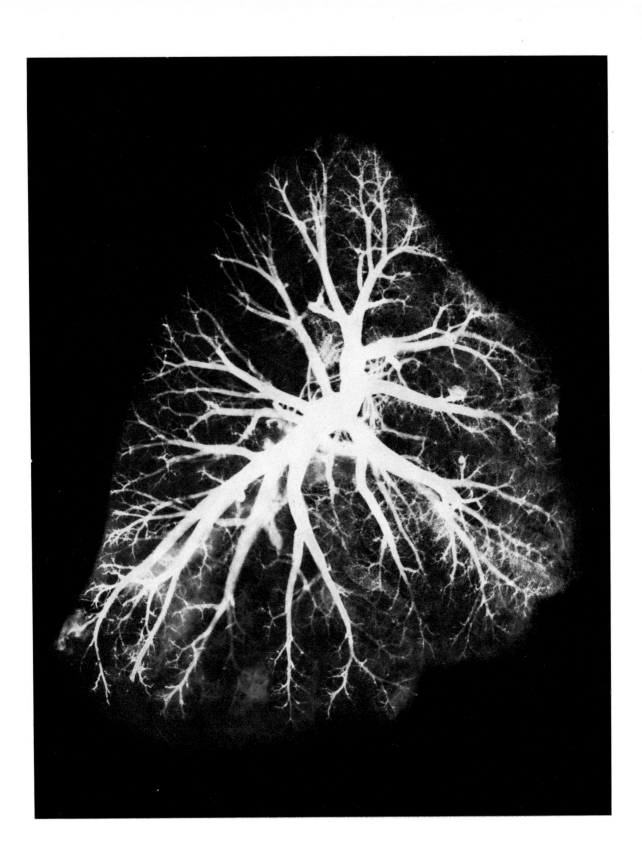

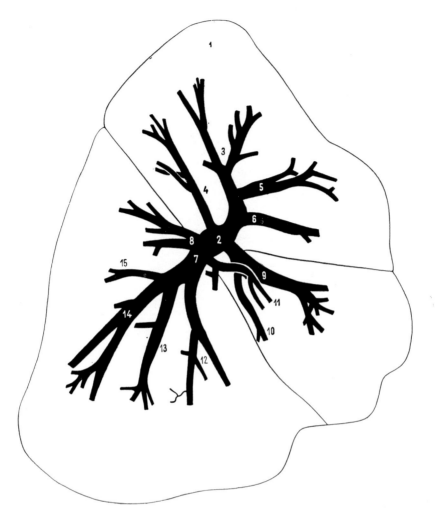

FIG. 53. The branches of the right pulmonary artery. Anatomical preparation.
Lateromedial view.

1. Right lung
2. Right pulmonary artery
3. Apical branch, A_1
4. Posterior branch, A_2
5. A_{3a}
6. A_{3b}
7. Basal part
8. Apical (superior) branch of inferior lobe, A_6
9. Medial branch of middle lobe, A_5
10. Lateral branch of middle lobe, A_4
11. Medial basal branch, A_7
12. Anterior basal branch, A_8
13. Lateral basal branch, A_9
14. Posterior basal branch, A_{10}
15. Subapical branch, A_x

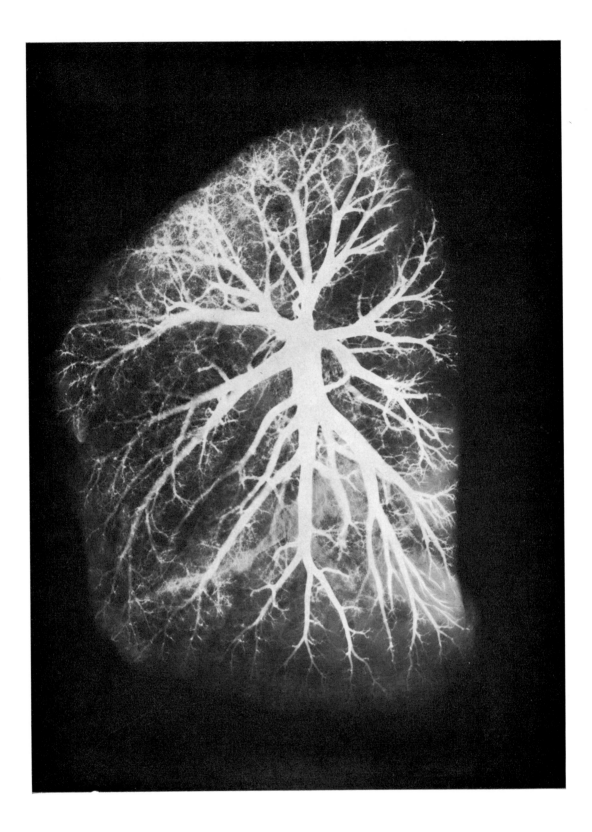

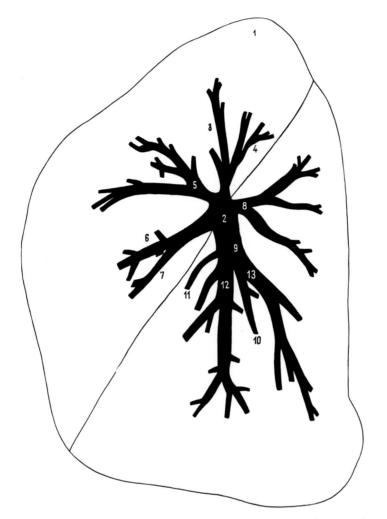

FIG. 54. The branches of the left pulmonary artery. Anatomical preparation.
Lateromedial view.

1. Left lung
2. Left pulmonary artery
3. Apical branch, A_1
4. Posterior branch, A_2
5. Anterior branch, A_3

6. Superior lingular branch, A_4
7. Inferior lingular branch, A_5
8. Apical (superior) branch of inferior lobe, A_6
9. Basal part

10. Medial basal branch, A_7
11. Anterior basal branch, A_8
12. Lateral basal branch, A_9
13. Posterior basal branch, A_{10}

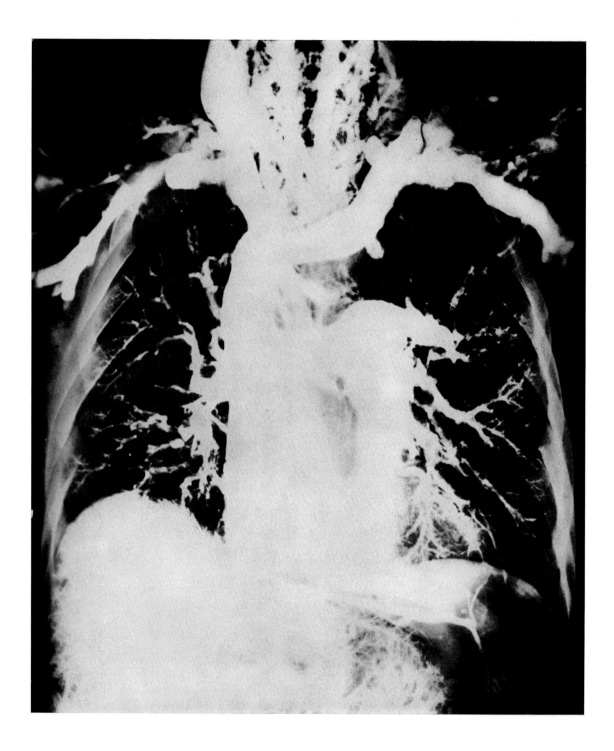

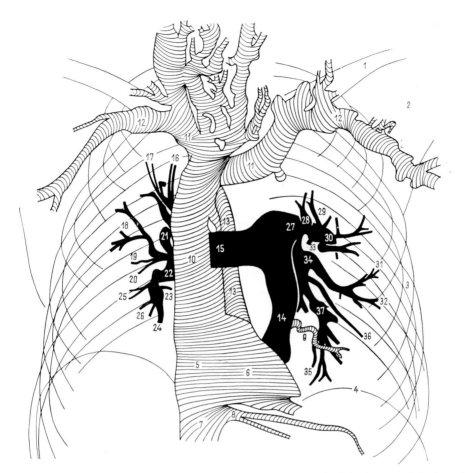

FIG. 55. The superior vena cava and its branches with the right half of the heart and the branches of the pulmonary trunk, I. Anteroposterior view.

1. Clavicle
2. Scapula
3. Ribs
4. Diaphragm
5. Right atrium
6. Right ventricle
7. Inferior vena cava
8. Hepatic veins
9. Venous branches of the heart
10. Superior vena cava
11. Brachiocephalic vein
12. Subclavian vein
13. Mediastinal veins and azygos vein

14. Pulmonary trunk
15. Right pulmonary artery
16. Apical branch, A_1
17. Posterior branch, A_2
18. Anterior branch, A_3
19. Lateral branch of middle lobe, A_4
20. Medial branch of middle lobe, A_5
21. Apical (superior) branch of inferior lobe, A_6
22. Basal part
23. Medial basal branch, A_7
24. Anterior basal branch, A_8
25. Lateral basal branch, A_9

26. Posterior basal branch, A_{10}
27. Left pulmonary artery
28. Apical branch, A_1
29. Posterior branch, A_2
30. Anterior branch, A_3
31. Superior lingular branch, A_4
32. Inferior lingular branch, A_5
33. Apical (superior) branch of inferior lobe, A_6
34. Basal part
35. Anterior basal branch, A_8
36. Lateral basal branch, A_9
37. Posterior basal branch, A_{10}

103

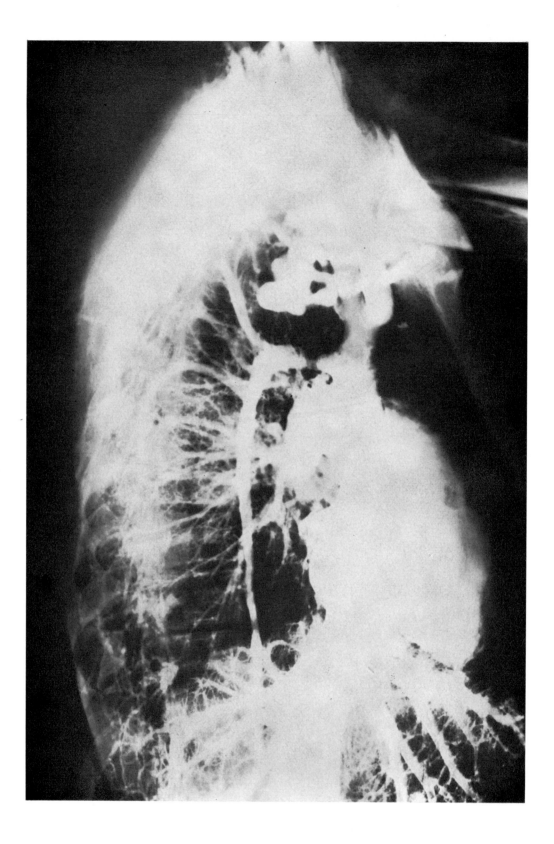

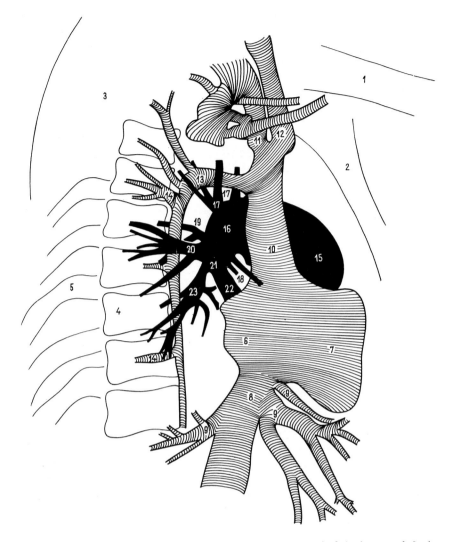

FIG. 56. The superior vena cava and its branches with the right half of the heart and the branches of the pulmonary trunk, II. Dextrosinistral view.

1. Humerus
2. Sternum
3. Scapula
4. Thoracic vertebrae
5. Costal angles
6. Right atrium
7. Right ventricle
8. Inferior vena cava
9. Hepatic veins
10. Superior vena cava
11. Right brachiocephalic vein
12. Left brachiocephalic vein
13. Azygos vein
14. Branches of azygos vein
15. Pulmonary trunk
16. Right and left pulmonary artery
17. Apical and posterior branches, A_1 and A_2
18. Middle lobar and lingular branches, A_4 and A_5
19. Left apical (superior) branch of inferior lobe, A_6
20. Right apical (superior) branch of inferior lobe, A_6
21. Basal parts
22. Medial and anterior basal branches, A_7 and A_8
23. Lateral and posterior basal branches, A_9 and A_{10}

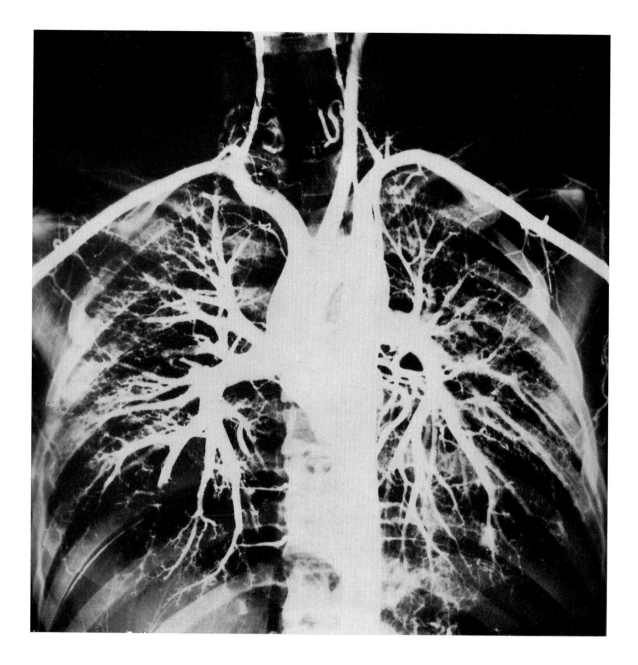

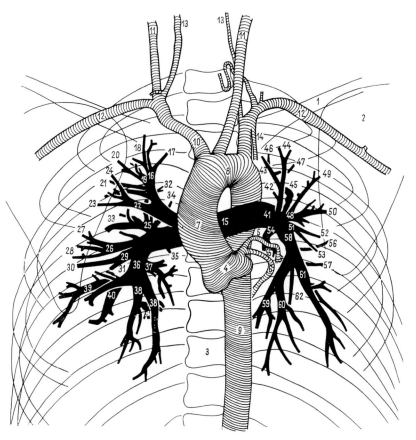

Fig 57. The thoracic aorta with the branches of the pulmonary arteries, I (pulmonary trunk ligated). Anteroposterior view.

1. Clavicle
2. Scapula
3. Thoracic vertebrae
4. Bulb of the aorta
5. Circumflex branch of left coronary artery
6. Anterior interventricular branch of left coronary artery
7. Ascending aorta
8. Arch of the aorta
9. Descending aorta
10. Brachiocephalic trunk
11. Common carotid artery
12. Subclavian artery
13. Vertebral artery
14. Left internal thoracic artery (ligated)
15. Right pulmonary artery
16. Apical branch, A_1
17. A_{1a}
18. A_{1b}
19. Posterior branch, A_2
20. A_{2a}

21. A_{2b}
22. Anterior branch, A_3
23. A_{3a}
24. A_{3b}
25. Apical (superior) branch of inferior lobe, A_6
26. Lateral branch of middle lobe, A_4
27. A_{4a}
28. A_{4b}
29. Medial branch of middle lobe, A_5
30. A_{5a}
31. A_{5b}
32. A_{2x}
33. A_{6a}
34. A_{6b}
35. A_{6c}
36. Basal part
37. Medial basal branch, A_7
38. Anterior basal branch, A_8
39. Lateral basal branch, A_9
40. Posterior basal branch, A_{10}

41. Left pulmonary artery
42. Apical branch, A_1
43. A_{1a}
44. A_{1b}
45. Posterior branch, A_2
46. A_{2a}
47. A_{2b}
48. Anterior branch, A_3
49. A_{3a}
50. A_{3b}
51. Lingular branch, A_{4+5}
52. Superior lingular branch, A_4
53. Inferior lingular branch, A_5
54. Apical (superior) branch of inferior lobe, A_6
55. A_{7x}
56. A_{6a}
57. A_{6b}
58. Basal part
59. Medial basal branch, A_7
60. Anterior basal branch, A_8
61. Lateral basal branch, A_9
62. Posterior basal branch, A_{10}

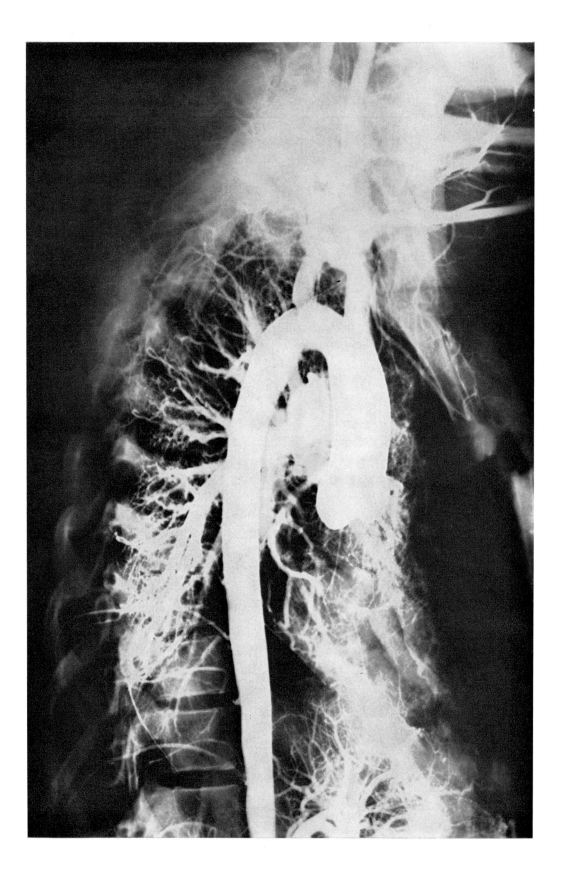

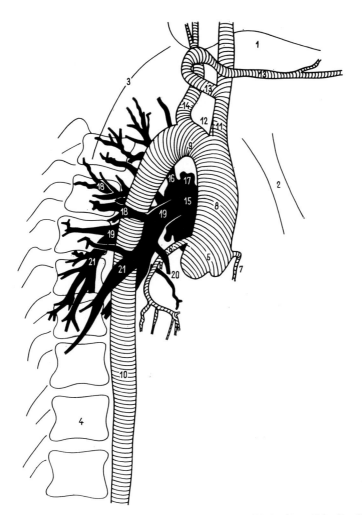

FIG. 58. The thoracic aorta with the branches of the pulmonary arteries, II
(pulmonary trunk ligated). Dextrosinistral view.

1. Humerus
2. Sternum
3. Scapula
4. Thoracic vertebrae
5. Bulb of the aorta
6. Circumflex branch of left coronary artery
7. Right coronary artery
8. Ascending aorta

9. Arch of the aorta
10. Descending aorta
11. Brachiocephalic trunk and left common carotid artery
12. Left common carotid artery
13. Right subclavian artery
14. Left subclavian artery
15. Right and left pulmonary artery

16. Apical and posterior branches A_1 and A_2
17. Anterior branches, A_3
18. Apical (superior) branches of inferior lobes, A_6
19. Basal parts
20. Lateral basal branches, A_9
21. Posterior basal branches, A_{10}

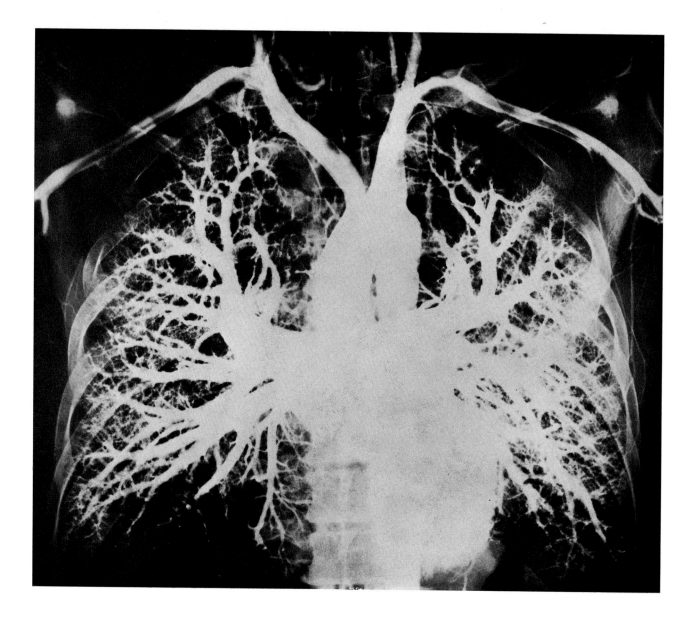

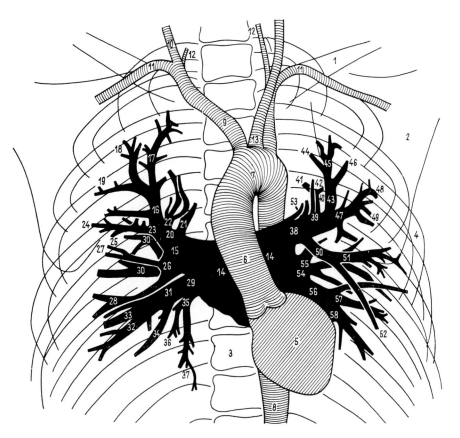

FIG. 59. The pulmonary veins, the left half of the heart and the branches of the thoracic aorta, I. Anteroposterior view.

1. Clavicle
2. Scapula
3. Thoracic vertebrae
4. Ribs
5. Left ventricle
6. Ascending aorta
7. Arch of the aorta
8. Descending aorta
9. Brachiocephalic trunk
10. Right common carotid artery
11. Subclavian artery
12. Vertebral artery
13. Left common carotid artery
14. Left atrium
15. Right superior pulmonary vein
16. Apical branch, V_1
17. V_{1a}
18. V_{1b}
19. V_{2x}
20. Posterior branch, V_2

21. V_{2a}
22. V_{2b}
23. Anterior branch, V_3
24. V_{3a}
25. V_{3b}
26. Branches of middle lobe, V_{4+5}
27. Lateral part, V_4
28. Medial part, V_5
29. Right inferior pulmonary vein
30. Apical (superior) branch, V_6
31. Superior basal vein
32. Anterior basal vein, V_8
33. V_9
34. V_{10}
35. Inferior basal vein
36. V_9
37. V_{10}
38. Left superior pulmonary vein

39. Apico posterior branches, V_{1+2}
40. V_1
41. V_{1a}
42. V_{1b}
43. V_2
44. V_{2a}
45. V_{2b}
46. V_{2c}
47. Anterior branch, V_3
48. V_{3a}
49. V_{3b}
50. Lingular branches, V_{4+5}
51. Superior part, V_4
52. Inferior part, V_5
53. Superior hilar vein
54. Left inferior pulmonary vein
55. Apical (superior) branch, V_6
56. Common basal vein
57. Superior basal vein, V_{9+10}
58. Inferior basal vein, V_8

111

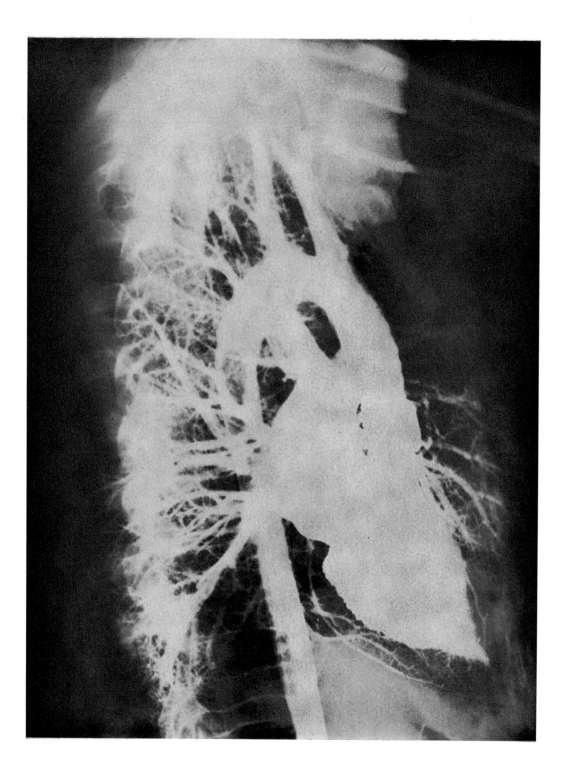

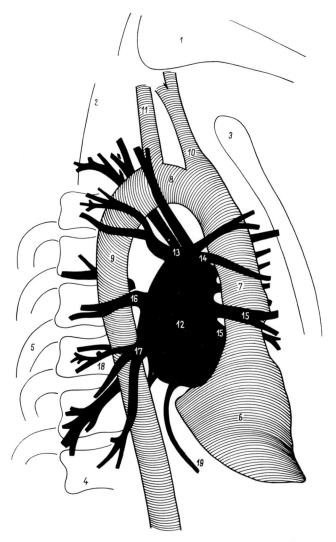

FIG. 60. The pulmonary veins, the left half of the heart and the branches of the thoracic aorta, II.
Dextrosinistral view.

1. Humerus
2. Scapula
3. Sternum
4. Thoracic vertebrae
5. Costal angles
6. Left ventricle
7. Ascending aorta
8. Arch of the aorta

9. Descending aorta
10. Brachiocephalic trunk and left common carotid artery
11. Left subclavian artery
12. Left atrium and trunks of pulmonary veins
13. Apical branch, posterior branch and apicoposterior branch, V_1, V_2

14. Anterior branches, V_3
15. Branch of middle lobe and lingular branch, V_4 and V_5
16. Apical (superior) branches, V_6
17. Basal veins
18. V_{10}
19. V_9

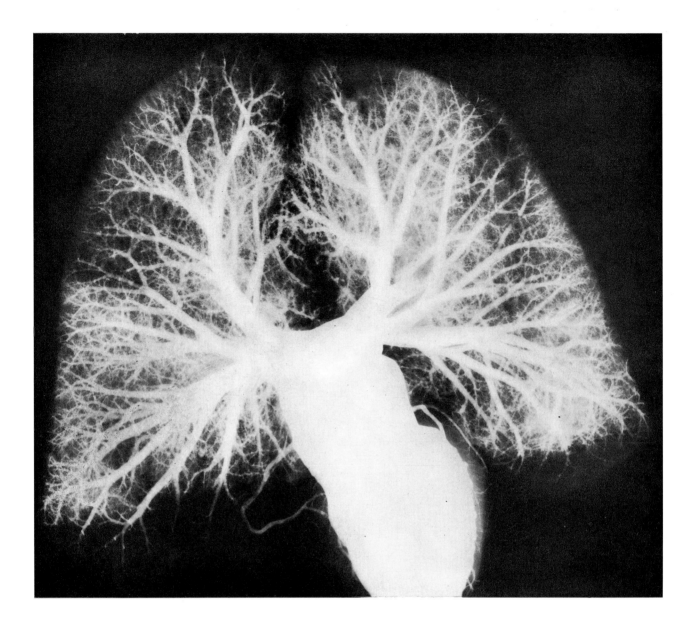

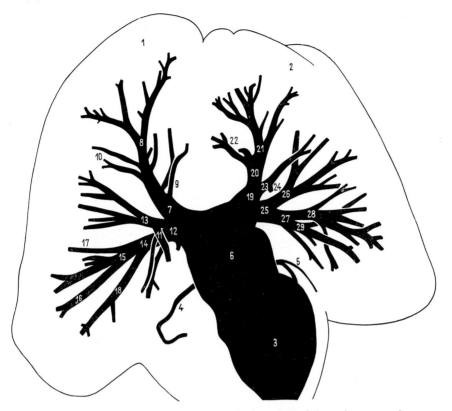
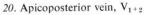

Fig. 61. The left half of the heart with the branches of the pulmonary veins.
Anatomical preparation. Anteroposterior view.

1. Right lung
2. Left lung
3. Left ventricle
4. Right coronary artery
5. Left coronary artery
6. Left atrium
7. Right superior pulmonary vein
8. Apical branch, V_1
9. Posterior branch, V_2
10. Anterior branch, V_3

11. Branch of middle lobe, V_{4+5}
12. Right inferior pulmonary vein
13. Apical (superior) branch, V_6
14. Common basal vein
15. Superior basal vein
16. Anterior basal branch, V_8
17. V_9
18. Inferior basal vein, V_{9+10}
19. Left superior pulmonary vein

20. Apicoposterior vein, V_{1+2}
21. V_1
22. V_2
23. Anterior branch, V_3
24. Lingular branch, V_{4+5}
25. Left inferior pulmonary vein
26. Apical (superior) branch, V_6
27. Common basal vein
28. Superior basal vein
29. Inferior basal vein

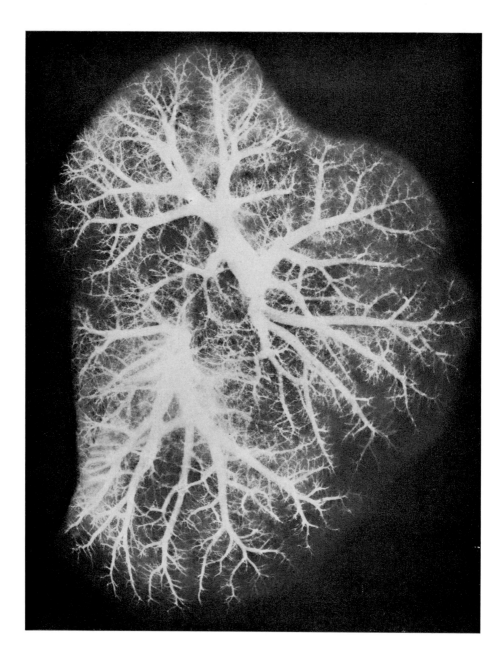

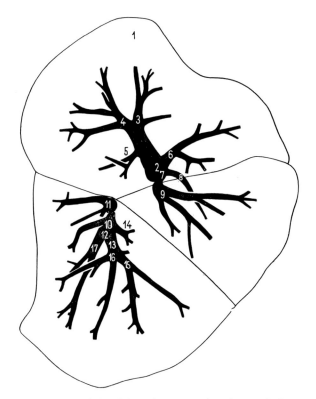

Fig. 62. The branches of the right pulmonary veins. Anatomical preparation.
Lateromedial view.

1. Right lung
2. Right superior pulmonary vein
3. Apical branch, V_1
4. Posterior branch, V_2
5. V_{2x}
6. Anterior branch, V_3

7. Branch of middle lobe,
   V_{4+5}
8. Lateral part, V_4
9. Medial part, V_5
10. Right inferior pulmonary vein
11. Apical (superior) branch, V_6

12. Common basal vein
13. Superior basal vein
14. V_7
15. Anterior basal vein, V_8
16. V_9
17. Inferior basal vein, V_{10}

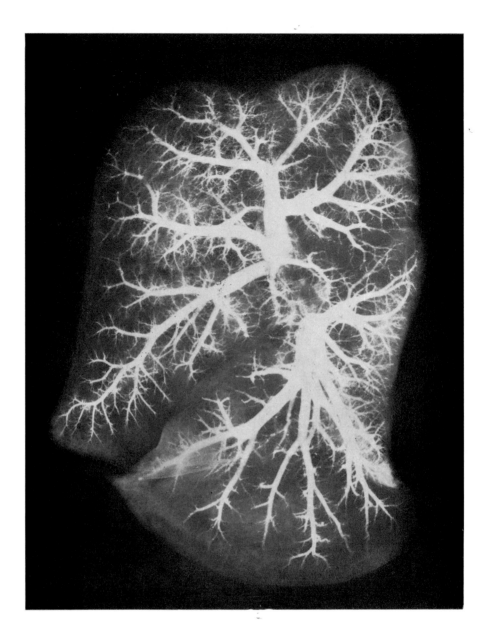

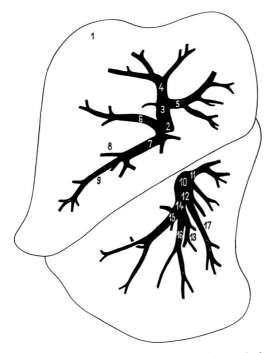

FIG. 63. The branches of the left pulmonary veins. Anatomical preparation.
Lateromedial view.

1. Left lung
2. Left superior pulmonary vein
3. Apicoposterior branch, V_{1+2}
4. V_1
5. V_2
6. Anterior branch, A_3

7. Lingular branch, V_{4+5}
8. Superior part, V_4
9. Inferior part, V_5
10. Left inferior pulmonary vein
11. Apical (superior) branch, V_6

12. Common basal vein
13. V_7
14. Superior basal vein
15. Anterior basal branch, V_8
16. V_9
17. Inferior basal vein, V_{10}

BLOOD VESSELS OF THE NECK AND THE HEAD

VASCULAR SYSTEM OF THE COMMON CAROTID
AND SUBCLAVIAN ARTERIES

The arteries of the head and neck constitute a functional unit. Communications between the subclavian and the common carotid arteries, both arising from the arch of the aorta, make the substitution of one by the other possible according to needs. As regards the architecture and mode of division, the arteries of the neck and face are similar to the other arteries, i.e., they form collateral connections in the shoulder girdle and in the cranial cavity. Their course and anastomoses are fairly constant. The arteries of the cranial cavity and the spinal cord have very thin walls resembling veins. Besides the internal elastic lamina they contain hardly any elastic elements, and they are poor in smooth muscles (Kirgis and Peebles 1961). Intracranial pressure is closely correlated with arterial expansion (Monro–Kelie's rule). There are numerous anastomoses on the surface of the brain, the morphologically and functionally most significant being the circulus arteriosus (circle of Willis). Branches penetrating into the cerebral tissue are practically terminal arteries (Elliott 1963). The functionallyl performed communications between extracraniae and intracranial vessels ensure circulation in casy of disturbed cerebral blood supply. Angiograph has revealed their morphology and function.

Common carotid artery

The common carotid artery arises on the right side from the brachiocephalic trunk, on the left from the aorta as its second branch (Figs 37/19, 38/18, 39/19, 40/11, 44/18, 45/17 and 18, 46/18, 57/11, 58/11 and 12, 59/10 and 13, 60/10, 64, 95/9 and 10, 96/10, 97/14 and 31, 98/7, 99/10, 100/9 and 20). The origin of the right artery is at the level of the sternoclavicular joint, that of the left at the height of the 6th thoracic vertebra. The height of origin may of course vary according to the configuration of the thoracic aorta. The trachea lies lmedial to, and the left subclavian artery to the left of the origin of the left common carotid artery. The eft braϲ hiocephalic vein crosses it obliquely from the front. The bilateral arteries, after becoming symmetrical at the height of the sternoclavicular joint, pass upward in the carotid sheath on both sides of the neck along the medial aspect of the internal jugular vein. They touch the thyroid gland and the pharynx from the front, and the longus colli and longus capitis in the back. Between and behind them lies the vagus nerve, in front of them the descending branch of the hypoglossal nerve. The commencement of the projection of the left common carotid artery extends upward and lateral to the median line as far as the sternoclavicular joint. From here after a slight divergence, the bilateral vessels run parallel upward. The common carotid artery divides in the carotid triangle into its two terminal branches, the external and the internal carotid arteries. The division is, according to Krayenbühl and Yasargil (1965), at the height of the 4th to 5th cervical vertebra (C1—C7) in 87 per cent of the cases. Bifurcation at a lower level is more frequent than at a higher level. The difference between the two sides may exceptionally exceed the width of a rib. Division at a lower point is more frequent on the left side. The bifurcation lies higher in short-necked than in long-necked individuals. There is often a bulbous dilatation at the bifurcation; it is usually bilateral, but frequently it occurs on the left side (Schwalbe 1878, Binswanger 1879). The dilatation usually extends to the external and the internal carotid arteries alike. The widest diameter of the dilatation occurs in the internal, less frequently in the common, and very rarely in the external carotid artery. The dilatation is usually pronounced in persons above 50, although Schäfer (1878) demonstrated its presence in a baby of 3 month. Krayenbühl and Yasargil (1965) registered a marked dilatation of the carotid sinus only in 1·8 per cent of their extensive material and exclusively in patients of advanced age. Two types of division are known. Division at an "acute angle" can mostly be found in individuals with long neck, while "arched" division is more characteristic of short-necked persons. The latter type is more frequently accompanied by bulb formation. Arch-shaped division is presently regarded as a sign of senescence.

The diameter of the common carotid artery averages 0·7 cm (0·6 to 0·9 cm). The two sides are frequently different. On the right side the artery is often wider than on the left. The length is 9·5 cm

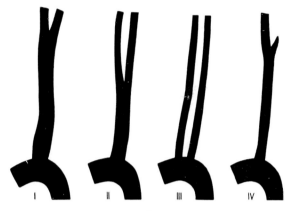

FIG. 64. Variable divisions of the common carotid artery I, normal type; II, deep division; III, division from the aorta; IV, internal carotid artery is absent.

(7 to 12 cm) on the right, 12·5 cm (10 to 15 cm) on the left side (Quain 1884). The difference in length between the two sides is about 3 cm, i.e., 1 cm less than the length of the brachiocephalic trunk.

Variations. Exceptionally the common carotid artery may be very short, only 1 to 2 cm (Fig. 64/II; Kantor, cit. Adachi 1928). The absence of the common carotid artery is very rare: its two branches spring off in such cases directly from the brachiocephalic trunk and the aorta, respectively (Fig. 64/III; Angermayer 1907, Fife 1921, Altmann 1947).

Supernumerary branches (e.g., inferior, superior and ima thyroid, lingual and occipital arteries) arise fairly often from the common carotid artery (Adachi 1928, Kukwa and Zbrodowski 1966).

External carotid artery and its branches

It is the frontal medial branch of the common carotid artery and supplies a considerable area of the face and neck (Figs 95/28, 96/12, 97/16 and 33, 98/9, 99/12, 100/10 and 21, 101/5). It has numerous anastomotic connections with the internal carotid and the subclavian arteries so that it participates in the collateral circulation of the brain. Covered by the platysma and the cervical fascia, the vessel arises from the medial side of the internal carotid artery in the carotid triangle on the anterior margin of the sternocleidomastoideus at the height of the third cervical vertebra (C1—C7; Krayenbühl and Yasargil 1965). After passing into the retromandibular fossa, it enters into the substance of the parotid gland where it divides into its terminal branches at the upper border of the gland. The length of the vessel is 7 to 8 cm (Paturet 1958), while its diameter is extremely variable (2·55 to 5·73 mm; Gyurkó and Szabó 1968).

Branches. It gives off anterior, medial, posterior and terminal branches. Anterior branches: superior thyroid, lingual and facial arteries. Medial branch: ascending pharyngeal artery. Posterior branches: occipital and posterior auricular arteries. Terminal branches: superficial temporal and maxillary arteries.

Variants are usually formed only by members of the same group. Variations apply to the origin, while the course of the branches is mostly typical. Handa et al. (1972) noted an external carotid artery coursing laterally from the internal carotid artery. Aaron and Chawaf (1967) observed a typical pattern of division only in 31 per cent.

Arising from the anterior aspect of the external carotid artery, the superior thyroid, lingual and facial arteries form common variations. Four alternatives are comparatively frequent. They arise separately (Fig. 65/I; Quain 1884: 79·1 per cent; Adachi 1928: 79·3 per cent). Rarely a thyrolingual trunk (Fig. 65/II) is present if the superior thyroid and lingual arteries arise together, a rare occurrence. A linguofacial trunk (Fig. 65/III) is present if the superior thyroid arises independently, while the other two vessels have a common origin (Quain 1884: 20·2 per cent; Adachi 1928: 18·7 per cent). The length of the trunk varies from 0·5 to 1·5 cm. The presence of a thyrolinguofacial trunk (Fig. 65/IV) is very rare (Adachi 1928: 0·3 per cent).

If the three trunks arise separately, the distance between their origins may be different. The lingual artery lies closer to the facial than to the superior thyroid artery. Their origins at the height of the third cervical vertebra are near if the common carotid artery divides high. If the division is low, the superior thyroid artery arises immediately above the origin of the external carotid artery and the

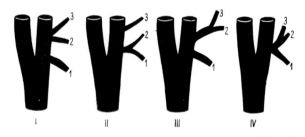

FIG. 65. Variable origins of the superior thyroid, lingual and facial arteries. I, normal type; II, thyrolingual trunk; III, linguofacial trunk; IV, thyrolinguofacial trunk. (*1*) Superior thyroid artery; (*2*) lingual artery; (*3*) facial artery.

121

lingual artery originates somewhat higher. These branches form no variants with the other branches of the external carotid artery.

The **superior thyroid artery** (Figs 66, 95/29, 96/13 and 19, 97/17 and 34, 98/10, 99/13) arises most fre-

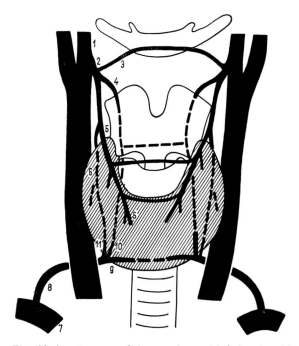

FIG. 66. Anastomoses of the superior and inferior thyroid arteries. (*1*) External carotid artery; (*2*) superior thyroid artery; (*3*) infrahyoid branch; (*4*) superior laryngeal artery; (*5*) anterior branch; (*6*) posterior branch; (*7*) subclavian artery; (*8*) inferior thyroid artery; (*9*) glandular branch (anastomosis with the contralateral branch); (*10*) inferior laryngeal artery; (*11*) glandular branch (anastomosis with the posterior branch of the superior thyroid artery).

quently 0·5 to 2 cm above the division of the common carotid artery (Livini 1900) from the anterior surface of the external carotid artery. It may exceptionally arise from the common carotid artery (Kukwa and Zbrodowski 1966). On its medial and forward course a deviating arch can be distinguished which ramifies into the terminal branches when it turns downward. The diameter of the superior thyroid artery is 0·2 cm (Djindjian et al. 1964), it supplies the larynx and the upper part of the thyroid gland. The artery has the following branches:

The *infrahyoid branch* (Figs 66/3, 96/14) runs to the root of the tongue and anastomoses with its contralateral partner.

The *sternocleidomastoid branch* (Fig. 96/15) runs toward the muscle of similar name.

The *superior laryngeal artery* (Figs 66/4, 95/30, 96/16, 98/11, 99/14) arises from the superior thyroid artery in 80 to 85 per cent of the cases, but it may

also originate from the external carotid, lingual, facial arteries and very rarely from the common carotid artery (Quain 1884, Bladt 1903, Adachi 1928). Running obliquely downward and medialward, the vessel enters the larynx where it anastomoses with the contralateral artery and the inferior laryngeal artery.

The *cricothyroid branch* is a significant small vessel as it runs between the thyroid and cricoid cartilage in front of the ligamentum conicum. Forming an anastomosis with the contralateral vessel, it gives off branches to the interior of the larynx.

At the upper pole of the thyroid gland the main trunk divides into the *anterior and posterior branches* (Figs 66/5 and 6, 95/31 and 32, 96/17 and 18, 98/12 and 13), which are functionally terminal arteries (Rauber and Kopsch 1951). The posterior branch is thinner; it ramifies on the posterior surface of the thyroid gland and communicates with the corresponding branch of the inferior laryngeal artery. It courses more laterally than the other terminal branch. The anterior branch runs downwards on the anterior surface of the gland and its side branch is in communication with the contralateral branch across the isthmus, therefore, it is significant from the viewpoint of collateral circulation (Djindjian et al. 1964). Although the anastomoses are anatomically well demonstrable, collateral circulation can hardly be observed in the thyroid vessels under normal conditions. Only a unilateral filling is achieved with in vivo angiography if only one of the four supplying arteries is injected with contrast medium. Full demonstration requires the simultaneous filling of the subclavian and external carotid arteries (Ormai and Szy 1962). Amistani (1950) considers extraglandular anatomoses more significant than intraglandular communications.

The **lingual artery** (Figs 95/33, 96/20 and 23, 97/18, 98/14, 99/15, 100/12 and 13), situated above the thyroid artery, is a direct branch of the external carotid artery. It may have sometimes common origin with the other two anterior branches. The vessel runs along the medial margin of the hyoglossus muscle towards the apex of the tongue. Its diameter measures 0·3 to 0·4 cm (Paturet 1958). The artery divides into its terminal branches at the level of the greater horn of the hyoid bone. It has the following *branches*:

The *suprahyoid branch* (Figs 95/34, 96/21, 98/18) runs along the upper border of the hyoid bone and anastomoses with its partner of the opposite side.

The *sublingual artery* (Figs 95/35, 96/24, 97/19, 98/17, 99/16) constitutes in exceptional cases a branch of the facial artery (Rauber and Kopsch 1951). Passing to the sublingual gland, it supplies the neighbouring muscles and the related part of the mucous membrane of the mouth. The vessel anastomoses with its contralateral partner as well as with the submental artery.

The *dorsal lingual branches* (Figs 95/36, 96/25, 97/20, 98/15, 99/18) run to the posterior part of the dorsum of the tongue and anastomose with the vessels of the opposite side. The vessels of the two sides sometimes unite to form a common trunk which pursues a sagittal course at the root of the tongue (arteria mediana linguae; Lenhossék 1922). The vessel may sometimes arise from the ascending palatine artery.

The *profunda linguae artery* (Figs 95/37, 96/22, 97/21, 98/16, 99/17). The largest artery of the tongue which courses on the exterior surface of the genioglossus muscle near the lower margin of the tongue towards the frenulum of the tongue. It is a terminal artery and does not communicate with the corresponding contralateral vessel.

Supernumerary branches are rare. The ascending palatine and the submental arteries may arise from the lingual artery (Rauber and Kopsch 1951).

The **facial artery** (Figs 95/38, 96/26, 97/22, 98/19, 99/19) arises above the lingual artery. Its function is taken over by the vessel of the opposite side or the transverse facial artery if the main trunk or one of its branches is underdeveloped (Hochstetter 1963). It is sometimes the infraorbital artery, the frontal branch or the buccal artery which becomes stronger in such cases (Grönross 1902). After origin, it curves upward and medially into the submandibular triangle, passes round the body of the mandible and appears at its outer surface in front of the masseter muscle. From here it runs obliquely to the medial palpebral commissure where its terminal branch communicates with the ophthalmic artery. The course of the vessel is tortuous. The *branches* of the facial artery are:

The *submental artery* (Figs 96/27, 99/22) runs forward on the mylohyoid muscle toward the mental protuberance where it divides into its two terminal branches. It may sometimes arise from the external carotid or the lingual artery. The vessel forms anastomosis with the sublingual artery.

The *ascending palatine artery* (Figs 67/3, 97/23, 98/20, 99/20) is of variable origin. The vessel is rarely double (Fig 67/II). In 10 per cent of the cases, it has a common origin with the ascending pharyngeal artery (Figs 67/III, V). If it arises alone, it may spring also from the external carotid (23 per cent), the occipital (Fig. 67/IV) or the lingual artery (Adachi 1928).

The *tonsillar and glandular branches* (Figs 99/21 and 23) are small branches running to the tonsil and the submandibular gland.

The *inferior and superior labial arteries* (Figs 98/21 and 22, 99/24 and 25) run in the lower and the upper lip, respectively. They form a vascular ring that is stronger above than below. The upper vessel usually gives off a branch to the septum of the nose (*arteria septi mobilis nasi*).

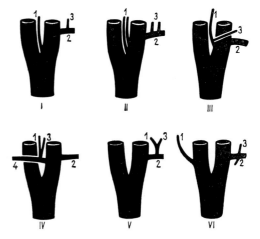

FIG. 67. Variations in the origin of the ascending pharyngeal and the ascending palatine artery. I, normal type; II, both vessels are duplicated; III, the ascending palatine arises from the ascending pharyngeal artery; IV, both vessels arise from the occipital artery; V, both vessels arise from the facial artery; VI, the ascending pharyngeal artery arises from the internal carotid artery. (*1*) Ascending pharyngeal artery; (*2*) facial artery; (*3*) ascending palatine artery; (*4*) occipital artery.

Angular artery (Figs 98/23, 99/26): this is the end branch of the main trunk, and anastomoses with the ophthalmic artery in the canthus.

As a supernumerary branch, the *ramus premassetericus* may accompany the anterior facial vein.

The **ascending pharyngeal artery** (Figs 67/1, 95/39, 96/28, 98/24, 99/27, 100/15) arises sometimes together with the ascending palatine artery (Figs 67/III and V). If it arises separately (91·9 per cent) it may spring from the occipital (Fig. 67/IV) or the internal carotid artery (Fig. 67/VI). In cases of joint origin it arises from the external carotid, the occipital or the facial artery. It is very thin and emerges from the medial surface of the external carotid in front of and medially to the internal carotid artery. It runs towards the base of the skull. It gives off *branches* to the pharynx, the tympanic cavity and the dura mater of the posterior cranial fossa: *pharyngeal branches* (Fig. 99/28), *posterior meningeal* (Fig. 99/30) and *inferior tympanic arteries* (Fig. 99/29).

The **occipital artery** (Figs 95/41, 97/25, 98/26, 99/32, 100/16) arises on the posterior surface of the external carotid artery above the origin of the facial artery. Its origin lies sometimes deeper (Livini

1900) and it may spring from the internal carotid (Krause 1880, Newton and Young 1968) or the thyrocervical trunk (Rauber and Kopsch 1951). Its common origin with the posterior auricular or the ascending pharyngeal artery has also been registered (Adachi 1928). Arriving below the sternocleidomastoid muscle, the artery runs backward in the groove to the occipital artery and ramifies into its *terminal branches* beneath the skin of the occiput. Here it anastomoses with the contralateral vessel as well as with the posterior auricular and the superficial temporal arteries. Moreover, the *descending branch* of the vessel (Figs 98/28, 99/34) communicates with the vertebral artery (Schechter 1964). This is clearly visible if this branch is strong. The *mastoid branch* (Fig. 99/33) enters the dura mater through the mastoid foramen, and the *meningeal branch* (Figs 98/27, 99/35) through the parietal foramen. The *auricular branch* ramifies on the back surface of the auricle; the *occipital branch* is the terminal twig of the vessel.

The **posterior auricular artery** (Figs 95/42, 97/26, 98/29, 99/36, 100/17) is weaker than the former and arises from the external carotid artery separately (85·5 per cent) together with the superficial temporal (0·6 per cent), or the occipital artery (13·9 per cent Adachi 1928). The vessel is sometimes rudimentary, in such cases its function is taken over by the occipital artery. It arises above the occipital artery covered by the parotid gland, and runs posterosuperiorly in the groove between the auricle and the mastoid process, where it divides into its two terminal branches.

Its first *branch*, the *stylomastoid artery*, enters the canal of the facial nerve through the stylomastoid foramen where it gives off side branches to the stapedius muscle (*ramus stapedius*), further to the tympanic cavity through the canaliculus of the chorda tympani (*posterior tympanic artery*) as well as to the mastoid process (*mastoid branches*). Anastomosis is formed with the tympanic branch of the maxillary artery. One of the terminal branches ramifies in the auricle (*auricular branch*), the other on the mastoid process (*occipital branch*) and both are in connection with the occipital artery.

Superficial temporal artery (Figs 95/43, 96/29, 97/28, 98/30, 99/37, 100/18), the more superficial terminal branch of the external carotid artery. It begins behind the ramus of the mandible in the parotid gland in the retromandibular fossa and runs straight upward. It bifurcates into the end branches on the temporal fascia above the root of the zygomatic arch. Its *branches* are:

The *parotid* (Figs 98/31, 99/38) and the *anterior auricular branches* are minute vessels to the parotid gland and the auricle, respectively.

The origin of the *transverse facial artery* (Fig. 99/39) is variable. It arises sometimes from the division of, or from the external carotid artery itself and in rare instances from the maxillary artery. It runs first covered by the parotid gland and then immediately below the zygomatic arch and above the parotid duct parallel with the latter it passes sagittally forward on the face. At times it is very strong, at times it is replaced by several minor trunks.

The *zygomaticoorbital artery* (Fig. 99/40) is in two-third of the cases a branch of the superficial temporal artery and in one-third a branch of the frontal branch (Adachi 1928). It runs towards the lateral margin of the orbit where it may form anastomosis with the branches of the ophthalmic artery.

The *middle temporal artery* (Figs 98/32, 99/41), is rarely a branch of the maxillary artery. It passes upwards in the groove for the temporal artery of the similarly named bone.

The *frontal and parietal branches* (Figs 98/33 and 34, 99/42 and 43) are terminal branches; the former is usually stronger. Their ramification is variable: they usually ramify above and less frequently below the zygomatic arch (Dall'Aqua 1900, Grote 1901). They supply the anterior and superior parts of the skull. They communicate with the supraorbital artery anteriorly, and with the branches of the occipital and posterior auricular arteries posteriorly.

The **maxillary artery** (Figs 68, 95/44, 96/30, 97/29, 98/35, 99/44, 100/19) is placed deeper and has a constant origin from the external carotid artery. Arising behind the neck of the mandible, it assumes a slightly curving "S" form, passes outside round the lateral pterygoid muscle and enters the pterygopalatine fossa. It may sometimes run within the lateral pterygoid muscle (Lauber 1901). Rarely it may arise from the facial artery. It may be divided into mandibular, pterygoid and pterygopalatine portions. Its *branches* are the following.

The *deep auricular* (Fig. 68/1) and the *anterior tympanic arteries* (Fig. 68/2) are small vessels running to the mandibular joint and the tympanic cavity, respectively.

The *middle meningeal artery* (Figs 68/4, 98/37, 99/46), the largest branch of the artery, may arise at different distances from the origin of the maxillary artery (Salamon et al. 1967). It may also originate from the ophthalamic artery (Raad 1964, Gabriele and Bell 1967). Below the lateral pterygoid muscle it reaches the inside of the base of the skull through the foramen spinosum. This artery is the main supplying artery of the meninges. It displays numerous variations within the skull (Giuffrida–

Ruggeri 1913). The *anterior branch* ramifies in the anterior cranial fossa, the *middle* and *posterior branches* divide in the middle cranial fossa, on the parietal, temporal and upper occipital parts of the skull cap. These branches are in communication

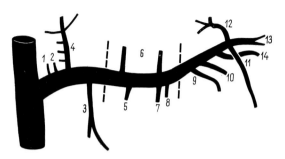

FIG. 68. The branches of the maxillary artery. (*1*) Deep auricular artery; (*2*) anterior tympanic artery; (*3*) inferior alveolar artery; (*4*) middle meningeal artery; (*5*) masseteric artery; (*6*) deep temporal arteries; (*7*) pterygoid branches; (*8*) buccal artery; (*9*) superior posterior alveolar artery; (*10*) infraorbital artery; (*11*) superior anterior alveolar arteries; (*12*) artery of the pterygoid canal; (*13*) splenopalatine artery; (*14*) descending palatine artery.

with one another, with their partners of the opposite side and also with the anterior meningeal artery. The branches of the anterior meningeal artery, ascending along the sagittal sinus, frequently form anastomoses in the shape of an 8 with the anterior branch of the middle meningeal artery. It is only through the anterior meningeal artery that communications are established in this area between the bilateral branches. The middle and posterior branches, which are considerably larger than the former branch, are in direct collateral connection with their contralateral partners. The branches of the anterior meningeal artery extending backward are in direct communications with the median portion of the middle meningeal artery. The arterial system is such that under normal conditions it can be demonstrated only by means of the subtraction technique (Salamon et al. 1967). Considerably more branches can be filled if a part of the arterial circulation is arrested (Nagy 1948). Outside the skull the middle meningeal artery has three minor branches: the *accessory meningeal branch* (Figs 98/38, 99/47) which enters the cranial cavity, the *superficial petrosal branch* which extends into the canal of the facial nerve, and the *superior tympanic branch* which passes into the tympanic cavity. A small vessel (*ramus anastomoticus cum arteria lacrimali*), forming anastomosis with the lacrimal artery, may be present as a supernumerary branch.

The *inferior alveolar artery* (Figs 68/3, 96/31, 97/30, 98/36, 99/45) arises from the lower surface of the maxillary artery either opposite or distal to the middle meningeal artery. The vessel is rarely double (Adachi 1928). Passing into the mandibular canal between the ramus of the mandible and the medial pterygoid muscle, the vessel runs through the canal to the mental protuberance. Emerging from the mental foramen, its terminal branch ramifies in the lower lip and anastomoses with the facial artery. The vessel gives branches to the teeth (*dental branches*) and to the mylohyoid muscle (*mylohyoid branch*).

Some of the branches arising from the middle portion of the maxillary artery (pars pterygoidea) run towards the muscles of similar name (*masseteric artery*, Figs 68/5, 99/48; *pterygoid branches*, Fig. 68/7; *buccal artery*, Fig. 68/8), while two other branches pass upwards to the temporal muscle (*deep temporal arteries*, Figs 68/6, 98/39, 99/49 and 50). As a rule, only the latter, i.e., the deep temporal arteries can be reliably identified, for the larger vessels make the demonstration of the other branches difficult.

Posterior superior alveolar artery (Figs 68/9, 98/40), runs vertically downward in the pterygopalatine fossa; passing along the surface of the tubercle of the maxilla and through the alveolar foramina the vessel reaches the posterior upper teeth, the maxillary sinus and the buccal mucous membrane.

The *infraorbital artery* (Figs 68/10, 98/43) reaches the orbit through the inferior orbital fissure; its terminal branch passes through the infraorbital canal and ramifies in the canine fossa. These ramifications extend as far as the anterior upper teeth (*anterior superior alveolar arteries*, Fig. 68/11). Anastomoses are formed with the terminal branches of the facial artery.

The *descending palatine artery* (Figs 68/14, 98/41) runs to the palate through the greater palatine canal. It gives small twigs to the pharynx, and to the auditory tube (*artery of the pterygoid canal*, Fig. 68/12) and the palate (*smaller palatine arteries*, Fig. 99/55). Its terminal branch, the *greater palatine artery* (Fig. 99/54), reaches the hard palate through the greater palatine foramen and communicates with the ascending palatine artery. If the canal is double, the artery is so too.

The *sphenopalatine artery* (Figs 68/13, 98/42, 99/56) extends to the nasal cavity through the sphenopalatine foramen and gives off branches which curve to the lateral wall (*posterior lateral nasal branches*) and to the posterior part of the septum (*posterior nasal septal branches*). Its terminal branch passes through the incisive canal and anastomoses with the greater palatine and superior labial arteries.

Angiography of the common carotid artery and external carotid artery

Angiography of the external carotid artery was much later adopted in clinical practice than cerebral angiography although technical facilities would have allowed its earlier introduction. The roentgen-anatomical descriptions and the radiological exploration of variants have only been published for about a decade (Schoenmackers and Scheunemann 1956, Ruggiero et al. 1963, Doyon 1966, Aaron and Chawaf 1967). For clinical practice angiograms representing collateral circulation between the intracranial vessels (see Section on the internal carotid artery), the contrast-filling of meningeal vessels (Salamon et al. 1967), the angiography of the jaw (Kettunen 1965) and of the thyroid gland (Djindjian et al. 1964) are the most significant.

On postmortem anteroposterior angiograms the common carotid arteries (Figs 44/18, 57/11, 59/10 and 13, 95/9 and 10, 98/7) show a similar course above the height of the sternoclavicular articulation on both sides. In the projection of the transverse processes of the vertebrae, the two parallelly upward running trunks divide slightly diverging at the height of the third cervical vertebra. The vertebral artery crosses the initial portion of the common carotid artery from behind at an acute angle. The inferior thyroid artery curves medially between the projection of the vertebral and the common carotid arteries, while the ascending cervical artery, following an approximately parallel course, courses upward laterally to the arteries of the skull. The larynx, thyroid gland and trachea are situated between the two major vessels. In the lateral view (Figs 45/17 and 18, 58/12, 60/10, 96/10, 99/10) the common carotid arteries are projected on each other, at the anterior border of the vertebral bodies. They are seen running upward behind the vertebral arteries. Separate projections of the bilateral arteries can be obtained in the oblique views (Figs 46/18, 97/14 and 31). In the first oblique view the right, in the second oblique view the left common carotid artery is seen in front of the column, while the contralateral artery is projected behind on the borders of the vertebrae. This way the trunks projected exclusively on the soft tissues can be better visualized in front of the corresponding vertebral arteries. The inferior thyroid and the ascending cervical arteries can be seen between the common carotid and the vertebral arteries. Lateral radiograms focused on the division of the common carotid (Fig. 100), if slightly rotated, show the overlapping projections of the bilateral vessels already separately, whereas a further rotation is necessary in order to distinguish the vertebral arteries. Because of cervical lordosis, the shadows of the forward curving vertebral arteries fall on the projection of the initial portion of the internal carotid artery.

Cervical pictures are suited for the visualization of the lower branches of the external carotid artery (superior thyroid and lingual arteries), while cranial roentgenograms are better suited for the visualization of the others. The shape of the skull must not be disregarded when judging the configuration of the vessels. Deep vessels are elongated in dolichocephaly and shortened in brachycephaly. Superficial vessels become tortuous if the skull is short. The course of the lingual and facial arteries vary with opening and closing of the mouth. The maxillary artery seems to be elongated in the angiograms of toothless individuals (Schoenmackers and Scheunemann 1956). Since the branches of the external carotid artery are closer to the sagittal than to the frontal plane, they can be better visualized in the lateral than in the anteroposterior view. Of course, the optimal view has to be changed according to possible anomalous anatomic situations.

In an anteroposterior view (Figs 95, 98) the main trunk of the external carotid artery (Figs 95/28, 98/9), appears in the lateral third of the distance between the angle of the mandible and the median line. The vessel intersects the lower border of the mandible obliquely and turns then in an "S" form laterally. Running medially, the trunk of the superior thyroid artery (Figs 95/29, 98/10) divides into a small, horizontally running hyoid branch and several branches descending on the two sides of the larynx. The superior laryngeal artery (Figs 95/30, 98/11), after curving toward the median line, forms a fork of two prongs, while the posterior branch is more laterally placed. The tortuous lingual artery (Figs 95/33, 98/14) falls upon the projection of the mandible: its initial segment appears to be shorter on account of its position. Running toward the median plane, the terminal branches intersect the projection of the vertebral artery. After curving round the body of the mandible, the facial artery (Figs 95/38, 98/19) passes obliquely upward and medially; its terminal branch extends to the medial canthus. The branches of this vessel run below and above the mandible (submental artery, superior and inferior labial arteries; Figs 98/22 and 21) in a medial direction and ramify in an approximately horizontal plane. The ascending palatine artery (Fig. 98/20), first curving medially in front of the projection of the main trunk of the external carotid artery, runs obliquely upward. The projection of its course appears somewhat medial to the ascending main trunk of the facial artery. The origin of the ascending pharyngeal artery (Figs 95/39, 98/24) is obscured by the internal carotid artery. Its pharyngeal branches pursue the same course as the ascending palatine artery. *Meningeal* and *tympanic branches* are hardly distinguishable in this projection. Arising posteriorly, the initial portion of the *occipital* (Figs 95/41, 98/26) and the *posterior auricular arteries* (Figs 95/42, 98/29) are obscured, and their further course can only partially be visualized since it runs in the proximity of the sagittal plane. The larger vessel, the occipital artery, runs on the medial, the posterior auricular artery on the lateral side of the apex of the mastoid process. The *superficial temporal artery* (Figs 95/43, 98/30) is the terminal branch of the external carotid artery and lies above the upper end of the ascending ramus of the mandible. Of its branches, the *zygomaticoorbital artery* seems to be short due to its location, and is hardly distinguishable; the *middle temporal artery* (Fig. 98/32), lying against the outer surface of the temporal bone, pursues a characteristic medially curved course which turns behind the zygomatic bone upward and laterally. The *frontal* and *parietal branches* (Figs 98/33 and 34), running upward along the projection of the border of the skull, reach the frontal and the parietal bones, respectively, after a tortuous course. Accordingly, their initial portion is difficult to distinguish, whereas two third of their courses are clearly visible in the projection of the cranial bones. The *maxillary artery* (Fig. 98/35) can, according to Aaron et al. (1966), be divided into two portions. While the proximal part, describing an "S" form, is curving medially, the distal portion lies in the pterygopalatine fossa where, forming a forward curve, the main trunk divides into its terminal branches. Arising from the proximal part of the maxillary artery, the *inferior alveolar artery* (Fig. 98/36) runs steeply downward in the mandibular canal and intersects the external carotid artery from the frontal side. The extracranial portion of the *middle meningeal artery* (Fig. 98/37) pursues a slightly curved medial course toward the foramen spinosum. After piercing it, the vessel may show variable arrangements according to its meningeal course. The *accessory meningeal artery* (Fig. 98/38), if present, enters the cranial cavity through the more medially placed foramen ovale. The minor branches (*deep auricular, anterior tympanic arteries*) are hardly distinguishable, whereas the ascending branches of the *deep temporal arteries* (Fig. 98/39) which cross the middle meningeal artery, can be well visualized. The three terminal branches of the maxillary artery have a fork-like division in the pterygopalatine fossa. The uppermost branch, bending into the nasal cavity, is the *sphenopalatine artery* (Fig. 98/42). The *infraorbital artery* (Fig. 98/43) runs along the groove of similar name so that its initial segment appears to be shortened. The steeply plunging initial portion of the *de-*

scending palatine artery (Fig. 98/41) lies in the projection of the margin of the nasal cavity. The lower portion of this vessel turns forward so that its projection along the palate is to a large extent in an orthoradiograde position.

In the **lateral view** (Figs 96, 99, 100), the *external carotid artery* (Figs 96/12, 99/12, 100/10 and 21) ascends in front of the internal carotid artery. It gives anterior and medial branches during its course to the angle of the mandible, while its other branches arise from the upper portion. The main trunk of the *superior thyroid artery* (Figs 96/13, 99/13) arising at the height of the hyoid bone runs steeply downward. Its branches can be easily identified in the soft tissues of the neck. Originating somewhat higher, the *lingual artery* (Figs 96/20 and 23, 99/15, 100/12 and 13) pursues a forward course. Its hyoid branch is approximately parallel with the corresponding portion of the superior thyroid artery. The *sublingual artery* (Figs 96/24, 99/16), a continuation of the main trunk, follows a forward path along the lower border of the body of the mandible. The *deep lingual artery* (Figs 96/22, 99/17) and the *rami dorsales linguae* (Figs 96/25, 99/18) cross the body of the mandible in an obliquely upward and forward course. Arising at the height of the mandibular angle, the *facial artery* (Figs 96/26, 99/19, 100/14) curves around the body of the mandible, runs forward and upward at an angle of approximately 45° and approaches the medial canthus in a tortuous course. It emits the *submental artery* (Fig. 96/27) below the mandible. Those parts of the facial artery which run to the lower and the upper lips follow a horizontal forward course. The hidden *ascending palatine artery* (Fig. 99/20), passes steeply upward in front of the external carotid artery, whereas behind it the *ascending pharyngeal artery* (Figs 96/28, 99/27, 100/15) courses steeply upward. The pharyngeal branches of the ascending pharyngeal artery emerge from behind the internal carotid artery. Only the lower portion of the *posterior meningeal artery* (Fig. 99/30), passing through the jugular foramen, and the lower part of the *inferior tympanic artery*, entering the tympanic cavity, are amenable to radiological visualization. The latter just like the other vessels of the petrous part of the temporal bone, cannot be distinguished from its surroundings because of its thinness. The situation is similar in respect of the backward curving *posterior auricular artery* (Figs 99/36, 100/17), whereas the *occipital artery* (Figs 99/32, 100/16) and its branches — crossing the lower third of the mastoid process — are clearly visible in their entire length in the projection of the parietal and occipital bones and in that of the soft cervical tissues. The *meningeal* and the *descending rami* (Figs 99/35 and 34) can usually be filled. Sheltered by the mandibular joint the *superficial temporal artery* (Figs 96/29, 99/37, 100/18) is projected upon the petrous portion of the temporal bone. The vessel emits two obliquely forward and slightly upward directed branches, namely the *transverse facial* (Fig. 99/39) and the *zygomatico-orbital arteries* (Fig. 99/40). It is in the projection of the squamae of the parietal and occipital bones, respectively, that the two terminal branches and the *middle temporal artery* (Fig. 99/41) can be distinguished from the meningeal arteries. In this projection, the *maxillary artery* (Figs 96/30, 99/44, 100/19) runs first forward and then obliquely upward and forward toward the pterygopalatine fossa. The *inferior alveolar artery* (Figs 96/31, 99/45), piercing the mandible, follows the course of this canal. Ascending opposite to it toward the foramen spinosum, the *middle meningeal artery* (Fig. 99/46) crosses the transverse facial and the zygomatico-orbital arteries. The projection of its intracranial portion coalesces with that of the frontal branch of the superficial temporal artery. The *masseteric artery* (Fig. 99/48) ramifies in the projection of the condylar process of the mandible. The terminal branches of the maxillary artery fork out like the twigs of a broom. The trunk of the *infraorbital artery* (Fig. 99/52), coursing forward at the base of the orbit, can be followed in its entire length in the infraorbital canal. Entering the nasal cavity, the forward running *sphenopalatine artery* (Fig. 99/56) ramifies into several branches. The *descending palatine artery* (Fig. 99/53) reaches the hard palate, turns forward almost at a right angle and ramifies.

The *external carotid arteries* (Fig. 97/16 and 33) the internal carotid as well as the more forward projected vertebral artery can be easily followed in pictures showing the **neck in an oblique view** (Fig. 97). Of the branches of the external carotid artery, the *superior thyroid artery* (Fig. 97/17) can be visualized more sharply than the *lingual* (Fig. 97/18) and *facial arteries* (Fig. 97/22).

The internal carotid artery and its branches

The internal carotid artery (Figs 95/27, 96/11, 97/15 and 32, 100/11 and 22, 101/6, 102/2, 104/8 and 9, 105/5, 107/5, 108/6, 109/6) is the larger branch of the common carotid. It usually arises in the carotid triangle at the height of the third cervical vertebra and the upper border of the thyroid cartilage.

Altmann (1947) distinguishes the following *variations in its origin.* Aplasia and hypoplasia, respectively (Flemming 1895, Töndury 1934, Galligioni et al. 1971, Fig. 64/IV), bilateral aplasia (Fisher 1954), bilateral aplasia on the cranial portion to the carotid siphon (Nishimoto and Takeuchi 1968) In case of the aplasia of the intracranial segment of the internal carotid artery the well-developed anterior communicating artery can form adequate collateral circulation (Mracek et al. 1971); independent origin from the aorta (Fig. 64/III) or the brachiocephalic trunk; unusually deep origin from the common carotid artery (Fig. 64/II); anomalous branches to replace the branches of the external carotid artery (Fig. 67/VI). It may even function as substitute for the entire external carotid artery (Seidel 1965).

The vessel ascends steeply toward the external opening of the carotid canal. Its cervical segment is situated in the groove between the pharynx and the deep muscles of the neck. In the lower portion of the internal carotid artery the internal jugular vein runs first on the external side of and then behind the artery. It lies lateral to and somewhat behind, and in its upper portion completely behind, the external carotid artery.

The internal carotid artery often shows a tortuous course at the level of the second cervical vertebra (Edington 1901, Rowlands and Swan 1902). The tortuosity may be spindle-shaped (coiling) or looped (kinking). Studying angiograms, Weibel and Fields (1965) observed such tortuosity in 60 per cent of the examined cases. It can be either unilateral or bilateral, and shows frequently a symmetrical arrangement. It is generally found at a distance of 3 to 4 cm (1 to 13 cm) from the bifurcation. Boström and Greitz (1967) regard this phenomenon as degeneration due to mechanical factors. Sometimes without being anatomically anomalous, the internal carotid artery is unusually wide (dolichomegal artery, Taptas 1948).

The internal carotid artery describes a characteristic curve in the carotid canal; its initial portion, inclining toward the median line, shows an upward convexity. In its position the artery is fixed by the carotid ligament. Emerging from the canal, the artery passes upward and forward while forming an "S" form in the carotid groove of the sphenoid bone. This segment lies in the cavernous sinus. In its further course, the vessel reaches the base of the brain across the meninx at the height of the tuberculum sellae, and gives off branches there. The part emerging from the canal passes directly into the cavernous sinus, and is likewise fixed there by ligaments (Platzer 1956). The segment between the entry of the artery into the carotid canal and its ramification has been termed carotid siphon (Fig. 69; Moniz 1940): it is "S", "Ω" or "U"-shaped (Krayenbühl and Richter 1952). Many anatomical variants have been described so far (Tartarini et al. 1955, Platzer 1956). The carotid siphon is usually open in children (Clara 1953, Schiefer and Vetter 1957). The diameter of the internal carotid artery

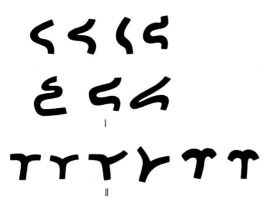

FIG. 69. Variations of the siphon of the internal carotid artery. I, lateral view; II, anteroposterior view (after Krayenbühl, H. and Yasargil, M. G.: Die zerebrale Angiographie. 2nd ed., Thieme, Stuttgart, 1965).

averages 0·9 cm (Paturet 1958) in 90 per cent of the cases, it is thicker than the external carotid artery. There is a difference in diameter between the bilateral internal carotid arteries in 40 per cent of the cases. From this fact conclusion may be drawn as to the wideness of the ipsilateral cerebral vessels (Lehrer 1968).

Variant branches. In the extracranial portion the internal carotid artery gives off branches only in exceptional cases. The ascending pharyngeal and the occipital arteries may sometimes have here supernumerary origins (Adachi 1928, Newton and Young 1968). Supernumerary branches, if present, form

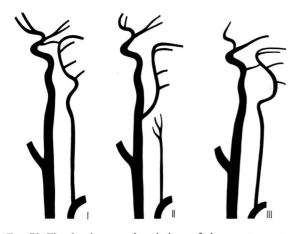

FIG. 70. The developmental variations of the anastomoses between the internal carotid and the vertebral arteries. I, normal type; II, primitive hypoglossal artery (rudimentary vertebral artery); III, primitive trigeminal artery (circle of Willis partially developed or defective).

anastomoses with the basilar artery; they are regarded as vestigial structures.

1. The primitive hypoglossal artery (Fig. 70/II) can be normally found in the human embryo measuring 0·9 to 1·1 cm, it connects the five cervical segmental arteries as far as the subclavian artery with the internal carotid artery. They subsequently undergo involution so that only a longitudinal anastomosis, the vertebral artery, remains (Törő and Csaba 1964). The course of the primitive hypoglossal artery follows that of the similarly named nerve. Its presence in adults is very rare; arising from the posterior part of the internal carotid artery, it reaches the base of the skull through the hypoglossal canal where the vessel unites with the basilary artery (Batujeff 1889, Oertel 1922, Lindgren 1950, Scott 1963, Handa et al. 1967, Keller and Weiss 1973.). Arnould and associates (1968) collected 24 cases from the literature until 1968.

2. The primitive acoustic (otic) artery is likewise a vestigial remnant information on which is scanty (Hyrtl 1836, Altmann 1947, Krayenbühl and Yasargil 1965).

3. The primitive trigeminal artery (Fig. 70/III) occurs more frequently than the preceding two arteries. In 3 mm long human embryos the trigeminal artery connects the portion of the internal carotid artery lying in the cavernous sinus with those paired vessels which are to develop into the basilar artery. It is then obliterated in 14 mm long embryos. We speak of the persistence of the trigeminal artery if it fails to disappear (Quain 1884, Blackburn 1907, Lindgren 1954, Hinck 1964, Wollschlaeger and Wollschlaeger 1964a, Lahl 1966). It occurs in 0·1 to 0·3 per cent of the cases. The vessel usually extends from the infraclinoid part of the internal carotid artery to the first portion of the basilar artery, perhaps to the superior cerebellar artery (Fiebach and Agnoli 1973. The posterior communicating artery is rudimentary in such cases. The vertebral arteries as well as the caudal portion of the basilar artery are narrow, too (Harrison and Luttreli 1953). Oertel (1922) described a case in which persistence of the trigeminal was associated with that of the hypoglossal artery.

4. The primitive olfactory artery connects the arteries of the nasal cavity with the anterior cerebral artery (Moffat 1967, Vogelsang 1968).

Typical **branches** of the internal carotid artery are the following:

Caroticotympanic branches are minor vessels running to the tympanic cavity through the canal of similar name.

The **cavernous branches** are likewise small twigs running to the tentorium, clivus, the internal auditory meatus, to the fourth and fifth cerebral nerves, the meninges and the orbit (Handa et al. 1966). These little branches are too small to be visualized with angiography. Those running to the tentorium could be demonstrated by subtraction (Peeters 1968).

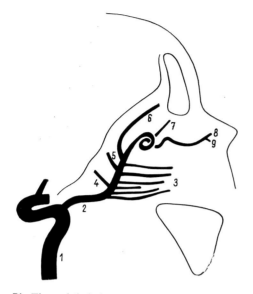

FIG. 71. The ophthalmic artery and its branches. Lateral view. (*1*) Internal carotid artery; (*2*) ophthalmic artery; (*3*) ciliary arteries; (*4*) posterior ethmoidal artery; (*5*) anterior ethmoidal artery; (*6*) supraorbital artery; (*7*) lacrimal artery; (*8*) supratrochlear artery; (*9*) dorsal artery of the nose.

If regular, the **ophthalmic artery** (Figs 71/2, 104/10, 105/6) springs from the medial side of the anterior convexity of the carotid siphon. As a variant, it may arise together with the middle meningeal artery (Raad 1964). Very rarely the ophthalmic artery arises on both sides from the middle meningeal artery (Harvey and Howard 1945). Hayrek and Dass (1962) found the origin to be from the middle meningeal artery in 3 per cent of 170 examined cases. As another variant it sometimes occurs that only the ciliary arteries and the central artery of the retina are given off by the internal carotid, while the others arise from the middle meningeal artery (Chanmugam 1936). Together with, or independent of this variation in origin, connection may exist with the maxillary artery. This anastomosis gains particular importance in case of occlusion of the internal carotid artery (Paillas et al. 1966). The ophthalmic artery lies on the lateral side of the anterior clinoid process and enters the orbital cavity through the optic foramen together with the optic nerve. A narrow bone strip may sometimes separate the artery from the nerve. Having entered the orbit, the vessel crosses the nerve from above and passes from the outer to its medial side. Rarely it may in such cases be situated below the optic nerve (Adachi

1928). The vessel runs forward at the medial side of the orbit below the superior oblique muscle of the eye and divides into end branches below the trochlea. Both its trunk and branches are tortuous, a property enabling the curvatures to straighten out when the eyes move (Lenhossék 1922). The diameter of the vessel is extremely variable but its length is 7 to 8 cm (Matushima 1970). It has the following *branches*:

The *central artery of the retina* (Fig. 104/11), a very small vessel, enters the optic nerve 6 to 20 mm behind the eyeball and reaches the latter in the axis of the nerve. It usually communicates with the ciliary arteries (Zinn's corona). In embryos, the vessel continues as the hyaloid artery in the vitreous body and runs as far as the posterior part of the capsule of the lens. It may persist in a vestigial form (Padget 1948). The diameter of the central artery of the retina is 0·3 mm (Vignaud et al. 1972).

The *lacrimal artery* (Figs 71/7, 104/12), arising on the boundary between the anterior and middle third of the ophthalmic trunk, runs to the lacrimal gland along the upper border of the lateral rectus of the eye. It may exceptionally arise from the middle meningeal or the deep temporal artery (Rauber and Kopsch 1951. The end branch of the vessel (*lateral palpebral artery*) supplies the upper eyelid. The lacrimal artery anastomoses with the middle meningeal artery through the inferior orbital fissure. The diameter of the lacrimal artery is 0·5 − 1·0 mm (Vignaud et al. 1972).

The *short and long posterior ciliary arteries* (Figs 71/3, 104/11) do not always spring from the main trunk but may arise from one of the side branches (posterior ethmoidal, supraorbital, lacrimal arteries). There are, at the beginning, 4 to 6 such arteries which divide into 10 to 16 branches and enter the eye around the optic nerve.

Muscular branches. The anterior ciliary arteries originate from them.

The *posterior and anterior ethmoidal arteries* (Figs 71/4 and 5, 104/15 and 16) start at the middle third of the main trunk and pass medially and upward. The posterior vessel runs to the ethmoidal cells across the similarly named canal. It is frequently a side branch of the anterior artery. The latter enters the cranial cavity through the anterior ethmoidal canal across the cribriform plate and supplies a twig to the meninges (*anterior meningeal artery*). A minor branch (*arteria falcea anterior*) to the anterior portion of the falx cerebri originates from here (Pollock and Newton 1968). This vessel may maintain a collateral circulation with the middle meningeal artery (Handa et al. 1971). There are anastomoses between the bilateral vessels to the ethmoidal cells (Kiss 1949). The terminal branches

130

enter the nasal cavity and divide on the anterior part of the lateral wall.

The *medial palpebral arteries,* arising from the third portion of the main trunk, supply the medial side of the upper and lower eyelids and are in connection with the lateral vessels (*superior and inferior palpebral arches*).

The *supraorbital artery* (Fig. 71/6) leaves the ophthalmic artery at its middle portion and runs toward the supraorbital foramen beneath the roof of the orbit. Having passed through the supraorbital notch, it ramifies on the forehead and communicates with the frontal branch of the temporal artery.

The *supratrochlear artery* (Figs 71/8, 104/13), a terminal branch of the ophthalmic artery, reaches the forehead across the frontal notch. It communicates medially with the corresponding contralateral vessel, laterally with the supraorbital and the superficial temporal arteries.

The *dorsal nasal artery* (Fig. 71/9), the other end branch, emerges from the orbit at the nasal canthus and communicates there with the terminal branch of the facial artery. Apart from the ethmoidal arteries, this vessel forms the most important anastomosis between the two sides.

The **anterior choroid artery** (Figs 85/11, 101/11, 102/14, 104/24, 105/21, 107/16, 108/13) arises from the posterior part of the carotid siphon immediately above the origin of the anterior communicating artery (Fig. 72/I). It springs off sometimes directly from the middle cerebral artery (Fig. 72/II). The vessel may further arise even from the bifurcation, the posterior communicating or the posterior cerebral artery (Cavatorti 1907, Sjörgen 1953, Carpenter et al. 1954, Mitterwallner 1955). It may be paired or absent (Hromoda 1957). Passing backward along the optic tract in the cisterna chiasmatis, the anterior choroid artery reaches the hippocampal sulcus; it supplies the choroid plexus of the inferior horn of the lateral ventricle and certain groups of basal ganglia. The vessel is notably larger if the posterior communicating artery is absent (Hasebe 1928). It may also replace the posterior cerebral artery (Blackburn 1907). Anastomoses are sometimes formed between the normally developed anterior and posterior choroid arteries; Krayenbühl and Yasargil (1958) call them "circulus arteriosus intracerebralis". Anastomosis may further exist with the main trunk of the posterior cerebral artery or with the middle cerebral artery.

A cerebral terminal branch of the internal carotid artery, which originates at the lateral side of the optic chiasma (Fig. 72/I), the **anterior cerebral artery** (Figs 72, 73/1, 85/2, 101/7, 102/3, 104/17, 105/7, 107/6, 108/7, 109/7) passes forward and medially

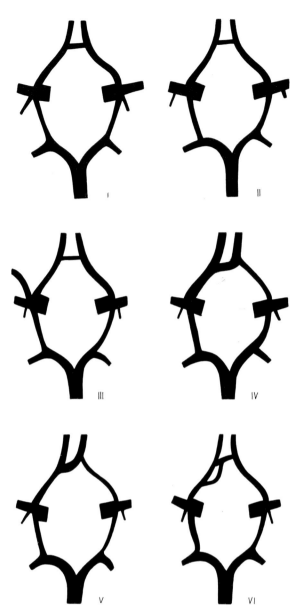

Fig. 72. Variations in the origin of the anterior choroid, middle cerebral and anterior cerebral arteries. I, normal type; II, anterior choroid arises from the middle cerebral artery; III, double middle cerebral artery; IV, asymmetric anterior cerebral artery; V, rudimentary anterior cerebral artery; VI, islet formation on the anterior cerebral artery.

above the optic nerve toward the longitudinal cerebral fissure to communicate there with the vessel of the opposite side (*anterior communicating artery*). It has a diameter of 0·75 to 2·75 mm (Ring and Waddington 1967b).

Variants are commonly seen. Aplasia occurs in 0·7 to 11 per cent (Mitterwallner 1955, Krayenbühl and Yasargil 1965). Hypoplasia (Fig. 72/V) has a frequency of 8 to 15 per cent (Cavatorti 1907, Mitterwallner 1955). A duplication of the vessel (Fig. 72/VI) is rare (Busse 1921, Stafford and Gonzalez 1957). The bilateral vessels may form a common trunk (anterior cerebral azygos artery). This variant is a phylogenetic remnant (LeMay and Gooding 1966). It may arise directly from the middle cerebral artery (Bullen and John 1890), or on the anterior side of the carotid siphon (Neumärker and Neumärker 1971).

Pericallosal artery (Figs 73/7, 85/3, 101/8, 102/6, 104/20, 105/8, 107/9, 108/10, 109/9). Three segments of this vessel can be distinguished (Lindgren 1954). The first extends from the origin to the genu of the corpus callosum (pars inferior); the second, passing round the genu of the corpus callosum, reaches the upper horizontal portion (pars anterior); the third

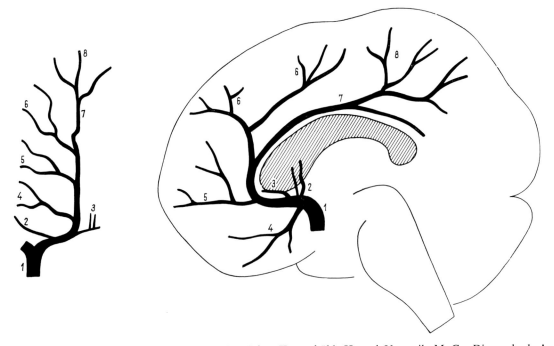

FIG. 73. Anterior cerebral artery and its branches (after Krayenbühl, H. and Yasargil, M. G.: Die zerebrale Angiographie. 2nd ed. Thieme, Stuttgart, 1965, modified). (*1*) Anterior cerebral artery; (*2*) striate branches; (*3*) middle anterior cerebral artery; (*4*) frontobasal branch; (*5*) frontopolar branch; (*6*) callosomarginal artery; (*7*) pericallosal artery; (*8*) posterior frontal artery.

The anterior cerebral artery curves round the genu of the corpus callosum in the longitudinal fissure of the cerebrum and terminates as the pericallosal artery (Fig. 73). The initial portion of the vessel constitutes the medial upper part of the characteristic T shape shown by the division of the carotid (Fischer-Brügge 1938 — "Carotisgabelung"). The diameter of the vessel is 0·1 to 0·3 cm. Its passage into the pericallosal artery has not been exactly located. Lindgren (1954) calls the whole segment after the anterior communicating artery, pericallosal artery. The anterior cerebral artery supplies the olfactory bulb, the gyrus rectus and gyrus cinguli, the medial part of the gyri orbitales and the medial surface of the frontal and parietal lobes as far as the parietooccipital sulcus to anastomose there with the posterior cerebral artery. The vessel may send off branches to the putamen, the internal capsule and the caudate nucleus (Strong and Elwyn 1948). The following *branches* arise from the artery:

runs along the upper horizontal portion (pars superior). Course and width of the vessel depend on the origin from the anterior cerebral artery and on its anastomosis with the corresponding contralateral artery. It may be replaced by several minor vessels (Krayenbühl and Yasargil 1965). The pars superior gives off branches to the corpus callosum and the medial side of the hemispheres, (*precentral branch, precuneal branch, parietooccipital branch, posterior frontal branch* Figs 102/7, 105/9, 10 and 11) but the callosomarginal artery usually supplies a larger area (*ramus parietooccipitalis*, Figs 102/7, 105/9 and 19).

Callosomarginal artery (Figs 73/6, 85/4, 101/3, 104/19, 105/12, 107/8, 108/9, 109/11). This artery arises from the first or second segment of the pericallosal artery at the level of the genu of the corpus callosum in two-third of the cases. It runs in the sulcus cinguli above the pericallosal artery and ramifies on the medial aspect of the hemisphere (*internal, medial and posterior frontal branches*).

Frontopolar branch (Figs 73/5, 85/5, 102/4 and 5, 104/18, 105/13, 107/10, 108/11, 109/10). This branch has a fairly constant course; it arises from the initial segment of the anterior cerebral artery, follows a path which, parallel to the base of the skull, runs along the median line at the medial side of the hemispheres toward the frontal pole. The vessel sends twigs to the frontal lobe.

lae. Its length is 0·3 to 0·5 cm (Jain 1964). *Insular part*: it bifurcates near the limen insulae in 90 per cent, and trifurcates in 10 per cent of the cases (Jain 1964). Coursing first horizontally and then upward, its branches reach the insula. Dilenge (1962) succeeded in identifying separately the various members of this interlaced vascular group. *Opercular part*: the temporal arteries ramify here downward. The

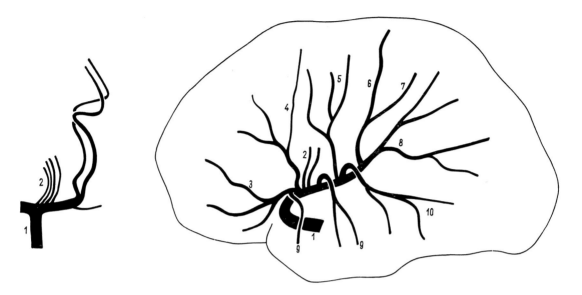

FIG. 74. Middle cerebral artery and its branches (after Krayenbühl, H. and Yasargil, M. G.: Die zerebrale Angiographie. 2nd ed., Thieme, Stuttgart, 1965, modified). (*1*) Middle cerebral artery; (*2*) striate branches; (*3*) orbitofrontal branch; (*4*) precentral branch; (*5*) central branch; (*6*) anterior parietal branch; (*7*) posterior parietal branch; (*8*) arteria gyri angularis; (*9*) anterior and middle temporal branches; (*10*) posterior temporal branch.

The *long central branch* (*recurrent artery*, Fig. 73/2) is not constant. It springs off from the initial part of the main trunk, gives off a few branches to the orbital surface, and reaches the head of the caudate nucleus, the putamen and the internal capsule through the anterior perforated substance. According to Lazorthes' (1961) measurement the vessel is 2 cm long.

The **middle cerebral artery** (Figs 74, 85/7, 101/10, 102/9, 104/21, 105/14, 107/11, 108/12, 109/12) is the other large branch arising at the division of the carotid artery; it is usually of the same diameter on both sides. The vessel pursues a lateral course at the base of the brain and forms then an upward curve in the lateral cerebral sulcus where it ramifies, so its branches were termed "the Sylvian group of vessels" by Moniz (1940). The artery may be doubled (Fig. 72/III). The diameter of the middle cerebral artery is 1·2 to 3·8 mm (Ring and Waddington 1967b).

Krayenbühl and Yasargil (1965) distinguish four segments. The *sphenoidal part* runs in a horizontal direction lateralward and backward to the limen insu-

angular artery runs obliquely backward. The ascending branches course upward at approximately right angles to anastomose with the *terminal* branches of the anterior cerebral artery. *Terminal part*: the terminal branches run downward (temporal branches), backward (angular artery) and upward (precentral, central, anterior and posterior parietal branches). The middle cerebral artery has the following *branches*:

The *striate branches* (Figs 74/2, 85/12, 102/10) are small twigs arising from the dorsal side of the initial portion of the middle cerebral artery, 2·5 cm to the side from the midline (Leeds et Goldberg 1970). Their number varies from 10 to 20. They enter the brain through the anterior perforated substance and ramifying they pass to the ventral part of the thalamus, the internal capsule, the lentiform nucleus, the head of the caudate nucleus and the globus pallidus (Kaplan and Ford 1966).

The *orbitofrontal branches* (*ascending frontal artery*, Figs 74/3, 85/6, 105/15, 107/12, 109/13) are the first branches emerging from the lateral cerebral sulcus; they pass forward and upward on the con-

133

vexity of the frontal lobe (Ring and Waddington 1967b).

Anterior, middle and posterior temporal branches (Figs 74/9 and 10, 85/10, 101/14, 102/11, 104/25, 105/17, 107/14, 108/14, 109/14 and 17), running downward from the main trunk supply the superior and middle temporal gyri. The anterior is sometimes a side branch of the posterior branch.

The *artery of the gyrus angularis* (Figs 74/8, 85/9, 101/12, 102/13, 104/23, 105/16, 107/15, 108/15, 109/15), a direct continuation of the main trunk, runs to the angular and supramarginal gyri.

The *anterior and posterior parietal branches* (Figs 74/6 and 7, 85/8, 101/13, 102/12, 104/22, 105/18, 107/13, 108/16, 109/16) supply the posterior part of the middle frontal and the central gyri as well as the parietal lobe.

The *precentral and central branches* (*pre-Rolandic, Rolandic arteries*, Figs 74/4 and 5, 105/19 and 20) are lodged in the precentral and central sulci, respectively. The branches plunging to the insula are called *ansae insulares*.

The *accessory middle cerebral artery* arises from the middle or the anterior cerebral artery (Crompton 1962). It pursues a lateral course to the lateral cerebral sulcus. It may occur on both sides, too (Handa et al. 1968).

The intracranial part of the vertebral artery, the basilar artery, the posterior celebral artery and their branches

The **intracranial portion of the vertebral artery** (Figs 75, 86/1, 95/11, 96/9, 97/8 and 35, 100/23 and 24, 101/21, 103/2, 104/34 and 35, 106/3, 107/26, 108/19, 109/18). Piercing the atlantooccipital membrane, it enters the cranial cavity through the foramen magnum. Its segment distal to this point is called the intracranial part. Its course in the cranial cavity is first lateral to and then in front of the medulla oblongata. It lies ventral to the 11th and ventromedial to the 12th cranial nerve. In about half of the cases the bilateral vessels unite to form the basilar artery on the margin of the medulla oblongata and the pons. Of 400 cases, Krayenbühl and Yasargil (1965) found the union at the lower margin of the pons in 66, cranial to it in 12, and caudal to it in 22 per cent.

Rickenbacher (1964) distinguishes three frequent *variations in the course* of the intracranial part of the vertebral artery. (1) Both vessels run from the upper part of the foramen magnum to the centre of the clivus (Fig. 103/2). They unite at the posterior margin of the clivus. The basilar artery follows a sagittal course forward in such cases (15 to 18 per cent). (2) One of the arteries pursues a straight course, the other runs forward forming the shape of an "S" (Fig. 108/19). The union takes place at the middle of the clivus. The basilar artery lies mostly in the midline, but may sometimes be asymmetrically situated (30 per cent). (3) Both vertebral arteries are curved (Fig. 95/11). If this curve has the same direction on both sides then the uniting vessels meet on the same side in which case a contralateral curve is formed by the basilar artery. If the two vessels form curves of opposite direction, they meet in the midline, and the basilar artery runs in a straight course (50 per cent).

The two vertebral arteries have the same diameter only in one third of the cases. In case of asymmetry the vessel of the left side is usually larger (Stopford 1916). When one of the vessels is as thin as a thread this difference may be striking (Krayenbühl and Yasargil 1965). The diameter of the vertebral artery averages 0·4 cm (Paturet 1958).

Variations are rare (Fig. 75). If present, they may assume the following forms: Cross anastomosis with the contralateral vessel (Schmiedel 1933, Fig. 75/II); islet formation (Stopford 1916, Fig. 75/III); absence on one side (Robinson, cit. Krayenbühl and Yasargil 1965, Fig. 75/IV); the absent vertebral artery is replaced by the primitive hypoglossal artery (Batujeff 1889, Fig. 75/V); the bilateral vessels do not unite (Fig. 75/VI) but one of them continues as the posterior inferior cerebellar artery (Berry and Anderson 1910).

Anomalies in the intracranial portion of the vertebral artery have been observed in 0·3 to 1·2 per cent of the cases (Hasebe 1928, Lindgren 1950, Mitterwallner 1955).

The vertebral artery has the following *branches*:

The *meningeal branch* arises with one or two trunks from the inner surface of the vertebral artery between the atlas and the foramen magnum (Hawkins and Melcher 1966). Having entered the cranial cavity, the vessel ramifies in the occipital portion of the dura mater and at the posterior end of the falx cerebri (Dilenge and David 1965). Greitz and Laurén (1968) observed with in vivo angiography an *anterior meningeal branch* ramifying in the cervical dura.

The *posterior spinal artery* arises from the vertebral artery above the foramen magnum and, lying against the posterior surface of the medulla oblongata, follows a downward course in the lateral angle between the spinal cord and the posterior roots of the spinal nerves as the *tractus arteriosus posterolateralis* (Lenhossék 1922). The vessel has the same calibre along its course to the conus terminalis; it is constantly reinforced by the segmental arteries of the spinal column. It can be visualized with in

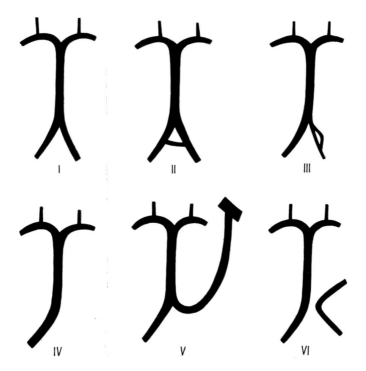

FIG. 75. Variations of the intracranial part of the vertebral artery. I, normal type; II, cross anastomosis; III, unilateral hypoplasia with islet formation; IV, unilateral aplasia; V, unilateral absence replaced by primitive hypoglossal artery; VI, the two vertebral arteries fail to unite and continue as the posterior inferior cerebellar artery.

vivo angiography (Doppman and Di Chiro 1968, Djindjian and Hurth 1970). In the blood supply of the 3 upper cervical segments also the intracranial branches of the vertebral artery participate (Chakravorty 1971). Stopford (1916) found the vessel to arise from the posterior inferior cerebellar artery in 73 per cent of the cases.

Anterior spinal branch: its origin lies on the inner surface of the vertebral artery, above that of the posterior spinal artery. Uniting with its contralateral partner in front of the anterior median fissure, it descends as the *tractus arteriosus anterior*. It may sometimes arise already from the basilar artery (Lenhossék 1922). If the vessel originates with several roots, they form a network of anastomoses (Hasebe 1928). There are several superficial arch-shaped anastomoses with the posterior spinal artery (*rami anastomotici arcuati*).

Posterior inferior cerebellar artery (Figs 76, 86/3, 101/22, 103/4, 104/33, 106/6, 107/24, 108/26, 109/24). It arises usually at the level of the anterior spinal branch from the vertebral (Fig. 76/I) or the basilar artery (Fig. 76/VI; Longo 1905). It may be absent unilaterally (Fig. 76/IV; Stopford 1916, Greitz and Sjörgen 1963) or double (Fig. 76/V; Mitterwallner 1955) or hypoplastic (Figs 76/II, and III; Lindgren 1950).

Greitz and Sjörgen (1963) distinguish three variants in origin: It springs off from the vertebral

artery and approaches the posterior pole of the tonsil (43 per cent). With the same origin, it reaches the anterior pole of the tonsil (40 per cent). It originates from the basilar artery (7 per cent). The artery is absent in 10 per cent of the cases. The diameter of the posterior inferior cerebellar artery measures between 0·25 to 1·9 mm (Ring and Waddington 1967b). After its origin, the artery runs

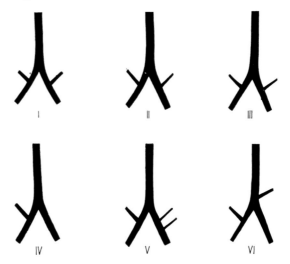

FIG. 76. Variations in the origin of the posterior inferior cerebellar artery. I, normal type; II, unilateral hypoplasia; III, bilateral hypoplasia; IV, unilateral aplasia; V, unilateral duplication; VI, the vessel of one side arises from the basilar artery.

135

between and below the medulla oblongata and cerebellum (cisternal portion) from where it curves into the fissure between the tonsil and the medulla oblongata (medullary portion). Here the artery usually bifurcates. The basal concave part (*medial branch*), taking a medial course, gets beneath the medulla oblongata, while the dorsal convex part (*lateral branch*) is directed toward the 1947, Boeri and Passerini 1964). The "S" form cannot be considered a deformity of old age for it has often been observed in the angiograms of young patients as well (Kuhn 1961, 1962). The distance between the basilar artery and the clivus is in the region of the clinoidal process 7·2 mm in adults; 2 cm behind the sella the distance is 2·9 mm. The distance in children over 10 years of

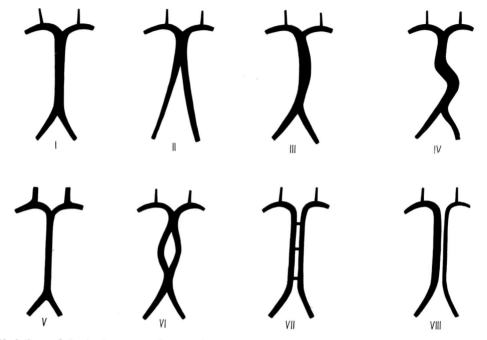

FIG. 77. Variations of the basilar artery. I, normal type; II, short; III, bent; IV, "S"-shaped; V, hypoplastic basila artery; VI, islet formation; VII, partial duplication; VIII, complete duplication

surface of the tonsil. There are numerous connections with the terminal branches of the superior cerebellar artery (Krayenbühl and Yasargil 1965).

The **basilar artery** (Figs 77, 86/2, 97/36, 98/46, 100/25, 101/20, 103/3, 104/30, 106/4, 107/25, 108/18) is the forward continuation of the two vertebral arteries united at the posterior end of the pons (Fig. 77/I). The vessel is considerably shorter if the bilateral vertebral arteries do not unite at the usual place (Fig. 77/II). Islet formation has been observed in 2 per cent of the cases (Fig. 77/VI; Cavatorti 1907, Stopford 1916). A partial or complete duplication may thus arise (Cavatorti 1907, Fields et al. 1965). It is only after a longer or shorter parallel course that the bilateral vessels unite in such cases, and one of the vessels is much larger than the other (Morris 1962). The course always depends on the position of the two vertebral arteries. A typical sagittal arrangement occurs only in 15 to 20 per cent of the cases. The course usually resembles the form of an "S" (Fig. 77/III and IV). "Megadolichobasilar anomaly" occurs if the "S" shape is very marked and a dilatation is also present (Dandy

age between the clivus and basilar artery, due to the great basal cisterns, is larger than in adults (Voigt et al. 1972). It is approximately above the posterior clinoid process that the basilar artery bifurcates into terminal branches: the two posterior cerebral arteries. The artery measures, on an average, 48·4 mm in length (males: 50·5, females, 46·4 mm) and 2·8 mm in diameter (males: 2·9, females: 2·7 mm; Salan and Astengo 1964). It has the following *branches:*

The *pontine branches* consist of three to five small vessels that are distributed in the pons. Gabrielsen and Amudsen (1969) described the radiological anatomy of the branches ramifying in the pons.

Artery of the labyrinth (Figs 86/7, 101/19, 107/21, 108/24) arises from the basilar artery as a solitary vessel in two-third and together with one of the cerebellar arteries in one-third of the cases (Stopford 1916). It originates more frequently from the posterior than from, or together with the anterior inferior cerebellar artery (Smaltino et al. 1971). Lelli (1939) found it double in 15 per cent in

136

adults and in 55·5 per cent in the foetus. It may give off a branch to the cerebellum (Hasebe 1928). Running together with the acoustic nerve, the artery enters the internal acoustic meatus and bifurcates in the pyramid (*vestibular* and *cochlear arteries*).

The *anterior inferior cerebellar artery* (Figs 86/6, 101/18, 104/32, 107/23, 108/25) may arise from the

The *superior cerebellar artery* (Figs 78, 86/8, 103/7, 104/31, 106/7, 107/22, 108/23, 109/23) arises near the division of the basilar artery behind the posterior cerebral artery (Fig. 78/I). It may be absent (Fig. 78/II) in 2 to 3 per cent, double on one side (Fig. 78/III) in 12 per cent, and double on both sides (Fig. 78/IV) in 3 per cent, origin from the posterior cerebral artery (Fig. 78/V, Krayenbühl

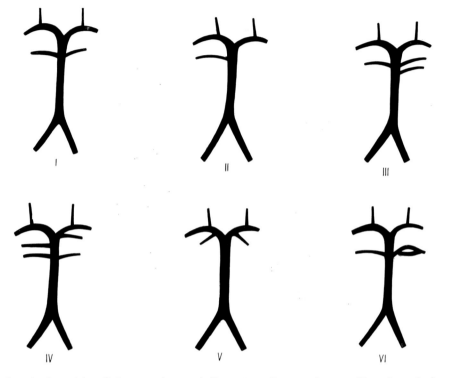

FIG. 78. Variations in the origin of the superior cerebellar artery. I, normal type; II, unilateral absence; III, unilateral duplication; IV, bilateral duplication (origin on one side from the posterior cerebral artery); V, origin on both sides from the posterior cerebral artery; VI, unilateral islet formation.

middle or lower part of the basilar artery (Rauber and Kopsch 1951). Its origin is usually above, or may be common with that of the artery of the labyrinth. Unilateral absence or duplication was observed by Blackburn (1907) in 3 per cent. The vessel is usually much smaller than the posterior inferior cerebellar artery. The diameter of the anterior inferior cerebellar artery is mostly less than 0·75 mm (Ring and Waddington 1967b). It supplies the anterior part of the lower surface of the cerebellum. It has 4 to 5 terminal branches. One runs to the 7th, 8th, 9th and 10th cranial nerve. One larger branch reaches the lateral part of the tegmentum, the flocculus and the lateral cerebellar hemisphere. Anastomosis is formed with the posterior inferior cerebellar artery (Atkinson 1949).

The *middle cerebellar artery* is a rare variant which occurs chiefly in the absence of one of the inferior cerebellar arteries.

and Yasargil 1965, Mani et al. 1968), or exceptionally, it forms an islet (Fig. 78/VI; Longo 1905, Cavatorti 1907). The diameter of the superior cerebellar artery is 0·5 to 1·7 mm (Ring and Waddington 1967b). Arising, the vessel follows the course of the posterior cerebral artery and winds round the cerebral peduncle; then passing along the pons it reaches the upper surface of the cerebellum. It gives off branches to the vermis (*medial branch*, Figs 86/10, 103/9, 106/8), to the upper surface of the cerebellar hemisphere (*lateral branch*, Figs 86/9, 103/8, 106/9) and to the choroid plexus (*medial choroid artery*). The latter runs as far as the pineal body (Pernkopf 1937, Lindgren 1950, Vieten 1964). Critchley and Schuster (1933) described two twigs of the lateral branch, one which runs to the pons (middle peduncular artery), and the other which reaches the anterior part of the flocculus (floccular branch).

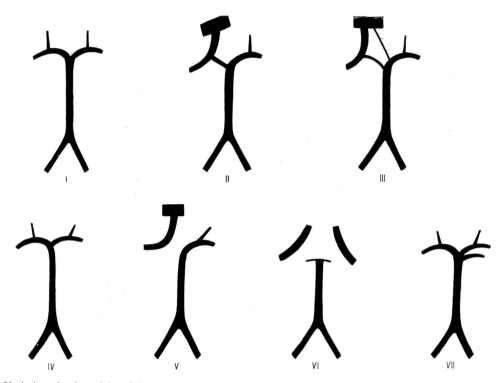

FIG. 79. Variations in the origin of the posterior cerebral artery. I, normal type; II, origin from the posterior communicating artery; III, origin from the anterior choroid artery; IV, origin from the contralateral posterior cerebral artery; V, origin on one side from the internal carotid artery; VI, origin on both sides from the internal carotid artery; VII, unilateral duplication.

Posterior cerebral artery (Figs 79, 80/3, 81/2, 85/14, 86/11, 101/15, 103/10, 104/27, 105/23, 106/11, 107/18, 108/20, 109/20), the terminal branch of the basilar artery.

It displays the following *variations in origin:* As a terminal branch of the basilar artery it reduces the importance of the posterior communicating artery (Fig. 79/I). The vessel may arise from the posterior communicating artery near the internal carotid artery (Figs 79/II, 83/IV). If the posterior communicating artery is rudimentary, the vessel arises from the anterior choroid artery (Hasebe 1928, Fig. 79/III). The vessel may spring off from the contralateral posterior cerebral artery (Hochstetter 1937, Fig. 79/IV). Both arise from one of the internal carotid arteries (Schiefer and Walter 1959, Figs 79/VI, 83/VI). One originates from the internal carotid, the other from the basilar artery (superior cerebral artery; Stopford 1916, Lindgren 1954, Fig. 79/V). The vessel may be unilaterally doubled (Gordon-Schaw 1910, Fig. 79/VII).

As regards morphological pattern, Salan and Astengo (1964) distinguish three types in the origin of the vessel. Angular is the most frequent form of origin. Although described in textbooks as typical, arched origin was found by these authors only in one third of the cases. Looped form of origin has been observed in about 13 per cent. The incidence

of the vessel's ramification from the internal carotid artery varies over a wide range (0.7 to 32 per cent) as observed by various authors (Fawcett and Blackford 1905/06, Longo 1905, Blackburn 1907, Sunderland 1948) in anatomical preparations, while angiograms in vivo showed a filling of the vessel via the internal carotid in 20 to 37 per cent (Moniz et al. 1933, Lange-Cosack et al. 1966). Therefore, it is evident that normal circulatory conditions depend

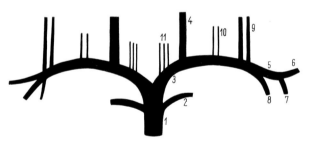

FIG. 80. Branches of the posterior cerebral artery (after Krayenbühl, H. and Yasargil, M. G.: Die Erkrankungen im Gebiet der Arteria vertebralis und Arteria basilaris. Thieme, Stuttgart, 1957, modified). (*1*) Basilar artery; (*2*) anterior inferior cerebellar artery; (*3*) posterior cerebral artery; (*4*) posterior communicating artery; (*5*) temporal branch; (*6*) anterior temporal branch; (*7*) posterior temporal branch; (*8*) occipital branch; (*9*) lateral and medial posterior choroid branches; (*10*) thalamic branches; (*11*) branches to the pons and quadrigeminal bodies.

138

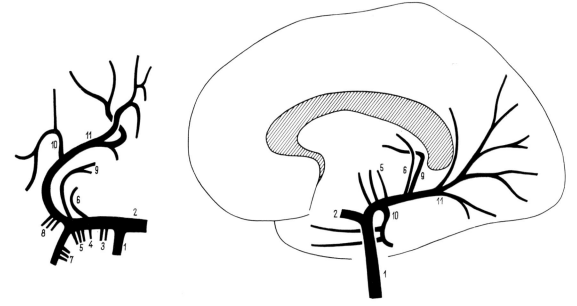

FIG. 81. Posterior cerebral artery and its branches (after Krayenbühl, H. and Yasargil, M. G.: Die zerebrale Angiographie. 2nd ed., Thieme, Stuttgart, 1965, modified). (*1*) Basilar artery; (*2*) posterior cerebral artery; (*3*) paramedian branches; (*4*) quadrigeminal branches; (*5*) thalamic branches; (*6*) medial posterior choroid branch; (*7*) premamillary branch; (*8*) peduncular branches; (*9*) lateral posterior choroid branch; (*10*) lateral temporal branches; (*11*) occipital branches.

not only on the morphological pattern but also on other factors that may determine collateral anastomoses.

Arising, the posterior cerebral artery winds round the cerebral peduncle or the pons to enter the medial portion of the subarachnoid cisterna located here; it divides at the anterior border of the cisterna at the approximate height of the tentorium. The artery supplies the medial surface of the occipital lobe, the inferior part of the temporal lobe, the quadrigeminal bodies and the tela choroidea media. Anastomoses are formed: with the superior cerebellar artery on top of the quadrigeminal bodies; with the pericallosal artery near the splenium of the corpus callosum; with the middle cerebral artery in the temporal and parietal lobes; via the posterior choroid with the anterior choroid artery in the area of the hippocampus (Strong and Elwyn 1948). Diameter of the posterior cerebral artery averages 1·2 to 2·2 mm according to Ring and Waddington (1967b).

The posterior cerebral artery has the following *branches:*

The *anterior and posterior temporal branches* (Figs 80/5, 81/10, 86/13, 101/16, 103/11, 104/28, 106/15, 107/19, 108/21, 109/22) are the anterior twigs of the posterior cerebral artery bifurcating in the subarachnoid cisterna. Arising as a common trunk which divides then into an anterior and a posterior part, they run to the lower side of the temporal lobe and to the lateral surface of the in-

ferior temporal gyrus, respectively. The two branches sometimes arise separately from the main trunk.

The *occipital (parietooccipital and calcarine) branches* (Figs 80/8, 81/11, 86/12, 103/12, 104/29, 106/16, 107/20, 108/22, 109/21) run to certain parts of the occipital and parietal lobes. The upper vessel supplies the medial and inferior surface of the occipital lobe; one of its twigs, the *posterior pericallosal artery,* winds to the corpus callosum above the splenium. The artery is frequently absent (Galloway et al. 1964). While the parietooccipital branch courses toward the parietooccipital sulcus, the calcarine branch runs toward the calcarine sulcus.

The *central branches (internal and external pontine arteries, arteries of the quadrigeminal bodies, internal and external thalamic arteries*; Figs 80/10 and 11, 81/4, 5, 7 and 8, 106/14) are small vessels running to the pons, quadrigeminal bodies and to the thalamus.

The *posterior lateral choroid branch* (Figs 80/9, 81/9, 86/14, 103/13, 106/13), often a multiple vessel, runs to the choroid plexus of the third and the lateral ventricle. It communicates with the anterior choroid artery in the lateral ventricle. Its side branches supply the basal ganglia.

The *posterior medial choroid branch* (Figs 80/9, 81/6, 86/14, 103/13, 106/12) curves round the brainstem and extends to the choroid plexus of the third ventricle (Galloway et al. 1964).

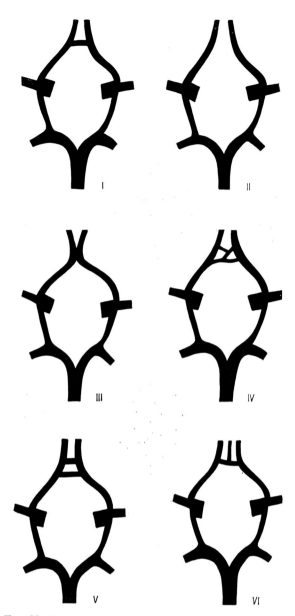

FIG. 82. Variations of the anterior communicating artery. I, normal type; II, absent; III, trunk formation; IV, plexiform connection; V duplication; VI, median artery of corpus callosum.

Arterial circle of Willis

The four cerebral arteries are joined to each other by the anterior communicating artery in front, and the posterior communicating arteries on the two sides. The vascular ring so formed (Circle of Willis) has many variations. Its pattern can be regarded as typical in half of the cases. Variations are of small significance under normal anatomical conditions, but may become extremely important in case of pathological circulation. Provided the circle of Willis is normal, the width of the anterior communicating artery amounts to a half or a third of

that of the anterior cerebral artery (Padget 1948), the diameter of the latter being half of the internal carotid artery. The posterior cerebral artery is twice as wide as the posterior communicating artery. The basilar artery is likewise twice the size of the posterior cerebral artery. Padget regards these measurements as characteristic of adults. The differences are less marked in the embryo and the newborn.

The **anterior communicating artery** (Figs 82, 107/7, 108/8, 109/8) is typical in 80 to 90 per cent (Riggs and Rupp 1963). De Almeida (1931) described 20 *variants* of the vessel. It is absent in about 0·3 per cent (Fig. 82/II; Fawcett and Blackford 1905/06, Blackburn 1907). The two anterior cerebral arteries may unite to form a common trunk and then separate once more, a configuration found in 1·2 per cent of the cases (Fig. 82/III; De Vriese 1905, Blackburn 1907). Duplication (Figs 82/IV and V) of the vessel, or its "V" or "Y" shape is of morphological but not of angiographic significance. Origin of the arteria mediana corporis callosi from the anterior communicating artery (Fig. 82/VI) has been observed in 2 to 23 per cent (Fawcett and Blackford 1905/06, Mitterwallner 1955, Curry and Culberth 1951).

The **posterior communicating artery** (Figs 83, 104/26, 105/22, 106/10, 107/17, 108/17) runs at the side of the hypothalamus in the interpeduncular cisterna and connects the two internal carotid arteries with the posterior cerebral artery. It is typical in 50 per cent of the cases only (De Vriese 1905). Surveying the material of several authors, Fields et al. (1965) estimated the frequency of the anomalies of the vessels at 59 per cent.

Padget (1947) described 21 possible *variations* of the posterior part of the arterial circle. Characteristic groups are the following. Normal type (Fig. 83/I). The posterior communicating artery of one side is rudimentary (Fig. 83/II). Unilateral absence of the posterior communicating artery and its replacement by the anterior choroid artery (Fig. 83/III). The posterior cerebral artery is rudimentary on this side, and blood is supplied here by the internal carotid artery. The posterior cerebral artery is rudimentary on one side. Blood is supplied as in the former case (Fig.83/IV).The posterior communicating artery is rudimentary on one side, the posterior cerebral artery on the other (Fig. 83/V). Blood is supplied instead of the posterior cerebral artery by the basilar and internal carotid arteries, respectively. The posterior communicating artery is bilaterally absent (Fig. 83/VI). There is no connection between the anterior and the posterior cerebral arteries at the base of the brain. Beside the circle of Willis also the primitive trigeminal, primitive hypoglossal and primitive otic arteries may form anastomoses between the basilar vessels.

From a clinical standpoint, morphological variations of the arterial circle may be divided into two groups: connection between the internal carotid and the basilar arteries remains adequate in the first and becomes inadequate in the second group. The importance of the latter becomes manifest if an artery at the base is insufficient. The function of the missing posterior communicating artery may be taken over by a fine arterial network passing through the mesencephalon (Ruggiero and Constans 1954, Krayenbühl and Yasargil 1965).

Based on angiographic studies, Lechi and Nizzoli (1964) distinguish three haemodynamic variants of the basilar circulation. (1) Blood flows from the carotid artery to the basilar artery through the well-developed posterior communicating arteries. (2) Blood flow is directed from the basilar artery to the internal carotid artery through the well-developed posterior communicating arteries. (3) The two arterial systems are in a state of equilibrium.

Blood supply of the basal ganglia and the internal capsule

The small arteries supplying blood to the basal ganglia are usually small and thus not amenable to angiographic visualization. Their demonstration by subtraction technique is partly successful (Hacker and Alonso 1968). Nevertheless, their clinical significance justifies their brief discussion. As regards origin, Strong and Elwyn (1948) classified these vessels into four categories.

The *anterolateral branches* (*striate arteries*) arise from the initial segment of the anterior cerebral and from the middle cerebral arteries. Passing through the anterior perforated substance they run to the head of the caudate nucleus, the putamen, the ventrolateral part of the thalamus, the globus pallidus and the anterior part of the internal capsule. These vessels are sometimes joined by the *middle striate artery*, a larger vessel arising from the anterior cerebral artery (Heubner 1872, Lazorthes 1961, Kaplan and Ford 1966).

The *anteromedial branches* originate from the anterior cerebral artery, the anterior communicating artery or the internal carotid artery. They enter the brain at the medial part of the anterior perforated substance and supply the anterior part of the hypothalamus including the preoptic and suprachiasmatic regions.

The *posteromedial branches* arise from the medial surface of the posterior cerebral and the posterior communicating arteries. They pass into the brain

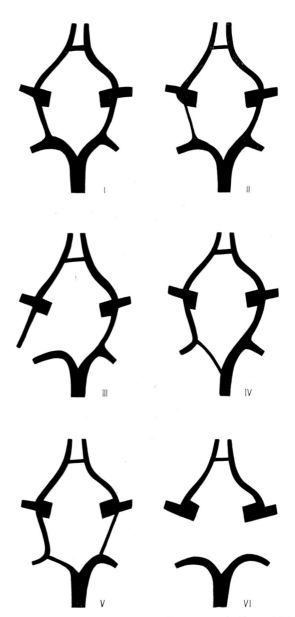

FIG. 83. Variations of the posterior communicating artery and the posterior cerebral artery. I, normal type; II, rudimentary; III, the absent posterior communicating artery is replaced by the anterior choroid artery; IV, posterior cerebral artery arises from the internal carotid artery; V, the posterior communicating artery of the one side and the posterior cerebral artery on the other side are rudimentary; VI, bilateral absence of posterior communicating artery.

through the tuber cinereum, the mamillary body and the interpeduncular fossa. Two groups of branches arise here. The vessels of the hypophysis, infundibulum and tuber cinereum constitute the rostral group. Some branches run to the medial and anterior part of the thalamus (*arteriae thalamoperforatae*). Yasusada (1964) succeeded in demonstrating these vessels angiographycally. The *arteries of the hypophysis* originate from the internal carotid

141

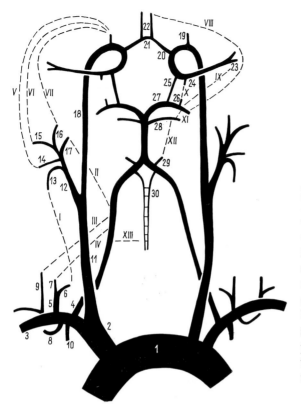

FIG. 84. Diagram of the cerebral collateral circulation (after Krayenbühl, H. and Yasargil, M. G.: Die Erkrankungen im Gebiet der Arteria vertebralis und Arteria basilaris. Thieme, Stuttgart, 1957, modified). I–II, anastomoses between the external carotid and the subclavian and between the external carotid and the vertebral arteries; III–IV, between the subclavian and the vertebral arteries; V–VII, between the external and internal carotid arteries; VIII–X, between the internal carotid and the vertebral arteries; XI–XII, between the vertebral and the basilar arteries; XIII, between the vertebral and the spinal arteries. (1) Aorta; (2) brachiocephalic trunk; (3) subclavian artery; (4) vertebral artery; (5) thyrocervical trunk; (6) inferior thyroid artery; (7) ascending cervical artery; (8) costocervical trunk; (9) deep cervical artery; (10) internal thoracic artery; (11) common carotid artery; (12) external carotid artery; (13) superior thyroid artery; (14) facial artery; (15) maxillary artery; (16) superficial temporal artery; (17) occipital artery; (18) internal carotid artery; (19) ophthalmic artery; (20) anterior cerebral artery; (21) anterior communicating artery; (22) pericallosal artery; (23) middle cerebral artery (parietooccipital branches); (24) anterior choroid artery; (25) posterior communicating artery; (26) posterior choroid artery; (27) posterior cerebral artery; (28) superior cerebellar artery; (29) posterior inferior cerebellar artery; (30) spinal arteries.

artery, and usually enter the gland forming an upper and a lower group. The posterior arteries play a part also in the blood supply to the anterior lobe (Szentágothai et al. 1957), as anastomoses exist between the arteries of the different lobes (Daniel and Prichard 1966). The caudal group supplies the mamillary body and the subthalamic portion of the hypothalamus. Some branches reach the inter-

thalamic adhesion, others extend to the raphe of the mesencephalic tegmentum. The terminal branches ramify in the red nucleus and in the medial part of the pes pedunculi.

The *posterolateral branches (thalamogeniculate arteries)* spring off from the lateral surface of the posterior cerebral artery, pass through the lateral geniculate body to the caudal half of the thalamus, to the pulvinar, and to the lateral posterior part of the nuclei of the brain stem.

The *anterior* and *posterior choroid arteries*, too, participate in the blood supply of the basal ganglia. Herewith only a summary of their respective area of supply is given. The anterior choroid artery gives off branches to the hippocampus, the medial and intermediary parts of the globus pallidus, to the anterior part of the posterior larger half of the internal capsule, the amygdaloid and caudate nuclei as also to the posterior part of the putamen. Certain branches extend as far as the pulvinar and the upper surface of the thalamus (Alexander 1942). The posterior choroid arteries have their division in the mesencephalon and the upper medial part of the thalamus.

Collateral circulation of the brain

Collateral circulation of the brain is important in pathological cases. It is necessary, therefore, to be familiar with the anatomical possibilities that must be considered if blood supply to certain areas is insufficient. Willis was the first to recognize as early as in 1684 the significance of collateral circulation when he described the anatomy of the arterial circle at the base of the brain. Numerous authors have described the anatomical and clinical aspects of the collateral circulation developing as a result of insufficient blood supply since routine angiography has been generally adopted in everyday practice (Sachs 1954, Kautzky and Zülch 1955. Mount and Taveras 1957, Lang et al. 1964, Zappe et al. 1965, Krayenbühl and Yasargil 1965, Fields et al. 1965, Kaplan and Ford 1966, Huber 1966, Hawkins 1966, Sindermann 1967, Gado and Marshall 1971).

Kaplan and Ford (1966) distinguish three types of collateral circulation according to their anatomical arrangement (Fig. 84).

1. Extracranial collaterals are connections between the internal and external carotid and the subclavian arteries outside the cranial cavity. These anastomoses form the following combinations: There is a significant connection between the external carotid and the subclavian arteries with the branches of the inferior and superior thyroid as

well as with the branches of the occipital and vertebral arteries (Figs 84/I and II). The subclavian artery is connected with the vertebral artery via the deep cervical and the ascending cervical arteries (Figs 84/III and IV). Collateral circulation between the bilateral subclavian arteries may be maintained via the communications of the two internal thoracic arteries (Fesani and Pellegrino 1968). The external and internal carotid arteries communicate via the ophthalmic, facial, maxillary and superficial temporal arteries (Figs 84/V to VII). A direct collateral circulation is possible between the maxillary artery and the internal carotid artery (Rabe 1970). The primitive otic and the primitive olfactory arteries may secure anastomosis between the external and internal carotid arteries.

2. Extracranial and intracranial collaterals like the primitive trigeminal, primitive hypoglossal and primitive otic arteries are only congenital vestiges. These vessels are extracranial branches of the internal carotid artery and anastomose with the basilar artery intracranially.

3. Intracranial collaterals maintain regional circulation between the branches of the vessels supplying the brain. They can be found in three regions.

a) Between the large vessels of the base of the brain: circle of Willis, between the anterior and posterior cerebral arteries (Fig. 84/VIII), between the middle and posterior cerebral arteries (Fig. 84/IX), between the anterior and posterior choroid arteries (Fig. 84/X), between the posterior cerebral and the superior cerebellar arteries (Fig. 84/XI), between the superior and posterior inferior cerebellar arteries (Fig. 84/XII), between the vertebral artery and the spinal arteries (Fig. 84/XIII);

b) Between the perforating branches of the basal ganglia: between the larger perforating branches of the anterior and middle cerebral arteries, the perforating branches of the anterior choroid artery and the proximal branches of the posterior cerebral artery. These anastomoses are formed at four points, viz., above the hypothalamus, above the geniculate body, in the choroid plexus of the lateral ventricle and on the medial surface of the temporal pole.

c) Pial (meningeal) arcades may be formed on the surface of the brain between the anterior and posterior cerebral arteries, between the middle and posterior cerebral arteries, between the posterior cerebral and the superior cerebellar arteries, between the superior and the posterior inferior cerebellar arteries. Connections between the external and internal carotid arteries and the vertebral artery via the meningeal arteries belong also to this group (Grisoli et al. 1969).

Cerebral angiography

Moniz (1927) made the first cerebral angiogram. He used cadavers for his initial experiments. After dog experiments he demonstrated the cerebral vessels in vivo by filling them via the common carotid artery. Moniz described subsequently (1934) the four phases of arteriography. Olivecrona (1934) improved his procedures. Loman and Myerson (1936) introduced the routine performance of percutaneous carotid and Takahashi (1940) that of the percutaneous vertebral angiography. Benedek and Hüttl (1938) called attention to the advantages of stereoangiography. The monographs by Ecker (1951) and Krayenbühl and Yasargil (1965) offered comprehensive morphological surveys of the cerebral vessels.

In *postmortem angiograms* from **anteroposterior view,** the lower part of the *internal carotid artery* can be visualized on both sides of the vertebral column (Figs 95/27, 101/6, 102/2). The vessel follows an "S"-shaped course from its origin to the base of the skull. The shadow cast by its portion running in the carotid canal lies in the projection of the apex of the pyramid. The siphon of the carotid occupies an orthodiagrade position and is, therefore, not visible in this view. In **lateral view** (Figs 96/11, 100/11 and 22, 104/8 and 9, 105/5, 109/6) the shadow of the vessel is projected either partly on or in front of the anterior border of the vertebral column. The segment situated in the carotid canal bends slighty forward. According to Tartarini et al. (1955) this is more pronounced when the petrous portion of the temporal bone is strongly developed. The siphon of the carotid is projected on the sella turcica in this view. Angiograms taken in **axial view** (Fig. 107/5) show the internal carotid in the projection of the base of the skull. It follows a slightly medial course. Its petrosal portion resembles the shape of an "S" and forms an angle of about 70° to the medial side; then it pursues a sagittal course again on the side of the sella turcica. The carotid siphon assumes the shape of a sheperd's crook in this view; it turns medially and divides into branches. The shape of the siphon is variable so that even a slightly oblique exposure may change it considerably (Gerlach and Viehweger 1955).

In the **anteroposterior view,** the *ophthalmic artery* appears at the lateral side of the internal carotid, at the middle of the distance between the middle cerebral artery and the intrapetrosal portion of the internal carotid artery (Raad 1964). Forming an elbow around the optic nerve, the vessel presents a characteristic picture. The further course and the branches of the main trunk are unidentifiable. The artery has been identified by means of angiography in vivo in 89 to 97 per cent of normal cases (Tartarini et al. 1955, Krayenbühl and Yasargil 1965). Pictures made by the subtraction method offer a clearer view. In the **lateral view** (Figs 104/10, 105/6), three portions of the ophthalmic artery can be distinguished according to Wheeler (1964). The first segment extends from the origin to the point where the first larger branches are given off. This portion, lying below the planum sphenoidale, is approximately straight. Windings right at the origin show a great number of variations. Dilenge and his associates (1961) distinguish along this portion a

jected on the cartilaginous nasal septum and the nasal bone. The *dorsal nasal artery* forms anastomosis with the end branch of the maxillary artery in the area of the nasal bones.

In the **anteroposterior view,** the *anterior choroid artery* (Figs 85/11, 101/11, 102/14) is seen to arise form the medial surface of the carotid siphon and to describe an ascending lateral curve. Its initial portion is crossed by the anterior cerebral artery, then the vessel forms another laterally convex arch in its upward course. The choroid plexus usually remains invisible in *postmortem* angiography, but

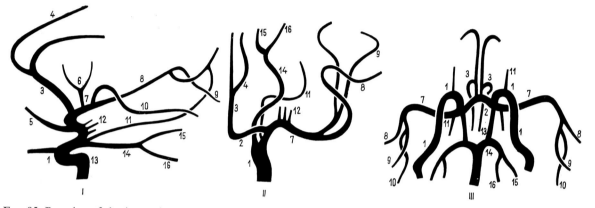

FIG. 85. Branches of the internal carotid artery in cerebral angiography (after Lindgren, E.: Cerebral Angiography. In: *Handbuch der med. Radiologie.* Ed. by L. Diethelm et al. X/3. vol. Springer, Berlin—Göttingen—Heidelberg, 1964, pp. 591—653, modified). I, lateral view; II, semiaxial view; III, axial view. (*1*) Internal carotid artery; (*2*) anterior cerebral artery; (*3*) pericallosal artery; (*4*) callosomarginal artery; (*5*) frontopolar branch; (*6*) ascending frontal branch; (*7*) middle cerebral artery; (*8*) posterior parietal branch; (*9*) artery of the gyrus angularris; (*10*) posterior temporal branch; (*11*) anterior choroid artery; (*12*) striate branches; (*13*) posterior communicating artery; (*14*) posterior cerebral artery; (*15*) occipital branch; (*16*) temporal branch

precanalicular, an intracanalicular and an extra-canalicular part. The middle portion extends to the line where the ciliary vessels divide into small twigs. The main trunk pursues here an upward course approximately parallel to and about 0·8 to 1·1 cm below the roof of the orbit. The *central artery of the retina* and the *ciliary arteries* (Fig. 104/11), though extremely thin, can be identified as parallel bands in the axis of the orbit. The *lacrimal artery* (Fig. 104/12) pursues a tortuous forward course in the upper part of the anterior third of the orbit. The *ethmoidal arteries* (Figs 104/15 and 16) arise from the dorsal surface of the main trunk and appear in the projection of the ethmoidal cells. The last portion extends to the terminal ramification of the ophthalmic artery. While the main trunk describes an arch in the initial course, the further course varies and depends on the shape of the orbit and on the position of the eyeball. The *supraorbital artery* arises usually from the middle portion and passes forward above the third portion along the upper wall of the orbit. The *supratrochlear artery* (Fig. 104/13), one of the terminal branches, is pro-

it can be demonstrated by angiography *in vivo* in 50 to 90 per cent of the cases (Sjörgen 1953, Krayenbühl and Yasargil 1965). In the **lateral view** (Figs 85/11, 104/24, 105/21), the anterior choroid artery is seen running and upward between the posterior and middle cerebral arteries. Its initial portion is frequently curved in an "S" shape. Identification is difficult because of the obscuring shadows of the middle cerebral branches. In the **axial view** (Figs 85/11, 107/16), the initial part of the vessel, though small, can be identified on both sides of the posterior communicating artery.

Anteroposterior pictures show the *anterior cerebral artery* (Figs 85/2, 101/7, 102/3) as constituting the medial upper bar of the characteristic "T" shape formed by the carotid division; it arches towards the midline. Its downward course appears to be concave in infancy and early childhood (Siqueira and Amador 1964, Paraicz 1965). The postcommunicant portion assumes an "S" or "SS" shape. Pictures made in the **lateral view** (Figs 85/2, 104/17, 105/7, 109/7) do not show the initial horizontal portion on account of the overlapping of the pro-

144

jections. The anteriorly convex second portion ascends parallelly with the contralateral vessel. This physiological convexity is sometimes hardly perceptible and sometimes pronounced (Bonnal and Legré 1958). In **axial view** (Figs 85/2, 107/6, 108/7), the initial part of the vessel shows a slight forward convexity where the artery turns into the medial direction, while its second portion courses forward parallelly with the midline.

Anteroposterior pictures show the *pericallosal artery* (Figs 85/3, 101/8, 102/6) to ascend along the medial plane. Its terminal branches spread laterally and upward. In **lateral view** (Figs 85/3, 104/20, 105/8, 109/9), the first part of the vessel curves forward, and then runs in a sagittal direction. Sometimes it first courses straight and bends upward thereafter. This forward running part may become convex if it turns downward. In **lateral view**, Horányi and Kárpáti (1959) found its arch to measure 0·8 to 1·3 cm under physiological conditions. In the **axial view** (Figs 85/3, 107/9, 108/10), the initial part of the vessel runs forward, the second part is usually orthodiagrade, while the third part, passing backward, crosses the circle of Willis somewhat laterally to the midline.

Anteroposterior pictures show the *callosomarginal artery* to lie slightly lateral to the pericallosal artery. In **lateral view** (Figs 85/4, 104/9, 105/12, 109/11) the vessel climbs steeply upward from the genu of the corpus callosum. Its frontal part ramifies passing further in this direction, while the other portions run backward above and approximately parallel to the pericallosal artery and divide into ascending terminal branches. In **axial view** (Figs 85/4, 107/8, 108/9), the initial portion of the main trunk as well as the frontal branches appear to be shorter, whereas its backward and somewhat laterally running part is more clearly visible.

The *frontopolar branch* can be hardly identified in the **anteroposterior view** (Figs 85/5, 102/4 and 5), but **lateral** (Figs 85/5, 104/18, 105/13, 109/10) and **axial** (Figs 85/5, 107/10, 108/11) exposures show its forward course along the midline as also its laterally running side branches quite clearly.

With angiography the *recurrent artery* has so far been demonstrated in a few cases only (Westberg 1963).

Middle cerebral artery. In **anteroposterior view** (Figs 85/7, 101/10, 102/9), the initial portion of the vessel is seen to pass horizontally toward the side. The steeply ascending branches form an arterial coil at the pars insularis. The *temporal branches* (Figs 85/10, 101/14, 102/11) follow then a downward and lateral course, while the *artery of the angular gyrus* (Figs 85/9, 101/12, 102/13), the *parietal* (Figs 101/13, 102/12), *precentral* and *central branches*

cannot be reliably distinguished. The demonstration of the *striate branches* (Fig. 102/10) in this view is successful only in one third of the cases. In the **lateral view** the main trunk (Figs 85/7, 104/21, 105/14, 109/12), pursues first a forward and slightly ascending and then a backward course. The *orbitofrontal branch* (Figs 85/6, 105/15, 109/13) coursing forward and upward branches off first from the main trunk. Describing first a downward arch, the *temporal branches* (Figs 85/10, 104/25, 105/17) continue as approximately parallel lines. The ascending trunks originate along the same line. If the two end points of this line (i.e., those of the first and the last arteries) are connected up and down, we obtain a triangular area called the "triangle of Sylvius" by Schlesinger (1953) and by Wollschlaeger and Wollschlaeger (1964b). According to Moniz (1940) the branches of the middle cerebral artery can be found on lateral cranial pictures in the backward continuation of the line connecting the carotid siphon and the incisive bone. In children Schiefer and Vetter (1957) found the course of the middle cerebral artery to run above this line. The same authors, using another auxiliary line which connects the sella turcica and the internal occipital protuberance, regard an angle of 36° to 44° as physiological in adults. Chase and Taveras (1963) drew a line between two points lying 2 cm above the anterior clinoid process and the lambdoid suture, respectively, and found that the branches of the middle cerebral artery were 1·0 cm above this line in adults, and 1·5 cm in children. In **axial view,** the main trunk of the *middle cerebral artery* (Figs 85/7, 107/11, 108/2) describes a forward curve in its lateral course. The *orbitofrontal branch* (Fig. 107/12) runs forward, while the other branches form an arterial coil similar to the anteroposterior pictures, in which the ascending and descending branches are superimposed.

The *vertebral artery* in the **anteroposterior view** can be seen (Figs 95/11, 100/23 and 24, 101/21, 103/2) running on the atlas in its groove and piercing the atlantooccipital membrane forming a medially convex arch. The bilateral vessels, after pursuing straight or tortuous courses according to the anatomical variants, meet in the midline in the projection of the clivus. In the **lateral view** (Figs 86/I 96/9, 100/23 and 24, 104/34 and 35, 106/3, 109/18), the projections of the bilateral vessels ascending from the foramen magnum, may appear to be superimposed. The distance between the bone and the artery sometimes measures 1·0 cm (Lindgren 1954). The point where the bilateral vessels unite to form the basilar artery cannot be accurately determined in this view. In the **axial view** (Figs 86/III, 107/26, 108/19), the vertebral artery piercing the atlantooccipital membrane is seen to cross the border of the foramen magnum between its posterior and middle third. From here the bilateral trunks pass toward each other in the projection of the foramen. They unite to form the basilar artery at variable points of the projection of the clivus.

It was in 25 per cent of their material that Dilenge and David (1965) succeeded in demonstrating the *meningeal branch* on angiograms in vivo. **Antero-posterior pictures** show its course quite clearly from the point where the vertebral artery enters

is projected below the foramen magnum. This portion appears sometimes in the projection of the vertebral canal. The upper portion of the caudal part is usually seen above the foramen magnum. Wolf and his co-workers (1962) determine the position of the apex of the *cranial part* in the lateral view that they measure the distance from the line connecting the dorsum sellae with the inner occipital protuberance. The projection of the cranial part is extremely variable. In the **anteroposterior view** (Figs 101/22, 103/4), it forms a medially

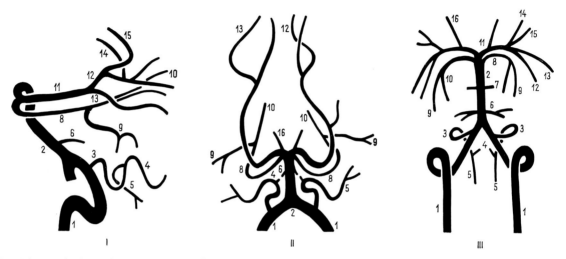

FIG. 86. Vertebral arteries and branches of the basilar artery in vertebral angiography (after Lindgren, E.: Cerebra Angiography. In: *Handbuch der med. Radiologie*. Ed. by L. Diethelm et al. X/3. vol. Springer, Berlin—Göttingen—Heidelberg, 1964, pp. 591—653, modified). I, lateral view; II, semiaxial view; III, submentovertical view. (*1*) Vertebral artery; (*2*) basilar artery; (*3*) posterior inferior cerebellar artery; (*4*) medial branch; (*5*) lateral branch; (*6*) anterior inferior cerebellar artery; (*7*) artery of the labyrinth; (*8*) superior cerebellar artery; (*9*) lateral branch; (*10*) medial branch; (*11*) posterior cerebral artery; (*12*) occipital branch; (*13*) temporal branch; (*14*) medial posterior choroid branch; (*15*) lateral posterior choroid branch; (*16*) posterior communicating artery

the cranial cavity. Sometimes its portion below the edge of the cranial bone can also be identified. It ascends steeply between the bilateral vertebral arteries. In the **lateral view,** the vessel runs on the inner side of the occipital bone toward the inner occipital protuberance.

The *anterior and posterior spinal branches* are too thin to be easily demonstrable. Schechter and Zingesser (1965) observed the anterior vessel *in vivo* in 50 per cent of the examined cases. *Postmortem* identification is often difficult on account of the larger vessels covering the spinal arteries.

It is usual to distinguish a caudal and a cranial portion on radiograms representing the *posterior inferior cerebellar artery*. The *caudal part* passing around the medulla oblongata, frequently at the lower border of the tonsil, goes around the tonsil in front of and medial to it. In **anterioposterior pictures** (Figs 86/3, 101/22, 103/4), this part lies laterally to the medulla, while in the **lateral view** (Figs 86/3, 104/33, 106/6) it

convex arch 1 to 2 mm from the midline, while, in the **lateral view** (Figs 104/33, 106/6), it shows a downward convex arch.

In the **anteroposterior view** (Figs 98/46, 101/20, 103/3), the *basilar artery* appears to be shorter than in reality, while it appears above the clivus in the **lateral view** (Figs 86/2, 100/25, 104/30, 106/4). Its course is not always parallel to the bone. It is in the **axial view** (Figs 86/2, 107/25, 108/18) that the position of the vessel on the clivus relative to the midline can best be observed.

The *artery of the labyrinth*, though sometimes identifiable on **anteroposterior pictures** (Fig. 101/19), is usually visualized only in the **axial view** (Figs 86/7, 107/21, 108/24). Frequently it cannot be filled.

The *anterior inferior cerebellar artery* is difficult to see in the **anteroposterior view** (Fig. 101/18), but is more clearly visible in the **lateral view** (Figs 86/6, 104/32). Seen in the **axial view** (Figs 86/6, 107/23, 108/35), the vessel can be distinguished from the

146

artery of the labyrinth by its backward and lateralward course followed by an arch directed medialward and backward. It can seldom be filled *in vivo*.

The *superior cerebellar artery* can usually be well filled. **Anteroposterior** (Fig. 103/7) and **axial pictures** (Figs 86/8, 107/22, 108/23) reveal its upward curving concavity. **Lateral pictures** (Figs 86/8, 104/31, 106/7) do not show the origin of the vessel. The trunk of the superior cerebellar artery runs below and parallel with the posterior cerebral artery.

In the **anteroposterior view,** the bilateral trunks of the *posterior cerebral artery* (Figs 101/15, 103/10) appear to be "U" shaped if the basilar artery is long, and "V" shaped if it is short (Lindgren 1954). Their further course is straight or curving downward or slightly "S" shaped, and then steeply ascending. In **lateral view** (Figs 85/14, 86/11, 104/27, 105/23, 106/11, 109/20), the initial portion of the artery is seen in front of the basilar artery if the latter is long, and behind it if it is short. It can be distinguished from the posterior communicating artery by its diameter. Seen in **axial view** (Figs 85/14, 86/11, 107/18, 108/20), the bilateral curved arteries, describing a great arch backward and lateralward, run parallel to and in front of the superior cerebellar artery.

In the **anteroposterior view** the *temporal branches* are placed laterally to the occipital branches passing upward and lateralward (Figs 101/16, 103/11). In the **axial view** they run backward and to the side (Figs 86/13, 107/19, 108/21). In the **lateral view** they course caudally from the occipital branches downward (Figs 86/13, 104/28, 106/15, 109/22).

Anteroposterior (Fig. 103/12) and **axial pictures** (Figs 86/12, 107/20, 108/22) show the *occipital branches* to ascend medially to the temporal vessels and to run backward. Seen in the **lateral view** (Figs 86/12, 104/29, 106/16, 109/21), the projection of the main trunk coincides with the line connecting the anterior clinoid process with the apex of the lambdoid suture.

The *posterior lateral and medial choroid branches* form a dorsalward concave arch in the **lateral view** (Figs 86/14 and 15, 106/12 and 13), but often are not demonstrable in the **anteroposterior** (Fig. 103/13) and **axial view** (Figs. 86/14 and 15).

It is only in the axial view that the *arterial circle of Willis* can be fully studied.

In the **anteroposterior view,** the *anterior communicating artery* is extremely variable because of the condition of projection, while in the **lateral view** (Fig. 109/8) it is obscured by the internal carotid and the anterior cerebral arteries. Its projection usually falls on or behind the anterior clinoid process. The trunk connecting the two anterior cerebral arteries can be clearly

seen in the **axial view** (Figs 107/7, 108/8). The *posterior communicating artery* is usually invisible in **anteroposterior angiograms,** while in **lateral view** (Figs 104/26, 105/22, 106/10), a slight dilatation (infundibulum) is observed in the initial portion in about one third of the cases. In the **axial view** (Figs 107/17, 108/17), the backward and somewhat medialward turning course of the bilateral trunks can be followed as far as the posterior cerebral artery.

The subclavian artery and its branches

The subclavian artery arises on the right side from the brachiocephalic trunk on the left from the aorta (Figs 37/20, 38/19, 40/12, 44/19, 45/19 and 20, 46/19, 57/12, 58/13 and 14, 59/11, 66/7, 87, 95/7 and 8, 97/7, 120/5). On the left side the vessel is so long as the right subclavian artery and the brachiocephalic trunk together. Here laterally its boundary is formed by the left lung, medially by the left common carotid artery. From its origin, it ascends steeply. Both subclavian arteries wind around the cupula pleurae and here from below it is bordered by the groove for the subclavian artery of the first rib, from the front by the anterior scalenus muscle and from behind by the middle scalenus muscle. Scarcely it may occur that it passes in front of the anterior scalenus muscle. As a rare *variant,* a vascular ring may surround this muscle (Krause 1880). In case of cervical rib, the subclavian artery is always seen above the uppermost rib. If, however, the cervical rib is rudimentary, the vessel appears above the fibrous bundle which extends from its apex to the sternum. The artery, in the hiatus scaleni, is separated from the corresponding vein by the anterior scalenus muscle. The brachial plexus lies partly above and partly behind the vessel. Having passed through the hiatus scaleni, the subclavian artery becomes superficial in the omoclavicular triangle and arrives then behind the clavicle. The vessel from the lower border of the clavicle is called axillary artery. The portion of the subclavian artery which forms an arch around the cervical pleura is projected above, the rest below the clavicle. Projection of its origin on the right appears between the second and third thoracic vertebrae, on the left in the middle or above the fourth thoracic vertebra. The diameter is 0·9 cm (0·6 to 1·1 cm) on the left, 0·7 to 0·8 cm (0·6 to 1·0 cm) on the right side (Adachi 1928).

The following 9 **branches** of the subclavian artery are distinguished: vertebral, internal thoracic, inferior thyroid, ascending cervical, superficial cervical arteries (thyrocervical trunk if the latter three vessels have a common origin), suprascapular artery (this, too, frequently forms part of the aforementioned trunk), deep cervical, supreme intercostal arteries (the latter two vessels form the costocervical trunk) and the transverse cervical artery.

The vertebral artery and the costocervical trunk display independent *variants in origin*. Adachi (1928) distinguished the following frequent types

thoracic, the suprascapular and the transverse cervical arteries arise separately, the others together (3·3 per cent; Fig. 87/VI). The internal thoracic and the inferior thyroid have separate origins, the other arteries arise together (3·3 per cent; Fig. 87/VII). The transverse cervical artery arises separately, while separate trunks are formed by the internal thoracic with the suprascapular

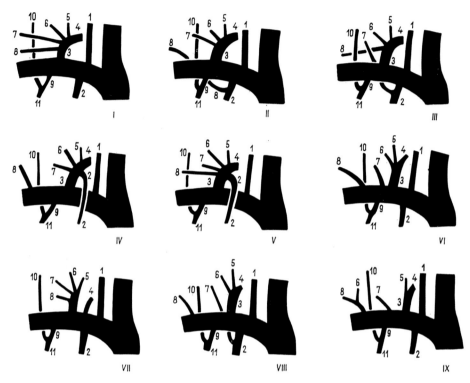

FIG. 87. Variations of the branches of the subclavian artery. I, normal type; II, the internal thoracic and the transverse cervical arteries arise together, and the others likewise originate together; III, the internal thoracic and the suprascapular arteries have a common origin, the other vessels arise likewise together; IV, the transverse cervical artery originates separately, the other vessels arise together; V, all six vessels have a common origin; VI, the internal thoracic, suprascapular and transverse cervical arteries arise separately, the others together; VII, the internal thoracic and the inferior thyroid arise separately, the other arteries have a common origin; VIII, the transverse cervical artery has a separate origin, the internal thoracic and the suprascapular artery arise together; IX, the internal thoracic and the suprascapular arteries arise separately, the inferior thyroid and the ascending cervical as well as the transverse cervical and superficial cervical arteries arise together. (1) Vertebral artery; (2) internal thoracic artery; (3) thyrocervical trunk; (4) inferior thyroid artery; (5) ascending cervical artery; (6) superficial cervical artery; (7) suprascapular artery; (8) transverse cervical artery; (9) costocervical trunk; (10) deep cervical artery; (11) highest intercostal artery.

regarding the origin of the other six vessels (Fig. 87). All vessels, save the internal thoracic artery, arise together (45·5 per cent; Fig. 87/I). There are two trunks: one is formed by the internal thoracic and the transverse cervical, the other by the remaining arteries (19 per cent; Fig. 87/II). One trunk is formed by the internal thoracic and the suprascapular arteries, the other by the remaining vessels (8·3 per cent; Fig. 87/III). All vessels, save the transverse cervical artery, arise together (4·1 per cent; Fig. 87/IV). All 6 vessels have a common origin (3·3 per cent; Fig. 87/V). The internal

artery as also by the inferior thyroid with the ascending cervical and the superficial cervical arteries (2·5 per cent; Fig. 87/VIII). Separate trunks are formed by the inferior thyroid, with the ascending cervical arteries and by the transverse cervical with the superficial cervical arteries, respectively, while the other two vessels arise independently (1·1 per cent; Fig. 87/IX). These 9 variations made up 90 per cent of the 121 cases, while the rest consisted of individual variants.

Vertebral artery (Figs 44/20, 45/23 and 24, 46/22, 57/13, 59/12, 88, 95/11, 96/9, 97/8 and 35,

100/23 and 24, 101/21, 103/2, 104/34 and 35, 106/3, 107/26, 108/19, 109/18). Adachi (1928) found the origin of this vessel at a distance of 2·5 cm (1·4 to 3·6 cm) from the first portion of the subclavian artery on the right side, and at a distance of 3·5 cm (1·6 to 5·0 cm) on the left. It may arise more proximally if the vessel enters the fifth or fourth foramen transversarium.

the superficial cervical artery (Fig. 88/VIII; Hirtel, cit. Krayenbühl and Yasargil 1965).

The vertebral artery arises always proximally to the internal thoracic artery and nearly always proximally to the thyrocervical trunk. Fiegel and Nadjmi (1971) found functional spasm at the initial segment of the vertebral artery in healthy individuals in 22 per cent. The vessel first ascends behind

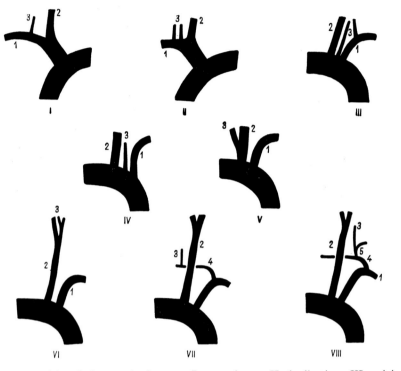

FIG. 88. Variations in the origin of the vertebral artery. I, normal type; II, duplication; III, origin of one member of the double artery from the aorta; IV, from the arch of the aorta; V, from the common carotid artery; VI, from the internal carotid artery; VII, from the inferior thyroid artery; VIII, from the superficial cervical artery. (*I*) Subclavian artery; (*2*) common carotid artery; (*3*) vertebral artery; (*4*) inferior thyroid artery; (*5*) superficial cervical artery.

Rabischong and his co-workers (1962) distinguish three types of the vertebral artery according to its origin, which may be: at the margin of the vertical and horizontal parts of the subclavian artery, in its horizontal or in its vertical portion.

Variations in origin (Fig. 88): Normal type (Fig. 88/I) in 94·6 per cent (Adachi 1928); from the subclavian artery with two roots (Fig. 88/II; Multanovsky 1928, Oblorca 1940); with one root, each, from the aorta and the subclavian artery, respectively (Fig. 88/III; Duret 1874, Lange 1939); from the arch of the aorta, especially on the left side (Fig. 88/IV; Duret 1874, Adachi 1928); from the common carotid artery (Fig. 88/V; Suzuki 1894, Rauber and Kopsch 1951); from the internal carotid artery (Fig. 88/VI; Batujeff 1889); with accessory roots from the inferior thyroid artery (Fig. 88/VII; Killian, cit. Krayenbühl and Yasargil 1965); from

the scalenus anterior muscle, passes then through one of the foramen transversarium and enters the canal formed by the foramens. The artery enters the foramen transversarium of the 6th cervical vertebra in 90 per cent of the cases, and that of the 5th or 7th vertebra in the other 10 per cent. Irregularity is more common in individuals in whom the origin is atypical. It follows a steeply upward course in the canal formed by the foramina transversia. Krayenbühl and Yasargil (1965) described a case in which a loop was formed at the height of the 3rd cervical vertebra. Passing through the foramen of the second cervical vertebra, the vessel curves backward and laterally (first bend) to arch into the foramen transversarium of the atlas (second bend). The vertebral artery curves then to the dorsal side of the lateral mass of the atlas to lie in the groove for the vertebral artery (third bend).

Winding medially, the vessel pierces the atlanto-occipital membrane and the dura mater to reach the foramen magnum (fourth bend) through which it enters into the cranial cavity. The formation of multiple loops shows so many individual variations

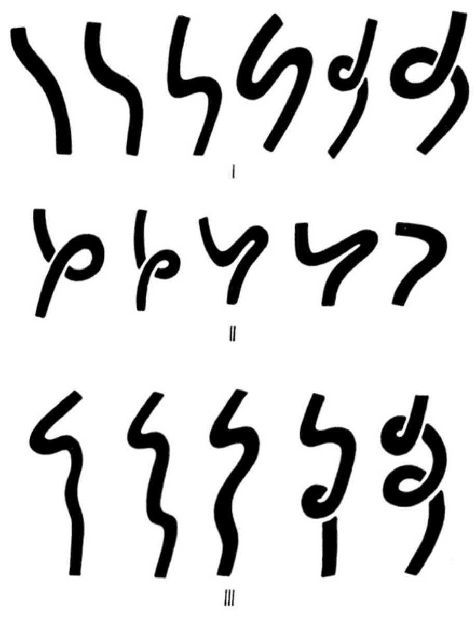

FIG. 89. Loops formed by the suboccipital part of the vertebral artery (after Krayenbühl, H. and Yasargil, M. G.: Die Erkrankungen im Gebiet der Arteria vertebralis und Arteria basilaris. Thieme, Stuttgart, 1957). I, loop at the axis; II, loop at the atlas; III, variations of loop between axis and atlas.

that it is difficult to differentiate the regular form (Fig. 89). Krayenbühl and Yasargil (1965) divide the different bends into four groups: Slight bends (5 per cent); loop formation only around the axis (8 per cent); large bend on the atlas, then a large and a small loop on the axis (40 per cent); large bends and loops all along (47 per cent).

The vertebral artery may be divided into three portions: from the origin to the foramen transversarium of the atlas (cervical part); the second portion extends as far as the atlantooccipital membrane (suboccipital part); the third portion is in the skull (intracranial part).

The *cervical portion* runs behind the inferior thyroid artery under normal conditions, but is placed in front of it if this segment enters the foramen of the fourth cervical vertebra. The inferior thyroid arises in exceptional cases from the vertebral artery (Quain 1884). The thoracic duct lies in front of the vertebral artery but may lie behind it if the vessel enters the fourth foramen (Adachi 1928). Inspection of the cervical vertebrae allows one to draw certain conclusions as to the anatomical pattern of the vessel. The vertebral artery often

enters the foramen of the 4th or 5th cervical vertebra if the anterior tubercle of the transverse process of the 5th vertebra is markedly protruding. The origin of the vessel is frequently irregular if the 1st rib is rudimentary or if a cervical rib exists. If the vertebral artery arises from the arch of the aorta there may be a supernumerary vessel which springs off from the subclavian artery and becomes rudimentary usually after the entry into the foramen (Adachi 1928). The large and the rudimentary vessels may exceptionally anastomose (Kemmetmüller 1911). Occasionally, the vertebral artery may have a branch which enters the vertebral canal through the intervertebral foramen and anastomoses with the meningeal branch of the ascending pharingeal artery (Minne et al. 1970). The artery of the left side is often stronger of the entry into the foramen is atypical. The left vertebral artery arising from the arch of the aorta is always smaller than the normally arising right artery (Adachi 1928). Vertebral process connected with old age may cause curves and unfixed constrictions on the vessel, which up to a certain limit are physiological (Harzer and Töndury 1966). Diameter of the vessel is 4·7 mm (3·7 to 7·2 mm) on the left, 4·6 mm (3·1 to 6·5 mm) on the right side (Brown and Tatlow 1963).

The second segment, the *suboccipital portion* is found in the suboccipital triangle. Massive connective tissue and muscles cover the artery. An osseous-fibrous canal is formed by the dorsal arch of the atlas and the posterior atlantooccipital membrane. This part of the artery is surrounded by the plexus of the vertebral vein and is accompanied by the vertebral nerve (from the cervicothoracic ganglion; Zolnai 1960). Between the atlas and the occiput the vertebral artery gives off often (but not always) a muscular branch which anastomoses with the occipital artery (Nierling et al. 1966). The groove for the vertebral artery is bridged by a piece of bone in about 10 per cent of the cases (Kimmerle 1930, Krayenbühl and Yasargil 1965). If the foramen transversarium of the atlas is missing, the vertebral artery curves into the vertebral canal below the arch of the atlas (Rickenbacher 1964).

The *third portion* of the vertebral artery was discussed already together with the circulation of the brain.

The internal thoracic artery (Figs 17/9, 44/21, 46/20, 57/14, 95/21) arises from the lower aspect of the subclavian artery, usually as an independent vessel. It has a common origin with other vessels in only 6 to 20 per cent of the cases (Quain 1884, Pellegrini 1904). In such cases, common origin is most frequent with the thyrocervical trunk and less frequent with the suprascapular or the thyroidea ima artery. *Variations* in origin may be from the brachiocephalic trunk, the aortic arch or the axillary artery (Rauber and Kopsch 1951). Also unilateral duplication of the artery has been observed (Pontes 1963). Arising, the internal thoracic artery runs forward and downward to pass after a short course behind the first rib and the clavicle. From here it courses downward between the costal cartilages and the costal pleura about 1·5 cm from the border of the sternum. The artery bifurcates into its terminal branches at the height of the sixth intercostal space. It supplies the anterior wall of the chest and abdomen, and gives off branches to the diaphragm and pericardium. It has the following *branches*:

The *pericardiacophrenic artery* (Figs 44/22, 45/25), a thin and long vessel, accompanied by the phrenic nerve, runs to the diaphragm where it communicates with other vessels supplying the muscle.

The *mediastinal branches* are small twigs to the thymus, the mediastinal connective tissue, muscles, lymph nodes and eventually to the bronchi.

Anterior intercostal branches. Arising with a common trunk in the upper 5th and 6th intercostal spaces, they run first below the pleura and then laterally, between the intercostal muscles near the border of the ribs. They anastomose with the posterior intercostal arteries.

The *perforating branches* are distributed in the 1st to 6th intercostal spaces, to the muscles, skin and to the breast.

The *musculophrenic artery* is the lateral terminal branch. It pierces the diaphragm at the height of the 6th or 7th rib and ramifies thereafter.

The *superior epigastric artery*, the medial terminal branch, runs between the sternal and the costal parts of the diaphragm and enters the sheath of the rectus abdominis muscle. It anastomoses with the inferior epigastric artery.

The lateral costal branch is a rare *variant* which runs along the lateral wall of the chest and supplies the area of the 2nd to 4th intercostal spaces.

The **inferior thyroid artery** (Figs 44/23, 46/23, 66/8, 95/14, 97/9) may arise from the thyrocervical trunk (88·5 per cent), the subclavian artery (4·5 per cent), the vertebral artery (0·8 per cent) or may be absent (6·2 per cent; Adachi 1928). Rauber and Kopsch (1951) found it to originate also from the common carotid artery and the arch of the aorta. If absent, it may be replaced by the thyroidea ima artery, the superior thyroid or the contralateral artery. It also may be doubled (Rossi et al. 1971). Its origin from the subclavian is usually distal to the vertebral artery. The artery runs an ascending convex course medially in front of the medial margin of the scalenus anterior muscle. Here it is situated in front of the vertebral artery. If the origin of the vertebral artery is irregular, it may run behind it (Yazuta, cit. Rauber and Kopsch 1951). The vessel is usually placed behind and only rarely in front of the sympathetic trunk. Its branches surround the inferior laryngeal nerve. The artery finally passes behind the common carotid artery to the lower pole of the thyroid gland and divides there. Situation in front of the common carotid artery is rare (Jenny 1910).

The inferior thyroid artery gives off *branches* to the thyroid gland (*glandular branches*), to the pharynx (*pharyngeal branches*), the esophagus (*esophageal branches*), the trachea (*tracheal branches*; Fig. 95/16) and to the larynx (*inferior laryngeal artery*; Fig. 95/15). The latter vessel, usually emerging from a glandular branch, ascends beside the trachea on the posterior surface of the thyroid gland. It anastomoses with the superior laryngeal artery. The glandular branches have two more twigs; one anastomoses at the isthmus with its partner of the opposite side, the other communicates with the posterior branches of the superior thyroid artery (Moreau 1965).

The **ascending cervical artery** (Figs 46/24, 95/17, 97/10) springs as a rule from the subclavian artery together with the inferior thyroid artery (thyrocervical trunk). It may exceptionally originate from the superficial cervical, suprascapular or subclavian arteries. The vessel is sometimes absent (Adachi 1928). It courses along the phrenic nerve in cranial direction.

Its *branches* enter the vertebral canal through the 4th to 6th intervertebral foramina (*spinal branches*; Fig. 95/18). Its muscular branches anastomose with the deep cervical artery at the level of the 5th cervical vertebra (Rauber and Kopsch 1951).

The **superficial cervical artery** (Figs 95/19, 97/11) never arises directly from the subclavian artery. It may originate from the thyrocervical trunk, the transverse cervical artery or together with the ascending cervical artery (Bean 1905). It pursues a superficial, upward course below the trapezius muscle.

The **suprascapular artery** (Figs 95/20, 97/12) may arise from the thyrocervical trunk, the subclavian, the internal thoracic or the transverse cervical artery. It passes above (sometimes between) the brachial plexus, crosses the subclavian artery and above the superior transverse ligament enters the supraspinous fossa. Following the neck of the scapula, the vessel enters the infraspinous fossa lying there on the bone. It anastomoses with the circumflex scapular artery. The *acromial branch* divides on the acromion and participates in the formation of the acromial network.

The **deep cervical artery** (Fig. 95/24) forms a common trunk with the highest intercostal artery in 80 to 90 per cent of the cases (costocervical trunk; Figs 44/24, 95/22). Furthermore, it may arise from the vertebral artery (Krayenbühl and Yasargil 1965), the transverse cervical or the suprascapular artery (Rauber and Kopsch 1951). It is sometimes missing. After its origin, the artery passes between the transverse process of the 7th cervical vertebra and the 1st rib, and runs toward the 2nd cervical vertebra. It sends off branches to the spine (*spinal branches*) and to the deep cervical muscles (*dorsal branches*).

The **highest intercostal artery** (Figs 44/25, 95/23) arises usually together with the deep cervical artery (costocervical trunk). It may exceptionally originate from the vertebral artery or the thyrocervical trunk (Krayenbühl and Yasargil 1957). Its absence was registered by Adachi (1928) in 0·3 per cent of the cases. The artery takes a descending course to take part in the supply of the first two intercostal spaces. It also gives off a branch to the vertebral canal.

The **transverse cervical artery** (Figs 44/26, 45/26, 46/21, 95/25, 97/13) may arise laterally to the scalenus anterior muscle as a direct branch of the subclavian artery, or originates exceptionally from the costocervical trunk and runs in this case between the trunks of the brachial plexus. The artery is a branch of the thyrocervical trunk if it arises medially to the scalenus anterior muscle. It is sometimes double. The vessel runs between the suprascapular and superficial cervical arteries at the bottom of the omoclavicular triangle, toward the medial angle of the scapula, where it bifurcates. Its *ascending branch* passes upward between the deep muscles of the neck, while the *descending branch* runs downward between the dorsal muscles along the vertebral border of the scapula.

Angiography of the subclavian artery and its branches

Angiography of the subclavian artery is of great clinical significance since the use of vertebral angiograms (Takahashi 1940). Study of the circulation of the thyroid gland made the observation of the thyrocervical trunk and its anastomoses indispensable (Djindjian et al. 1964). Recently, attempts have been made also, to study the internal mammary artery (Feldman et al. 1967). The roentgenological significance of the main trunk of the subclavian artery becomes particularly evident in connection with the variants of the aortic arch (cf. pp. 37).

Postmortem angiograms in the **anteroposterior view** (Figs 44, 57, 59, 95) show the projection of the origin of the *subclavian artery* (Figs 44/19, 57/12, 59/11, 95/7 and 8) in the space between the 2nd and 3rd thoracic vertebrae on the right side, and at the height of the 3rd or the 4th vertebra on the left. The right artery arches behind the clavicle; its projection hardly extends beyond the upper border of the clavicle. The left subclavian artery ascends steeply to the left of and parallel with the left carotid artery. It begins to turn left at the lower border of the space of the sternoclavicular joint. Its further course is parallel with the contralateral vessel. The *vertebral artery* (Figs 44/20, 57/13, 59/12, 95/11, 103/2) runs medially and upward from its origin until its entry into the foramen transversarium of the cervical vertebrae. This segment may be slightly "S"-shaped in adults and arched in children (Radner 1955). Having reached the foramen transversarium, the vessel usually ascends in a straight line. The suboccipital portion turns laterally at a right angle (first bend) and continues in a cranial direction (second bend). The vessel then describes a medially directed curve (third bend). The projection of this bend depends to a great extent on the direction of the central beam. It is with a downward convex arch (fourth bend) that the vessel enters the vertebral canal. The initial segment of the vertebral artery crosses the projection of the common carotid artery. The transverse course of the inferior thyroid artery can be seen between these two vessels approximately at the height of the 1st thoracic vertebra. The further course of the vertebral artery can be found first medially to the common and then medially to the internal carotid artery. It is crossed here by the branches of the superior thyroid and lingual arteries. The second and third bends of the suboccipital segment or its upper and lower horizontal portions are visible in the projection of the internal carotid artery. Arising from the inferior surface of the subclavian artery, the *internal thoracic artery* (Figs 44/21, 57/14, 95/21) descends along the border of the sternum and gives off branches in its downward course. The short *thyrocervical trunk* (Figs 44/23, 95/13) arises in front of the internal mammary artery and runs a parallel course with the common carotid then arches backwards and divides into several branches. The *inferior thyroid artery* (Fig. 95/14) describes a curve medially between the common carotid and the vertebral arteries and turns then downward. Since its terminal branches turn once more upward, the course of the vessel resembles a horizontally placed "S". The steeply ascending main trunk of the *ascending cervical artery* (Fig. 95/17) runs a parallel course with the large cervical vessels. Sometimes its upper per segment cannot be distinguished from these major vessels. The variable arrangement in the soft tissues of the neck makes the identification of the *superficial cervical artery* (Fig. 95/19) difficult, for its origin is frequently behind the common carotid artery. The *suprascapular artery* after its origin (Fig. 95/20) crosses the subclavian artery and then turns toward the supraspinous fossa. Pictures focused on the shoulder may sometimes show its course surrounding the neck of the scapula. The *deep cervical artery* (Fig. 95/24), provided it arises from the costocervical trunk, intersects the subclavian artery and runs toward the 2nd cervical vertebra. Its position is more lateral than that of the ascending cervical artery. The distribution of the *highest intercostal artery* (Figs 44/25, 95/23) in the intercostal spaces sometimes cannot be visualized because of the obscuring major vessels. As the initial segment of the *transverse cervical artery* (Figs 44/26, 95/25) describes a tortuous backward course, its portion is most orthoroentgenographic. Its ascending branch appears along the projection of the major vessels, its descending branch appears at the medial border of the scapula.

In the **lateral view** (Figs 45, 58), the ascending segment of the *subclavian artery* (Figs 45/19, 58/14) — the last branch of the aortic arch — is distinguishable separated from the other two main vessels. The segment behind the clavicle is slightly curved backward on both sides. The place of its projection depends to a great extent on the actual position of the upper arm. The cervical segment of the *vertebral artery* (Figs 45/23, 97/8 and 35, 104/34 and 35, 106/3) is seen in the projection of the transverse process of the vertebrae behind the common carotid and then behind the internal carotid arteries. Its position adopts to the physiological lordosis of the vertebral column. The suboccipital portion runs backward after the first bend and once more upward after the second bend. Another backward turn constitutes the third bend. The fourth bend may be projected in the third bend or appear above it. The segment which enters the vertebral canal is directed steeply upward and forward. In the lateral view are the anastomoses between the vertebral and external carotid arteries best distinguishable (Nierling et al. 1966). Bending

forward after its origin, the *internal thoracic artery* is seen behind the projection of the sternum, with which its further course is parallel. The *pericardiacophrenic artery* (Fig. 45/25) with its long, oblique course is directed toward the pericardium from above downward and forward. It crosses the projection of the left subclavian artery, the brachiocephalic trunk, the left common carotid, the anterior part of the arch of the aorta and sometimes the ascending aorta. Because of the superposition of the bilateral projections, the branches of the subclavian artery cannot be seen separately in the cervical segment. Chest angiograms show the *descending branch* of the *transverse cervical artery* (Fig. 45/26) in the region of the upper thoracic vertebrae in the form of an obliquely back and downward running trunk.

The first **oblique view** is especially suitable for demonstrating the *right subclavian artery*, while the second oblique for the main trunk of the *left subclavian artery* (Fig. 46/19). In this view (Figs 46, 97), the subclavian artery of the corresponding side lies more parallel to the plane of the film, thus its entire course as well as the origin of the vertebral artery are well visualizable. The *cervical segment* of the *vertebral artery* (Figs 46/22, 97/8 and 35) runs behind the common carotid artery. The *inferior thyroid, ascending cervical* (Fig. 97/10) and sometimes also the *superficial cervical arteries* (Fig. 97/11) can be seen between the aforementioned two vessels, while the other minor branches are not demonstrable in this view. The *suboccipital portion* of the *vertebral artery* (Fig. 97/8 and 35), in the second oblique view, turns on the left side forward, upward and backward before spreading out, while its contralateral partner ascends obliquely backward. The position is reversed in the first oblique view.

Axial pictures of the base of the skull (Fig. 107) show the *vertebral artery* (Fig. 107/26) turning laterally after the first bend. The arrangement of the bends referring to the atlas is easily identified in this projection. The trunk winds backward after the second bend to take then a medial course (third bend). The arch of the fourth bend crosses the cervical part before passing into the vertebral canal.

THE INTERNAL JUGULAR VEIN AND ITS AREA
OF DRAINAGE

The veins of the neck and head form a harmonic unit, their principal function being the drainage of the brain. Despite individual variations, anastomoses between the intracerebral and extracerebral veins show a generally uniform pattern, whereas communications of the neck and shoulder girdle with the thoracic veins are more variable. The collateral network plays a more subordinate clinical role in this area, since the cervical organs are less sensitive to circulatory disturbances than the nervous tissue.

The course of the cerebral veins is independent of the arteries. Arising from the brain, their delicate branches form pial plexuses. The major venous trunks which open into the sinuses, lined with endothelium developed from the two layers of the dura mater, arise from here. The internal jugular vein drains mainly the sinuses. It is capable of receiving blood from both sides (Woodhall 1939). Variations are numerous but less easily demonstrable than those of the arteries, for this reason comparatively few authors have studied this subject (Johanson 1954, Lindgren 1954, Dilenge 1962, Wolf et al. 1963, Wolf and Huang 1964, De Dominicis et al. 1964, Krayenbühl and Yasargil 1965). From the viewpoint of topography and contrast filling, the veins of the brain are divided into external and internal, the sinuses into upper and lower groups. Owing to the communications among them as well as connections with the extracranial vessels, the veins of the head and the neck represent a functional unit. There are no valves demonstrable by angiography in the cerebral veins (Krayenbühl and Yasargil 1965). Anatomical examinations have shown, however, that all cerebral veins are provided with a single but strong valve of connective tissue at the orifice into the sinus (Kiss 1957).

Internal jugular vein and its extracerebral area of drainage

The internal jugular vein (Figs 47/18, 92/13, 94/13, 110/8, 111/8 and 9, 112/4, 113/7, 115/7) carries the largest part of the venous blood of the neck and head to the superior vena cava. It begins with a dilatation in the posterior larger part of the jugular foramen (upper bulb of jugular vein). The vein runs downward within the carotid sheath, first along the posterior, then the lateral side of the internal carotid artery; it pursues afterward a course laterally and somewhat in front of the common carotid artery. Together with the subclavian vein, it empties into the brachiocephalic vein behind the sternoclavicular articulation. It has a second dilatation at the orifice (lower bulb of jugular vein). Caudally to this bulb the vein contains a valve which, according to Tenchini (1900), is composed of three cusps in 5 per cent of the cases. The vein has a length of 15 cm, and a diameter of 0·9 to 1·0 cm at the base of the skull, and 1·2 to 1·3 cm at the orifice (Paturet 1958). The right vein is often thicker. If rudimentary, the left internal is replaced by the external jugular vein. Duplication (Rodriguez and Adriao 1931) and also islet formation (Kessel 1928) have been observed.

Its *extracranial branches* are:

The vein receives, while still in the bulb, small branches from the internal ear (*vein of the cochlear canaliculus*) and the meninges (*meningeal veins*).

The *pharyngeal veins* (Fig. 113/34) drain the *pharyngeal plexus* (Figs. 110/16, 113/33), situated on the posterior and lateral wall of the pharynx, into the internal jugular vein. They are in communication with the pterygoid and the vertebral plexuses.

The *lingual vein* is often a multiple vessel. The *dorsal lingual veins* empty usually into the lingual and sometimes into the retromandibular vein, while the large trunk of the *sublingual vein* empties into the lingual vein or exceptionally into the retromandibular vein (Rauber and Kopsch 1951). Anastomoses are established with the superior thyroid vein and the pharyngeal plexus. A small branch accompanies the hypoglossal nerve.

The *superior thyroid vein* accompanies the corresponding artery and receives the *superior laryngeal vein*. It opens into the facial or directly into the internal jugular vein. The *middle thyroid vein* crosses the common carotid artery frontally and opens into the internal jugular vein (Moreau 1965). Their calibre is variable. A vein connects the posterior surface of the thyroid gland with the pharyngeal plexus which may often be better developed than the thyroid veins (Chevrel et al. 1965).

The *facial vein* runs obliquely behind the facial artery across the face to join the retromandibular vein below the angle of the mandible where it opens into the internal jugular vein. The *angular vein*, a branch of the vessel, commencing at the nasal canthus forms an important anastomosis with the superior ophthalmic vein. The frontal branches (*supratrochlear* and *supraorbital* veins) form arched anastomoses with the superficial temporal vein. Their course and size are variable (Süsse and Kunits 1966). The veins of the eyelids empty into the main trunk from a lateromedial, those of the nose and upper lip from the opposite direction (*upper* and *lower palpebral*, *external nasal* and *superior labial veins*). The *inferior labial* usually unites with the *submental vein* (Fig. 113/37) before opening into the facial vein. The *deep facial vein* forms an important anastomosis with the pterygoid plexus. The vessel receives the *external palatine vein* from the soft palate and the tonsillar area.

The *retromandibular vein* (Figs 111/14, 113/36, 115/23), a large vessel descending in the parotid gland, joins the facial vein below the angle of the mandible and opens into the internal jugular vein. Its *superficial* and *middle temporal branches* communicate with the vessels of the forehead and the occiput. After the union with the *maxillary veins*, these branches form the main trunk of the retromandibular vein. The maxillary veins drain partly the powerful *pterygoid plexus* (Figs 111/13, 113/35, 115/22). This network drains the regions of the skull, mouth, nose, pharynx and orbit (*middle meningeal* and *deep temporal veins; vein of the pterygoid canal; anterior auricular, parotid, temporomandibular articular, tympanic* and *stylomastoid veins* (Kádár and Kocsis 1959).

The *external jugular vein* (Figs 110/9, 113/38, 115/24), formed behind the auricle by the union of the *occipital* and the *posterior auricular veins*, pursues a superficial downward course and opens into the brachiocephalic or the internal jugular or the subclavian vein (Rauber and Kopsch 1951). In the middle and above its orifice the vessel is provided with a valve. The portion between the valves is fusiformly dilated. Absence of the vein and islet formation have also been observed (Drewes 1963). The diameter measures 0·5 to 0·9 cm (Paturet 1958). It forms an anastomosis with the retromandibular vein and receives moreover the *anterior jugular vein* (Fig. 110/10) which descends from the chin. The latter bilateral veins uniting in the median may form the *median cervical vein*. An arched union may take place above the jugular notch of the sternum (*jugular venous arch*; Fig. 110/13). The size of this arch is variable; it communicates with the surrounding veins. The external jugular vein also chains the *suprascapular* and the *transverse cervical veins*. Anastomosis is sometimes formed with the cephalic vein (Drewes 1963).

Veins and sinuses of the brain, veins of the orbit and veins of the cranial bones

Most cortical and subcortical **veins of the brain** (Figs 90, 91, 92) open directly into the sinuses. Certain veins of the lower surface of the frontal and temporal lobes are drained by the basal vein.

1. *External veins of the brain.*

The *superior cerebral veins* (Fig. 115/11) run toward the midline along the convexity of the brain. This group of ascending vessels consists of 12 to 15 pairs of veins (*frontal veins*, Figs 90/2, 91/2, 112/10, 113/23, 114/5; *central veins*, Figs 91/3, 113/25, 114/6; *parietal veins*, Figs 91/4, 113/24, 114/7; *occipital veins*, Figs 91/5, 113/26, 114/8). These veins run between the gyri in the subarachnoid space toward the interhemispheric fissure, pierce the arachnoid mater of the brain near the sinus, and reach the inner surface of the dura mater. They empty into the superior sagittal sinus. While the course of the veins of the forehead follows the direction of blood flow in the sinus, they open into the sinus at backward increasing angles (occipitally, at an angle of 180°) in the opposite direction. This is due to the "sinus principle", i.e., that the increasing negative pressure of the backward widening sinus is balanced by the oppositely directed orifice and the tortuosity of the veins (Kiss 1957). The orifice of the frontal veins is more lateral than that of the more posteriorly placed vessels, a phenomenon especially marked in children (Krayenbühl and Yasargil 1965). The smaller occipital veins empty into the transverse sinus. Another group of the superficial cerebral veins follows a descending course. The *superficial middle cerebral vein* (Figs 91/13, 112/14, 113/22) begins in the region of the lateral cerebral sulcus and pursues a descending forward course. It empties into the sphenoparietal or the cavernous sinus. The veins of the group sometimes pass below the temporal lobe to the superior petrosal or the transverse sinus. One to three veins can be found in this region. The *temporooccipital veins* (Figs 91/14, 113/27, 114/14) carry the blood from the lateral surface of the temporal lobe to the transverse sinus in an arched backward course.

The *inferior cerebral veins*, which are the veins of the lower surface, collect blood in the medial region of the frontal lobe from the *gyri olfactorii vein* and the *anterior cerebral veins;* they are drained by the basal vein. The medial veins of the temporal lobe open into the basal vein, its lateral veins into the temporooccipital vein, the transverse or the superior petrosal sinus.

The superficial cerebral veins display a great number of *variations* and are in anastomosis with one another (Delmas et al. 1951, Dilenge 1962, Krayenbühl and Yasargil 1965). Around the pole of the insula due to anastomoses between the precentral, parietal, superficial middle cerebral and temporooccipital veins (*anastomotic vein;* Fig. 91/6 and 15) their development is always a function of the others. Delmas and his associates (1951)

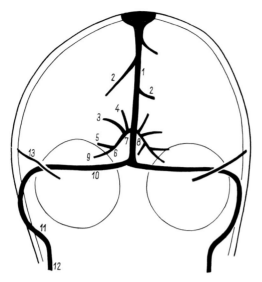

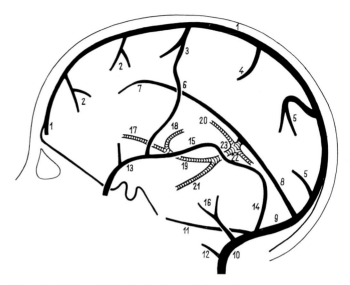

FIG. 90. Veins of the brain. Anteroposterior view. (1) Superior sagittal sinus; (2) frontoparietal veins; (3) thalamostriate vein; (4) posterior septal vein; (5) hippocampal vein; (6) basal vein; (7) vein of the septum pellucidum; (8) internal cerebral vein; (9) lenticulostriate veins; (10) transverse sinus; (11) sigmoid sinus; (12) internal jugular vein; (13) sphenoparietal sinus.

FIG. 91. Veins of the brain. Lateral view. (1) Superior sagittal sinus; (2) frontal veins; (3) precentral veins; (4) parietal veins; (5) occipital veins; (6) superior anastomotic vein; (7) inferior sagittal sinus; (8) straight sinus; (9) transverse sinus; (10) sigmoid sinus; (11) superior petrosal sinus; (12) inferior petrosal sinus; (13) superficial middle cerebral vein; (14) temporooccipital vein; (15) inferior anastomotic vein; (16) temporal vein; (17) vein of the septum pellucidum; (18) thalamostriate vein; (19) internal cerebral vein; (20) posterior vein of the corpus callosum; (21) basal vein; (22) superior cerebellar veins; (23) great cerebral vein.

brought this into connection with the dominant and nondominant hemispheres. The superficial middle cerebral vein sometimes empties into the superior petrosal sinus.

De Dominicis and his co-workers (1964) distinguish the following four types of the superficial cerebral veins: few veins with abundant communications (23 per cent), uniform veins with medium diameters (38 per cent), few large vessels with scanty collateral network (13 per cent), vessels of various size (26 per cent). The authors demonstraed these variations with serial angiography.

The *superior* (Figs 91/22, 113/29) and *inferior* (Fig. 112/15) *cerebellar veins*, vessels of the upper surface, run to the transverse sinus, the straight sinus or, below the tentorium, to the great cerebral vein. The postero-latero-inferior veins (Fig. 114/20) pass toward the sigmoid sinus or, ascending, toward the superior petrosal and transverse sinuses. From the flocculus, the *petrosal vein* empties into the inferior or the superior petrosal sinus (Krayenbühl and Yasargil 1965, Mine 1971).

2. *Internal veins of the brain.*

Centrally placed, these vessels drain the basal ganglia. It is by the confluence of the following three vessels that the *internal cerebral vein* (Figs 90/8, 91/19, 113/18) is formed by the union of three veins around the interventricular foramen.

Vein of the septum pellucidum (Figs 90/7, 91/17, 113/20, 114/10) drains the septum pellucidum and the caudate nucleus. It is often double. The vein courses from the front backward and upward to the interventricular foramen. Passing 1 mm laterally to the midline, it has a length of about 15 mm (Baumgartner et al. 1963).

The *thalamostriate vein* (Figs 90/3, 91/18, 112/11, 113/19, 114/11) returns blood from the internal capsule and the striatum from behind forward along the stria terminalis, parallel with the internal cerebral vein.

The *choroid vein* drains the choroid plexus. It courses from behind forward in the lateral ventricles (Ben Amor et al. 1971). The internal cerebral vein runs parallel with its contralateral partner in the tela choroidea of the third ventricle. Besides the above veins it also receives the *internal occipital vein* and unites with the basal vein to open into the great cerebral vein.

The *basal vein* (Figs 90/6, 91/21, 112/12, 113/21, 114/13) returns the blood from the base of the brain (insula, hippocampus, olfactory gyrus, peduncles and pons) to the great cerebral vein (*venae insulares, hippocampi;* Fig. 90/5; *venae gyri olfactorii, cerebrales anteriores, pedunculares, pontis*). The *lateral mesenchephalic vein*, originating from the confluence of the venae pontis, posterior inferior cerebellar

156

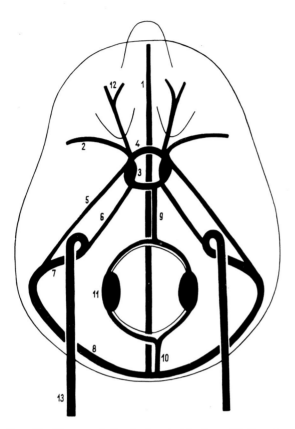

FIG. 92. Sinuses of the brain. Axial view. (*1*) Superior sagittal sinus; (*2*) sphenoparietal sinus; (*3*) cavernous sinus; (*4*) anterior and posterior intercavernous sinuses; (*5*) superior petrosal sinus; (*6*) inferior petrosal sinus; (*7*) sigmoid sinus; (*8*) transverse sinus; (*9*) basilar plexus; (*10*) occipital sinus; (*11*) vertebral venous plexuses; (*12*) superior ophthalmic vein; (*13*) internal jugular vein.

transverse sinus (Krayenbühl and Yasargil 1965). The vena anastomotica mesencephali lateralis persistens is a rare variation. It is the continuation of the basal vein in the superior petrosal sinus and has been observed in 0·1 to 0·2 per cent (Wolf et al 1963).

Sinuses of the brain. Certain sinuses (cavernous and sigmoid) are compressible, others have rigid walls. The connection between their dilatation in the direction of blood flow and the thoracic sucking action has already been referred to above.

1. *Superior sinus group.* The *superior sagittal sinus* (Figs 90/1, 91/1, 92/1, 112/8, 113/13, 114/4, 115/10) runs backward above the hemispheres from the crista galli to the internal occipital protuberance. Its cross-section is triangular; the sinus becomes wider in its backward course. The diameter measures 0·95 cm (0·5 to 1·35 cm) at the beginning, and 2·23 cm (1·7 to 2·8 cm) at the orifice (Portela-Gomes 1964). There are dilatations (lacunae) in the middle portion. The Pacchonian granulations protrude into these venous lacunae. The sinus receives the superior cerebral veins and, veins from the pericranium, furthermore, through the lacunae, the meningeal and diploic veins.

The *inferior sagittal sinus* (Figs 91/7, 112/8, 113/12, 114/9, 115/10) describes a great curve at the inferior concave border or at a distance of 1 cm at most of the falx cerebri and courses until its juncture with the tentorium (Hempel and Elmohamed 1971). The anterior part of the sinus does not always run along the border of the falx cerebri. It collects several small veins from the falx cerebri and the attached parts of the hemispheres.

The *straight sinus* (Figs 91/8, 113/11, 114/16) runs from the union of the inferior sagittal sinus and the great cerebral vein in the tentorium toward the internal occipital protuberance. It meets the superior sagittal sinus in the confluence of the sinuses. Its

veins and petrosal vein, opens into the basal vein (Wackenheim et al. 1971). The basal vein winds round the cerebral peduncle and follows from below an upward medial course.

The *great cerebral vein* (Figs 91/23, 113/17, 114/12) is a 1 cm long solitary trunk, which forms a convex arch downward below the splenium of the corpus callosum and continues in the straight sinus. The frequently calcified pineal body is situated below the vessel. It receives tributaries also from the posterior part of the corpus callosum and the upper surface of the cerebellum (*posterior veins of the corpus callosum*, Figs 91/20, 113/28; *superior*, Figs 91/22, 113/29; and *precentral cerebellar veins*).

Variations are rare among the larger internal cerebral veins, but the minor branches show great variability (Johanson 1954). The basal vein is sometimes rudimentary. The great cerebral vein may be absent or very short. In the latter case there may be a dilatation at its orifice (Hempel and Elmohamed 1971). The superior petrosal sinus may open into the superficial middle cerebral vein or the

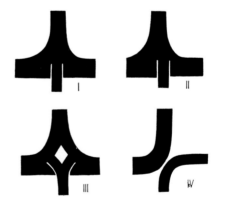

FIG. 93. Variations of the confluence of sinuses. I, normal type; II, slightly lateral opening of the superior sagittal sinus; III, bifurcation of the end of the superior sagittal and the straight sinuses; IV, the superior sagittal sinus joins the right, the straight sinus the left transverse sinus.

157

cross-section forms an equilateral triangle with the apex pointing upward. The diameter at the orifice of the straight sinus is 0·4 to 0·5 cm (Paturet 1958).

The *confluence of the sinuses* (Figs 93, 112/7) is formed by the union of the straight and the superior sagittal sinuses. It is drained by the transverse sinus. The confluence presents, according to Clara (1953), the typical reversed "T" shape in the midline in 20 per cent of the cases (Fig. 93/I). The orifice of the superior sagittal sinus is slightly displaced to the right in 50 per cent (Fig. 93/II). In 30 per cent the superior sagittal and the straight sinuses divide resembling a fork in shape. Sinuses so formed unite in the transverse sinus of the same side (Fig. 93/III). The straight sinus continues frequently in the left transverse sinus (Fig. 93/IV). Variations cover a wide range (Elmohamed and Hempel 1966). In case of bilateral rudimentary transverse sinus, the superior sagittal sinuses open into the internal jugular vein mediated by the two occipital sinuses (Chiriac et al. 1972). The transverse sinus and the internal jugular vein are often wider on the right than on the left side (Gejrot and Lauren 1964).

The *transverse sinus* (Figs 90/10, 91/9, 92/8, 112/6, 113/9, 114/17, 115/9) extends laterally from the internal occipital protuberance, in the transverse groove to the posterior border of the petrous part of the temporal bone. Its diameter measures 0·8 cm (0·5 to 1·2 cm) on the right, and 0·65 cm (0·3 to 1·2 cm) on the left side (Gejrot and Lauren 1964). It drains the occipital, superior cerebellar and some diploic veins. The transverse sinus may be unilaterally absent (Lindgren 1954). It sometimes receives an accessory sinus (parasinus sagittalis) from the occipital area (Elmohamed and Hempel 1966).

The *sigmoid sinus* (Figs 90/11, 91/10, 92/7, 112/5, 113/8, 114/18, 115/8) is the continuation of the transverse sinus, courses with an "S" curve from the margin of the tentorium cerebelli in the grooves of the occipital and petrosal bones in the direction of the jugular foramen and terminates there at the beginning of the internal jugular vein. The cross-section of the sinus is semicircular, its length and shape are variable. The superior petrosal sinus opens into the initial portion of the sinus. The sigmoid sinus communicates with the external veins of the skull via the mastoid emissary and the posterior condylar emissary veins.

The *occipital sinus* (Figs 92/10, 112/16, 114/19), the smallest of the superior sinuses, runs from the confluence of the sinuses to the foramen magnum. Bifurcating there, it winds round the foramen and empties into the superior bulb of the internal jugular vein. The occipital sinus is in communication with the internal vertebral venous plexus (Fig.

92/11; Zolnai 1960). Das and Hasan (1970) studying 200 cadavers found it in 64·5 per cent, and in 22·5 per cent the occipital sinus was doubled.

2. *Inferior sinus group.* The *cavernous sinus* (Figs 92/3, 113/16, 115/14) is the main area of drainage for the inferior sinuses and, in particular, for the base of the brain. Placed at the root of the greater wing of the sphenoid bone on the sides of the sella turcica, the sinus has an oval cross-section and extends from the superior orbital fissure to the petrous part of the temporal bone. The cranial nerves III, IV and V/1 run along the outer wall of the sinus, and its course traverses the internal carotid artery, cranial nerve VI and the sympathetic plexus. The average length of the cavernous sinus is 2 cm, its width 1 cm (Paturet 1958). The sinus may be missing on one side (Elliott 1963). The bilateral cavernous sinuses are in communication anteriorly and posteriorly at the bottom of the hypophyseal fossa and behind the dorsum sellae via the *intercavernous sinus* (Figs 92/4, 115/15). Further communications exist with the pterygoid plexus and the internal carotid venous plexus by means of the venous plexus of the foramen ovale, with the facial vein by means of the superior ophthalmic vein, and with the internal vertebral venous network via the network of basilar sinuses. The cavernous sinus receives the sphenoparietal sinus anterolaterally, while the petrosal sinuses emerge from its posterolateral apex. It is via the latter that a greater part of the blood is carried from the cavernous to the sigmoid sinus. The other way of venous return is via the network of basilar sinuses. The cavernous sinus is more compressible from the outside than the other sinuses because only one of its walls consists of bone (Tönnis and Schiefer 1959).

The *sphenoparietal sinus* (Figs 90/13, 92/2, 112/13, 115/16) courses medially along the posterior edge of the greater wing of the sphenoid bone to the cavernous sinus. It collects the blood from the dural veins.

The *superior petrosal sinus* (Figs 91/11, 92/5, 112/9, 113/14, 115/13) runs from the cavernous sinus backward and laterally at the upper border of the pyramid in an approximately horizontal plane to the sigmoid or to the transverse sinus. It forms a significant communication between the inferior and the superior sinuses; it receives some of the inferior cerebellar and cerebral veins.

The *inferior petrosal sinus* (Figs 91/12, 92/6, 113/15, 115/12) represents another important communication joining the cavernous and sigmoid sinuses and the internal jugular vein. It may occur that the inferior petrosal sinus opens into the vertebral veins (Shiu et al. 1968). The inferior petrosal sinus pursues a backward and downward lateral course toward the jugular foramen from the posteroinferior part of the cavernous sinus along the posteroinferior border of the petrous portion of the temporal bone. It terminates in front of the cranial nerves IX, X and XI. The inferior petrosal sinus receives the *veins of the labyrinth* and some of the inferior superficial veins of the pons and cerebellum. It is in communication with the *venous network of the hypoglossal canal* (Krayenbühl and Yasargil 1965).

The network of basilar sinuses (*basilar plexus*, Fig. 92/9) consists of interconnecting venous channels in the dura mater; it extends from the cavernous and inferior petrosal sinuses to the internal vertebral venous plexus.

Ophthalmic veins. The functional role of the orbital veins lies in anastomoses maintaining collateral circulation. They have no valves, thus allowing blood to flow in any direction. They communicate anteriorly with the facial vein, inferiorly with the pterygoid plexus, medially (via the ethmoidal veins) with one another, and posteriorly with the cavernous sinus.

The *superior ophthalmic vein* (Figs 92/12, 115/17), running backward in the upper part of the orbit, enters the cranial cavity through the superior orbital fissure and opens into the cavernous sinus. Its diameter is 0·2 to 0·3 cm at the origin. Aron-Rosa and his associates (1966b) distinguish three segments of the vein. The first, bending obliquely upward and backward, the second, bending upward and outward, form an arch. The third segment, bending from the lateral to the medial direction, enters the cranial cavity. It drains the greater part of the veins of the orbit (*ethmoidal veins*, Fig. 115/18; *lacrimal, vorticose veins; central vein of the retina*). It has several communications with the inferior ophthalmic vein.

The *inferior ophthalmic vein* (Fig. 115/20) is considerably thinner than the corresponding superior vessel. It is formed by the union of the obliquely running veins at the base of the eyeground and opens into the superior ophthalmic vein or directly into the cavernous sinus. Besides the connection with the superior orbital vein, it anastomoses with the facial and lacrimal veins and, through the inferior orbital fissure, with the pterygoid plexus (Fig. 115/21).

The **diploic veins,** the veins of the cranial bones, are situated in the cancellous bone. They communicate with the external veins through the inner and the outer tables of the skull. After forming numerous anastomoses with one another, the diploic veins open into the sinuses or into the veins of the epicranial aponeurosis (*frontal, anterior* and *posterior temporal, occipital diploic veins*).

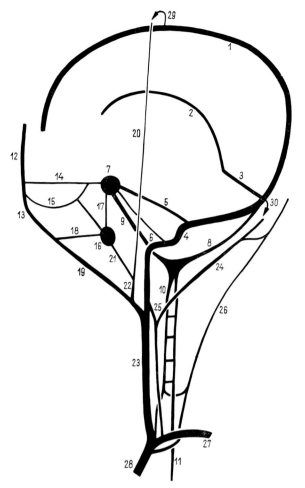

FIG. 94. Diagram showing the collateral circulation of the cerebral veins. (*1*) Superior sagittal sinus; (*2*) inferior sagittal sinus; (*3*) straight sinus; (*4*) transverse and sigmoid sinuses; (*5*) superior petrosal sinus; (*6*) inferior petrosal sinus; (*7*) cavernous sinus; (*8*) occipital sinus; (*9*) basilar plexus; (*10*) vertebral vein; (*11*) internal and external vertebral plexuses; (*12*) nasofrontal vein; (*13*) angular vein; (*14*) superior ophthalmic vein; (*15*) inferior ophthalmic vein; (*16*) pterygoid plexus; (*17*) venous plexus of the foramen ovale; (*18*) deep facial vein; (*19*) facial vein; (*20*) superficial temporal vein; (*21*) maxillary vein; (*22*) retromandibular vein; (*23*) internal jugular vein; (*24*) occipital vein; (*25*) external jugular vein; (*26*) deep cervical vein; (*27*) subclavian vein; (*28*) brachiocephalic vein; (*29*) parietal emissary vein; (*30*) occipital emissary vein.

Collateral circulation of the cranial veins

The system of cranial veins maintains a balanced circulatory condition via the intracranial and extracranial communications (Fig. 94).

1. The internal communications ensure harmonic communication between the superior and inferior groups of sinuses (superior and inferior petrosal sinus), between the various external veins (superior and inferior anastomic veins) as also between the internal and external veins (basal vein).

2. The external communications maintain collateral circulation between the intracranial and pericranial network of veins. The following vessels serve the purposes of external communication: a) The emissary veins (Figs 94/29 and 30) consist of veins (parietal, mastoid, condylar and occipital emissary veins) and venous plexuses which pass through the openings of the cranial wall (venous plexus of the hypoglossal canal, the foramen ovale and the internal carotid). The latter maintain a significant communication with the pterygoid plexus. The emissary veins have a valvular function if the intracranial vessels are overfilled. In contrast to the intracranial veins, they fill up to 70 to 90 per cent in cases of carotid and vertebral angiographies (Rabinov 1964). b) Superior and inferior ophthalmic veins (Fig. 94/14 and 15). Devoid of valves, these vessels are able to bring about collateral circulation not only between the cavernous sinus and the facial vein but also between each other. c) The internal vertebral plexus (Fig. 94/11), via its connection with the inferior and superior systems of sinuses (basilar plexus, occipital sinus), maintains extensive communications with the veins of the spinal cord.

Phlebography of the head and neck

In the "venous phase" of carotid and vertebral angiographies, the cerebral veins fill between 2 to 20 seconds in various succession. Simultaneously with the improving methods, the route of the contrast material can be followed bringing thus forward the functional study of this venous system. Of the collateral vessels, the internal vertebral plexus and the emissary veins can be most frequently visualized. The orbital veins fill mostly through the facial or frontal veins (Déjean and Boudet 1951, Lombardi and Passerini 1968). Despite its numerous communications, the ophthalmic vein can be demonstrated only by angular puncture or via the frontal vein (Nebauer and Süsse 1966, Aron-Rosa et al. 1966b). Demonstration of the pterygoid plexus requires retrograde filling through the retromandibular vein (Scheunemann and Schrudde 1964). The facial veins do not fill with carotid angiography on account of the numerous anastomoses (Bargman 1957). The veins of the face can be visualized if the facial vein is filled (Süsse and Kunits 1966). A better visualization of the posterior sinuses is achieved by retrograde sinography than by vertebral angiography (Gejrot and Lauren 1964). Retrograde filling of the internal jugular vein is suitable for the filling and demonstration of the anastomoses of the cavernous sinus (Wende and Ciba 1968). The cavernous sinus can be filled via

the orbital veins as well (Aron-Rosa et al. 1966a). Being of slight practical use, diplography has not found wide acceptance (Fischgold et al. 1952).

In *postmortem phlebography* the sinuses appear to fill wider according to their anatomical shape. Identification is made difficult by the superposition of their intensive shadows and the synchronous filling of the superficial and deep cerebral veins. However, axial projection allows good orientation and makes up for the limitations of the other two directions.

Anteroposterior pictures of the neck (Fig. 110) show the bilateral shadow of the *internal jugular vein* (Fig. 110/8) along the vertebral column. The upper segment appears in the projection of the mandible, while the further course is free. The inferior bulb of the vein is visible behind the sternoclavicular articulation. The *vertebral veins* (Fig. 110/14) pursue a slightly curved outward course in the projection of the vertebral column. Their lower end is lost behind the internal jugular vein. The *vertebral plexuses*, covering the vertebral column, further the *esophageal veins*, *tracheal veins* (Fig. 110/16) and *impar thyroid plexus* cannot be separated from each other. Only the transverse course of the *intervertebral veins* (Fig. 110/15) can be observed separate from the others. Lying laterally to the internal vein, the *external jugular vein* (Fig. 110/9) follows a downward course in the soft tissues.

In the **lateral view** (Fig. 111) the *internal jugular vein* (Figs 111/8 and 9) is situated in the plane of the transverse processes. The bilateral shadows are usually superimposed. The various parts of the *facial* and *retromandibular veins* (Fig. 111/14) cannot be distinguished. The *pterygoid plexus* (Fig. 111/13) appears in the projection of the upper end of the ascending mandibular ramus. It can rarely be filled completely. The *external jugular vein* and the *anterior external vertebral plexus* (Fig. 111/12) appear in front of the vertebral column, while the deep cervical veins show together with the posterior venous plexus behind it.

Anteroposterior pictures of the skull (Fig. 112) show the course of the *superior sagittal sinus* (Fig. 112/8) to fall on the calvaria orthodiagraphically, thus its characteristic triangular cross-section is always visible. The cerebral veins and sinuses projected in the median sagittal planes owing to their sheltered position, cannot be identified, whereas the laterally turning branches of the deep veins (*thalamostriate, hippocampal, basal* and *lenticulostriate veins*, Fig. 112/11 and 12) show a characteristic course between the superior cerebral veins and the confluence of the sinuses on both sides of the midline. The bilateral *internal cerebral veins*, forming a semicircle, pursue a "V" or "U" shaped course at the side of the pineal body (Wolf et al. 1963). The medially turning section of the postnasal segment of the *superior ophthalmic vein* can sometimes be filled. The *inferior ophthalmic vein* courses downward in a lateromedial direction (Aron-Rosa et al. 1966b). The *transverse sinus* (Fig. 112/6), crossing the orbit transversely, runs laterally, to continue as the *sigmoid sinus* (Fig. 112/5) which, forming a right angle, runs downward and medially to terminate in the *internal jugular vein* (Fig. 112/4). The latter begins its steep descending course with a slight lateral bend. The *superficial middle cerebral vein* (Fig. 112/14) and the *sphenoparietal sinus* (Fig. 112/13) can sometimes be followed above the upper bend of the sigmoid sinus. Wolf and his co-workers (1963) demonstrated *in vivo* the various superficial cerebral veins in 55 to 70 per cent. The *vertebral plexus* (Fig. 112/18) lying in front of the vertebral column, partly obscures from view the course of the *vertebral veins*. The *occipital sinus* (Fig. 112/16) and the *network of the basilar sinuses* appear in the projection of the base of the cranium, in the area of the clivus.

In **lateral view** (Fig. 113), the *superior sagittal sinus* (Fig. 113/13) and the characteristic course of the *superior cerebral veins* (Figs 113/23 to 26) are easily recognizable. The superior sagittal sinus, forming a right angle at the confluence of sinuses, continues into the transverse sinus. Because of the overlapping their shadows, the *sigmoid sinuses* (Fig. 113/8) cannot be easily separated. The *cavernous sinus* (Fig. 113/16) can rarely be filled in in *vivo* cerebral angiograms (Krayenbühl and Yasargil 1965). The negative shadow of the carotid siphon is sometimes visible in the cavernous sinus if it is filled (Gvozdanović 1952). The *superior ophthalmic vein* can be visualized only when directly filled (Aron-Rosa et al. 1966b). The intensive bone shadow makes it difficult to differentiate the *inferior* (Fig. 113/15) and *superior* (Fig. 113/14) *petrosal sinuses* at the inferior and superior borders of the petrous part of the temporal bone. The *straight sinus* (Fig. 113/11) and the curved *inferior sagittal sinus* (Fig. 113/12) traverse the cranial cavity from above downward and backward. The juncture of the sickle-shaped inferior sagittal sinus and the straight sinus clearly reveals the site of the orifice of the *great cerebral vein* (Fig. 113/17). The latter together with the *internal cerebral vein* (Fig. 113/18) describe a mildly curved "S" shape (Krayenbühl and Yasargil 1965). The internal cerebral vein is identifiable by its dorsally convex course. The *basal vein* (Fig. 113/21) forming a slightly downward convex arch, passes upward from the front. The venous angle formed by the *vein of the septum pellucidum*

(Fig. 113/20) and the *thalamostriate vein* (Fig. 113/19) is clearly visible (Krayenbühl and Richter 1952). Several methods have been suggested for the reliable identification of the interventricular foramen (Curry and Culberth 1951, Schmidt-Wittkamp and Roscher 1966). The *temporooccipital vein* (Fig. 113/27) describes a backward curve in the angle formed by the straight and transverse sinuses. The *superficial middle cerebral vein* (Fig. 113/22) forms a forward convex arch downward to the projection of the sella turcica. Of the veins of the face the branches of the *facial* and *retromandibular veins* (Fig. 113/26) as well as the large *pterygoid plexus* (Fig. 113/35) are projected upon the ascending portion of the mandible and upon the area of the sphenoid bone. The *ophthalmic veins* converge backward on the roof and the floor of the orbit.

In the **axial view** (Fig. 115) the *internal jugular vein* (Fig. 115/7) pursues a downward course from the jugular foramen along the vertebral column; it crosses first the *sigmoid sinus* (Fig. 115/8) and then the *transverse sinus* (Fig. 115/9). A characteristic bilateral double loop resembling the shape of an "8" is thus formed in the temporooccipital region. The *superior sagittal sinus* (Fig. 115/10), dividing the skull sagittally, commencing in front in the projection of the septum of the nose, courses backward. As in anteroposterior view, the sinus obscures all other structures lying in the median sagittal plane. The *cavernous* (Fig. 115/14) and *intercavernous sinuses* (Fig. 115/15) form in this projection a ring around the sella. The *superior* (Fig. 115/13) and *inferior petrosal sinuses* (Fig. 115/12) are more clearly visible in the projection of the upper and lower border of the pyramid than in the other two projections. The anteriorly convex course of the *sphenoparietal sinus* (Fig. 115/16) which follows the lesser wing of the sphenoid bone as well as the lateral temporal veins can be separately identified, whereas the smaller deep veins around the median plane are not differentiable. The three segments and most side branches of the *superior ophthalmic vein* (Fig. 115/17) are clearly visible. The *external jugular vein* (Fig. 115/24) crosses first the projection of the transverse sinus, then that of the sigmoid sinus. It unites from two branches behind the projection of the mandibular angle. The projection of the *pterygoid plexus* (Fig. 115/22) and its communications with the orbital veins appear behind the wall of the orbit. The *vertebral veins*, the *vertebral plexus* and the *suboccipital plexus* (Fig. 115/25) appear in the area of the occipital bone and the foramen magnum. The branches of the suboccipital plexus cannot be identified separately.

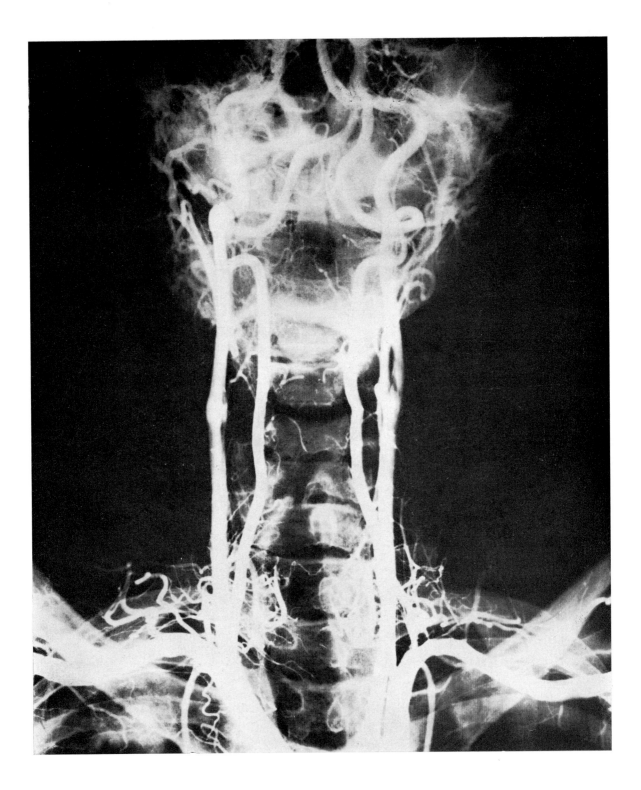

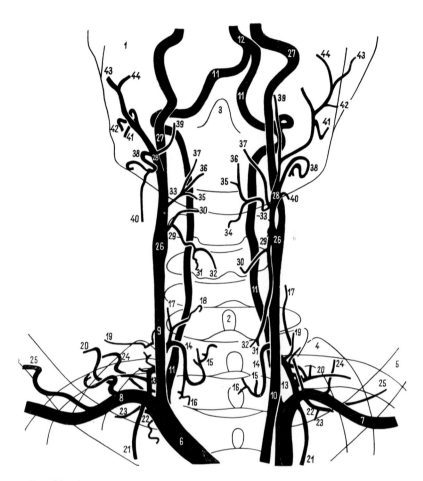

FIG. 95. The common carotid artery, subclavian artery and their branches, I.
Anteroposterior view.

1. Mandible
2. Cervical vertebrae
3. Dens axis
4. 1st rib
5. Clavicle
6. Brachiocephalic trunk
7. Left subclavian artery
8. Right subclavian artery
9. Right common carotid artery
10. Left common carotid artery
11. Vertebral arteries
12. Basilar artery
13. Thyrocervical trunk
14. Inferior thyroid artery
15. Inferior laryngeal artery

16. Esophageal and tracheal branches
17. Ascending cervical artery
18. Spinal branches
19. Superficial cervical artery
20. Suprascapular artery
21. Internal thoracic artery
22. Costocervical trunk
23. Highest intercostal artery
24. Deep cervical artery
25. Transverse cervical artery
26. Carotid sinus
27. Internal carotid artery
28. External carotid artery
29. Superior thyroid artery

30. Superior laryngeal artery
31. Posterior branch
32. Anterior branch
33. Lingual artery
34. Suprahyoid branch
35. Sublingual artery
36. Dorsal lingual branches
37. Deep lingual artery
38. Facial artery
39. Ascending pharyngeal artery
40. Sternocleidomastoid branch
41. Occipital artery
42. Posterior auricular artery
43. Superficial temporal artery
44. Maxillary artery

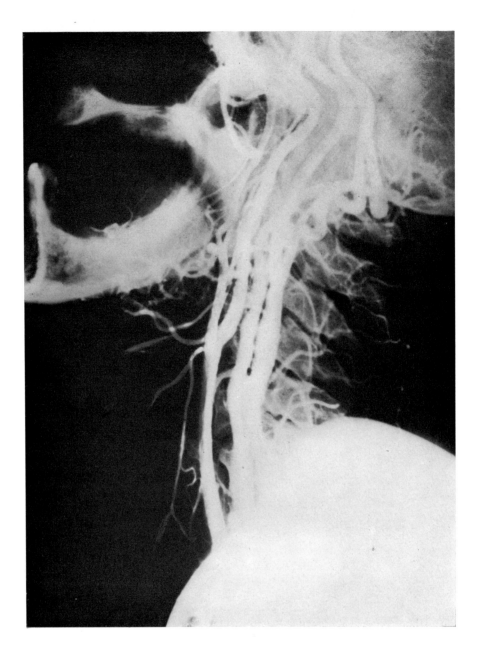

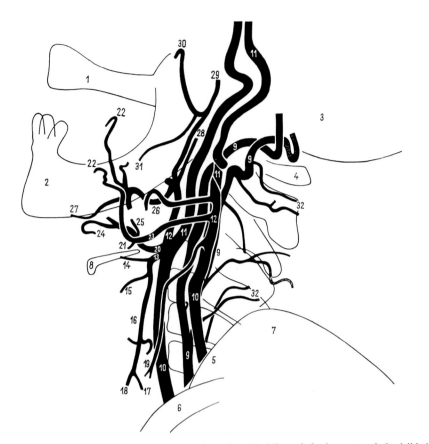

FIG. 96. The common carotid artery and its branches, II. (The subclavian artery is invisible.)
Sinistrodextral view.

1. Maxilla
2. Mandible
3. Occipital bone
4. Arch of the atlas
5. Spinous process of vertebra C7
6. Clavicle
7. Acromion
8. Hyoid bone
9. Left and right vertebral arteries
10. Left and right common carotid arteries
11. Left and right internal carotid arteries
12. Left and right external carotid arteries
13. Right superior thyroid artery
14. Infrahyoid branch
15. Sternocleidomastoid branch
16. Superior laryngeal artery
17. Posterior branch
18. Anterior branch
19. Left superior thyroid artery
20. Right lingual artery
21. Suprahyoid branch
22. Deep lingual artery
23. Left lingual artery
24. Sublingual artery
25. Dorsal lingual branches
26. Left and right facial arteries
27. Submental artery
28. Ascending pharyngeal artery
29. Superficial temporal artery
30. Maxillary artery
31. Inferior alveolar artery
32. Spinal branches of vertebral artery

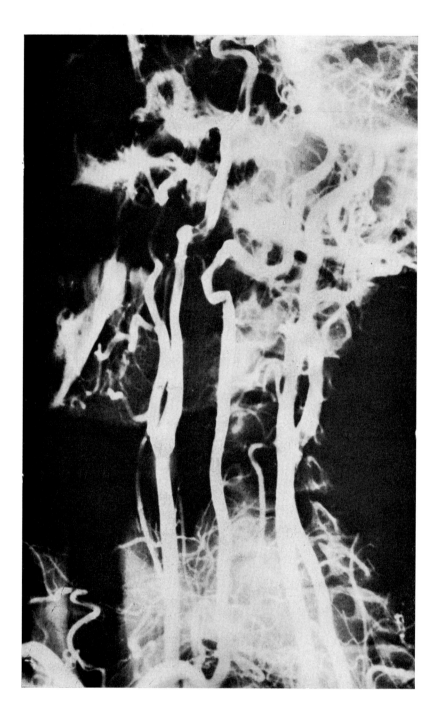

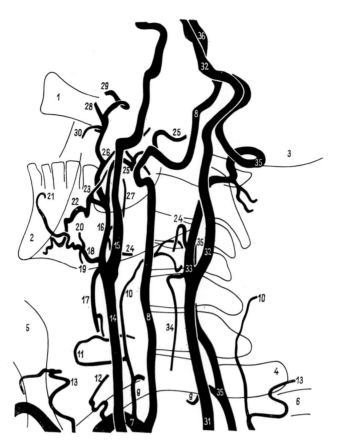

FIG. 97. The common carotid artery, subclavian artery and their branches.
III. Second oblique view.

1. Maxilla
2. Mandible
3. Occipital bone
4. Vertebra C7
5. Clavicle
6. 1st rib
7. Left subclavian artery
8. Left vertebral artery
9. Right and left thyrocervical
   trunks
10. Ascending cervical artery
11. Superficial cervical artery

12. Suprascapular artery
13. Transverse cervical artery
14. Left common carotid artery
15. Left internal carotid artery
16. Left external carotid artery
17. Left superior thyroid artery
18. Lingual artery
19. Sublingual artery
20. Dorsal lingual branch
21. Deep lingual artery
22. Facial artery
23. Ascending palatine artery
24. Sternocleidomastoid branch

25. Occipital artery
26. Posterior auricular artery
27. Ascending pharyngeal artery
28. Superficial temporal artery
29. Maxillary artery
30. Inferior alveolar artery
31. Right common carotid artery
32. Right internal carotid artery
33. Right external carotid artery
34. Right superior thyroid artery
35. Right vertebral artery
36. Basilar artery

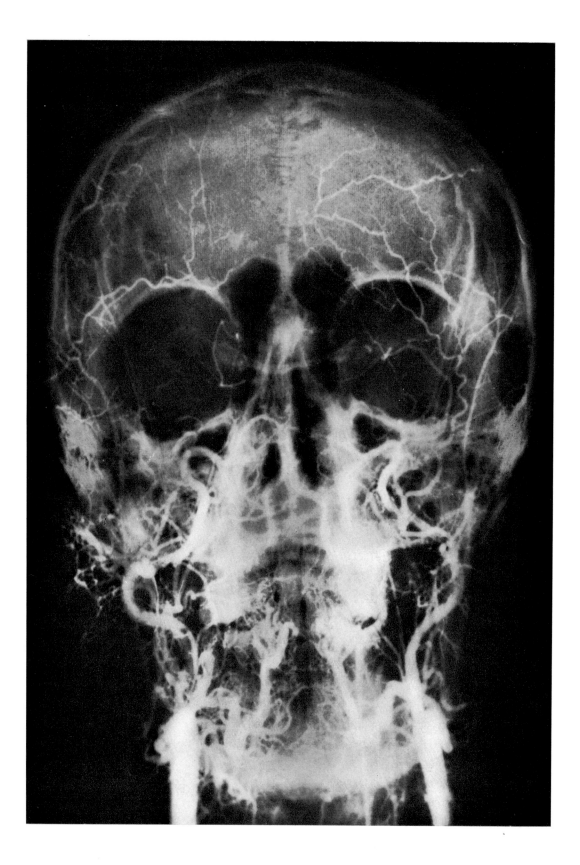

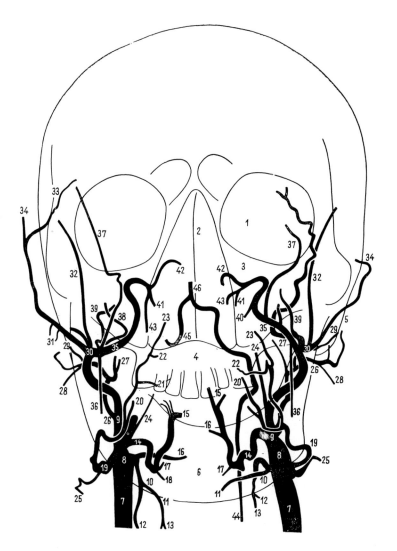

FIG. 98. The external carotid artery and its branches, I. (The internal carotid artery is ligated.)
Anteroposterior view.

1. Orbit
2. Nasal cavity
3. Maxillary sinus
4. Superior alveolar process
5. Mastoid process
6. Mandible
7. Common carotid artery
8. Carotid sinus
9. External carotid artery
10. Superior thyroid artery
11. Superior laryngeal artery
12. Posterior branch
13. Anterior branch
14. Lingual artery
15. Dorsal lingual branches
16. Deep lingual artery

17. Sublingual artery
18. Suprahyoid branch
19. Facial artery
20. Ascending palatine artery
21. Inferior labial artery
22. Superior labial artery
23. Angular artery
24. Ascending pharyngeal artery
25. Sternocleidomastoid branch
26. Occipital artery
27. Meningeal branch
28. Descending branch
29. Posterior auricular artery
30. Superficial temporal artery
31. Parotid branches

32. Middle temporal artery
33. Frontal branch
34. Parietal branch
35. Maxillary artery
36. Inferior alveolar artery
37. Middle meningeal artery
38. Accessory meningeal branch
39. Deep temporal artery
40. Posterior superior alveolar artery
41. Descending palatine artery
42. Sphenopalatine artery
43. Infraorbital artery
44. Left vertebral artery
45. Right vertebral artery
46. Basilar artery

169

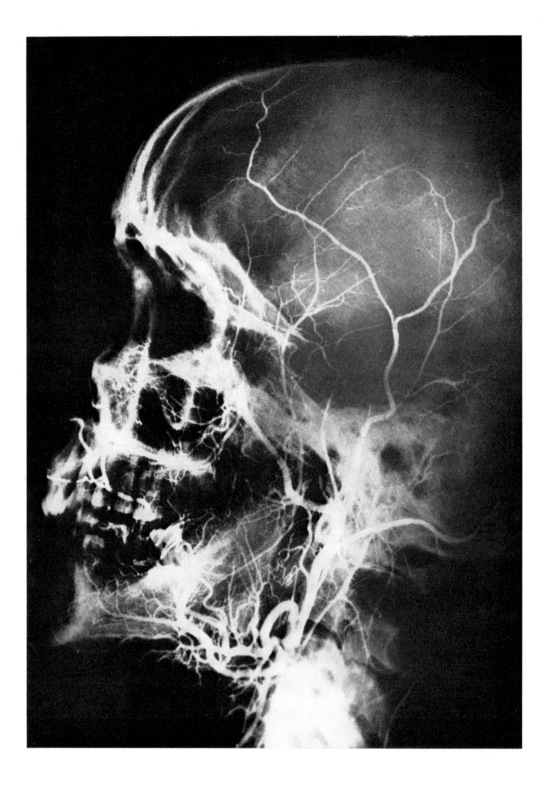

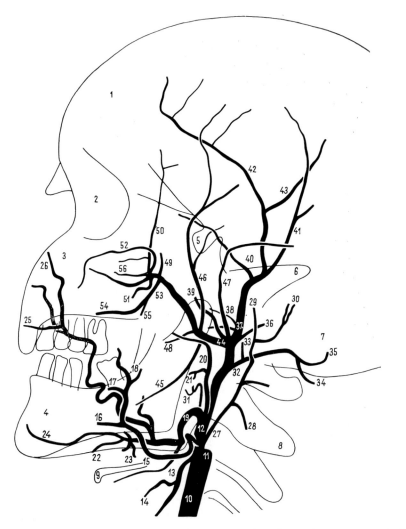

FIG. 99. The external carotid artery and its branches, II. (The internal carotid artery is ligated.)
Sinistrodextral view.

1. Frontal bone
2. Orbit
3. Maxilla
4. Mandible
5. Sella turcica
6. Temporal bone
7. Occipital bone
8. Spinous process of the axis
9. Hyoid bone
10. Right common carotid artery
11. Ligated internal carotid artery
12. External carotid artery
13. Superior thyroid artery
14. Superior laryngeal artery
15. Lingual artery
16. Sublingual artery
17. Deep lingual artery
18. Dorsal lingual branches
19. Facial artery

20. Ascending palatine artery
21. Tonsillar branch
22. Submental artery
23. Glandular branches
24. Inferior labial artery
25. Superior labial artery
26. Angular artery
27. Ascending pharyngeal artery
28. Pharyngeal branches
29. Inferior tympanic artery
30. Posterior meningeal artery
31. Sternocleidomastoid branch
32. Occipital artery
33. Mastoid branch
34. Descending branch
35. Meningeal branch
36. Posterior auricular artery
37. Superficial temporal artery
38. Parotid branches
39. Transverse facial artery
40. Zygomaticoorbital branch

41. Middle temporal artery
42. Frontal branch
43. Parietal branch
44. Maxillary artery
45. Inferior alveolar artery
46. Middle meningeal artery
47. Accessory meningeal branch
48. Masseteric artery
49. Anterior deep temporal artery
50. Posterior deep temporal artery
51. Posterior superior alveolar artery
52. Infraorbital artery
53. Descending palatine artery
54. Greater palatine artery
55. Smaller palatine arteries
56. Sphenopalatine artery, lateral, posterior and septal nasal arteries

171

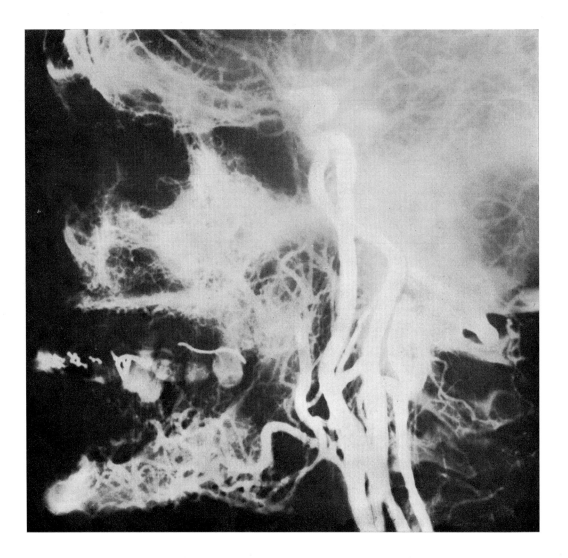

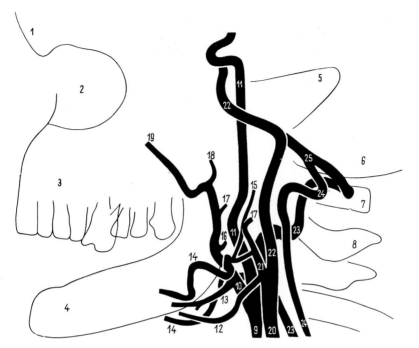

FIG. 100. Division of the common carotid artery.
Sinistrodextral view.

1. Frontal bone
2. Orbit
3. Maxilla
4. Mandible
5. Temporal bone
6. Occipital bone
7. Arch of the atlas
8. Spinous process of the axis
9. Right common carotid
   artery
10. Right external carotid
    artery
11. Right internal carotid
    artery
12. Left lingual artery
13. Right lingual artery
14. Facial artery
15. Left ascending pharyngeal
    artery
16. Occipital artery
17. Posterior auricular artery
18. Superficial temporal artery
19. Maxillary artery
20. Left common carotid ar-
    tery
21. Left external carotid artery
22. Left internal carotid artery
23. Right vertebral artery
24. Left vertebral artery
25. Basilar artery

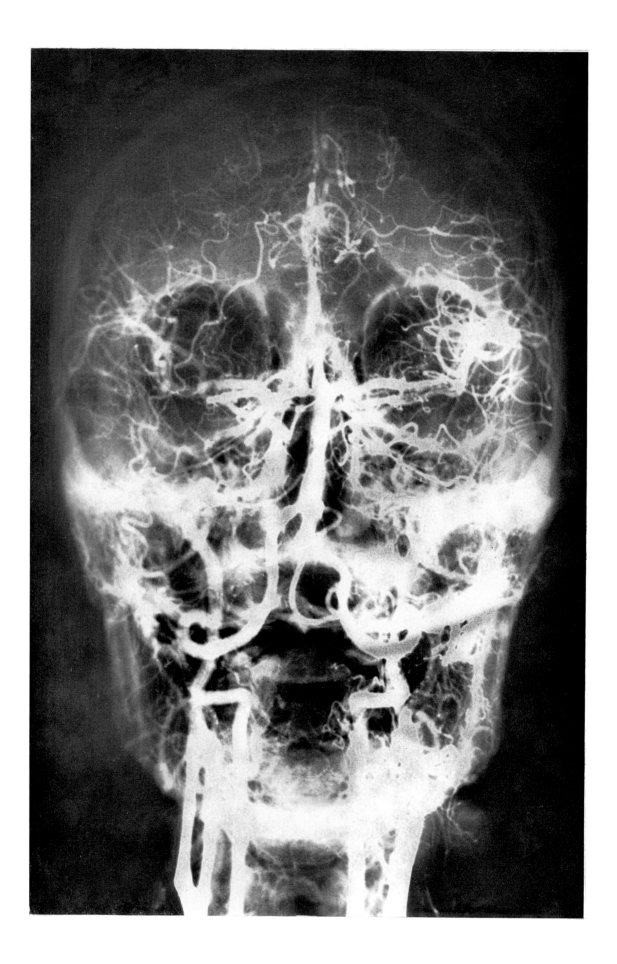

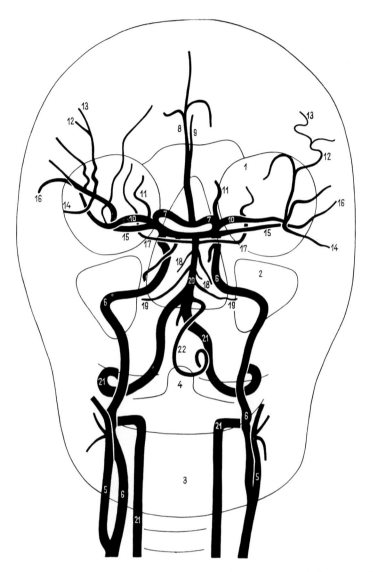

FIG. 101. The internal carotid artery, vertebral artery and their branches, I.
Anteroposterior view.

1. Orbit
2. Maxillary sinus
3. Mandible
4. Dens axis
5. External carotid artery
6. Internal carotid artery
7. Anterior cerebral artery
8. Pericallosal artery
9. Callosomarginal artery
10. Middle cerebral artery
11. Anterior choroid artery
12. Artery of the angular gyrus
13. Posterior parietal branches
14. Posterior temporal branches
15. Posterior cerebral artery
16. Temporal branches
17. Superior cerebellar artery
18. Anterior inferior cerebellar artery
19. Artery of the labyrinth
20. Basilar artery
21. Vertebral artery
22. Posterior inferior cerebellar artery

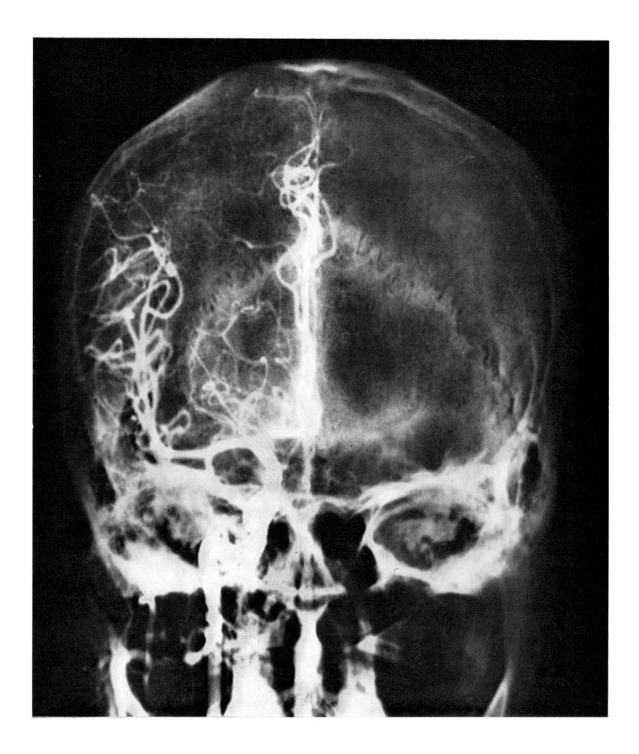

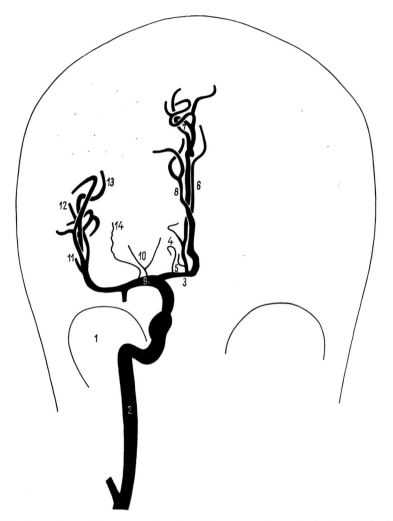

Fig. 102. The internal carotid artery and its branches, I. (Angiography in vivo by I. Gorácz.)
Anteroposterior view (20° craniocaudal inclination).

1. Orbit	*6.* Pericallosal artery	*10.* Striate branches
2. Internal carotid artery	*7.* Precentral and precuneal	*11.* Posterior temporal branches
3. Anterior cerebral artery	branches	*12.* Posterior parietal branches
4. Frontobasal artery	*8.* Callosomarginal artery	*13.* Artery of the angular gyrus
5. Frontopolar artery	*9.* Middle cerebral artery	*14.* Anterior choroid artery

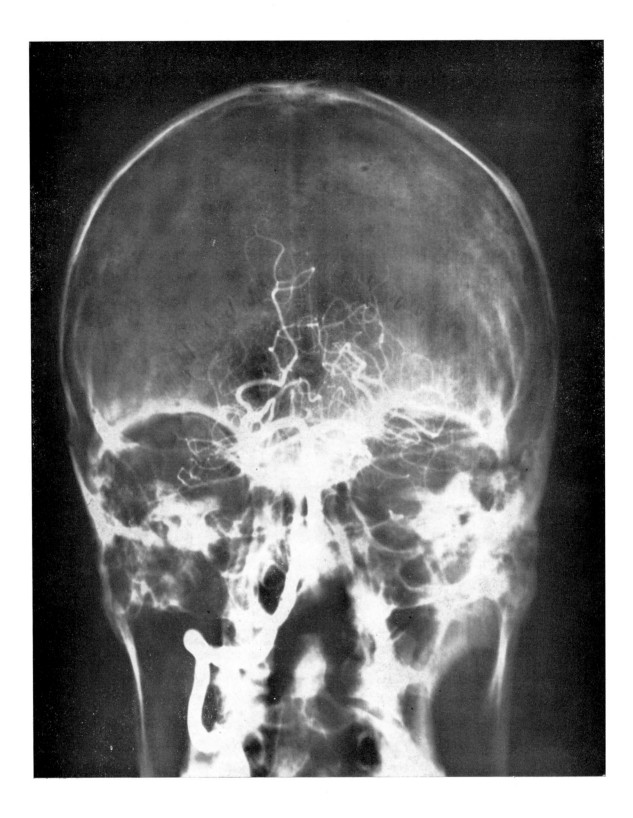

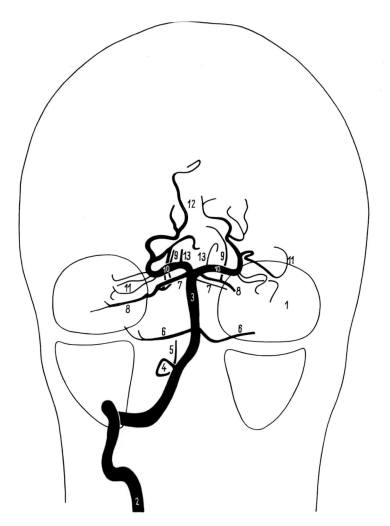

Fig. 103. The vertebral artery, basilar artery and their branches, I. (Angiography in vivo by I. Gorácz.) Anteroposterior view (20° craniocaudal inclination).

1. Orbit
2. Vertebral artery
3. Basilar artery
4. Posterior inferior cerebellar artery
5. Medial branch
6. Anterior inferior cerebellar artery
7. Superior cerebellar artery
8. Lateral branches
9. Medial branches
10. Posterior cerebral artery
11. Temporal branches
12. Occipital branches
13. Lateral and medial posterior choroid branches

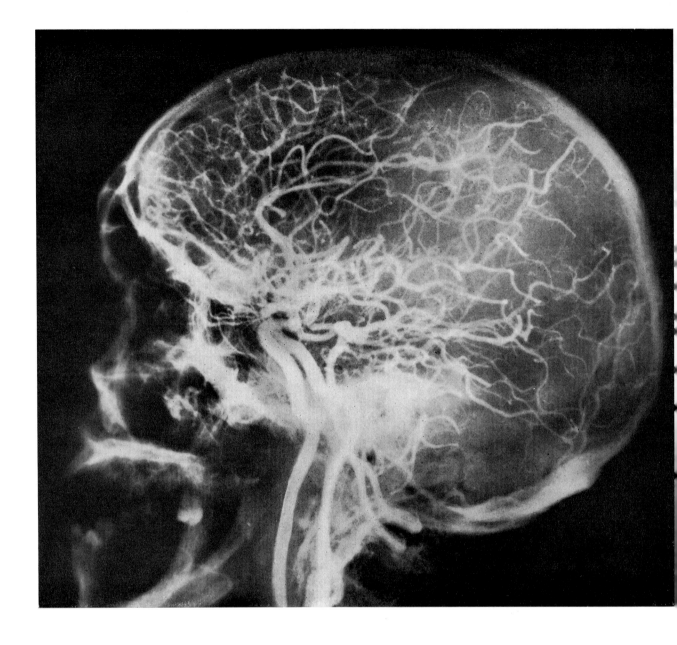

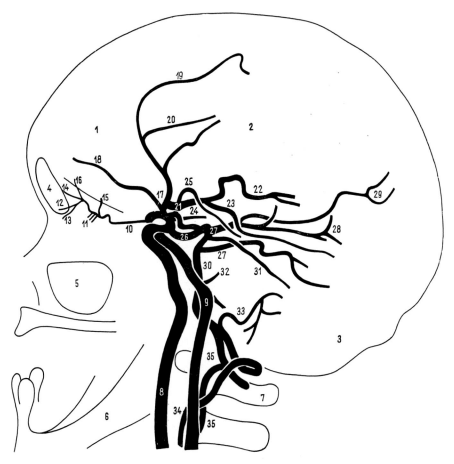

FIG. 104. The internal carotid artery, vertebral artery and their branches, II.
Sinistrodextral view.

1. Frontal bone
2. Parietal bone
3. Occipital bone
4. Frontal sinus
5. Maxillary sinus
6. Mandible
7. Arch of the atlas
8. Right internal carotid artery
9. Left internal carotid artery
10. Ophthalmic artery
11. Ciliary arteries and central artery of retina
12. Lacrimal artery
13. Supratrochlear artery
14. Supraorbital artery
15. Posterior ethmoidal artery
16. Anterior ethmoidal artery
17. Anterior cerebral artery
18. Frontopolar branch
19. Callosomarginal artery
20. Pericallosal artery
21. Middle cerebral artery
22. Posterior parietal branch
23. Artery of the gyrus angularis
24. Anterior choroid artery
25. Posterior temporal branch
26. Posterior communicating artery
27. Posterior cerebral artery
28. Temporal branches
29. Occipital branches
30. Basilar artery
31. Superior cerebellar artery
32. Anterior inferior cerebellar artery
33. Posterior inferior cerebellar artery
34. Left vertebral artery
35. Right vertebral artery

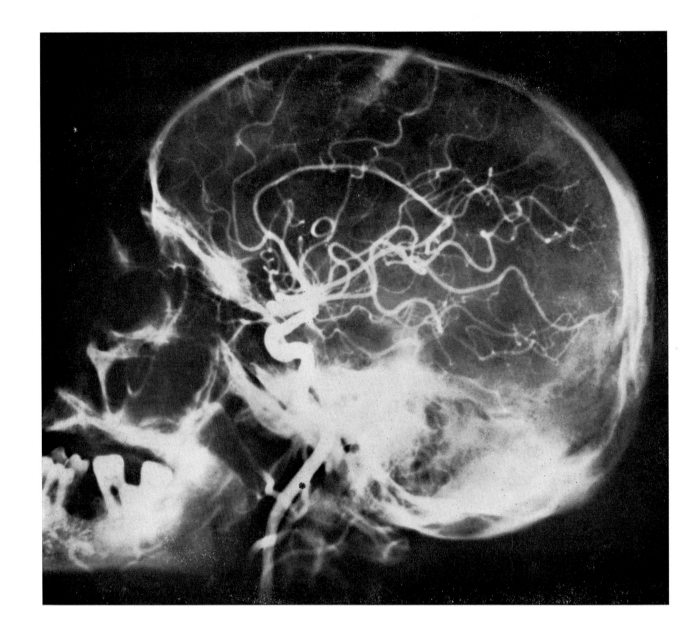

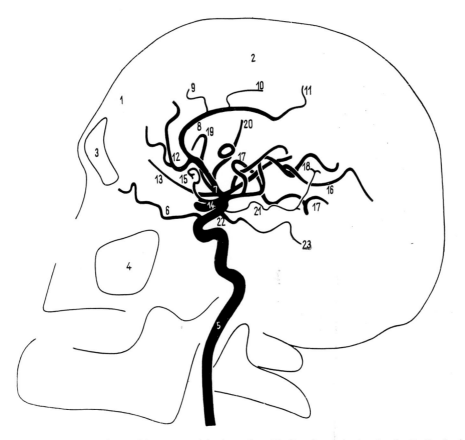

FIG. 105. The internal carotid artery and its branches, II. (Angiography in vivo by I. Gorácz.) Sinistrodextral view.

1. Frontal bone
2. Parietal bone
3. Frontal sinus
4. Maxillary sinus
5. Internal carotid artery
6. Ophthalmic artery
7. Anterior cerebral artery
8. Pericallosal artery

9. Precentral branches
10. Precuneal branches
11. Parietooccipital branches
12. Callosomarginal artery
13. Frontopolar branch
14. Middle cerebral artery
15. Ascending frontal branch
16. Artery of the angular gyrus

17. Posterior temporal branches
18. Posterior parietal branches
19. Precentral branch
20. Central branch
21. Anterior choroid artery
22. Posterior communicating artery
23. Posterior cerebral artery

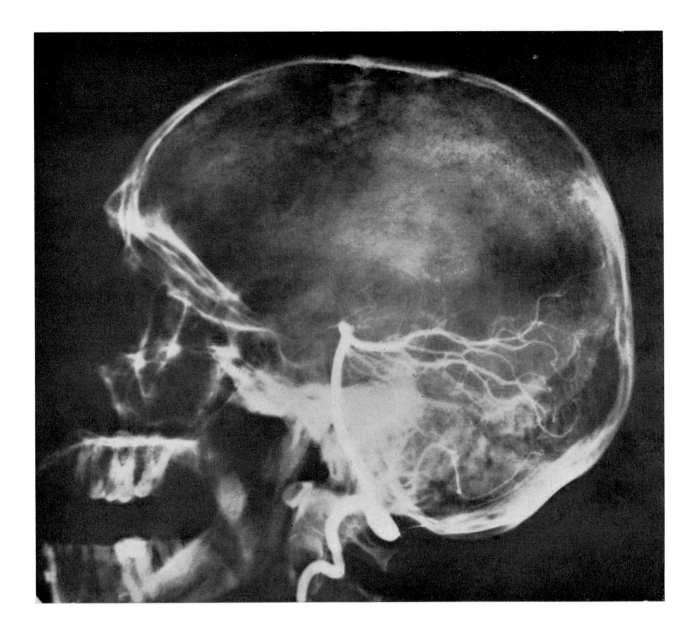

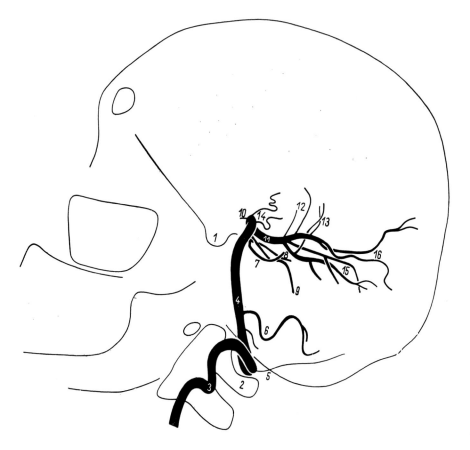

FIG. 106. The vertebral artery, basilar artery and their branches, II. (Angiography in vivo by I. Gorácz.) Sinistrodextral view.

1. Sella turcica
2. Arch of the atlas
3. Vertebral artery
4. Basilar artery
5. Extracerebral branch
6. Posterior inferior cerebellar artery, medial branch
7. Superior cerebellar artery
8. Medial branch
9. Lateral branch
10. Posterior communicating artery
11. Posterior cerebral artery
12. Medial posterior choroid branch
13. Lateral posterior choroid branch
14. Central branches
15. Temporal branches
16. Occipital branches

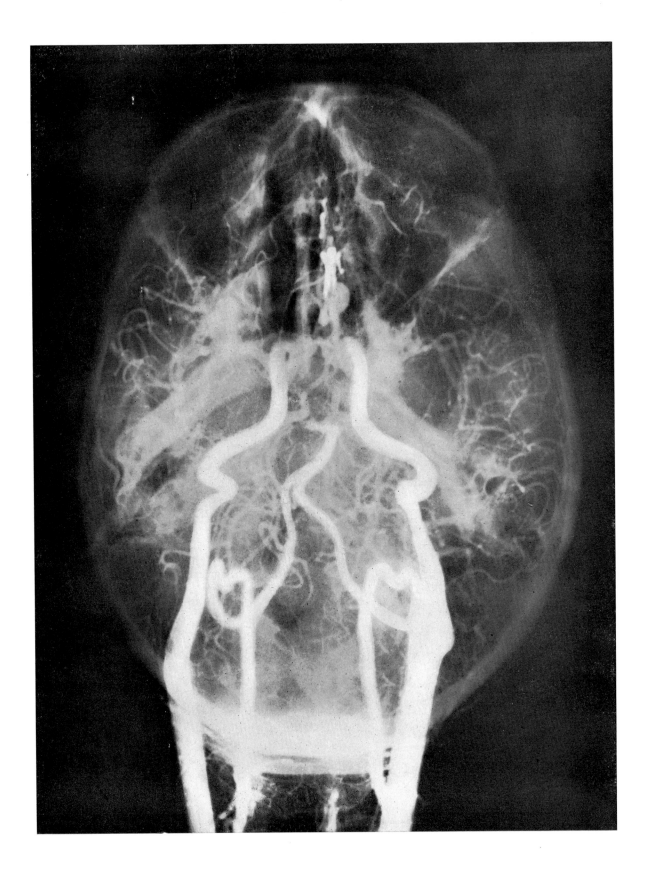

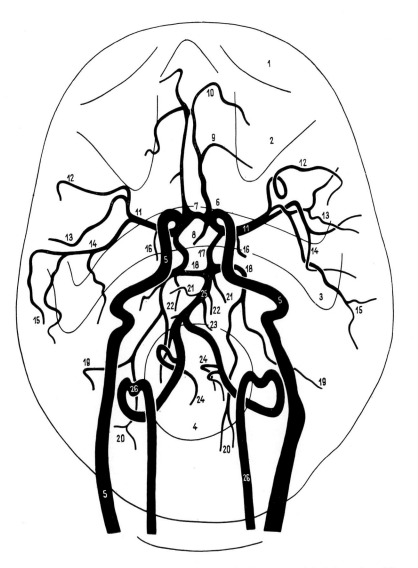

FIG. 107. The internal carotid artery, vertebral artery and their branches, III.
Submentovertical view (position Welin IV).

1. Orbit
2. Maxillary sinus
3. Mandible
4. Foramen magnum
5. Internal carotid artery
6. Anterior cerebral artery
7. Anterior communicating artery
8. Callosomarginal artery
9. Pericallosal artery
10. Frontopolar branch
11. Middle cerebral artery
12. Orbitofrontal branches
13. Parietal branches
14. Temporal branches
15. Artery of the gyrus angularis
16. Anterior choroid artery
17. Posterior communicating artery
18. Posterior cerebral artery
19. Temporal branches
20. Occipital branches
21. Artery of the labyrinth
22. Superior cerebellar arter
23. Anterior inferior cerebellar artery
24. Posterior inferior cerebellar artery
25. Basilar artery
26. Vertebral artery

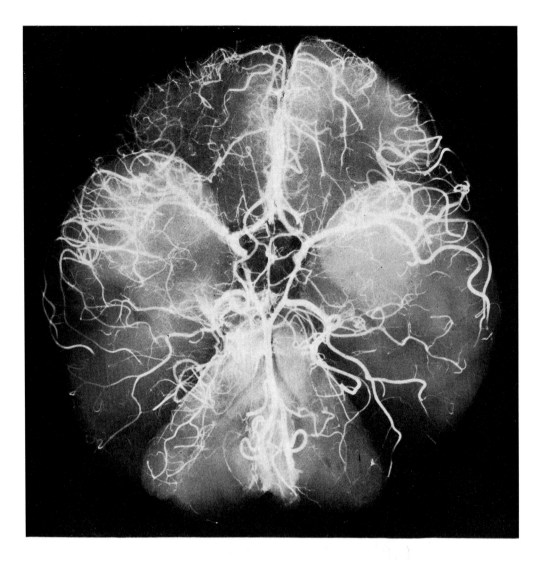

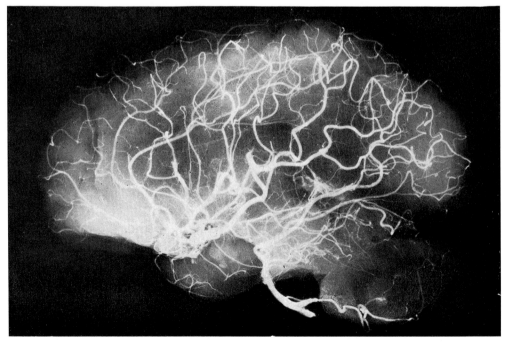

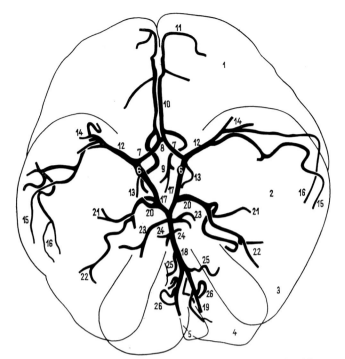

FIG. 108. Arteries of the cerebrum, cerebellum and the medulla oblongata, I.
Anatomical preparation. Craniocaudal view.

1. Frontal lobe
2. Temporal lobe
3. Occipital lobe
4. Cerebellum
5. Medulla oblongata
6. Internal carotid artery
7. Anterior cerebral
   artery
8. Anterior communicat-
   ing artery
9. Callosomarginal artery
10. Pericallosal artery
11. Frontopolar branch
12. Middle cerebral artery
13. Anterior choroid artery
14. Temporal branches
15. Artery of the angular
    gyrus
16. Parietal branches
17. Posterior communicat-
    ing artery
18. Basilar artery
19. Vertebral artery
20. Posterior cerebral artery
21. Temporal branches
22. Occipital branches
23. Superior cerebellar artery
24. Artery of the labyrinth
25. Anterior inferior cere-
    bellar artery
26. Posterior inferior cere-
    bellar artery

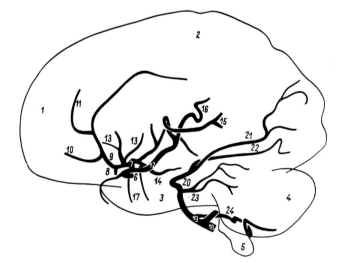

FIG. 109. Arteries of the cerebrum, cerebellum and the medulla oblongata, II. Anatomical preparation, sagittal hemi-
section. Mediolateral view.

1. Frontal lobe
2. Parietal lobe
3. Temporal lobe
4. Cerebellum
5. Medulla oblongata
6. Internal carotid artery
7. Anterior cerebral artery
8. Anterior communicating
   artery
9. Pericallosal artery
10. Frontopolar branch
11. Callosomarginal artery
12. Middle cerebral artery
13. Ascending frontal branch
14. Posterior temporal
    branch
15. Artery of the angular gyrus
16. Parietal branch
17. Anterior and middle
    temporal branches
18. Vertebral artery
19. Basilar artery
20. Posterior cerebral artery
21. Occipital branches
22. Temporal branches
23. Superior cerebellar artery
24. Posterior inferior cere-
    bellar artery

189

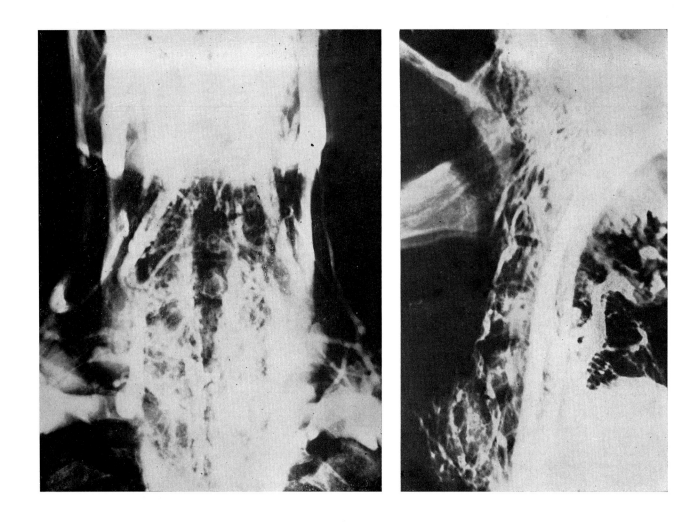

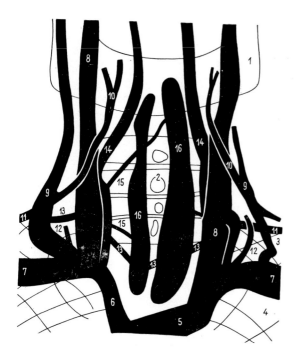

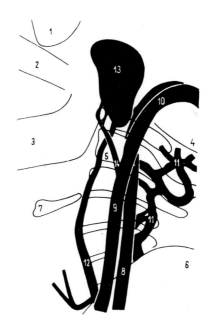

FIG. 110. The internal jugular vein and its branches,
I. Anteroposterior view.

FIG. 111. The internal jugular vein and its branches,
II. Sinistrodextral view.

1. Mandible
2. Cervical vertebrae
3. Clavicle
4. 1st rib
5. Left brachiocephalic vein
6. Right brachiocephalic vein
7. Subclavian vein
8. Internal jugular vein
9. External jugular vein
10. Anterior jugular vein
11. Transverse scapular vein
12. Superficial cervical vein
13. Venous jugular arch
14. Vertebral vein
15. Intervertebral veins
16. Internal and external vertebral venous plexuses and pharyngeal plexus

1. Maxillary sinus
2. Maxilla
3. Mandible
4. Occipital bone
5. Axis
6. Acromion
7. Hyoid bone
8. Left internal jugular vein
9. Right internal jugular vein
10. Sigmoid sinus
11. Posterior vertebral venous plexuses
12. Anterior vertebral venous plexuses
13. Pterygoid plexus
14. Retromandibular vein

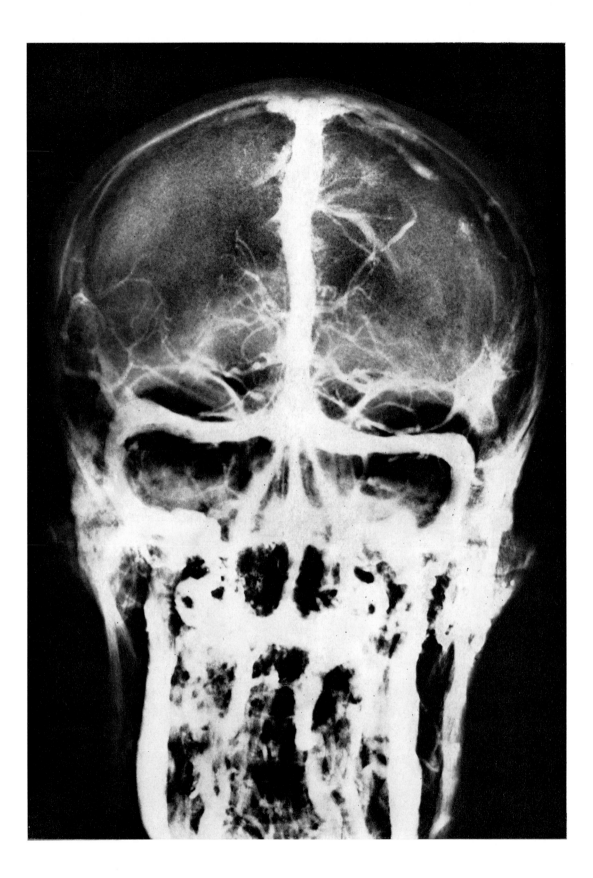

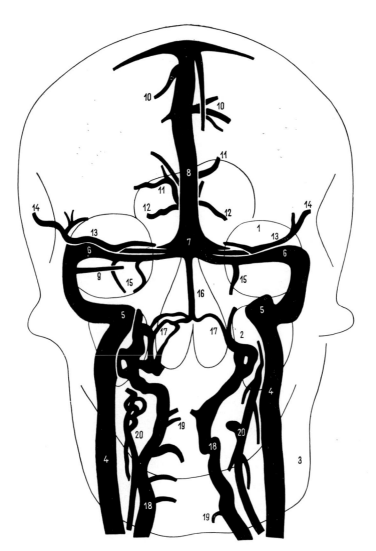

FIG. 112. The jugular vein; sinuses of the dura mater; the internal and external veins
of the cerebrum and cerebellum, I. Anteroposterior view.

1. Orbit
2. Maxillaɪy sinus
3. Mandible
4. Internal jugular vein
5. Sigmoid sinus
6. Transverse sinus
7. Confluence of sinuses

8. Superior and inferior
   sagittal sinuses
9. Superior petrosal sinus
10. Frontoparietal veins
11. Thalamostriate vein
12. Basal vein
13. Sphenoparietal sinus

14. Superficial middle cerebral vein
15. Inferior cerebellar veins
16. Occipital sinus
17. Suboccipital venous plexus
18. Vertebral vein
19. Intervertebral veins
20. Deep cervical vein

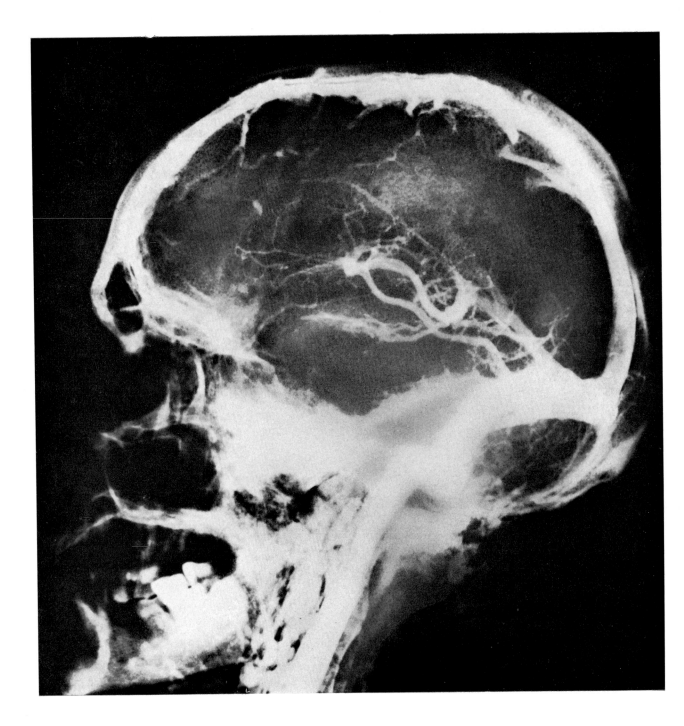

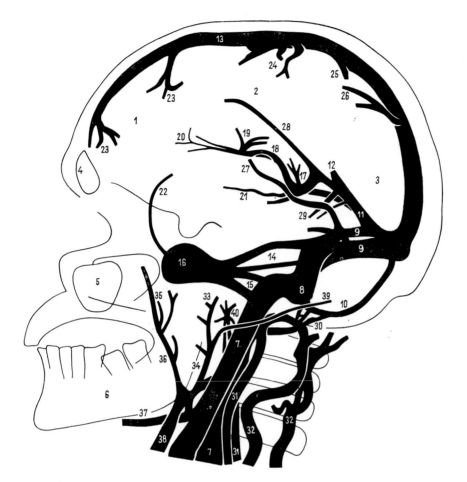

FIG. 113. The internal and external jugular vein; sinuses of the dura mater; the internal and external veins of the cerebrum and cerebellum, II. Sinistrodexral view.

1. Frontal bone
2. Parietal bone
3. Occipital bone
4. Frontal sinus
5. Maxillary sinus
6. Mandible
7. Internal jugular vein
8. Sigmoid sinus
9. Transverse sinus
10. Occipital sinus
11. Straight sinus
12. Inferior sagittal sinus
13. Superior sagittal sinus
14. Superior petrosal sinus
15. Inferior petrosal sinus
16. Cavernous sinus
17. Great cerebral vein
18. Internal cerebral vein
19. Thalamostriate vein
20. Vein of the septum pellucidum
21. Basal vein
22. Middle cerebral veins
23. Ascending frontal veins
24. Frontoparietal veins
25. Central vein
26. Ascending occipital veins
27. Temporooccipital vein
28. Posterior vein of corpus callosum
29. Superior cerebellar veins
30. Suboccipital venous plexus
31. Vertebral vein
32. Deep cervical vein
33. Pharyngeal plexus
34. Pharyngeal vein
35. Pterygoid plexus
36. Retromandibular vein
37. Submental vein
38. External jugular vein
39. Occipital vein
40. Prevertebral venous plexuses

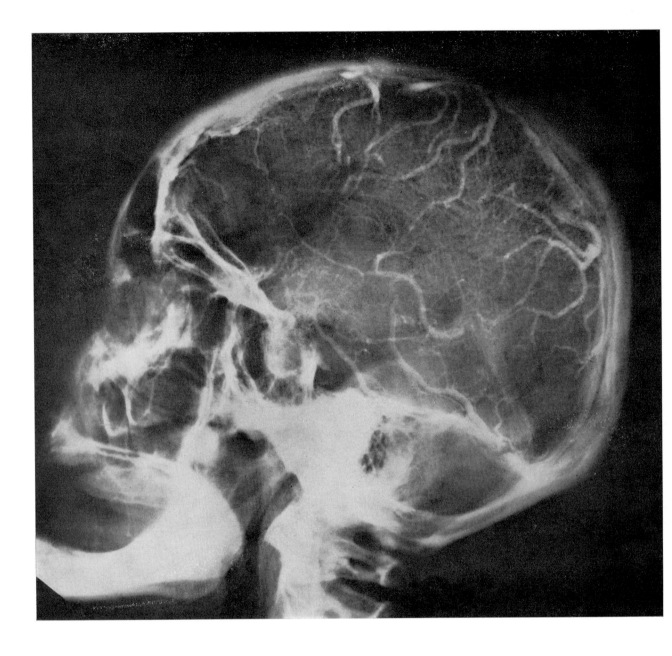

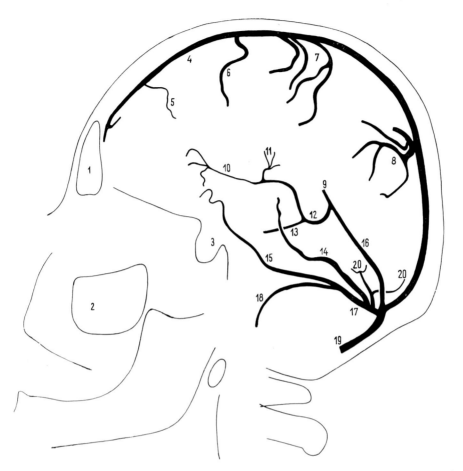

FIG. 114. The sinuses of the dura mater; the internal and external veins of the cerebrum and cerebellum. (Venography in vivo by I. Gorácz.) Sinistrodextral view

1. Frontal sinus
2. Maxillary sinus
3. Sella turcica
4. Superior sagittal sinus
5. Ascending frontal veins
6. Central vein
7. Parietal veins
8. Occipital veins
9. Inferior sagittal sinus
10. Vein of the septum pellucidum
11. Thalamostriate vein
12. Great cerebral vein
13. Basal vein
14. Temporooccipital vein
15. Temporal vein
16. Straight sinus
17. Transverse sinus
18. Sigmoid sinus
19. Occipital sinus
20. Posterior cerebellar veins

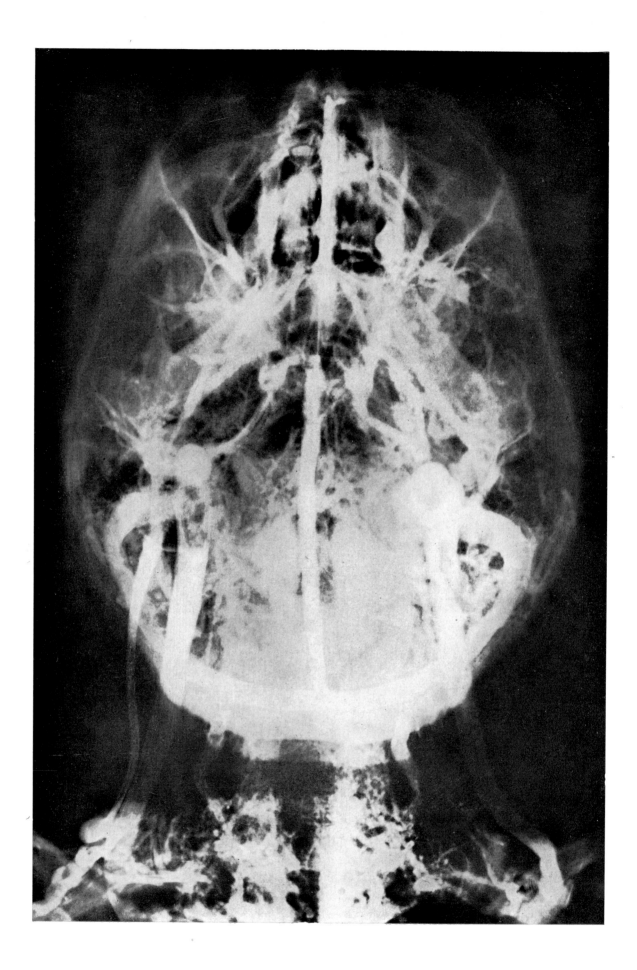

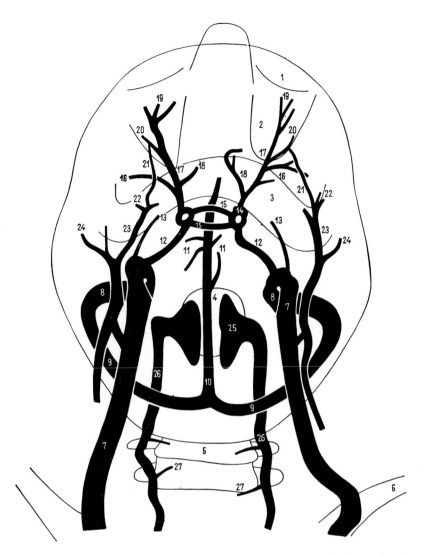

FIG. 115. The internal and external jugular vein; sinuses of the dura mater; the internal and external veins of the cerebrum and cerebellum, III. Submentovertical view (position Welin IV).

1. Orbit
2. Maxillary sinus
3. Mandible
4. Foramen magnum
5. Cervical vertebrae
6. Clavicle
7. Internal jugular vein
8. Sigmoid sinus
9. Transverse sinus
10. Superior and inferior sagittal sinuses
11. Superior and internal cerebral veins
12. Inferior petrosal sinus
13. Superior petrosal sinus
14. Cavernous sinus
15. Intercavernous sinuses
16. Sphenoparietal sinus
17. Superior ophthalmic vein
18. Ethmoidal veins
19. Branches of the superior ophthalmic vein
20. Inferior ophthalmic vein
21. Anastomosis between the inferior ophthalmic vein and pterygoid plexus
22. Pterygoid plexus
23. Retromandibular vein
24. External jugular vein
25. Suboccipital venous plexus
26. Vertebral vein
27. Intervertebral veins

BLOOD VESSELS OF THE UPPER EXTREMITIES

THE AXILLARY ARTERY AND ITS BRANCHES

In comparison to the circulation of the lower extremities that of the upper extremities shows an abundance of collateral communications. Normal blood pressure is here 40 to 60 mm Hg lower than in the vessels of the lower extremities. Since vascular diseases are comparatively rare in this region, anatomical and functional morphological research of these systems are of less clinical significance.

Axillary, brachial, ulnar, radial arteries and their branches

The **axillary artery** (Figs 116/1, 120/6, 121 and 122/6), as the continuation of the subclavian artery, begins below the inferior margin of the clavicle and runs as far as the lower edge of the pectoralis major muscle (the level of the surgical neck of the humerus). Its entire course lies in the axillary fossa, lateral to and deeper than the axillary vein. Anteriorly, the vessel is covered by the pectoralis major muscle. The pectoralis minor muscle covers only the middle third of the artery. The vessel is surrounded by the upper third of the brachial plexus. The plexus surrounds its middle third and encircles its lower third from behind and from two sides. The course of the axillary artery depends on the position of the arm. It descends obliquely when the arm is hanging, runs horizontally if the arm is in a horizontal position, and describes an ascending concave arch if the arm is raised. The length of the axillary artery is 8 to 12 cm, the diameter 0·6 to 0·8 cm (Paturet 1958). *Branches:*

The *highest thoracic artery* (Figs 116/3, 120/7), a vessel of variable strength, supplies the upper two intercostal spaces.

The *thoracoacromial artery* (Figs 116/4, 120/8), is a wide trunk which trifurcates after a short course. Its acromial branch (*ramus acromialis*) participates in the formation of the acromial network, the two other segments run to the deltoid muscle (*deltoid branch*) and the pectoralis major muscle (*pectoral branches*).

The *lateral thoracic artery* (Figs 116/5, 120/12) arises from the middle third of the axillary artery.

It runs along the lateral side of the chest toward the muscles of the chest wall and to the breast (*lateral mammary branches*).

The *subscapular artery* (Figs 116/6, 120/14, 121 and 122/7) descends along the subscapularis muscle and bifurcates. One branch (*thoracodorsal artery*, Figs 120/16, 121/9) ramifies in the muscles at the posterolateral border of the thorax, the other forms an arterial arch with the suprascapular artery around the lateral border of the scapula (*scapular circumflex artery*, Figs 120/15, 121/8).

The *anterior* and *posterior circumflex humeral arteries* (Figs 116/8 and 7, 120/17 and 18, 121 and 122/10 and 11) encircle the surgical neck of the humerus. The anterior vessel is thinner, but its importance in the supply of the head at the humerus is greater (Neihardt and Spanta 1969).

The most frequent *variation* is that the branches of the axillary artery and certain branches of the brachial artery arise with a common trunk formed by the union of five vessels (Fig. 116/II; subscapular, posterior humeral circumflex, radial and medial collateral, ulnar collateral arteries). This variation occurs in 6·6 per cent among Europeans, and in 39·8 per cent among the Japanese (Adachi 1928). The deep brachial artery springs often from this trunk. The posterior humeral circumflex artery may originate from the deep brachial artery. From the axillary artery may moreover commence the radial artery which arises at a high level (Fig. 116/III) as also the common interosseous artery (Gray 1954). The anterior humeral circumflex artery arises together with another vessel in 10 per cent of the cases (Quain 1884)

The **brachial artery** (Figs 116/2, 117/1, 120/19, 121 and 122/12, 123 and 124/5) extends from the lower border of the pectoralis major muscle to the cubital fossa to divide into terminal branches before the neck of the radius (1 cm below the elbow joint). The vessel runs in the medial bicipital groove between the brachial veins together with the nerves. The median cubital vein crosses the brachial artery frontally in the bend of the elbow where the vessel runs the most superficially. Its projection lies along the straight line drawn from the middle of the axil-

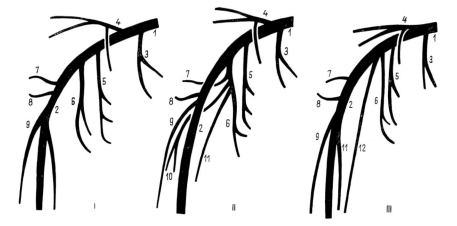

FIG. 116. Variations in the division of the axillary artery. I, normal type; II, the subscapular, posterior circumflex humeral, radial and middle collateral and the superior collateral ulnar arteries arise with a common trunk; III, high origin of radial artery. (*1*) Axillary artery; (*2*) brachial artery; (*3*) highest thoracic artery; (*4*) thoracoacromial artery; (*5*) lateral thoracic artery; (*6*) subscapular artery; (*7*) posterior circumflex humeral artery; (*8*) anterior circumflex humeral artery; (*9*) deep brachial artery; (*10*) radial and middle collateral arteries; (*11*) superior collateral ulnar artery; (*12*) radial artery.

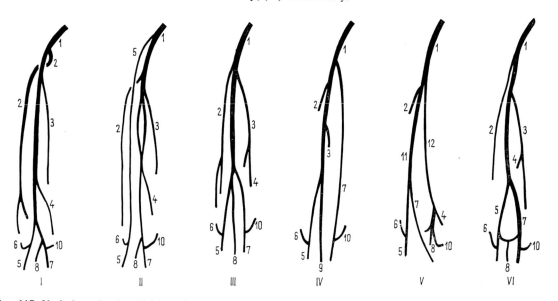

FIG. 117. Variations in the division of the brachial artery. I, normal type; II, high division of radial artery (islet formation on the brachial artery); III, high division of radial and interosseous arteries; IV, high division of ulnar artery (rudimentary deep brachial artery); V, separation of deep and superficial brachial arteries; VI, high division with transverse anastomosis. (*1*) Brachial artery; (*2*) deep brachial artery; (*3*) superior collateral ulnar artery; (*4*) inferior collateral ulnar artery; (*5*) radial artery; (*6*) radial recurrent artery; (*7*) ulnar artery; (*8*) common interosseous artery; (*9*) median artery; (*10*) ulnar recurrent artery; (*11*) superficial brachial artery; (*12*) deep brachial artery.

lary fossa to the centre of the line connecting the epicondyles of the humerus. The length of the brachial artery, varying with the site of division, amounts to 15 to 30 cm, its diameter is 0·5 to 0·6 cm (Paturet 1958).

Variations of the brachial artery (Fig. 117). 1. Variations in course. The upper segment of the artery sometimes forms an islet (Fig. 117/II); or it may run anteriorly in relation to the median nerve or may be situated behind the "supracondylar proc-

ess" (Rauber and Kopsch 9511). 2. Division at a high point. In one-eighth of the cases the brachial artery divides above the elbow joint. More distal than the typical division is extremely rare. High division usually occurs in the proximal, less frequently in the distal and still more rarely in the middle third of the arm. Occasionally already the axillary artery may bifurcate. In three-fourth of the cases the radial artery originates at a high point (Figs 116/III, 117/II). In such cases the further portion of the brachial artery divides into the ulnar and the interosseous arteries. Exceptionally the radial artery arises together with the interosseous artery (Fig. 117/III). Even more seldom the ulnar artery and the interosseous artery originate separately at a high point (Fig. 117/IV; Quain 1884, McCormack et al. 1953). The artery, originating high, descends in front of the median nerve (superficial brachial artery (Fig. 117/V; Loetzke and Kleinau 1968). Transverse anastomosis is sometimes formed in the region of the elbow between the divided vessels (Fig. 117/VI; Kadanoff and Balkansky 1966). The aberrant radial artery may give off anomalous branches. High division is bilateral in one-fifth of the cases (Quain 1884). *Branches:*

The *deep brachial artery* (Figs 116/9, 117/2, 120/21, 121 and 122/13), arising at a high point from the medial side of the brachial artery, goes around the humerus from behind accompanied by the radial nerve and reaches the lateral aspect of the humerus (*nutrient branches to the humerus*), the deltoid muscle (*deltoid branch*, Figs 120/20, 121 and 122/14), while one of its terminal branches (*middle collateral artery*, Figs 116/10, 121 and 122/15) reaches the arterial rete of the elbow joint. The other terminal branch (*radial collateral artery*, Figs 116/10, 121 and 122/16) anastomoses with the radial recurrent artery and is then lost in the rete of the elbow joint. The ulnar collateral artery may be a supernumerary branch (Adachi 1928).

The *superior and inferior ulnar collateral arteries* (Figs 116/11, 117/3 and 4, 121 and 122/17 and 18) spring off from the middle and the lower third of the arm and run to the rete of the elbow joint. The upper vessel accompanies the ulnar nerve.

The **radial artery** (Figs 117/5, 123 and 124/6, 125/7, 126 and 127/6) arises at the bend of the elbow at the level of the neck of the radius. It describes a straight line in the direction of the styloid process of the radius below the brachioradialis muscle. The vessel passes directly along the bone in the lower third of the forearm. Bending sharply round the radius after having reached the carpus, the vessel passes into the radial foveola, gains the palm through the muscle of the 1st interosseous space and forms the deep palmar arch by uniting with the deep branch of the ulnar artery. Its course may be characterized by a straight line connecting the midpoint of the line between the epicondyles with the styloid process of the radius. *Branches:*

The *radial recurrent artery* (Figs 117/6, 123 and 124/7) winds back from the beginning of the trunk to the arterial network of the elbow.

The *palmar carpal branch* (Fig. 125/9) is a small vessel to the rete carpi volare.

The *superficial palmar branch* (Figs 123 and 124/8, 125/8) is the radial root of the superficial palmar arch.

The *dorsal carpal branch* (Fig. 125/10), the strongest carpal vessel, is the most important artery in the formation of the dorsal carpal arch. It gives off the *dorsal metacarpal* and *dorsal digital arteries* of the hand.

The *principal artery of the thumb* (Figs 125/11, 126 and 127/8) is a terminal branch of the radial artery. It originates as it turns medially on gaining the palm; it descends on the palmar aspect of the first metacarpal bone. The artery supplies the thumb and the radial aspect of the forefinger (*radial artery of the index finger*, Figs 125/12, 126 and 127/11).

The *deep palmar arch* (Figs 125/20, 126 and 127/7) is the other terminal branch of the radial artery. It gives off four *palmar metacarpal arteries* (Figs 125/21, 126 and 127/9) which run along the interosseous muscles toward the fingers. They join the common digital branches of the superficial palmar arch at the clefts of the fingers. They anastomose with the dorsal metacarpal arteries via the *perforating branches*.

The **ulnar artery** (Figs 117/7, 123 and 124/9, 125/13, 126 and 127/13) is the larger terminal branch of the brachial artery. From its origin it runs obliquely, covered by the flexor muscles, to the ulna reaching it at the boundary between the upper and the middle third of the bone. The vessel, covered now by a few muscles only, follows a straight course toward the pisiform bone and reaches the palm on the lateral side of the bone below the ligamentum volare. The artery ends below the palmar aponeurosis in the superficial volar arch. *Branches:*

The *ulnar recurrent artery* (Figs 117/10, 123 and 124/10), a short and thick vessel, originates at the commencement of the main trunk. Its *anterior branch* anastomoses with the inferior ulnar collateral artery, while the *posterior branch* ends in the network of the elbow joint.

The *common interosseous artery* (Figs 117/8, 123 and 124/11), a larger vessel, arises somewhat distally to the ulnar recurrent artery and divides into two branches. The posterior branch (*posterior interosseous artery*, Figs 123 and 124/13), after piercing the interosseous membrane, forms a communication between its ascending branch (*recurrent interosseous artery*, Figs 123 and 124/14) and the middle collateral artery. The descending branch ends in the deep extensor muscles on the posterior side of the interosseous septum. The anterior branch of the artery (*anterior interosseous artery*, Figs 123 and 124/12) follows a similar course on the palmar side. The common interosseous artery is sometimes the largest artery of the forearm (median artery, Fig. 117/9). The diameter of the common interosseous artery is two-third of the ulnar artery. The posterior interosseous artery is larger than the anterior interosseous artery (Kenesi and Honnart 1969).

The *palmar and dorsal carpal branches* (Fig. 125/14 and 15) are small vessels to the carpus.

The *deep palmar branch* (Fig. 125/16) the smaller terminal branch of the main trunk, together with the radial artery, takes part in the formation of the deep palmar arch (Fig. 125/20).

The *superficial palmar arch* (Figs 125/17, 126 and 127/10) is the larger of the two terminal branches. The three *common palmar digital arteries* (Fig. 125/18) commencing there, bifurcate at the fingers and supply the inner surfaces between the second to fifth fingers (*palmar digital arteries*, Figs 125/19, 126 and 127/12). The radial border of the forefinger is supplied by the principal artery of the index finger and the ulnar border of the fifth finger by a separate artery.

Blood supply of the fingers. The proximal phalanges are supplied by both the dorsal and palmar arteries, the distal phalanges mainly by the palmar vessels. These arteries form superficial arches on the dorsal aspect of the distal phalanges at the height of the superficial base, and form proximal and distal arches beneath the nails (Figs 126, 127/14, Flint 1955).

Variations of the arteries of the forearm and the hand. The *radial artery* (Figs 116/III, 117/II) has a highly placed origin in 12 per cent of the cases (Gray 1954). The superficial palmar branch arises sometimes from the forearm. In such cases the main trunk bends over to the dorsal side in its middle third (Kiss 1963). The radial recurrent artery is sometimes very large or double (Adachi 1928). High origin of the *ulnar artery* (Fig. 117/IV) is about 8 per cent (Gray 1954). Its course is fairly constant if its origin is normal, and superficial if the origin is placed high. The *arteries of the hand* show numerous variations. The three variations of the superficial arterial arch are the ulnar (60·7 per cent), the radioulnar (31·3 per cent) and the medianoulnar (8 per cent) arches (Jaschtschinski 1897). Insufficient development of the superficial arch is compensated by the deep arterial arch so that in such cases blood is supplied to the fingers by the deep palmar arch alone. Sometimes the radial artery contributes only to the formation of the superficial arch (Rauber and Kopsch 1951). Edwards (1960) described 11 important variations of the palmar arterial arches. The variations of the vessels of the *fingers*, and particularly those of the forefinger are numerous (Weatherby 1955).

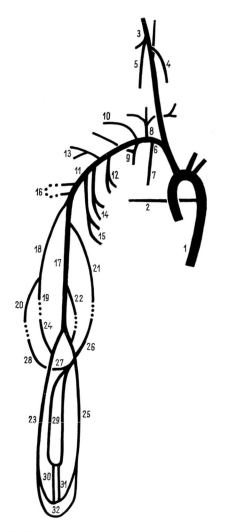

Fig. 118. Collateral arterial network of the upper extremities. (*1*) Aorta; (*2*) posterior intercostal artery; (*3*) external carotid artery; (*4*) superior thyroid artery; (*5*) occipital artery; (*6*) subclavian artery; (*7*) internal thoracic artery; (*8*) thyrocervical trunk; (*9*) costocervical trunk; (*10*) transverse cervical artery; (*11*) axillary artery; (*12*) highest thoracic artery; (*13*) thoracoacromial artery; (*14*) lateral thoracic artery; (*15*) subscapular artery; (*16*) posterior and anterior circumflex humeral arteries; (*17*) brachial artery; (*18*) deep brachial artery; (*19*) radial collateral artery; (*20*) middle collateral artery; (*21*) superior ulnar collateral artery; (*22*) inferior ulnar collateral artery; (*23*) radial artery; (*24*) radial recurrent artery; (*25*) ulnar artery; (*26*) ulnar recurrent artery; (*27*) common interosseous artery; (*28*) interosseous recurrent artery; (*29*) posterior and anterior interosseous arteries; (*30*) carpal branches; (*31*) deep palmar arch; (*32*) superficial palmar arch.

Collateral circulation of the upper extremities

The abundant collateral network of the upper extremities (Fig. 118) ensures adequate circulation even if a major artery becomes insufficient. Brantigan (1963) classifies the anastomotic systems into three groups:

1. The scapular anastomoses connect with each other the vascular systems of the aorta (intercostal artery), the external carotid (occipital and superior thyroid arteries), the subclavian artery (all branches excepting the vertebral artery), the axillary artery (all branches) and the brachial artery (deep brachial artery).

2. Anastomoses around the elbow ensure good collateral circulation between the branches coming from above (superior and inferior ulnar collateral arteries, deep brachial artery) and those coming from below (interosseous, radial and ulnar recurrent arteries).

3. The anastomoses of the forearms and hand form arterial arches through the two arteries of the forearm and the interosseous arteries as also through the palmar and dorsal carpal and the superficial and deep palmar arches.

Arteriography of the upper extremities

The vascular anatomy of the upper extremities is of considerably less clinical significance than that of the lower extremities. Haschek and Lindenthal (1896) were the first to make a postmortem angiogram of an amputated limb, an achievement of historical significance. The first to report on angiography in vivo were Berberich and Hirsch (1923). Even large textbooks on angiology discuss but briefly the anatomical aspects because, thanks to the abundant peripheral circulation, vascular insufficiency occurs practically only on the fingers (Ratschow 1959, Abrams 1961). McCormack et al. (1953) described variations in the arterial supply of the arm and forearm, Flint (1955) those of the fingers, and Edwards (1960) those of the hand. Technical developments will surely facilitate such examinations on a larger scale (Strickland and Urquhart 1963, Soila et al. 1963, Zsebők 1969).

Postmortem angiograms of the **shoulder** in the **anteroposterior view** (Fig. 120) show the *axillary artery* (Fig. 120/6) to form a slightly upward curving arch beginning at the 1st rib and pursuing an oblique course and to cross the projection of the scapula. Its lower border is situated in the projection of the neck of the scapula. Here the artery lies medially to the surgical neck of the humerus. As already noted, the shape of the artery depends on the position of the arm. Of the descending branches the *highest thoracic artery*, (Fig. 120/7), begins at the approximate height of the border of the 2nd rib. The *lateral thoracic artery* (Fig. 120/12) is projected on the border of the costal arches. The origin of the *subscapular artery* (Fig. 120/14) is often overlapping with the projection of the circumflex humeral artery;

it is nevertheless easily identifiable by its characteristic downward winding course. The *thoracodorsal artery* (Fig. 120/16) descends along the lateral border of the scapula. The *circumflex scapular artery* (Fig. 120/15) runs medially and communicates with the terminal branches of the suprascapular artery. The two *circumflex humeral arteries* (Figs 120/17 and 18) usually form a large bend at their origin which allows their elongation when the arm has been abducted.

Anteroposterior pictures of the upper arm (Fig. 121) show the projection of the *brachial artery* (Fig. 121/12) next to the medial border of the humerus. Its last segment appears in the projection of the elbow joint where it ramifies. The *deep brachial artery* (Fig. 121/13) intersects obliquely the projection of the humerus in its middle third. The *collateral arteries* (Figs 121/15 to 18) descend on the corresponding sides of the humerus. There are often several arterial communications between them and the main trunk.

In **lateral view** (Fig. 122), the projection of the *brachial artery* (Fig. 122/12) on the humerus or in front of the elbow joint appears in a slight "S" shape. The *deep brachial artery* (Fig. 122/13) arises from the backward convex upper part of the brachial artery; its shadow, together with most of its branches, appears behind the humerus. The *collateral arteries* (Figs 122/15 to 18) descend partly in and partly behind the projection of the humerus. The arterial arches can be seen in this projection as well.

Anteroposterior angiograms of the forearm (Fig. 123) show (as noted in the anatomical description) the *radial* (Fig. 123/6) and the *ulnar* (Fig. 123/9) *arteries* in the projection of the bones, while the *common* (Fig. 123/11) and *posterior* (Fig. 123/13) *interosseous arteries* appear between the bones. The *recurrent interosseous arteries* (Figs 123 and 124/14) begin their ascending course between the projections of the radius and the ulna.

Lateral pictures (Fig. 124) show the two major vessels in front of the bones. The upper two third of the *radial artery* (Fig. 124/6) is more superficially placed, while its lower third which crosses the *ulnar artery* (Fig. 124/9) lies closer to the bone. The *interosseous arteries* (Figs 124/11 to 14) show a descending and ascending course, respectively, in the projection of the bones. The *radial recurrent artery* (Fig. 124/7) ascends in front of the bones in the projection of the soft tissues.

Dorsopalmar angiograms of the hand (Fig. 125) show the respective courses of the *radial* (Fig. 125/7) and the *ulnar artery* (Fig. 125/13) above the projections of the corresponding bones. The first describes a radially directed curve, the latter passes downward in a straight and likewise somewhat radially directed line. The carpal arteries and the arterial arches are observable in accordance with the extent of their development. The *superficial palmar arch* (Fig. 125/17) extends more distally than the *deep palmar arch* (Fig. 125/20). The tortuous course of the *arteries of the metacarpus and the fingers* (Figs 125/18, 19 and 21) makes their elonga-

tion possible on occasion of different hand movements.

Pictures of the thumb, taken from two directions (Figs and 126, 127), show the *principal artery of the thumb* (Figs 126 and 127/8) and its ramification, further the *arterial arches* (Figs 126 and 127/14) at the level of the proximal and distal phalanges, connecting the bilateral arteries.

THE AXILLARY VEIN AND ITS AREA OF DRAINAGE

The double venous system of the arm is well suited for the maintenance of good collateral circulation. Numerous communications connect the deep veins accompanying the arteries with the superficial veins. The cephalic vein, with its high orifice and its numerous connections with the neck and the chest wall, is able to replace also the circulation of the lower segment of the axillary vein. Blood flow is regulated by valves in both systems. Venous tension is low in them so that, in contrast to the lower extremities, the muscles of the arm have no pumping effect. Certain muscular actions do, however, accelerate the centripetal flow of blood. This phenomenon is of considerably less significance here than in the lower extremities (Moberg 1960). The veins of the muscles of the arm empty freely into the superficial veins. The dorsal veins of the hand and the veins of the forearm are filled if the arm is hanging, but in contrast to the lower extremities, they do not empty when the muscles are in active movement. Negative thoracic pressure facilitates the flow of blood in the region of the shoulder girdle. The patency of veins against the pumping effect is ensured by the "lever" action of the surroundings (Brecher 1956).

The axillary vein and its branches

The **axillary vein** (Figs 119/2, 128/5, 129 and 130/7), formed by the union of the two brachial veins, begins at the level of the lower border of the pectoralis major muscle and extends to the clavicle where it is continuous with the subclavian vein. Its course runs medially to the corresponding artery. The vessel is provided with one valve. Its length is 4·1 cm (3 to 5 cm), its diameter 1·3 cm (0·8 to 1·9 cm; Garusi and Moretti 1963). Doubling of the vein has been observed in 1 per cent (Drewes 1963). In such cases one of the double veins, a small vessel which frequently accompanies the artery, extends from the middle brachial to the subclavian

vein (Kaldyi 1877). Islet formation is rare around the axillary artery (Bile 1935). The vessel sends *branches* to the chest wall, further to the deep and upper layers of the arm.

Branches the chest wall: The *lateral thoracic vein* and the *thoracoepigastric veins* drain the blood of the chest wall into the axillary vein, the latter veins are able to maintain important collateral circulation between the inferior and the superior vena cava.

The deep veins of the arm (*brachial veins*, Figs 119/3, 128/6, 129 and 130/8, 131 and 132/5; *ulnar veins*, Figs 131 and 132/8; *radial veins*, Figs 131 and 132/8), usually two, accompany the corresponding arteries, and their division is similar to that of the arteries. They form multiple anastomotic communications. Besides, they are in communication with the superficial veins, especially in the vicinity of the joints. The veins of the forearm contain 8 to 15, those of the upper arm, 6 to 12 valves. The veins of the forearm drain the hand.

Superficial veins of the arm: The *cephalic vein* (Figs 119/4, 128/7, 129 and 130/9, 131 and 132/10) begins in the radial part of the dorsal venous network of the hand, winds upward around the radial border of the forearm through the radial foveola and reaches the cubital fossa. Here it communicates with the basilic vein via the median cubital vein, then it curves through the lateral bicipital groove into the fossa between the deltoid and the pectoralis major muscle. Turning then medially, it opens into the axillary vein 2 to 3 cm below the clavicle. It has a spindle-shaped dilatation before the orifice. It collects the superficial veins of the radial side of the arm. There are 6 to 10 valves in it. It has an important role in collateral circulation if the axillary vein is insufficient, for it is in connection with the subclavian vein through its anastomoses. Numerous *variations* of the cephalic vein have been observed (Fig. 119). It is rarely absent but more frequently rudimentary (Fig. 119/II), in which case it is replaced by the

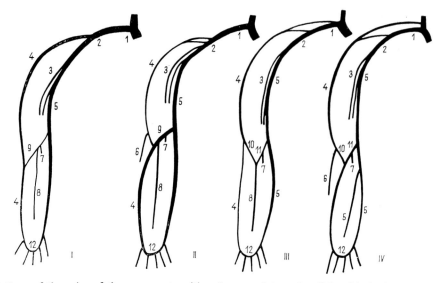

Fig. 119. Variations of the veins of the upper extremities. I, normal type (medial cubital vein: "N"); II, cephalic vein small, divided (median cubital vein: "Y"); III, cephalic vein partly opens into subclavian vein; low orifice of basilic vein (median cubital vein: "M"); IV, accessory cephalic vein; double basilic vein; cephalic vein opens into the axillary and the internal jugular vein (median cubital vein: "W"). (1) Subclavian vein; (2) axillary vein; (3) brachial veins; (4) cephalic vein; (5) basilic vein; (6) accessory cephalic vein; (7) anastomosis between superficial and deep veins; (8) median vein of forearm; (9) median cubital vein; (10) median cephalic vein; (11) median basilic vein; (12) dorsal venous network of the hand.

basilic vein (Sobotta 1911). Its upper segment may have a double orifice into the axillary vein or, else, may form an islet in 1 to 15 per cent of the cases (Rominger 1958, Drewes 1964). One branch of the bifurcating cephalic vein may open into the sub-clavian vein (Fig. 119/III) or into the concomitant axillary vein. Communications may be formed with the external and the internal jugular veins (Drewes 1964). The vein is often doubled in the forearm. The *accessory cephalic vein* (Fig. 119/IV) runs on the dorsal side and opens into the cephalic vein around the elbow (Rauber and Kopsch 1951). The cephalic vein sometimes receives the thoracoacromial vein or one of its branches.

The *basilic vein* (Figs 119/5, 128/8, 129 and 130/11, 131 and 132/9) runs from the ulnar part of the dorsal venous network of the hand to the bend of the elbow where it communicates with the cephalic vein. It passes then in the medial bicipital groove, penetrates into the deeper layers and opens into the medial brachial vein. The vessel has 4 to 8 valves. Of the *variations*, its doubling in the forearm (Fig. 119/IV, Rauber and Kopsch 1951) and its variable orifices in the arm (Fig. 119/III, Rominger 1958, Drewes 1964) deserve to be mentioned.

The *median vein of the forearm* (Figs 119/8, 131 and 132/11) passes superficially along the front of the forearm; dividing below the elbow into two branches, the *median basilic vein* (Fig. 119/11) and the *median cephalic vein* (Fig. 119/10), it opens into the two larger trunks. Its oblique connecting branch

at the elbow, the *median cubital vein* (Figs 119/10, 131 and 132/6), is directly connected with the deep veins. The *variations* of the cubital veins can be classified into three main groups (Kadanoff et al. 1966): 1. The median cubital vein (Fig. 119/I) connects the two major veins obliquely. 2. The cephalic vein opens obliquely into the basilic vein, when the cephalic vein originates as a small branch from the median cubital vein. 3. The cubital anastomosis of the three veins of the forearm resembles the shape of an "M" which continues evenly on the arm. Paturet (1958) distinguishes the following patterns formed by the cubital veins: "N" shape (8 per cent, Fig. 119/I) "Y" shape (30 per cent, Fig. 119/II); "M" shape (60 per cent, Fig. 119/III), and "W" shape (2 per cent, Fig. 119/IV).

As regards the anatomy and variations of the superficial veins of the hand, reference should be made to the work by Saïfi (1967).

Phlebography of the upper limbs

The phlebography is less frequently applied with respect to the upper limbs than to the lower extremities. Since the phlebographic study of Sgalitzer et al. (1931) only few authors have studied the radiological anatomy of the veins of the arm (Lavizzari and Ottolini 1955, Rominger 1958, Drewes 1963, Garusi and Moretti 1963). Knowledge is comparatively more extensive concerning the veins of the arm and the shoulder girdle. Lack of shadow and the so-called pelott phenomenon (Tagariello 1952, Drewes 1963), observed in the roentgenograms of the axillary and subclavian veins, have proved to be just haemodynamic variations depending on the actual position of the joints and muscles of the arm. We observed this phenomenon before the orifice of the cephalic vein.

In vivo, the veins of the forearm can be filled with intraarterial injection (Zsebők 1969) and the veins of the arm and shoulder girdle via the cubital vein (Fischer 1951).

In case of *postmortem anterograde phlebography* the **anteroposterior pictures of the forearm** (Fig. 131), filled through the hand, show the *basilic vein* (Fig. 131/9) on the medial side, the *cephalic vein* (Fig. 131/10) on the lateral aspect of the forearm. They form numerous anastomoses along their entire course. Visualization is difficult on account of the approximately synchronous filling of the deep veins. The superficial veins at the bend of the elbow usually provide the most abundant communications between the deep veins and the two veins of the skin.

In the **lateral view** (Fig. 132) the *basilic vein* above the wrist from the dorsal side (Fig. 132/9) turns to the dorsal margin of the radius, and the *cephalic vein* (Fig. 132/10) to the palmar side of the forearm. Differentiation of the superficial from the deep veins is usually easier in this view. The course of the deep veins is paired.

Anteroposterior phlebograms of the (abducted) **arm** (Fig. 129) show the *brachial veins* (Fig. 129/8) to run along the medial side of the humerus. Their division corresponds to that of the arteries. It is usually difficult to separate the *basilic vein* (Fig. 129/11) from the paired brachial veins. The *cephalic vein* (Fig. 129/9) ascends in the projection of the humerus laterally to the brachial veins. Typically, it opens into the axillary vein in the projection of the scapula, above the head of the humerus. Several transverse anastomoses are formed in the arm between the cephalic vein and the deep veins.

Lateral pictures (Fig. 130) show the *cephalic vein* (Fig. 130/9) separately in front of the humerus, whereas the projections of the other veins are mostly superimposed in the axis of the bone. Anastomoses between the superficial and the deep veins are clearly visible.

Anteroposterior roentgenograms of the shoulder (Fig. 128) show the *brachial veins* (Fig. 128/6): they turn medially and upward in the upper third of the arm and unite in the *axillary vein* (Fig. 128/5). Lateral to them, the *cephalic vein* (Fig. 128/7) appears in the projection of the humerus; it turns medially above the brachial veins and opens into the axillary vein in a slightly arched form.

It is only by means of intraosseous phlebography (i.e., by injections into the ribs) that the branches of the axillary vein situated in the chest wall can be demonstrated *in vivo* (Szücs 1964).

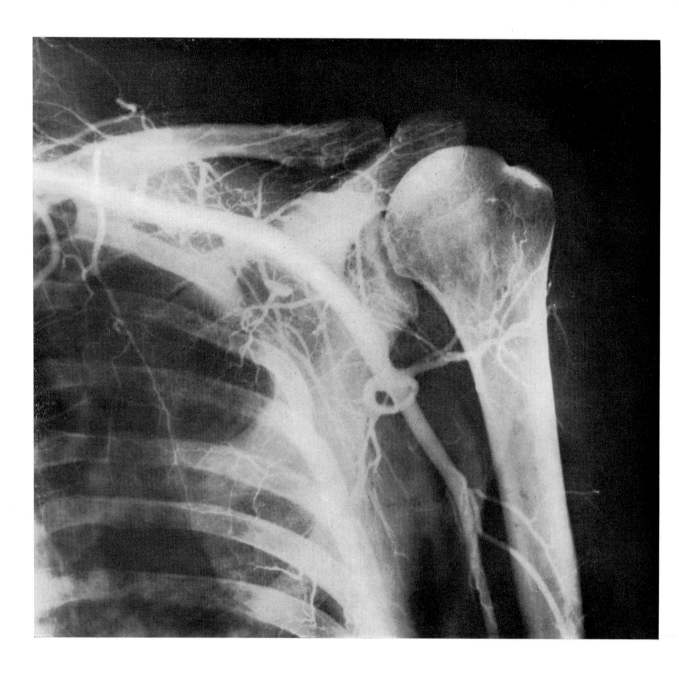

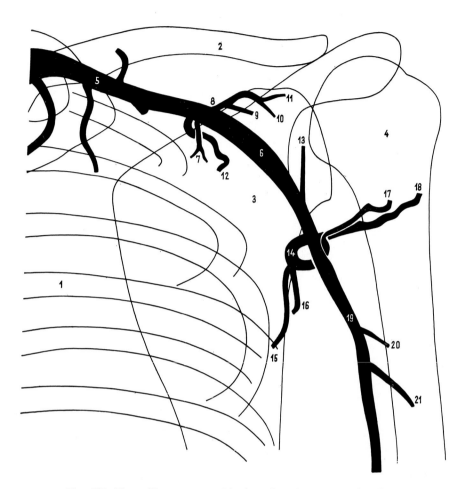

FIG. 120. The axillary artery and its branches. Anteroposterior view.

1. Ribs
2. Clavicle
3. Scapula
4. Humerus
5. Subclavian artery
6. Axillary artery
7. Highest thoracic artery
8. Thoracoacromial artery
9. Pectoral branch
10. Deltoid branch
11. Acromial branch
12. Lateral thoracic artery
13. Subscapular branch
14. Subscapular artery
15. Circumflex scapular artery
16. Thoracodorsal artery
17. Anterior circumflex humeral artery
18. Posterior circumflex humeral artery
19. Brachial artery
20. Deltoid branch
21. Deep brachial artery

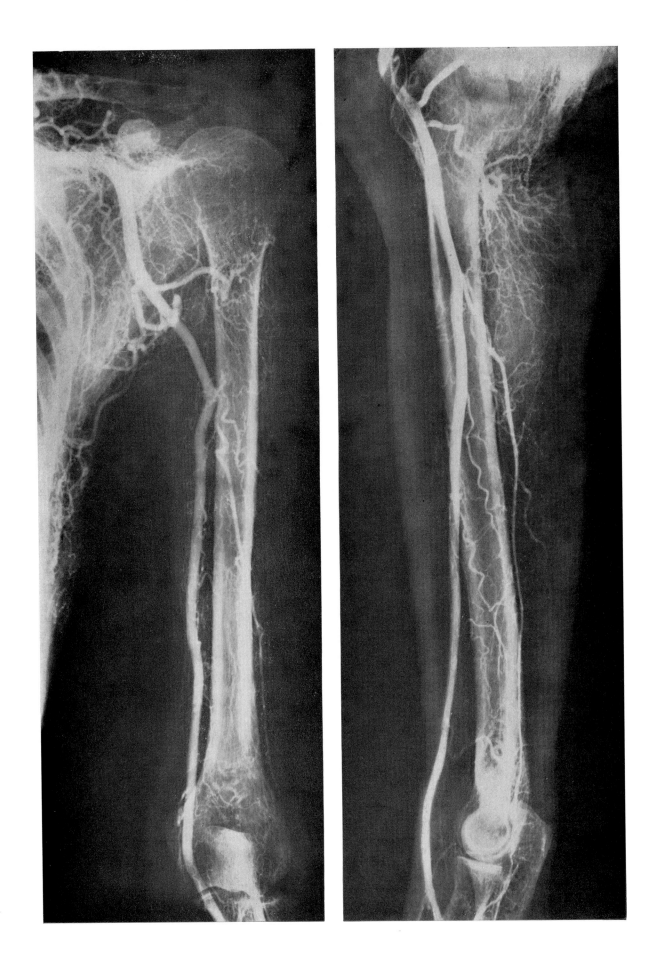

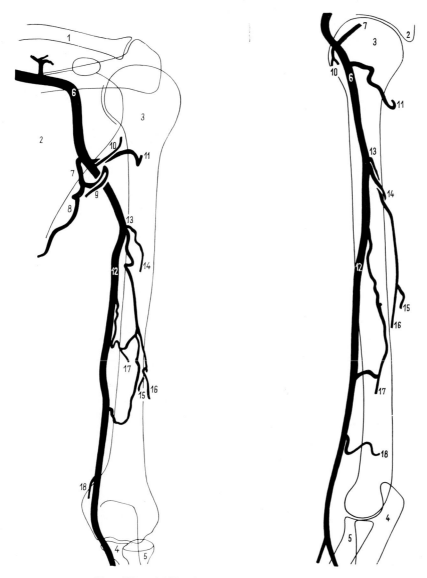

FIGS 121 and 122. The brachial artery and its branches.
Anteroposterior view (Fig. 121) and lateromedial view (Fig. 122).

1. Clavicle
2. Scapula
3. Humerus
4. Ulna
5. Radius
6. Axillary artery
7. Subscapular artery
8. Circumflex scapular artery
9. Thoracodorsal artery
10. Anterior circumflex humeral artery
11. Posterior circumflex humeral artery
12. Brachial artery
13. Deep brachial artery
14. Deltoid branch
15. Middle collateral artery
16. Radial collateral artery
17. Superior ulnar collateral artery
18. Inferior ulnar collateral artery

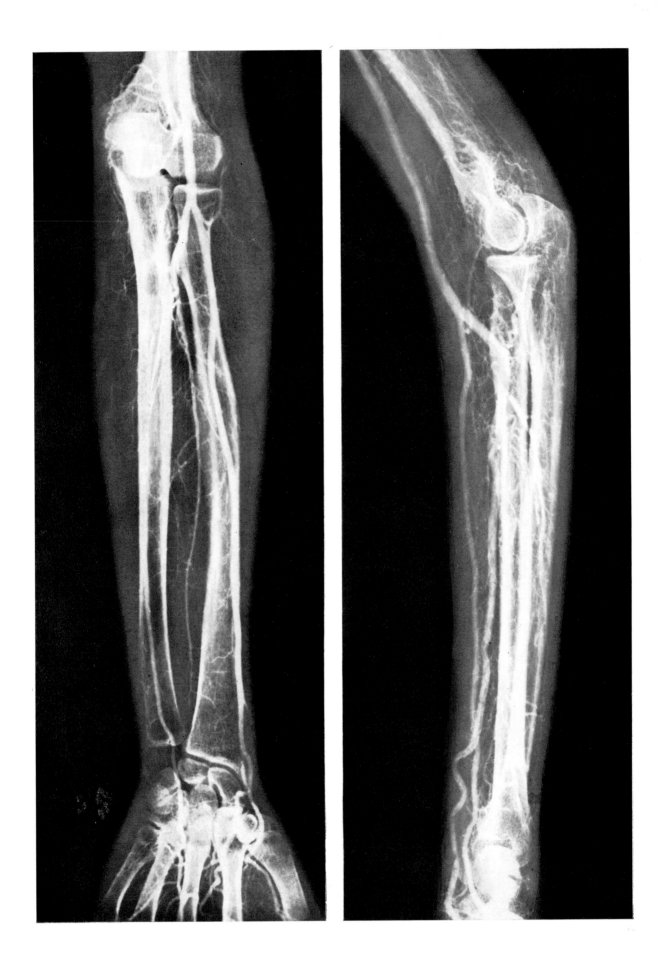

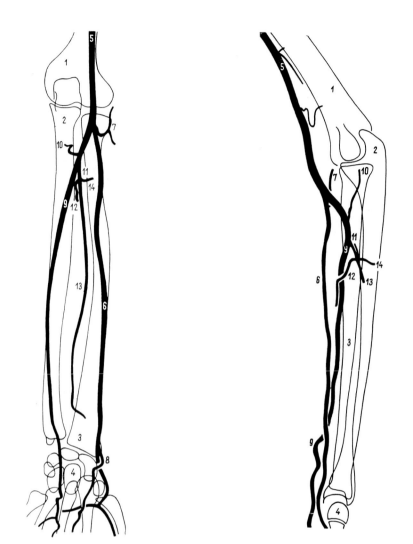

FIGS 123 and 124. The radial artery, ulnar artery and their branches. Anteroposterior view (Fig. 123) and lateromedial view (Fig. 124).

1. Humerus
2. Ulna
3. Radius
4. Bones of the carpus
5. Brachial artery
6. Radial artery
7. Radial recurrent artery
8. Superficial palmar branch
9. Ulnar artery
10. Ulnar recurrent artery
11. Common interosseous artery
12. Anterior interosseous artery
13. Posterior interosseous artery
14. Interosseous recurrent artery

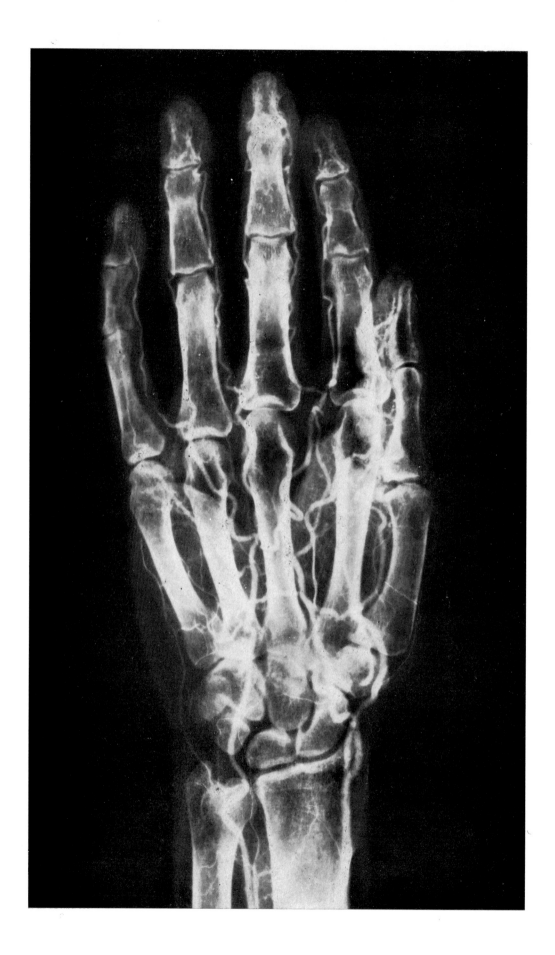

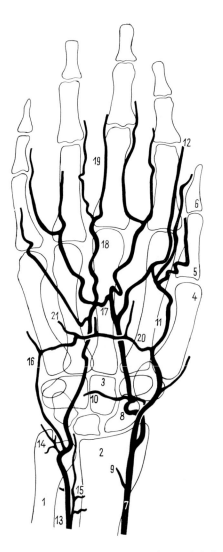

FIG. 125. The superficial and deep palmar arches and their branches.
Dorsopalmar view.

1. Ulna
2. Radius
3. Bones of the carpus
4. Metacarpal bones
5. Proximal phalanges
6. Distal phalanges
7. Radial artery
8. Superficial volar branch

9. Palmar carpal branch
10. Dorsal carpal branch
11. Principal artery of the thumb
12. Radial artery of the index finger
13. Ulnar artery
14. Dorsal carpal branch

15. Palmar carpal branch
16. Deep palmar branch
17. Superficial palmar arch
18. Common palmar digital arteries
19. Palmar digital arteries
20. Deep palmar arch
21. Palmar metacarpal arteries

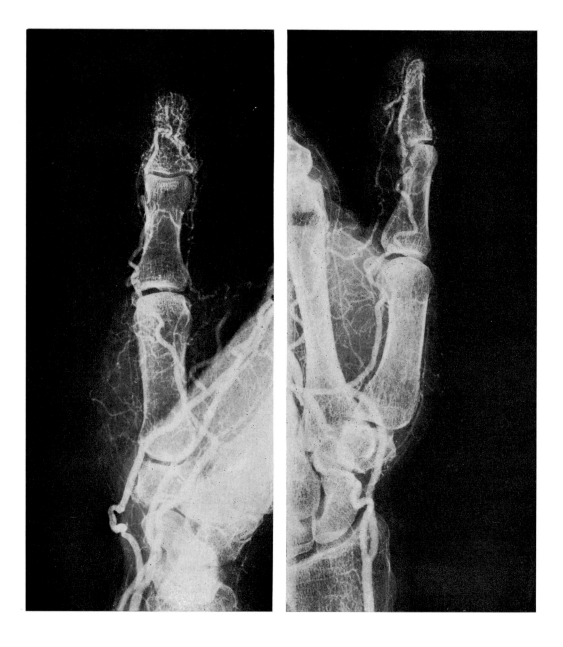

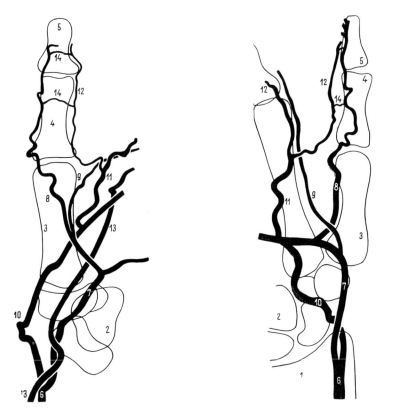

Figs 126 and 127. Principal artery of the thumb and its branches. Anteroposterior view
(Fig. 126) and mediolateral view (Fig. 127).

1. Radius	6. Radial artery	11. Radial artery of the index finger
2. Bones of the carpus	7. Deep palmar arch	12. Palmar digital arteries
3. Metacarpal bones	8. Principal artery of thumb	13. Ulnar artery
4. Proximal phalanx	9. 1st dorsal metacarpal artery	14. Arcus digitorum
5. Distal phalanx	10. Superficial palmar arch	

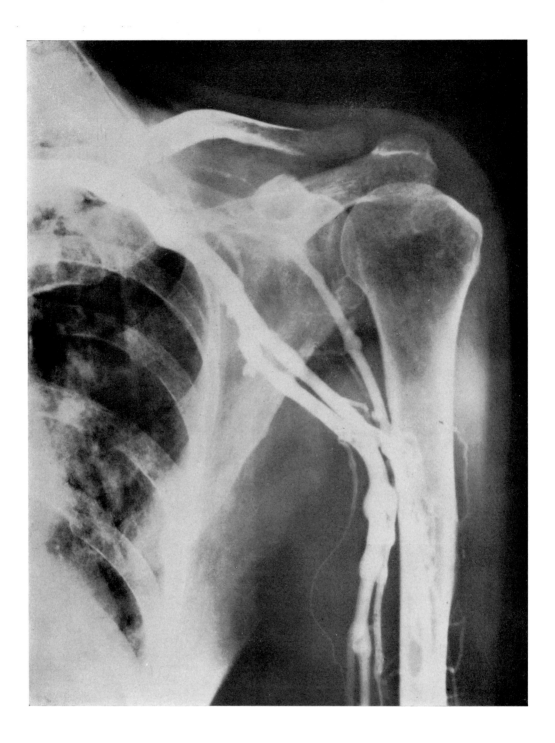

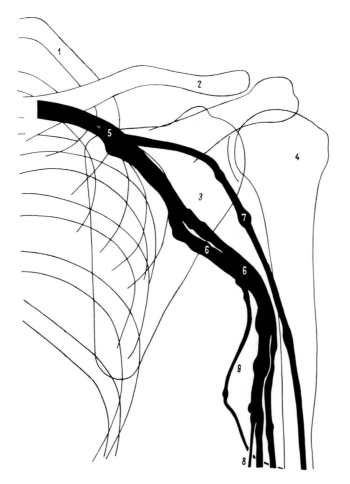

FIG. 128. The axillary vein and its branches. Anteroposterior view.

1. Ribs
2. Clavicle
3. Scapula
4. Humerus
5. Axillary vein
6. Brachial veins
7. Cephalic vein
8. Basilic vein
9. Superior ulnar collateral
   vein

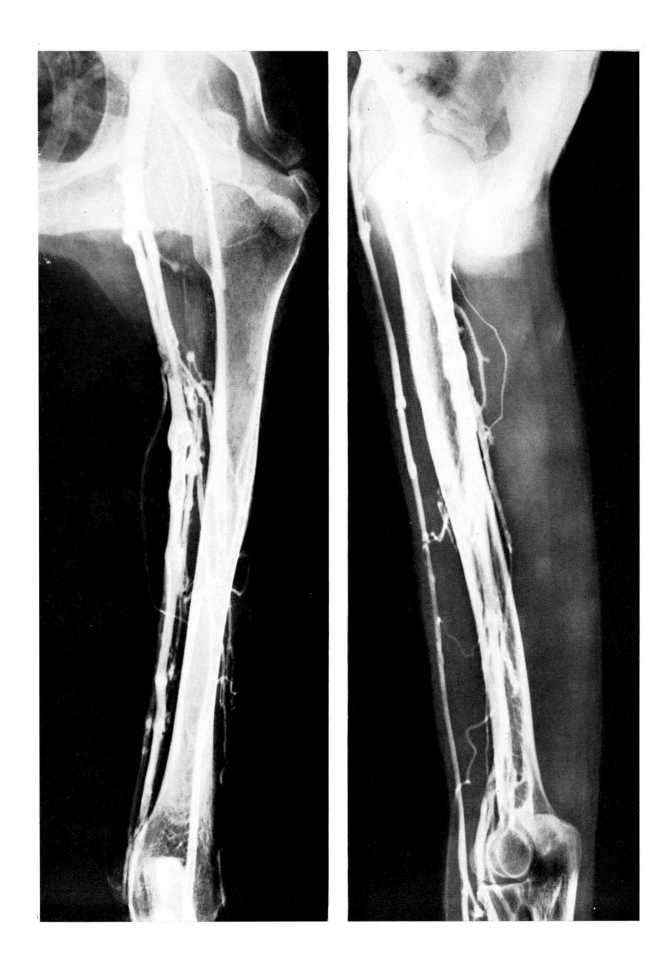

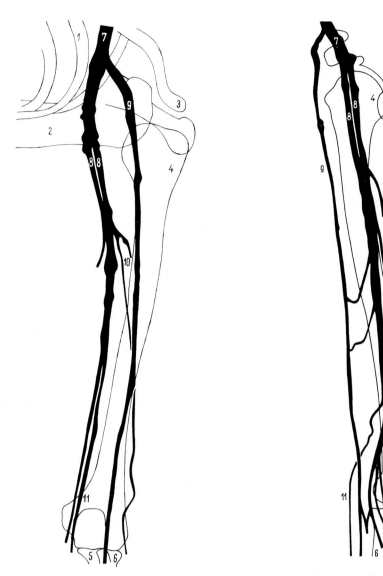

FIGS 129 and 130. The brachial veins, cephalic vein, basilic vein.
Anteroposterior view (Fig. 129) and lateromedial view (Fig. 130).

1. Ribs	*5*. Ulna	*9*. Cephalic vein
2. Scapula	*6*. Radius	*10*. Deep brachial
3. Clavicle	*7*. Axillary vein	veins
4. Humerus	*8*. Brachial veins	*11*. Basilic vein

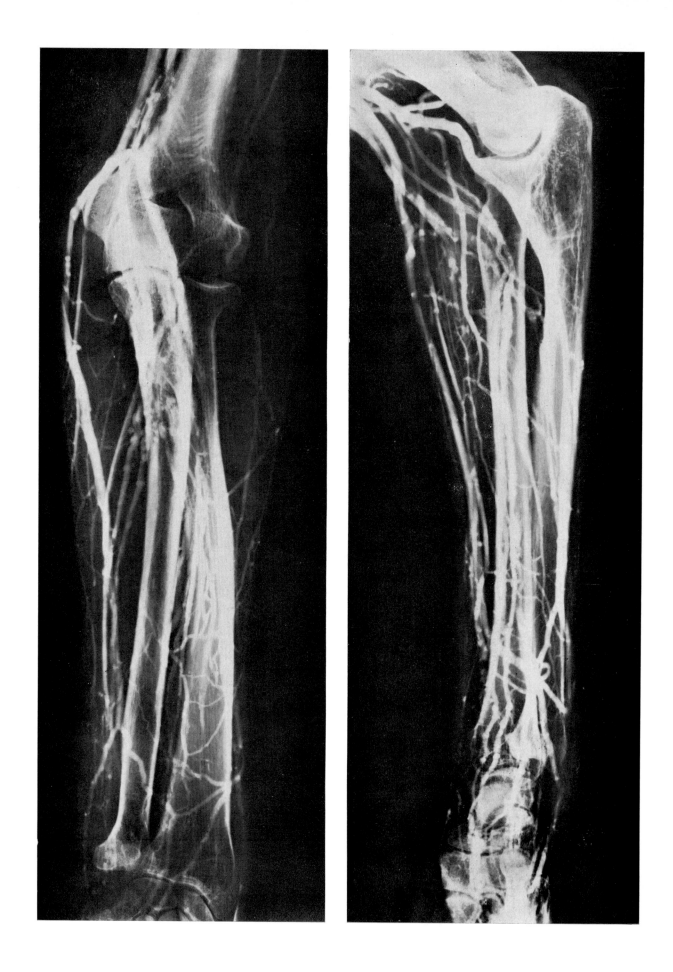

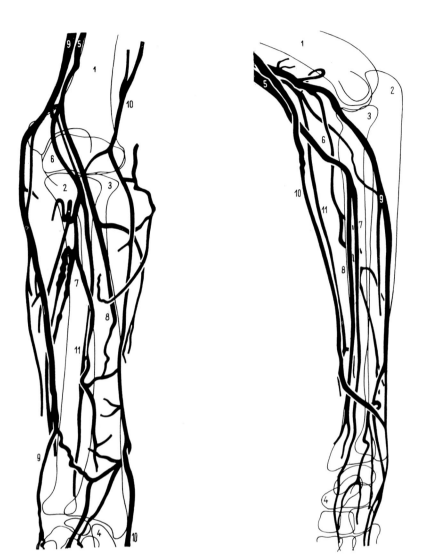

FIGS. 131 and 132. The radial and ulnar veins, basilic vein, cephalic vein.
Anteroposterior view (Fig. 131) and lateromedial view (Fig. 132).

1. Humerus
2. Ulna
3. Radius
4. Bones of the carpus

5. Brachial veins
6. Median cubital vein
7. Ulnar veins
8. Radial veins

9. Basilic vein
10. Cephalic vein
11. Median vein of the
forearm

BLOOD VESSELS OF THE ABDOMINAL CAVITY

THE ABDOMINAL AORTA AND ITS BRANCHES

The trunk and collateral circulation of the abdominal aorta

The abdominal aorta (Figs 133, 151/5, 152/4, 153/9, 156/3, 157/2) passes through the aortic opening of the diaphragm and enters the abdominal cavity in the midline at the level of the 12th thoracic vertebra. Its whole course is in prevertebral position, either in the midline (7 per cent) or somewhat to the left (70 per cent). Only in exceptional cases (5 per cent) does the vessel run to the right of the spinal column. Sometimes it describes a mild curve and is in such cases mostly on the left side (De Luca and De Serio 1960). The arched course bears an influence also upon the height of division (Mercier and Vanneuville 1968). The sympathetic plexus surrounds the entire length of the abdominal aorta. The inferior vena cava lies to the right of the aorta. The two vessels are in contact in the lower half of the abdomen, while, in the upper half of the abdominal cavity, the inferior vena cava deviates to the right from the aorta. The initial portion of the thoracic duct is placed behind and to the right, the ascending lumbar veins to the left of the aorta. In front of it, below the diaphragm, lie the omental bursa, the pancreas, the splenic vein, the lower segment of the duodenum, the root of the mesentery, the left renal vein and the intestines. The abdominal aorta is pressed along its entire abdominal course against the posterior abdominal wall and the spine by the parietal portion of the peritoneum. The left suprarenal gland and the renal capsule are placed to the left of the vessel.

The abdominal aorta divides into its two terminal branches (common iliac arteries) at the lower border of the 4th (3rd to 5th) lumbar vertebra. Division at the height of the 2nd lumbar vertebra is exceptional (Adachi 1928, De Luca and De Serio 1960). The division is deeper in advanced age. The angle of division is 65° to 75°. The length of the abdominal aorta is 20 to 23 cm, the diameter 2·3 cm (1·5 to 3·0 cm; De Luca and De Serio 1960).

The *median sacral artery* (Figs 133/12, 151/38, 192/8, 194/5), the rudimentary continuation of the abdominal aorta, begins at the division in the mid-line. It may arise from either of the two common iliac arteries. From this small artery, passing in front of the sacrum, originates at the level of the 5th lumbar vertebra the *fifth lumbar artery* (Fig. 133/13) and the *sacral branches*. These latter communicate with the branches of the iliolumbar artery.

The abdominal aorta gives off branches to the abdominal wall and the viscera. The branches of the abdominal aorta may be paired or unpaired. In the order of origin, the following typical ramifications (Fig.133) can be seen.

Name of branch	Level of origin	Localization
1. Inferior phrenic arteries	12th thoracic	frontal, bilateral
2. Lumbar arteries	1st–4th lumbar	behind, bilateral
3. Celiac trunk	12th thoracic–1st lumbar	frontal
4. Middle suprarenal artery	1st–2nd lumbar	bilateral
5. Superior mesenteric artery	1st–2nd lumbar	frontal
6. Renal artery	1st–2nd lumbar	bilateral
7. Testicular artery (ovarian artery)	2nd–3rd lumbar	frontal, bilateral
8. Inferior mesenteric artery	3rd–4th lumbar	frontal

The **collaterals** of the abdominal aorta (Fig. 134) maintain circulation via communication between the subclavian and the external iliac arteries or the abdominal aorta and the external iliac artery, respectively. The routes are as follows: (1) Subclavian artery—internal thoracic artery—superior and inferior epigastric arteries—external iliac artery (Figs 134/2, 3, 16 and 15). (2) Abdominal aorta—posterior intercostal artery (XII) and lumbar arteries—deep circumflex iliac artery—external iliac artery

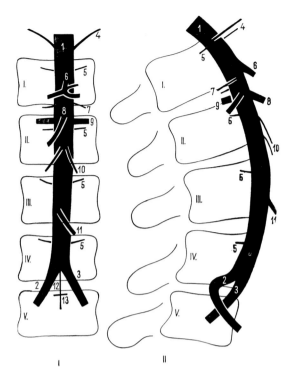

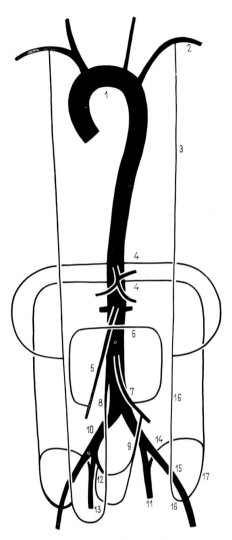

Fig. 133. Localization of the branches from the abdominal aorta. I, anteroposterior view, II, lateral view. (*1*) Aorta; (*2*) right common iliac artery; (*3*) left common iliac artery; (*4*) inferior phrenic artery, (*5*) 1st to 5th lumbar arteries; (*6*) celiac trunk; (*7*) middle suprarenal artery; (*8*) superior mesenteric artery; (*9*) renal artery; (*10*) testicular (ovarian) artery; (*11*) inferior mesenteric artery; (*12*) median sacral artery; (*13*) lumbalis ima (5th lumbar) artery.

(Figs 134/4, 17 and 15). (3) Abdominal aorta—lumbar arteries—iliolumbar artery—internal iliac artery—external iliac artery (Figs 134/4, 14, 11 and 15). (4) Abdominal aorta—superior mesenteric artery—Riolan's arch—inferior mesenteric artery—superior and inferior rectal arteries—internal pudendal artery—internal iliac artery—external iliac artery (Figs 134/5, 6, 7, 9, 13, 12, 11 and 15). (5) Abdominal aorta—testicular artery (ovarian artery)—anterior scrotal branches (anterior labial branches)—external iliac artery (Figs 134/8 and 15).

For clinical purposes, Gottlob (1956) grouped the circulation through the collateral pathways into two categories, namely upper circulation when the obstruction is immediately below the origin of the renal artery and lower, when the lumen is occluded immediately above the bifurcation. Upper circulation is maintained according to the aforesaid grouping heads as under (1), (4) and (5); lower circulation as under (2), (3) and the lower tract of (4). According to Göbbeler and Löhr (1968) regional blood flow may be secured independently through the visceral or parietal arteries.

Fig. 134. Collaterals of the abdominal aorta. (*1*) Aorta; (*2*) subclavian artery; (*3*) internal thoracic artery; (*4*) 12th posterior intercostal artery; lumbar arteries; (*5*) superior mesenteric artery; (*6*) Riolan's arcade; (*7*) inferior mesenteric artery; (*8*) testicular (ovarian) artery; (*9*) superior rectal artery; (*10*) common iliac artery; (*11*) internal iliac artery; (*12*) internal pudendal artery; (*13*) inferior rectal artery; (*14*) iliolumbar artery; (*15*) external iliac artery; (*16*) inferior epigastric artery; (*17*) deep circumflex iliac artery.

Inferior phrenic artery, lumbar arteries, middle suprarenal artery, testicular artery and their branches

The **inferior phrenic artery** (Figs 133/4, 135/7, 136/2, 153/15 and 16), a paired vessel, arises from the anterior surface of the aorta immediately below the diaphragm at the level of the 12th thoracic vertebra (Fig. 135/7A). It may also originate from the celiac trunk (Fig. 135/7B), the left gastric artery (Figs 135/7C, 153/15), the common hepatic artery (Fig. 135/7D) and the renal artery (Fig. 135/7E;

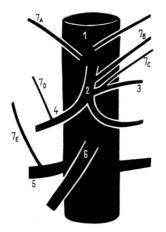

FIG. 135. Variations in the origin of the inferior phrenic artery. (*1*) Aorta; (*2*) celiac trunk; (*3*) left gastric artery; (*4*) common hepatic artery; (*5*) right renal artery; (*6*) superior mesenteric artery; (*7*) inferior phrenic artery (7_A arising from the aorta, 7_B from the celiac trunk, 7_C from the left gastric, 7_D from the common hepatic, 7_E from the right renal artery).

Pick and Anson 1940, Kahn 1967). The accessory inferior phrenic artery is extremely rare (Paturet 1958). Following the shape of the domes of the diaphragm, the inferior phrenic artery describes a curve on both

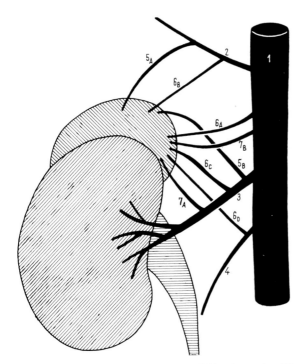

FIG. 136. Variations of the suprarenal blood supply. (*1*) Aorta; (*2*) inferior phrenic artery; (*3*) renal artery; (*4*) testicular artery; (*5*) superior suprarenal artery (5_A arising from the inferior phrenic, 5_B from the renal artery); (*6*) middle suprarenal artery (6_A arising from the aorta, 6_B from the inferior phrenic, 6_C from the renal, 6_D from the testicular artery); (*7*) inferior suprarenal artery (7_A arising from the renal artery, 7_B from the aorta).

sides. Its length measures 4·8 cm before the division, its diameter is 0·83 mm (De Luca and De Serio 1960). Together with the superior, the inferior phrenic artery supplies the diaphragm and the suprarenal glands. Its *branches:*

The *superior suprarenal artery*, the upper branch to the suprarenal gland (Figs 136/5A, 140/3, 153/43, 154/5, 156/15), is frequently a multiple artery (Gagnon 1957). A small branch from the main trunk, curves down to the renal capsule (Boijsen 1959). It originates from the renal artery in one-sixth of the cases (Fig. 136/5B).

The superior capsular artery and the middle suprarenal artery may arise, as supernumerary vessels, from the inferior phrenic artery (Adachi 1928, Anson et al. 1947).

The **lumbar arteries** (Figs 133/5, 152/26), four paired arteries, arise from the posterior side of the abdominal aorta at the level of the middle segment of the bodies of the lumbar vertebrae. Running laterally they enter the psoas muscle. The first two arteries are covered by the crura of the diaphragm. All vessels of the right side pass behind the inferior vena cava. The 5th lumbar artery arises from the iliolumbar artery. The average diameter of the lumbar arteries is 0·14 cm (De Luca and De Serio 1960). Each artery gives off a *dorsal branch* at the level of the intervertebral foramen which also furnishes a *spinal branch*. In their further curving course, they communicate with the branches of the inferior epigastric artery, above with the anterior intercostal arteries and below, with the iliolumbar, the deep and superficial circumflex iliac arteries (Paturet 1958).

The **middle suprarenal artery** arises in 70 per cent of the cases from the aorta (Figs 133/7, 136/6A, 140/5, 156/14) below the origin of the superior mesenteric artery. It may also originate from the left gastric, splenic, common hepatic, 1st lumbar, inferior phrenic (Fig. 136/6B), renal (Fig. 136/6C) and the testicular (Fig. 136/6D) arteries (Boijsen 1959, Gagnon 1964, Kahn 1967). After reaching the suprarenal gland, the artery ramifies into numerous branches and forms communications with the superior and inferior suprarenal arteries.

The **testicular (ovarian) arteries** (Figs 133/10, 137, 156/19, 194/27, 198/4, 199/8) arise on the anterior side of the aorta below the origin of the renal artery, at the height of the 2nd to 3rd lumbar vertebra (Fig. 137/I). They may commence with a common trunk from the aorta (Fig. 137/II, Rauber and Kopsch 1951), from the renal (Fig. 137/III) or the supernumerary renal artery (Anson and Kurth 1955) as well as from the middle suprarenal artery (Fig. 137/IV, Adachi 1928). Variations in the origin occur in 10 to 15 per cent. The length of the *testicular*

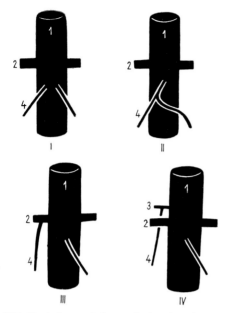

FIG. 137. Variations of the testicular (ovarian) artery. I, normal type; II, common trunk; III, origin from the renal artery; IV, origin from the middle suprarenal artery. (*1*) Aorta; (*2*) renal artery; (*3*) middle suprarenal artery; (*4*) testicular (ovarian) artery.

artery is 21·7 cm (17 to 30 cm), its average diameter 0·8 mm (De Luca and De Serio 1960). The vessel crosses the ureter and the external iliac artery obliquely on the musculus psoas major; then it enters the inguinal canal and ramifies in males in the testicle. The *ovarian artery* is shorter. It turns medially at the boundary of the true pelvis. Passing through the ligament of the ovary, it divides between the folds of the broad ligament. In its initial course, the ovarian (testicular) artery often gives off several small branches to the renal capsule or the ureter (*capsular* and *ureteric branches;* Fig. 140/11; Schmerber 1896).

The renal arteries, their branches and their collateral circulation

The renal arteries (Figs 133/9, 138, 139, 140, 151/35, 152/24 and 25, 153/40, 154/2, 155/2, 156/10 and 11, 157/32) arise bilaterally from the sides of the abdominal aorta, somewhat behind its middle plane, at the level of the 1st or 2nd lumbar vertebra. The origin of the vessel is at the level of the lower half of the 1st lumbar vertebra in more than 50 per cent, between the 1st and 2nd in about 25 per cent, and sometimes at the height of the 2nd lumbar vertebra (Edsman 1957, De Luca and De Serio 1960, Olsson 1964). The artery of the right side usually originates somewhat higher than its contralateral partner. Heidsieck (1928) found the right renal

artery 1·41 cm and the lett 1·51 cm below the origin of the superior mesenteric artery. Sabbagh et al. (1970) found the origin of both renal arteries in one case at the division of the aorta. Edsman (1957) found correlation between the position of the kidneys and the origin of the renal arteries. He was able to determine the site of origin of the individual renal arteries with a 95 per cent accuracy on the left and with one of 70 per cent on the right side by means of his diagram. Arising, the renal arteries run toward the hilum. The right artery lies behind the inferior vena cava. Both arteries are frontally covered by the corresponding veins.

The right artery has a length of 4·5 cm (3·7 to 7·0 cm), the left artery one of 4·0 cm (2·5 to 5·0 cm; De Luca and De Serio 1960a, b, c, d). The length depends on the point of ramification. The average diameter: on the right, 0·43 cm; on the left, 0·45 cm (0·2 to 0·6 cm for both sides). The course of the renal arteries may be ascending, horizontal or descending (Augier 1923, Narath 1951). Boijsen (1959) registered ascending arteries in 40·1 per cent on the left, in 8·6 per cent on the right side; horizontal courses in 43·4 per cent on the left, in 39·0 per cent on the right side; descending vessels in 16·5 per cent on the left, in 51·9 per cent on the right side. In cases of renal artery with a straight course the increase in blood pressure influences the kidney's position on account of the stiffening of the vessel (Hayek 1935). If the vessel is tortuous, the position of the kidney is displaced laterally or downward in similar cases (Mörike 1965).

The renal artery bifurcates usually either before the hilum of the kidney or in the sinus; these branches, giving off further branches, ramify like terminal arteries in the kidney (Graves 1954, Boijsen 1959, Olsson 1964). It is usual to divide the kidney into segments belonging to certain larger vessels. Running in front of and behind the renal pelvis, respectively, the anterior and the posterior main trunks divide into further branches. Boijsen (1959) distinguishes 4 or 5, Graves (1954) and Sykes (1964) 5, Serov (1959) 4, Ternon (1959) 3, Faller and Ungvári (1962) 7 segments.

Löfgren (1949) distinguishes in each kidney seven dorsal (D) and seven ventral (V) pyramids. The kidney has three parts: the superior part contains the three pairs of upper pyramids (1V, 1D, 2V, 2D, 3V, 3D), the intermediate part contains the 4th and the 5th pair (4V, 4D, 5V, 5D), the inferior part contains the 6th and the 7th pair (6V, 6D, 7V, 7D). Considering pyramidal distribution, Boijsen (1959) presents the vascular supply of the four segments, described by him, as follows.

The *posterior branch* (Figs 155/4, 156/10) is usually a continuation of the posterior branch of the

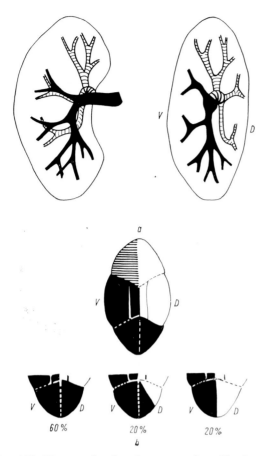

FIG. 138. Diagram showing the segmental ramification of the renal arteries (after Olsson, O. and Jönsson, G.: Roentgen examination of the kidney and the ureter. In: Handbuch der Urologie. Vol. V/1. Springer, Berlin—Göttingen—Heidelberg, 1962. pp. 1—365). *V*, ventral artery; *D*, dorsal artery, *a*, scheme of the most frequent blood supply, *b*, variation of blood supply of the inferior pole (black: from the front; white: from behind; striped: segments of mixed supply).

renal artery. In 80 per cent it arises from the renal artery outside the hilum, and in 5 to 10 per cent directly from the aorta (Fine and Keen 1966). The vessel turns behind the calyces toward the hilum; in 20 per cent of the cases it supplies a part of the posterior portion of the lower segment, and in 20 per cent it supplies blood to the entire posterior part of the kidney (Olsson and Jönsson 1962). Beside permanently supplying the pyramids 4D and 5D, the area of supply of the vessel may include the whole apex in which case the entire dorsal part of the kidney relies on this branch for blood supply (Fig. 138).

The *anterior branch* (Figs 155/3, 156/1) gives off an upper and a middle branch to the medial part of the anterior side of the kidney (*superior anterior*, Fig. 156/12 and *inferior anterior segmental arteries*, Fig. 156/20). The latter artery has an extrahilar origin in 7 per cent, the anterior superior in 25 per

cent of the cases (Fine and Keen 1966). The vessel entering the parenchyma winds around the upper calyces or around the neck of the calyces and divides. course of the arteries of the anterior surface is usually parallel with the neck of the middle calyces, but may run crosswise as well (Mátyus 1965). The vessel supplies pyramids 4V and 5V but may supply also the pyramid 3V, and more frequently (60 per cent) the apex of the inferior pole (6V, 6D, 7V, 7D, Olsson and Jönsson 1962).

The *inferior segmental* (*polar*) *artery* is a direct branch of the aorta in 60 per cent, and arises from the anterior branch of the main trunk in 40 per cent of the cases. Its area of supply covers the pyramids 6V, 6D, 7V and 7D. The posterior branch supplies half of the posterior part of the kidney in 20, the whole of it in another 20 per cent of the cases.

The *superior segmental* (*polar*) *artery* (Figs 153/41, 154/3, 156/12) has many variations. It may arise from the hilar or the proximal segment of the main trunk of the renal artery (80 per cent) or from the aorta. The vessel frequently divides before entering the parenchyma, in which case it may cause compression by encircling the neck of the superior calyces. The vessel supplies the pyramids 1V, 1D, 2V, 2D and in 10 per cent of the cases 3V and 3D (Graves 1954).

Multiple renal arteries (Figs 139, 153, 154, 156). The renal arteries have numerous variations; they are of clinical importance partly because they are frequently associated with pathological processes and partly because they can easily be confused with other vessels (Olsson 1964).

The incidence of multiple renal arteries is estimated at 26 per cent (Boijsen 1959, Edsman 1957, Vogler and Herbst 1958, Geyer and Poutasse 1962). Supernumerary arteries occur in approximately the same proportion on both sides. Duplication of the renal artery (Figs 139/IV, 153/40 and 41, 156/10 and 11) has been observed in 24 to 25 per cent, triplication (Figs 139/VII, 156/10 and 11) in 1 to 2 per cent, quadruplication in 0·1 per cent (Hellström 1928, Boijsen 1959). Even 6 renal arteries have been described on one side (Kyaw and Newman 1971).

Hellström ordered the variations of the renal arteries in the following scheme:

1. Renal artery without polar arteries (normal type)

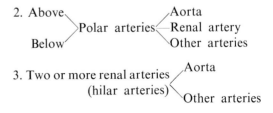

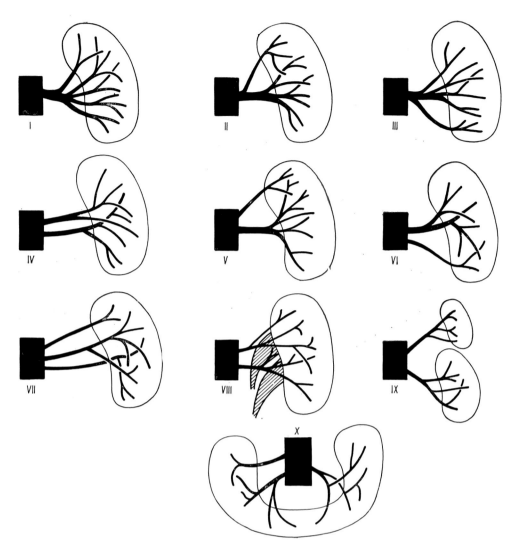

FIG. 139. Variations of the renal arteries. I, normal type; II, one artery + superior polar artery; III, one artery + inferior polar artery; IV, two arteries; V, two arteries (superior polar artery arises from the aorta); VI, two arteries (inferior polar artery arises from the aorta); VII, three arteries (superior polar artery arises from the aorta); VIII, two arteries (double renal pelvis); IX, two arteries (double kidney); X, horseshoe kidney.

Supernumerary origin of the upper and lower polar arteries is the most frequent. Evaluating the blood supply of 11,000 kidneys, Merklin and Michels (1958) registered the origin of the superior segmental artery from the renal artery (Fig. 139/II) in 12 per cent, from the aorta (Fig. 139/V) in 7 per cent; origin of the inferior segmental artery from the renal artery (Fig. 139/III) in 1·4 per cent and from the aorta in 5·5 per cent (Fig. 139/VI). If not from the aorta, the supernumerary renal arteries may spring from the common hepatic artery, the celiac trunk, the superior and inferior mesenteric artery and the internal iliac artery (Rauber and Kopsch 1951, Tille 1961, Mlynarczyk et al. 1966). A supernumerary renal artery may originate also from the contralateral renal artery (Libshitz et al. 1972). The superior polar artery arises more frequently from the renal artery, while the less frequent in-

ferior polar artery commences more often in the aorta. The upper vessels begin above the main renal arteries, before reaching the renal sinus. The origin of the lower supernumerary vessel is more variable. As a rule, it runs to the hilum of the kidney from where it pursues a normal further course. The middle segments are less frequently supplied by supernumerary arteries than the two poles. Bálint and Palkovich (1952) divided the anomalous renal vessels into two groups. Arteries of the first group have their special area of supply, those of the second group form anastomoses with the renal artery without supplying any particular segment. The latter arise mainly from the muscle arteries or from the extrarenal segment of the renal artery.

Kápolnási and Végh (1972) found a solitary renal artery which supplied both kidneys with one branch each.

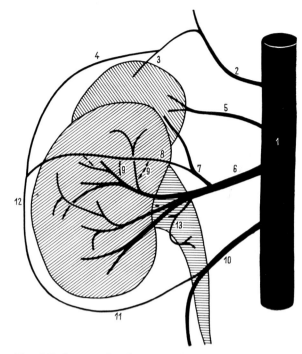

Fig. 140. Intrarenal and extrarenal collaterals of the renal artery. (*1*) Aorta; (*2*) inferior phrenic artery; (*3*) superior suprarenal artery; (*4*) superior capsular artery; (*5*) middle suprarenal artery; (*6*) renal artery; (*7*) inferior suprarenal artery; (*8*) middle capsular artery; (*9*) perforating arteries (*10*) testicular artery; (*11*) inferior capsular artery; (*12*) perirenal arterial arch; (*13*) pelvic and ureteric branches.

Variations in the development of the kidneys. Variations in the development of the kidneys are accompanied by changes in their vascular system. Olsson (1964) distinguishes from a clinical viewpoint the following categories: Variations in number (agenesis, supernumerary kidneys). Irregular position (ectopia, rotation). Irregular shape or size (hypoplasia, hyperplasia, fusion). Structural anomalies. Only supernumerary kidneys and certain forms of fusion are the anatomical variations of normal functioning. Double kidneys (Fig. 139/IX) are supplied by one or more renal arteries. Archlike communications in the sinus may exist among multiple vessels (Babics 1945). The blood supply of fused kidneys (horseshoe kidney, Fig. 139/X) shows great variability (Vogler and Herbst 1958, Pirlet and Delvigne 1965). The frequently occurring supernumerary renal arteries arise besides the aorta mainly from the common iliac artery (Boatman et al. 1971). There is no correlation between the variability of the calyces and the renal pelvis on the one hand, and the number of renal arteries, on the other. In cases with double pelves (Fig. 139/VIII) there are supernumerary vessels in about 50 per cent (Boijsen 1959).

Intrarenal vascular structure (Figs 154, 155, 156). A close correlation exists between the above-mentioned types of division of the renal artery, the segmental and subsegmental (*interlobar*) arteries running between the pyramids, and the lobation of the kidney (Sykes 1964). After giving off small branches to the calyces and the renal pelvis, every interlobar artery runs toward the cortex along the side of the pyramid. At the margin of the cortex and the medulla dichotomy takes place. The vessels running at right angles to the surface turn so that the further course runs parallel to the surface (*arcuate arteries*). From them the *interlobular arteries*, from which the *vasa afferentia* are derived, course toward the cortex (Gray 1954). The medulla is supplied with blood by the *arteriolae rectae verae* which originate from the arcuate arteries, and by the *arteriolae rectae spuriae* which commence in the *vasa efferentia*.

Extrarenal branches of the renal artery:

The *inferior phrenic artery* (Fig. 135/7$_E$) arises sometimes on the right side from the renal artery (Kahn 1967).

The *superior suprarenal artery* (Fig. 136/5$_B$) arises, frequently in multiple form, from the renal artery in one-sixth of the cases (Gagnon 1957).

The *middle suprarenal artery* (Figs 136/6$_C$, 156/14) originates sometimes from the renal artery (Boijsen 1959).

The *inferior suprarenal artery* (Figs 136/7$_A$, 151/36, 154/6, 156/13), branch of the renal artery in 97 per cent of the cases, gives off a small branch to the capsule of the kidney (superior capsular artery). The vessel may originate from the aorta (Fig. 136/7B), the testicular artery (Fig. 137/IV), the inferior capsular as well as from the ureteral artery (Gagnon 1966).

Capsular arteries. The *superior capsular artery* (Figs 140/4, 153/42, 154/4, 156/16) may arise from the inferior capsular artery, the renal artery, the aorta or from the inferior phrenic artery (Anson et al. 1947). The *middle capsular artery* (Figs 140/8, 154/7, 156/17), winding round the hilum of the kidney from the front and from behind, runs to the convex border of the kidney. It communicates with the interlobar and interlobular arteries by way of its perforating branches (Schmerber 1895). It may arise from the lumbar arteries, the superior mesenteric, the left colic and the renal arteries (Schmerber 1896). The *inferior capsular artery* (Figs 140/11, 156/18) is usually a branch of the testicular artery. It describes an arch which extends below the inferior pole of the kidney and communicates with the superior capsular artery.

The testicular (ovarian artery) (Figs 137/III, 156/19) sometimes arises from the renal artery or a supernumerary renal vessel (Anson and Kurth 1955).

The *pelvic and ureteric branches* (Fig. 140/13) are small vessels to the pelvis and the ureters (Douiville and Hollinshead 1955).

Collateral circulation of the kidney (Fig. 140).

The segmental arteries of the kidney are terminal vessels (Graves 1954) so that there is no collateral arterial circulation in this organ. Nephrography is nevertheless feasible by the isolated filling of a segmental artery (Mátyus 1965). This is made possible by venous or arteriovenous anastomoses (Gömöri et al. 1965). Extrarenal and intrarenal anastomoses may, however, maintain collateral circulation to a certain extent.

1. Most significant of the extrarenal communications is the arched anastomosis between the inferior and the superior capsular arteries formed on the convex aspect of the kidney (arcus arteriosus perirenalis, Figs 140/12, 154/8). Also the inferior suprarenal, the pelvic and ureteric branches, possibly the inferior phrenic, the superior and middle suprarenal, the subcostal as well as the testicular arteries may contribute to the maintenance of collateral circulation (Habighorst et al. 1966, Suhler et al. 1966, Tongio et al. 1971). Anastomoses have been registered via the superior and the inferior mesenteric arteries (Camerini and Scagnol 1967).

2. Intrarenal anastomoses may be formed through the perforating arteries (Fig. 140/9) which connect the interlobar and interlobular arteries with the capsular vessels (Merklin and Michels 1958, Graves 1954, Boijsen 1959). Two groups of these vessels are known: the glomerular and aglomerular branches. Under normal condition, blood in the perforating branches circulates from the kidney to the perirenal vessels (Eliska 1968). According to clinical observations, the normally imperceptible small vessels are capable of maintaining adequate blood supply if the main trunk becomes insufficient (Haage and Rehm 1964).

The celiac trunk and its branches

The *celiac trunk* (Figs 133/6, 141, 143/6, 151/11, 152/8, 153/13, 157/6) arises from the aorta immediately below the aortic opening. The projection of

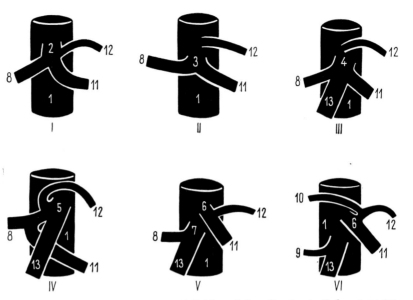

Fig. 141. Variations in the origin and division of the celiac trunk. I, hepatogastrolienal trunk (celiac trunk); II, hepatolienal trunk; III, hepatolienomesenteric trunk; IV, celiacomesenteric trunk; V, gastrolienal and hepatomesenteric trunks; VI, gastrolienal trunk. (*1*) Aorta; (*2 to 7*) various types of division of the celiac trunk; (*8*) common hepatic artery; (*9*) right accessory hepatic artery; (*10*) left accessory hepatic artery; (*11*) splenic artery; (*12*) left gastric artery; (*13*) superior mesenteric artery.

its origin is usually seen at the level of the intervertebral space between the 12th thoracic and the 1st lumbar vertebrae (Rossi and Cova 1904, Adachi 1928, Ödman 1958). The vessel may originate deeper if it arises together with the superior mesenteric artery. With reference to the anterior wall of the aorta, the vessel commences to the left of the midline in 25 per cent and in the midline in 75 per cent of the cases. Its origin on the right side is exceptional. Related to the renal artery, the distance of the origin is 1 to 4 cm (Boijsen and Olin 1964) and to the superior mesenteric artery, it originates at a distance of 0·92 cm (0·2 to 3·0 cm; Michels 1955). The celiac trunk usually follows a downward course to the right (Rossi and Cova 1904), although it may exceptionally run upward to the right (Ödman 1958). It gives off branches to the stomach, liver, gall bladder, duodenum, pancreas and spleen. In the course of their ramification, they form several anastomoses with the branches of the superior mesenteric artery. The celiac trunk measures 2·48 cm (1·1 to 3·5 cm) in length and 1·01 cm (0·6 to 1·3 cm) in width (Michels 1955).

Adachi (1928) distinguishes six types of division of the celiac trunk (Fig. 141): Truncus hepatogastrolienalis (celiac trunk; Fig. 141/I) is formed by the union of the common hepatic, the left gastric and the splenic arteries. This type occurs in 73 to 90 per cent of the cases (Rossi and Cova 1904, Piquand 1910, Adachi 1928). Truncus hepatolienalis (Fig.

231

141/II) is present if the left gastric artery arises separately which occurs in 7·5 per cent of the cases (Piquand 1910, Adachi 1928). Truncus hepatolienomesentericus (Fig. 141/III) is present if, in addition to the common hepatic and splenic arteries, also the superior mesenteric artery arises with the common trunk which occurs in 1·2 per cent (Adachi 1928). Truncus celiacomesentericus (Fig. 141/IV) is formed by the common origin of the three standard vessels and the superior mesenteric artery (1·3 per cent, Rossi and Cova 1904, Rio Branco 1912, Eaton 1917). Communication may be formed also between the celiac trunk, superior and inferior mesenteric arteries (Zwerina and Poisel 1966). The truncus gastrolienalis is formed by the common origin of the left gastric and the splenic arteries, the truncus hepatomesentericus by that of the common hepatic and the superior mesenteric arteries. This type (Fig. 141/V) is seen in 0·4 per cent of the cases (Adachi 1928). Truncus gastrolienalis (Fig. 141/VI) is present if the left gastric and the splenic arteries arise together. The common hepatic artery is absent, and its function is taken over by the left accessory hepatic artery (emitted by the left gastric artery) or the right accessory hepatic artery (emitted by the superior mesenteric artery). The incidence of this variation is 2 to 4 per cent (Rio Branco 1912, Adachi 1928). The lack of the celiac trunk and the superior mesenteric arteries have been described in which case they were replaced by the well developed inferior mesenteric artery (Witt and Kourik 1969). Numerous combinations of the six main types are possible owing to the variable origin of the side branches.

The celiac trunk gives off the following *branches:* left gastric, common hepatic (right accessory hepatic, left accessory hepatic, left accessory gastric), right gastric, cystic, gastroduodenal and splenic arteries. In addition, the celiac trunk may have the following variations in division: dorsal pancreatic, right inferior phrenic, middle colic and accessory middle colic arteries (Adachi 1928, Michels 1955, Ödman 1958).

The **left gastric artery** (Figs 141/12, 143/20, 151/25, 152/15, 153/14, 157/7, 158/3, 165/14) usually originates from the celiac trunk but springs off in 6 per cent of the cases directly from the aorta (Michels 1955). Its origin is at the level of the 2nd lumbar vertebra (Th 12—L 2) (De Luca and De Serio 1960). If arising directly from the aorta, it originates 0·5 cm higher. The inferior phrenic artery (Fig. 153/15) may commence in such cases in the left gastric artery. The main trunk runs to the upper end of the lesser curvature of the stomach between the layers of the lesser omentum. It forms an arterial arch with the right gastric artery along the lesser curvature of the stomach. The artery sometimes bifurcates along the curvature. Its side branches (6 to 12) run at right angles to the axis of the stomach on the anterior and posterior wall of this organ. The left gastric artery supplies a larger area in the upper two-third of the stomach than the branches of the left gastroepiploic artery which extends to this area from the greater curvature. The left gastric artery has a length of 6 cm (3 to 10 cm) and a diameter of 0·3 cm (0·2 to 0·7 cm De Luca and De Serio 1960). Collateral circulation is established mainly via the esophageal and the short gastric branches (Sundergren 1970). It anastomoses with the terminal branches of the left gastroepiploic artery behind the stomach and intraparietally (Levasseur and Couinaud 1968).

The **common hepatic artery** (Figs 141/8, 143/7, 151/12, 152/9, 153/17, 157/8) originates from the eliac trunk (93 per cent), the superior mesenteric artery (4 per cent) or from the aorta (3 per cent; Adachi 1928, Morino 1959). Its origin is usually at the level of the 1st lumbar vertebra (Th 12—L 2; De Luca and De Serio 1960). The common hepatic artery and its continuation, the hepatic artery, run in the hepatoduodenal ligament to the porta hepatis. The bile duct lies to the right of the vessel, while the portal vein is between and behind these vessels. The length of the hepatic artery is 5·3 cm (3 to 8 cm; De Luca and De Serio 1960), its diameter 0·4 to 1·2 cm (Michels 1955, Ödman 1958). Collateral circulation chiefly provided by the gastroduodenal, cystic and right gastric arteries, is quite varied.

Adachi (1928) distinguished the following *variations in the types of division* of the common hepatic artery: 1. After a course of 2 to 3 cm the common hepatic artery divides into the hepatic artery and the gastroduodenal artery (91 per cent). 2. The main trunk divides into three branches. Two are distributed to the liver, while the third continues as the gastroduodenal artery (5 per cent). 3. The main trunk gives off a first and a second branch to the liver, further the gastroduodenal artery (3·5 per cent). 4. After giving off three branches to the liver the vessel continues as the gastroduodenal artery (0·5 per cent).

The **hepatic artery** (Figs 142/1, 151/13, 153/18, 157/9, 162/4, 163/5, 183/15) is the continuation of the common hepatic artery. It is the main source of hepatic blood supply. Its length is 0·5 to 4 cm, its diameter 0·3 to 0·7 cm (Ödman 1958).

The vessel usually enters the liver with three *branches* (middle, right and left branches). The following arteries are, according to Michels (1957), most frequently present in the porta hepatis: 1. right, left and middle branches (from the hepatic artery); 2. right and middle branches (from the

232

hepatic artery); left branch (from the left gastric artery); 3. left and middle branches (from the hepatic artery); right branch (from the right accessory hepatic artery). 4. Right, left and middle branches (from the hepatic artery); left accessory hepatic artery. 5. Right, left and middle branches (from the hepatic artery); right accessory hepatic artery. 6. There are sometimes five branches of the hepatic artery in the hilum (Kiss 1926). 7. The right or left accessory hepatic artery may exist also or may be present together without any branches of hepatic artery. This possibility is rare.

The *middle branch* (Figs 162/12, 163/11, 183/21), is an arterial segment, that enters and supplies the quadrate lobe of the liver. It courses along the anterior side of the left branch of the portal vein. It arises together with the left and right branches in 50, with the right branch in 40, and with the left branch in 10 per cent of the cases (Adachi 1928). Exceptionally, it may commence directly in the hepatic artery. It may also be absent (2 per cent). The diameter measures 0·36 cm (0·2 to 0·6 cm; Michels 1955).

The *right branch* (Figs 142/7, 143/8, 151/14, 153/20, 157/10, 162/5, 163/6, 183/16) courses usually in front of and rarely behind the hepatic duct. It sends off discrete branches to the anterior and posterior sides of the right branch of the portal vein; sometimes both branches are on the anterior side. It is absent in 10 per cent, when its function is taken over by the left or the right accessory hepatic artery. It has a diameter of 0·64 cm (0·4 to 0·9 cm; Michels 1955).

The *left branch* (Figs 142/2, 143/9, 151/15, 153/19, 157/12, 162/6, 163/7, 183/17) enters the porta hepatis behind the left branch of the portal vein in two-third and in front of it in one-third of the cases. If absent (20 per cent), it is replaced by the right or exceptionally by the left accessory hepatic artery. The diameter measures 0·5 (0·3 to 0·7 cm; Michels 1955).

The branches of the hepatic artery are segmentally distributed to the liver (Healey et al. 1953, Couinaud 1954a). There are, according to Couinaud's grouping, eight segments in the liver. The branches of the hepatic artery, portal vein and hepatic duct ramify during their parallelly running courses. The arteries are often tortuous even in normal cases (Alfidi et al. 1968).

Segmentation of the arteries of the liver according to Couinaud (1954; Fig. 142):

1. *Left lobe of the liver.* In case of one bifurcating artery the first branch (*medial segmental artery*, A_4; Figs 142/6, 162/12, 163/11, 183/21) supplies mainly the lower surface of the liver (*superficial branch*, A_{4a}) and sometimes also the triangular part of the

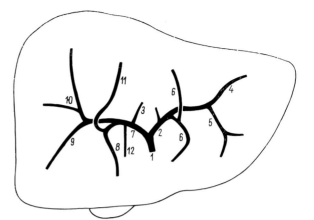

Fig. 142. Division of the hepatic artery in the liver. (*1*) Hepatic artery; (*2*) left branch; (*3*) arteries of the caudate lobe, A_1; (*4*) superior lateral segmental artery, A_2; (*5*) inferior lateral segmental artery, A_3; (*6*) medial segmental artery, A_4; (*7*) right branch; (*8*) inferior anterior segmental artery, A_5; (*9*) inferior posterior segmental artery, A_6; (*10*) superior posterior segmental artery, A_7; (*11*) superior anterior segmental artery, A_8; (*12*) cystic artery.

liver's convexity to the right of the left lobar border (*deep branch*, A_{4b}). The other branch (*lateral segmental artery*, A_{2+3}) divides promptly into two side branches: the *superior lateral segmental artery*, A_2 (Figs 142/4, 162/10, 163/9, 183/19) and the *inferior lateral, segmental artery*, A_3 (Figs 142/5, 162/11, 163/10, 183/20) which supply the corresponding portions of the left segment of the liver. Variations of two arteries: A_{2+3}, A_4; A_{2+3+4a}, A_{4b}; A_2, A_{3+4}. Variations of the three arteries: A_{2+3}, A_1, A_4; A_{1+2}, A_3, A_4.

2. *Right lobe of the liver.* One branch, the *anterior segmental artery*, A_{5+8}, bifurcating, supplies the antero-inferior part of the middle one-third of the right lobe (*inferior anterior segmental artery*, A_5; Figs 142/8, 162/13, 163/12, 183/22) as also its antero-superior part (*superior anterior segmental artery*, A_8; Figs 142/11, 162/16, 163/16, 183/25). The other branch (*posterior segmental artery*, A_{6+7}) supplies the inferolateral part of the right border of the lobe (*inferior posterior segmental artery*, A_6; Figs 142/9, 162/14, 163/14, 183/23), further its posterosuperior part (*superior posterior segmental artery*, A_7; Figs 142/10, 162/15, 163/15, 183/24), Variations: A_{6+7}, A_5, A_8; A_6, A_{5+7+8}; A_{7+8}, A_5, A_6; $A_{5+6+7+8}$.

3. *Caudate lobe of the liver.* The artery which supplies the caudate lobe (*segmental artery to the caudate lobe*, A_1; Figs 142/3, 162/8, 163/8, 183/18) may originate from both the right and the left branches (70 per cent), from the right branch (14 per cent), the left branch (8 per cent), from both the right branch and the hepatic artery (3 per cent), from both the left branch and the hepatic artery (2 per cent) or from the left gastric artery (3 per cent).

233

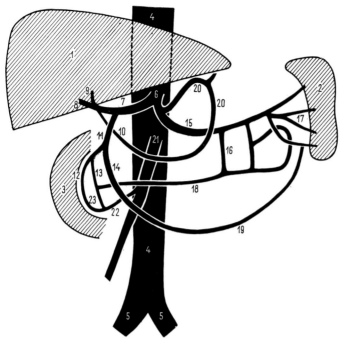

FIG. 143. Principal branches of the celiac trunk (diagram showing blood supply of the pancreas). (*1*) Liver; (*2*) spleen; (*3*) duodenum; (*4*) aorta; (*5*) common iliac artery; (*6*) celiac trunk; (*7*) common hepatic artery; (*8*) right branch of the hepatic artery; (*9*) left branch; (*10*) right gastric artery; (*11*) gastroduodenal artery; (*12*) retroduodenal artery; (*13*) superior supraduodenal artery; (*14*) right gastroepiploic artery; (*15*) splenic artery; (*16*) arteries of the tail of pancreas; (*17*) splenic branches; (*18*) dorsal pancreatic artery; (*19*) left gastroepiploic artery; (*20*) left gastric artery; (*21*) superior mesenteric artery; (*22*) inferior pancreaticoduodenal artery; (*23*) pancreaticoduodenal arches.

The segmental branches are in anastomosis in half of the cases. Extrahepatic communications exist between the larger hepatic arteries and the left gastric, gastroduodenal and cystic arteries (Michels 1955).

The *right accessory hepatic artery* (Fig. 141/9) may arise from the superior mesenteric artery (10 per cent) and less frequently from the celiac trunk, the aorta, the cystic or the pancreaticoduodenal artery (Michels 1955). The vessel runs behind the portal vein and the bile duct to the porta hepatis and supplies as a rule the right lobe of the liver. In the porta hepatis it is situated between the bile duct and the right branch of the portal vein. Here it may anastomose with the hepatic artery or the right branch. The length of the right accessory hepatic artery is 8 cm (7 to 10 cm), its diameter 0·7 cm (0·6 to 0·8 cm; Michels 1955).

The *left accessory hepatic artery* (Figs 141/10, 162/7) may originate from the left gastric artery (17 per cent), or from the aorta, the splenic and the superior mesenteric arteries (Piquand 1910, Michels 1955). From its origin the artery runs between the membranes of the lesser omentum, courses in an

arch to the right and enters the left lobe of the liver. In the porta hepatis it is situated on the posterior (rarely on the anterior) side of the left branch of the portal vein. It may replace the left branch of the hepatic artery. The diameter of the left accessory hepatic artery measures 0·44 cm (0·4 to 0·5 cm; Michels 1955).

The *left accessory gastric artery* is actually similar to the left accessory hepatic artery, only the direction of their courses is reversed, so that they can replace each other. They may establish a connection between the left gastric artery and the arteries of the left hepatic lobe. Between the layers of the lesser omentum is the circulus arteriosus hepatogastricus formed (Adachi 1928). From this ring of vessels arise the hepatic, the left gastric, the right gastric, the gastroduodenal and the inferior phrenic arteries.

The **right gastric artery** (Figs 143/10, 151/16, 153/26, 157/14, 158/4), which runs on the right side of the lesser curvature of the stomach, is smaller than the left gastric artery (Yakubi 1920). It arises from the proper hepatic artery (50 per cent), from the right or left branch (40 per cent), or from the common hepatic artery (10 per cent; Piquand 1910). It branches off from the arterial arch which exists between the gastroduodenal and the hepatic arteries. According to Browne (1940) the artery is missing in 10 per cent of the cases. It runs between the layers of the lesser omentum along the lesser curvature to the left gastric artery. With the latter it forms the superior arterial arch of the stomach. In the region of the pylorus its terminal branches anastomose with the supraduodenal arteries, branches of the gastroduodenal artery.

Cystic artery (Figs 153/21, 157/11, 162/9, 163/13, 183/26). The artery of the gallbladder is usually from the right (61 to 82 per cent) or the left (1 to 13 per cent) branch of the hepatic or from the right accessory hepatic artery (12 per cent), but it may also arise from the hepatic artery, from the vessels A_8 and A_6, from the common hepatic artery, the gastroduodenal artery, the celiac trunk, the superior mesenteric artery or the retroduodenal artery (Rubaschewa 1930, Anson 1951, Couinaud 1954a, Kourias and Peveretos 1972). Doubling of the vessel occurs in 12 to 25 per cent (Rio Branco 1912, Daseler and Cutter 1948, Hess 1961, Deutsch 1967). Triplication is extremely rare (Hess 1961). According to Rubaschewa (1930) the cystic artery divides into a right and a left branch at the junction of the body and the neck of the gall bladder. The main branches are subserous. The left branch supplies the inferior surface and the fundus, the right branch the anterior surface. There are abundant communications between the two branches (Habighorst et al. 1965). Anastomoses are moreover formed with the subcapsular arteries of the right lobe and the quadratus lobe. Kádár and Bálint (1953) in the corrosion preparations found the left branch to provide the principal communication between the arteries of the gall-bladder and the liver. Arteriovenous shunts may be formed here with the portal vein. Also the vascular network of the cystic and hepatic ducts is in communicaton with the branches of the cystic artery (Lang 1947). The length of the cystic artery is 1·7 cm (0·2 to 3·0 cm), its diameter 0·27 cm (0·2 to 0·4 cm; Michels 1955).

The **gastroduodenal artery** (Figs 143/11, 151/17, 152/10, 153/22, 157/13), arising at the beginning of the common hepatic artery, curves downward, then divides into its terminal branches medial to the descending part of the duodenum before the head of the pancreas. It gives off branches to the head of the pancreas, the duodenum and to a part of the omentum. The length of the gastroduodenal artery is 6 cm; its diameter, 0·53 cm (0·4 to 0·7 cm; Michels 1955, Ödman 1958). *Branches:*

The *superior supraduodenal arteries* (Figs 143/13, 152/12, 153/25, 157/17) are small trunks or a single branch to give off branches to the head of the pancreas (*pancreatic branches*) and to the duodenum (*duodenal branches*). They first curve in front of the head of the pancreas then they pursues a mediodorsal course. They often communicate with the arteries of the dorsal side (secondary pancreaticoduodenal arcades; Michels 1955). They form finally the *anterior pancreaticoduodenal arch* (Fig. 151/8) with the inferior (anterior) pancreaticoduodenal artery (Pierson 1943).

The *retroduodenal artery* (Figs 143/12, 153/24, 157/16), the posterior artery of the head of the pancreas, is often a multiple vessel. It may arise also from the hepatic artery, from the right or middle branch and the right gastric artery (Michels 1955). First, it courses dorsolaterally behind the head of the pancreas, winds then medially and forms the *posterior pancreaticoduodenal arch* with the inferior (posterior) pancreaticoduodenal artery (Falconer and Griffiths 1950, Anson 1951). The diameter of the retroduodenal artery is 0·1 to 0·2 cm (Ödman 1955).

Kokas and Kubik (1954) distinguish four types of pancreaticoduodenal arcades. On the anterior arch they observed tortuous or pointed or dented type resembling a "U" in shape. Communication

in this case is provided by the forward curving branches of the posterior arch. On the posterior arch they found a U-shaped, pointed, angular or irregularly shaped formation. The vessels pursue an oblique course to the lumen of the intestine. According to Moretti (1965), the anterior arch may be composed of 1 to 3, the posterior of 1 to 4 vessels.

The *right gastroepiploic artery* (Figs 143/14, 151/19, 152/11, 153/23, 157/15, 158/6) is the direct continuation of the gastroduodenal artery. It may furthermore spring off from the right and left accessory hepatic, the splenic or the superior mesenteric arteries (Adachi 1928). Crossing the superior horizontal part of the duodenum from behind, it runs in front of the pancreas to the greater curvature of the stomach and communicates between the layers of the greater omentum with the left gastroepiploic artery, a branch of the splenic artery (arcus arteriosus ventriculi inferior). The diameter of the right gastroepiploic artery measures 0·2 to 0·4 cm (Ödman 1958). Its branches ramify in the omentum and the greater curvature of the stomach (*epiploic branches*). The right gastroepiploic artery communicates intraparietally with the superior arterial arch of the stomach. Collateral circulation is ensured by the anastomoses between the omental branches (Levasseur and Couinaud 1968).

The **splenic artery** (Figs 143/15, 151/20, 152/16, 153/27, 157/18, 164/4, 165/4, 166 and 167/2) is the largest branch of the celiac trunk. It arises sometimes from the aorta (Rossi and Cova 1904) or the superior mesenteric artery (Kupic et al. 1967). The origin of the vessel is at the level of the 1st lumbar vertebra (Th 12—L 2; De Luca and De Serio 1960). It follows a horizontal or slightly upward tortuous course to the left, along the upper border of the pancreas (groove for the splenic artery) above the splenic vein, in 90 per cent of the cases. The vessel is situated behind the pancreas in 8 per cent, and in front of it in 2 per cent (Henschen 1928). Passing through the phrenicolienal fold, the artery reaches the spleen to divide there into its terminal branches. It supplies the body and tail of the pancreas, the spleen, the left half of the greater omentum, the greater curvature of the stomach and a part of the fundus. The length of the splenic artery is 9·5 cm (7 to 14 cm), its diameter 0·55 cm (0·4 to 0·8 cm; Ödman 1958). The splenic artery may be doubled (Kupic et al. 1967). Its *branches:*

The *pancreatic branches* (Figs 151/21, 153/28) supply the body and tail of the pancreas. The splenic artery gives off 6 to 10 minor arteries to the gland (Anson 1951). The *dorsal pancreatic artery* (Figs 143/18, 165/6) may sometimes originate from the splenic artery immediately after its origin (Muller and Figley 1957). Running to the posterior side, the dorsal pancreatic artery anastomoses with the retroduodenal and the inferior pancreaticoduodenal arteries (Ödman 1958). The anastomosis assumes the form of a thick trunk in 5 per cent of the cases (Chérigié et al. 1967). The *inferior pancreatic artery* arises from the distal portion of the splenic artery and contributes to the supply of the tail. It occurs in 10 per cent of the cases that all arteries of the pancreas unite to form a common trunk, the so-called *arteria pancreatica magna*, which runs on the inferior surface parallel with the splenic and may have a width of 0·2 to 0·4 cm (Michels 1955). A minor branch (*arteria caudae pancreatis*; Figs 143/16, 157/20, 165/7), mostly a multiple vessel, arises from the main trunk of the splenic artery and runs to the tail of the pancreas.

The *short gastric arteries* (Figs 151/22, 157/21, 164/5, 165/5) are small vessels that run from the splenic artery to the fundus of the stomach to anastomose there with the other arteries.

The *left gastroepiploic artery* (Figs 143/19, 151/23, 153/29, 157/19, 158/5, 164/6, 165/13, 166 and 167/3) arises together with the inferior terminal branch of the splenic artery, and courses in the gastrosplenic part of the greater omentum then in the gastro-mesocolic part about 1·5 cm below the greater curvature of the stomach and anastomoses with the right gastroepiploic artery. The vessel at issue is larger than the right artery. Its branches run to the greater curvature of the stomach and the greater omentum (*epiploic branches*), sometimes to the lower pole of the spleen (*inferior polar artery*). Their number totals 16 to 20. In the upper part of the body of the stomach the supply by the left gastric artery is considerably more than by the left gastroepiploic artery, while they have an equal share in the supply of the lower half of the corpus and the antrum. The left gastroepiploic artery may form anastomosis with Riolan's arch. Often this anastomosis is demonstrable only in pathological conditions (Luzsa 1963, Kahn and Abrams 1964).

The *splenic branches* (Figs 143/17, 151/24) are terminal branches of the splenic artery. Diverging in a brushlike form, they supply the spleen segmentally. The number of segments varies from 2 to 5. The *superior polar artery*, A_1 (Figs 164/7, 165/9, 166 and 167/4), the *superior terminal artery*, A_2 (Figs 164/8, 165/10, 166 and 167/5), the *middle terminal artery*, A_3 (Fig. 164/9), the *inferior terminal artery*, A_4 (Figs 164/10, 165/11, 166 and 167/6) and the *inferior polar artery*, A_5 (Figs 164/11, 165/12, 166 and 167/7) divide the spleen into segments arranged stepwise in a downward direction (Kikkawa 1966a). Gyurkó and Szabó (1966) found the spleen to be supplied by two arteries in 10·77, by three in 40, by four in 38·46 and by five in 10·77

per cent of the examined cases. The ramification may take place in the hilum (marginal type) or earlier from the main trunk (diverging type). The superior polar vessel sometimes arises separately from the splenic, and the inferior polar vessel from the left gastroepiploic artery (Ödman 1958). Anastomosis between the various segmental arteries is demonstrable outside the spleen in 15·1, and within the spleen in 7·1 per cent (Kikkawa 1966b). In cases of an accessory spleen (Haberer 1901) the supplying artery may be independent or emitted by a segmental branch (Fig. 165/8). Kádár (1950) demonstrated by microcorrosion that blood flow in the spleen is uninterrupted because the branches of the arteries open directly into the sinuses. The lumina of the vessels are in free contact with the pulp of the spleen across the wall of the sinuses.

The superior mesenteric artery and its branches

The superior mesenteric artery (Figs 133/8, 141/13, 143/21, 144/6, 151/26, 152/18, 153/31, 157/22) arises from the anterior wall of the aorta at the height of the 1st to 2nd lumbar vertebra (Th. 12—L. 2.; Michels 1955, Ödman 1959). Its distance from the celiac trunk is 0·5 to 2 cm, from the bifurcation of the aorta 11·5 cm (Jackson 1963), from the inferior mesenteric artery 5·3 cm (3·5 to 7·0 cm; Gillot et al. cit. Handbook of Circulation 1959).

Variations in origin are possible if the vessel arises together with the celiac trunk (Adachi 1928) or the inferior mesenteric artery (Gwyn and Skilton 1966), further in cases of duplication (Delannoy 1923).

Arising, the superior mesenteric artery is placed in front of the horizontal part of the duodenum to the left of the superior mesenteric vein, between the two layers of the mesentery. Its initial portion is obliquely crossed from behind by the left renal vein and from the front by the boundary between the splenic vein and the head of the pancreas. Emerging from beneath the pancreas, it takes a steeply descending course. Its further course is, according to our observations, of three types. Most frequently the artery curves to the right and divides on the right side of the aorta (Type I; Fig. 144/I). Less often it winds to the left and starts to give off branches on the left side already (Type II; Fig. 144/II) to follow thereafter a course toward the right. Type III begins with a course resembling the shape of an "S" to the left, but ramifies only having wound over to the right side of the aorta.

The length of the superior mesenteric artery from its origin to the emission of the first branch measures 4·3 cm (3 to 6 cm). The diameter is 0·5 cm (0·4 to 0·6 cm) according to De Luca and De Serio

1960), and 0·8 to 1·4 cm according to Michels (1955).

Its *branches* supply the small intestine and the colon as far as the splenic flexure, and contribute moreover to the supply of the pancreas and duodenum.

The *inferior pancreaticoduodenal arteries* (Figs 143/22, 153/32) arise from the superior mesenteric artery in 93, from the celiac trunk in 1 per cent, and are replaced by the retroduodenal arteries in 6 per cent of the cases (Adachi 1928). If originating from the superior mesenteric artery, it arises from the right side or from the posterior wall of the superior mesenteric artery independently, or from its left side together with the jejunal arteries. They supply the inferior horizontal part of the duodenum (*anterior branch;* Fig. 157/24) on the other hand they ramify on the posterior part of the head and the lower border of the body of the pancreas (*posterior branch;* Fig. 157/23). They anastomose with the retroduodenal arteries on the inner side of the descending part of the duodenum. The duodenojejunal flexure is supplied already by the jejunal arteries.

The *jejunal* and *iliac arteries* (Figs 151/27, 152/19, 153/33, 157/25, 159/2) are vessels of the small intestine, and their number varies from 6 to 20 (Dwight 1903). After their division they run between the layers of the mesentery to the jejunum and ileum while numerous arch-shaped anastomoses are formed among their branches. The arches generally follow each other in five segments (Fig. 159/3). The segment without anastomoses is the longest in the jejunum and the shortest in the ileocecal portion. Anastomoses are the most frequent around Meckel's diverticulum (Lardennois and Okinczyc 1910).

The *ileocolic artery* (Figs 151/30, 153/34, 157/26, 160/4) arises together with the right colic artery in one third of the cases (Steward and Rankin 1933). At its origin, the vessel often forms an anastomosis with the 12th right posterior intercostal artery (Jackson 1963). It follows an obliquely descending course to the right. Its proximal part is placed retroperitoneally. The vessel crosses from the front the right ureter, the testicular artery and the psoas major muscle. It ramifies before reaching the ileocecal region. Its branch winding to the left, communicates with the terminal ileal artery (*ramus iliacus;* Fig. 160/5). Supplying the cecum, the trunk divides into two branches, the *anterior* and *posterior cecal arteries* (Fig. 160/6 and 8). The *artery of the appendix* (Fig. 160/7), the artery of the vermiform process, courses behind the ileum and runs before its orifice into the ileocecal valve to the mesentery of the appendix. Passing along the posterior border of the latter, the artery of the appendix gives off

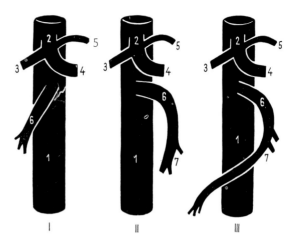

FIG. 144. Variations in the course of the superior mesenteric artery. I, turn to the right; II, turn to the left; III, "S"-shaped type. (*1*) Aorta; (*2*) celiac trunk; (*3*) common hepatic artery; (*4*) splenic artery; (*5*) left gastric artery; (*6*) superior mesenteric artery; (*7*) branches of superior mesenteric artery.

4 to 6 branches which are in no essential communication with one another. It commences only in about one third of the cases from the ileocolic artery. It may furthermore arise from the ramus iliacus, the anterior or posterior cecal arteries and from the right colic artery. The vessel may be doubled (Inamura 1923). The *ascending artery* of the ileocolic artery (Fig. 160/9) is in communication with the right colic artery. The artery of the appendix usually ends as a terminal vessel (Solanke 1968).

The *right colic artery* (Figs 151/29, 153/35, 157/27) emerges from the right side of the superior mesenteric artery. It may arise independently (38 per cent), together with the middle colic artery (52 per cent), as a branch of the ileocolic artery (8 per cent) or may be absent (2 per cent; Michels et al. 1965). The artery supplies the ascending colon and the right flexure of the colon. It forms an arched anastomosis with the ileocolic artery at the margin of the ascending colon and another with the middle colic near the flexure.

The *middle colic artery* (Figs 151/28, 153/36, 157/28, 158/7) arises in 44 per cent of the cases about 1 cm below the inferior pancreaticoduodenal artery. It commences in 52 per cent together with the right colic artery or may, as aberrant vessel, arise cranially to the origin of the jejunal arteries (4 per cent; Michels et al. 1965). Rarely it originates directly from the aorta (Steward and Rankin 1933). The middle colic artery courses to the right toward the right flexure of the colon. It gives off branches upward to the transverse colon and to the left flexure of the colon. The artery supplies the right flexure and the transverse colon. The extent of its contribution to the supply to the left flexure is variable. In

237

general, the arteries of the colon communicate with one another by forming one or two arches. Thus, the arches between the main trunks are less than the arches of the small intestine. Two to three cm before the lumen of the intestine there is no anastomosis between the vessels coursing at right angles to the intestinal wall.

The *right accessory hepatic artery* and the *left superior accessory colic artery* can be the branches of the superior mesenteric artery (Adachi 1928, Mercier and Vanneuville 1968).

The inferior mesenteric artery and its branches

The inferior mesenteric artery (Figs 133/11, 151/31, 152/20, 153/37, 157/29) arises from the left side of the anterior surface of the aorta at the level of the upper third of the 4th (L3—4) lumbar vertebra. It may have a common origin with the superior mesenteric artery (Gwyn and Skilton 1966). The origin of the artery is at a distance of 5 to 6 cm from the bifurcation of the aorta (Michels 1955) and 5·3 cm (3·5 to 7·0 cm) from the superior mesenteric artery (Gillot et al. cit. Handbook of Circulation 1959). Rarely the inferior mesenteric artery may be missing (Bernardi et al. 1971). The artery supplies the left flexure, the descending and sigmoid colons, furthermore, the oral two-third of the rectum. Its branches communicate with the middle colic artery around the left flexure and with the internal pudendal artery in the rectum. The length of the inferior mesenteric artery is 12 cm (4 to 22 cm); its diameter 0·23 cm (0·08 to 0·5 cm; De Luca and De Serio 1961). Michels et al. (1965) described three types of division: into two branches in 56, into three branches in 38, into two branches with transverse anastomosis in 6 per cent of the cases. It has the following *branches*:

The *left colic artery* (Figs 151/32, 152/21, 153/38, 157/30, 161/2) is the first branch of the main trunk which divides after a course of scarcely 1 cm into 2 to 6 twigs. It courses to the left retroperitoneally at the height of the 4th lumbar vertebra. Its ascending portion, in front of the left ureter and the psoas muscle, runs toward the left flexure where it communicates with the middle colic artery. Sometimes a connecting branch is given off here to the splenic or the left gastroepiploic artery (Luzsa 1963, 1965, Kahn and Abrams 1964). The horizontal or slightly descending portion of the vessel supplies the descending colon and anastomoses with the arteries of the sigmoid colon.

The *sigmoid arteries* (Figs 151/33, 152/22, 153/39, 157/31), branches of the main trunk, course to the

sigmoid colon and divide into 2 to 5 parts. First they run retroperitoneally and then in the sigmoid mesocolon after intersecting the common iliac artery and vein. They anastomose upward with the left colic artery and downward with the superior rectal artery.

The *superior rectal artery* (Figs 151/34, 152/23), a continuation of the main trunk, has a steeply downward directed retroperitoneal initial course. Usually divided into two branches it supplies the oral two-third of the rectum. The vessel anastomoses with the sigmoid arteries as also with the middle rectal artery (from the internal pudendal artery). The diameter of the superior rectal artery measures 0·2 to 0·3 cm (Michels et al. 1965).

The extent to which the superior mesenteric artery contributes, via the marginal arteries, to the *blood supply of the left flexure of the colon* is greater than what could be expected on the basis of the anatomical examinations (Drummond 1913). Michels et al. (1965) found the anastomotic communication between the two colic arteries to be good in 61, poor in 32 and absent in 7 per cent of the cases. With angiography in vivo from the inferior mesenteric artery, only the aboral half of the descending colon is filled in 18, its aboral two-third in 25, the left flexure in 44, the section above the flexure in 10, and the aboral third of the transverse colon in 3 per cent of the cases (Kahn and Abrams 1964).

Michels et al. (1965) found that the left flexure of the colon may receive a variant blood supply from the middle colic artery which springs from the celiac trunk (celiacocolic trunk), the splenic artery (splenocolic trunk), the right accessory hepatic artery (hepatocolic trunk), the dorsal pancreatic artery (pancreatocolic trunk), the right gastroepiploic artery (gastrocolic trunk) and from the posterior omental artery (omentocolic trunk).

Collateral circulation of the unpaired abdominal arteries

Collateral circulation plays an important part in the blood supply of the abdominal viscera. Riolan (1649) was the first to describe the anastomoses which connect the abdominal vessels. Haller (1759) described the more important communications among the vessels of the internal organs, of which he named Riolan's arch the arch-shaped intercommunicating vascular system of the colon. The clinically significant collaterals of the three unpaired abdominal vessels are as follows (Fig. 145).

1. The anterior pancreaticoduodenal arch (Fig. 145/16 and 23) forms anastomosis between the celiac trunk and the superior mesenteric artery. This rela-

tively small anastomosis consists of the superior supraduodenal and the inferior pancreaticoduodenal arteries. If necessary its diameter may increase many times (Diemel and Schmitz-Dräger 1965, Schmidt and Schimanski 1967).

2. The posterior pancreaticoduodenal arch (Fig. 145/15 and 22) connects the retroduodenal and the inferior pancreaticoduodenal arteries. It is less significant than the anterior arch (Diemel and Schmitz-Dräger 1965).

3. The dorsal pancreatic artery (Fig. 143/18) may communicate with the pancreaticoduodenal arches. It may maintain a regional circulation with the splenic and the gastroduodenal arteries via its anastomoses with the smaller arteries of the pancreas (Reuter and Olin 1965).

4. The constant communications along the lesser and the greater curvature of the stomach (arcus arteriosus ventriculi superior et inferior; Fig. 143/10 and 20) maintain good conditions of blood flow between the left gastric and the hepatic arteries as also between the splenic and the gastroduodenal arteries. Anastomoses may be formed also with the esophageal arteries and the left inferior phrenic artery (Michels et al. 1968).

5. Anastomoses may be formed between the various vessels of the hilum of the liver (hepatic artery—gastroduodenal artery; hepatic artery—right accessory hepatic artery; Michels 1953). Intrahepatic anastomoses may exist among the branches of the hepatic artery, further among these branches and the cystic artery (Schorn et al. 1957, Düx et al. 1966).

6. Via its communications with the middle and left colic arteries, the Riolan's arch (Fig. 145/26) connects the superior and the inferior mesenteric arteries. The connection may be dilated if the inferior mesenteric artery is insufficient when blood flows from the direction of the middle colic artery (type I; Baylin 1939, Diemel et al. 1964). The stream of blood takes an opposite course if the superior mesenteric artery becomes constricted (type II;

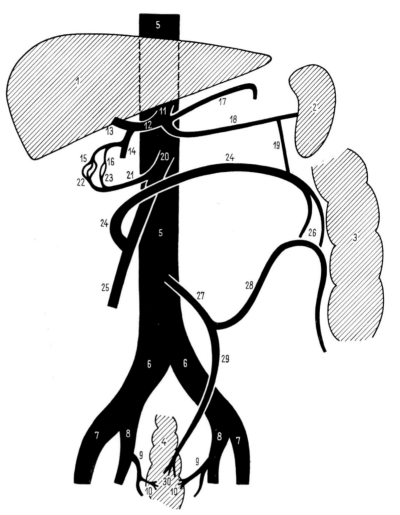

FIG. 145. Principal collaterals of the unpaired abdominal arteries. (1) Liver; (2) spleen; (3) descending colon; (4) rectum; (5) abdominal aorta; (6) common iliac artery; (7) external iliac artery; (8) internal iliac artery; (9) internal pudendal artery; (10) inferior rectal artery; (11) celiac trunk; (12) common hepatic artery; (13) hepatic artery; (14) gastroduodenal artery; (15) retroduodenal artery; (16) supraduodenal artery; (17) left gastric artery; (18) splenic artery; (19) anastomosis between the splenic and the middle colic arteries; (20) superior mesenteric artery; (21) inferior pancreaticoduodenal artery; (22) posterior branch; (23) anterior branch; (24) middle colic artery; (25) right colic and ileocolic arteries; (26) anastomosis between the middle and the left colic arteries; (27) inferior mesenteric artery; (28) left colic artery; (29) superior rectal artery; (30) anastomosis between the superior and the inferior rectal arteries.

Debray et al. 1961, Carucci 1963, Diemel et al. 1964). The middle and left colic arteries can be regarded as functional terminal vessels if their communication is insufficient (Jackson 1963).

7. The superior and middle rectal arteries (Fig. 145/30) ensure collateral circulation between the inferior mesenteric and the internal pudendal arteries, an anastomosis of minor clinical significance (Barbaccia and Pompili 1960, Edwards and Lemay 1955, Bellmann and Herwig 1964).

8. Kahn and Abrams (1964) demonstrated the existence of an anastomosis between the inferior mesenteric and splenic arteries around the left

flexure of the colon under pathologic conditions. We, on the other hand, found such arterial communication under normal anatomical conditions (Luzsa 1963, 1965; Figs 145/19, 153/30).

9. Communications exist sometimes between the 12th right posterior intercostal artery and the ileocolic artery (Jackson 1963); besides, the lumbar arteries may be in communication with the right colic or the splenic artery (Bücheler et al. 1966). An arched anastomosis may be found between the inferior phrenic and the celiac trunk (Fry and Kraft 1963).

Arteriography of the abdominal aorta and its branches

Visualization in vivo of the abdominal vessels has become possible since 1931 when Dos Santos and his co-workers elaborated the percutaneous angiography of the abdominal aorta. X-ray anatomy of the abdominal arteries was systematically summarized by Mercier and Vanneuville (1968). Neither the retrograde (Seldinger 1953) nor the intravenous method (Steinberg et al. 1959) gives a uniform and clear view of the entire vascular apparatus of the abdomen. Identification is difficult owing to the great number of the filling vessels, and because the minor vessels with a rapid rate of circulation cannot all be simultaneously visualized. Functional study of the vessels and the consequent evaluation of their morphological properties became possible only by selective methods, by the isolated filling of certain vessels. (Renal artery: Alken and Sommer 1950, celiac trunk: Ödman 1958, superior mesenteric artery: Ödman 1959, inferior mesenteric artery: Ström and Winberg 1962, splenic artery: Rösch and Bret 1963, suprarenal arteries: Ludin 1963, lumbar arteries: Van Voorthuisen 1964, hepatic artery: Dreyfuss et al. 1967, inferior phrenic artery: Kahn 1967, capsular arteries: Meyers et al. 1967, ovarian artery: Thomas 1966.) The superselective arteriography of the celiac trunk enables the more exact filling of the side branches (Rösch 1971).

In *postmortem angiography*, all abdominal vessels are simultaneously and intensively filled with contrast material through the abdominal aorta. **Summation pictures,** made in the **anteroposterior view** (Figs 151, 153), are therefore suitable only for the study of the larger vessels because the numerous vascular crossings and the superposition of shadows disturb the clear view. The upper third of the *abdominal aorta* (Fig. 151/5) lies in or somewhat to the left of the midline. Its further course is straight or slightly curved. The thickness of the vessel decreases uniformly as far as the division. It divides

at the 4th lumbar vertebra into the bifurcating right and left common iliac arteries. The *inferior phrenic arteries* (Figs 153/15 and 16) describe upward and laterally directed arches from their origin. Of the *suprarenal arteries* (Figs 153/43, 156/13 to 15), the upper arteries often begin from the phrenic artery; the middle and inferior suprarenal arteries are difficult to fill after death. The laterally directed segmental branches of the *lumbar arteries* run toward the vertebral column along the border of the vertebrae (*dorsal branches*), and their projection is frequently orthoroentgenographic. Selective filling of the *testicular artery* yields a more reliable visualization of its steeply descending course along the vertebral column. The courses of the right and left *renal arteries* (Figs 151/35, 153/40) differ according to the position of the kidneys. Their initial portion is crossed on one or the other side by the superior mesenteric artery depending on the course the latter follows. The thin network and the anastomoses of the extrarenal branches may form multiple bends (Palubinskas 1964). Their filling is variable. The identification of the segmental branches of the renal arteries, as well as of the interlobar, interlobular and arcuate arteries is often difficult on account of the simultaneously filling gastric and intestinal vessels. The *celiac trunk* (Figs 151/11, 153/13) is hardly distinguishable from the intensive shadow of the aorta. The ascending and sinistrolaterally running course of the *left gastric artery* (Figs 151/25, 153/14) crosses the beginning of the splenic artery. Winding to the left, the *splenic artery* (Figs 151/20, 153/27) runs toward the hilum of the spleen in front of the projection of the 10th and 11th vertebrae, first in a transverse and then in an ascending direction. From its origin, the *left gastroepiploic artery* (Figs 151/23, 153/29) describes a downward curve and turns to the right. The *common hepatic artery* (Figs 151/12, 153/17) follows a right and somewhat upward course. It ramifies at the right border of the spine between the projections of the 12th thoracic and 2nd lumbar vertebrae. The *gastroduodenal artery* (Figs 151/17, 153/22) descends steeply 1·5 to 5·5 cm to the right of the midline (Ödman 1958). Provided the conditions are favourable, its terminal branches can be followed as far as the inferior pancreaticoduodenal artery. Crossing the aorta, the *right gastroepiploic artery* (Figs 151/19, 153/23) runs over to the left side. The *hepatic artery* (Figs 151/13, 153/18) gives off the *right gastric artery* to the lesser curvature (Figs 151/16, 153/26) in its initial course. The right gastric artery crosses the aorta above the gastroepiploic artery between the 11th thoracic and 3rd lumbar vertebrae. The right gastric artery is usually smaller than the right gastroepiploic artery. Showing variable origins and

240

courses, the *hepatic branches* intersect the projections of the lower ribs and those of 9th to 12th posterior intercostal arteries. The *cystic artery* (Fig. 153/21) follows a tortuous course along the axis of the gall bladder. The portion of the *superior mesenteric artery* (Figs 151/26, 153/31) that extends beyond the border of the aorta crosses one of the renal arteries. In case the superior mesenteric artery curves to the left, the *inferior pancreaticoduodenal artery* (Figs 151/18, 153/32), coursing to the right after its origin, is situated in the projection of the aorta. The latter artery is shorter and divides immediately after its origin if the superior mesenteric artery belongs to the right-turning type. The *jejunal* and *iliac arteries* (Figs 151/27, 153/33) coursing to the intestines come off in succession from the main trunk to be distributed in a broom-like pattern among the intestines. Because of their superimposed projections, the anastomoses existing between these vessels show a tangled network. While the *ileocolic artery* (Figs 151/30, 153/34) follows a downward course to the right, the *right colic artery* (Figs 151/29, 153/35) runs more horizontally above it. The course of the *middle colic artery* (Figs 151/28, 153/36) depends on the size of the right colic artery. In general, its branches cannot be followed as far as the left flexure of the colon. The thin initial portion of the *inferior mesenteric artery* (Figs 151/31, 153/37) is intersected by the branches of the superior mesenteric artery. Its steeply ascending and laterally running as well as its descending trunks can nevertheless be separated from the superior mesenteric artery. The *superior rectal artery* (Fig. 151/34) and its characteristic intersection with the common iliac artery are clearly distinguishable.

Lateral pictures (Fig. 152) reveal only the larger vascular trunks. Their relative positions and their origin are, however, clearer in the lateral aspect than in the sagittal view. The *abdominal aorta* (Fig. 152/4) follows the physiological lordosis of the vertebral column. Its division is not clearly visible because the projections of the initial part of the bilateral common iliac arteries are superimposed. The *lumbar arteries* (Fig. 152/26) commencing in segments and the *renal arteries* (Figs 152/24 and 35) beginning from the aorta, pass backward. The lower part of the branches of the left renal artery usually falls into the projection of the upper part of the right kidney. The actual pattern depends, of course, on the position of the kidneys. The entire *celiac trunk* (Fig. 152/8) is visible in this view. Also its position relative to the superior mesenteric artery and their possible communication can be visualized (Fig. 152/17). The *left gastric artery* runs first upward in a straight line, makes then a turn of nearly 180° to follow a descending course (Fig. 152/15).

It is only at its origin that the *splenic artery* (Fig. 152/16) can be identified because of its orthoroentgenographic course to the left, slightly upward and backward. The *common hepatic artery* (Fig. 152/9) descends forward to the liver. Its first branch is the *gastroduodenal artery* (Fig. 152/10) which pursues a steeply descending forward course. The *right gastroepiploic artery* (Fig. 152/11) courses forward in a downward convex arch then turns upward. The *hepatic artery* (Fig. 152/13) gives off segmental branches in front of the anterior border of the spine at a distance exceeding the width of a vertebral body. The angle formed by the main trunk of the *superior mesenteric artery* (Fig. 152/18) and the abdominal aorta depends on the repletion of the bowels and the adiposity of the abdomen. The angle is smaller in asthenic and much greater in pyknic individuals. The smaller branches are indistinguishable in this view. Origin and beginning of the *inferior mesenteric artery* (Fig. 152/20) are usually projected behind the aorta so that only the further course of its branches is seen in this direction. The *left colic artery* (Fig. 152/21) courses backward and upward, the *sigmoid artery* (Fig. 152/22) forward and downward, while the *superior rectal artery* (Fig. 152/23) follows a steep downward course.

Anatomical preparations of the entire abdominal complex, in **anteroposterior view** (Fig. 153), yield good visualization even of the minor branches of the abdominal arteries without the disturbing shadows of the bones and soft tissues. This way it is possible to observe on the same picture organs of different vascular structures, such as the liver, spleen, kidneys, intestines. Identification of anastomoses can be visualized according to their anatomical development.

Roentgenograms of the kidneys either with the adjacent tissues (Figs 154, 156) or devoid of their fatty capsules (Fig. 155) make it possible to study the relative positions of the *renal* (Figs 154/2, 155/2, 156/10 and 11), *suprarenal* (Figs 154/5 and 6, 156/13 to 15) and *testicular arteries* (Fig. 156/19). The suprarenal arteries ramify in a brush-like manner into about 50 small branches and form a superficial network from where they pass into the gland with a radial course (Anson et al. 1947). The *arcus arteriosus perirenalis* (Fig. 154/8), formed by the *capsular arteries* (Figs 154/4, 156/16 to 18), the minute branches of the *pelvic branches* and the communications of the *testicular artery* can be individually differentiated. The extra- and intrarenal anastomoses can be filled also under normal conditions. The intrarenal segmental divisions can be followed as far as the arcuate arteries. In contrast to in vivo angiography, the multiple renal and the polar arteries can be filled completely.

Centred anteroposterior angiograms of the unpaired vessels (Fig. 157) are best suited for the visualization of the communications between the celiac trunk and the superior mesenteric artery. The size and the course of the anastomoses connecting the branches of the *gastroduodenal artery* (Fig. 157/13) with the *inferior pancreaticoduodenal artery* (Figs 157/23 and 24; *arcus pancreaticoduodenalis anterior* and *posterior*) can be observed free of interfering shadows.

In **centred pictures of the stomach in anatomical preparations** (Fig. 158), the configuration of the *arcus arteriosus ventriculi superior* (Figs 158/3 and 4) and *inferior* (Figs 158/5 and 6) shows, in spite of the overlapping projections of the anterior and the posterior walls, the extent to which the various arteries contribute to the blood supply. The *middle colic artery* (Fig. 158/7) runs parallel to the greater curvature. The *omental branches* cross the gastroepiploic arteries from behind.

In the **isolated angiograms of the intestinal loops** (Fig. 159), the vascular structure of the small intestine shows differently developed arcades in the various parts of the ileum and jejunum. No major anastomoses are visible 1 to 2 cm from the intestinal wall. (Submucosal arterial plexuses cannot be filled by this method.)

Pictures of the cecum (Fig. 160) show variously developed anastomoses connecting the *ileocolic artery* (Fig. 160/4) with the right colic artery and the arteries of the small intestine. The *cecal arteries* (Figs 160/6 and 8) surround the cecum. The *artery of the appendix* (Fig. 160/7) runs first to the right and — according to the actual position of the appendix — turns away to divide into its segmental terminal branches. There are no macroscopically perceptible significant communications among them.

Pictures centred on the large intestine (Fig. 161) reveal that its arched anastomoses are less numerous than those of the small intestine. Communications between the minor branches cease to exist at some distance from the intestinal wall already.

Anteroposterior roentgenograms of the liver (Fig. 162) show the left-curving path of the *left branch* (Fig. 162/6). The *medial segmental artery*, A_4 (Fig. 162/12) forms a loop and ramifies. The *superior lateral segmental artery*, A_2 (Fig. 162/10), continuous with the main trunk, follows a course toward the left border of the liver. The *inferior lateral segmental artery*, A_3 (Fig. 162/11) deviates slightly downward. The *right branch* (Fig. 160/5) pursues a straight course to the right. Usually it gives off a descending branch; the *cystic artery* (Fig. 162/9) from its initial portion. The *superior anterior segmental artery*. A_8 (Fig. 162/16) runs upward to the right in the direction of the convex line of the liver, whereas the *inferior anterior segmental artery*, A_5 (Fig. 162/13) pursues a steeply descending course. The further course of the main trunk lies in the direction of the right border of the liver, and it divides into the ascending *superior posterior segmental artery*, A_7 (Fig. 162/15) and the descending *inferior posterior segmental artery*, A_6 (Fig. 162/14). The *segmental arteries to the caudate lobe*, A_1 (Fig. 162/8) usually follow an upward course from the origin of the right and the left main branches. In **craniocaudal** roentgenograms of the liver (Fig. 163) the *left branch* (Fig. 163/7) runs with a convex course backward to the left. The *medial segmental artery*, A_4 (Fig. 163/11) runs first forward and then, forming a loop, passes backward. Thus its projection intersects the arteries of the lateral segments. The *superior lateral segmental artery*, A_2 (Fig. 163/9) passes laterally backward, the *inferior lateral segmental artery*, A_3 (Fig. 163/10) laterally forward. The *right branch* (Fig. 163/6) courses sideways and divides after a short course. The *cystic artery* (Fig. 163/13) runs in a straight forward line along the border of the gall bladder. The *inferior anterior segmental artery*, A_5 (Fig. 163/12) courses forward, the *superior anterior segmental artery*, A_8 (Fig. 163/16) crosses the arteries of the lateral segment in its forward course. The *posterior inferior segmental artery*, A_6 (Fig. 163/14) pursues a lateral course, the *superior posterior segmental artery*, A_7 (Fig. 163/15) runs obliquely backward. If the major branches of the *segmental artery of the caudate lobe*, A_1 (Fig. 163/8) are filled they are seen to pass backward from the bifurcating right and left main branches. The type of division of the arteries in the hepatic area is dychotomic. The terminal branches form a subcapsular plexus. With suitable technique even vessels of $0 \cdot 1$ mm can be identified. Simultaneous filling of the bile ducts shows that their division is similar to that of the arteries.

Pictures of the spleen (Figs 164, 165, 166 and 167) and its surroundings reveal the types of division in the *splenic artery* (Figs 164/4, 165/4) and its relation to the adjacent organs. The tail of the pancreas is usually supplied by the *arteriae caudae pancreatis* (Fig. 165/7) which arise before the division of the splenic artery. Its connection with the arteries of the left flexure of the colon may be visualized in this way. The *left gastroepiploic artery* (Figs 164/6, 165/13) describes a descending curve to the right. The *short gastric arteries* (Figs 164/5, 165/5) run to the lateral and posterior aspects of the fundus of the stomach. Division of the *splenic branches* and their relation to the possibly existing *supernumerary spleen* (Fig. 165) are clearly visible also in unidirectional pictures because the intrasplenic ramification is fairly uniform from above downward. Crossing of the larger trunks is rarely seen in the anteroposterior direction. Two-directional roentgenograms of anatomical preparations of the isolated organ show the entire course and arrangement of the various segmental branches: the *superior polar artery*, A_1 (Figs 164/7, 165/9, 166 and 167/4); the *superior terminal artery*, A_2 (Figs 164/8, 165/10, 166 and 167/5), *middle terminal artery*, A_3 (Fig. 164/9) *inferior terminal artery*, A_4 (Figs 164/10, 165/11, 166 and 167/6) and the *inferior polar artery*, A_5 (Figs 164/11, 165/12, 166 and 167/7). The typical brushlike division does not obscure the vessels of the adjacent vascular bed from either direction.

THE INFERIOR VENA CAVA AND ITS BRANCHES

The inferior vena cava and its branches besides their own area of drainage, are in close connection with the portal circulation. If the latter is insufficient, they are able to take over its role partially. The clinical significance of the segmentally arranged hepatic veins was increased by angiography. The branches of the inferior and superior venae cavae form a collateral network that can replace each other reciprocally.

Anatomy of the inferior vena cava and its branches

The inferior vena cava (Figs 146, 147/11, 168/5, 169/5, 170/4, 180/4, 181/5, 182/4, 208/7, 209/4) is formed at the level of the 4th to 5th lumbar vertebrae by the junction of the common iliac veins. It drains the lower extremities, the pelvis and the abdominal cavity. From its origin, the vessel courses — forming a slight curve laterally — in front of the right margin of the vertebral column as far as the 2nd to 3rd lumbar vertebrae. Here it turns slightly to the right and forward, perforates the diaphragm and opens after a short thoracic course into the right atrium. The initial portion of the vein passes to the right of and behind the right common iliac artery. The psoas major muscle is behind this portion, while the renal, suprarenal, lumbar and right phrenic arteries are situated above it. The inferior vena cava is crossed obliquely from the front by the right testicular artery. The mesentery, the descending part of the duodenum, the pancreas, the superior mesenteric artery and the liver lie in front of the inferior vena cava. The portal vein runs first in front and to the left, and crosses then its course obliquely from forward passing to the right side of the inferior vena cava. The aorta is to the left, the right ureter, kidney, and suprarenal gland to the right of the inferior vena cava. It is impressed from behind by the right renal artery and from the front by the caudate lobe. The thoracic portion of the vein consists of an extrapericardial and an intrapericardial segment. The vessel is devoid of valves. The length of the inferior vena cava averages 24 cm (20 cm abdominal + 0.5 cm phrenic + 3.5 cm thoracic por-

tions). The diameter is 2·2 cm in the initial portion, 3 cm at the level of the renal veins, and 3·3 cm above the hepatic veins (Paturet 1958). The frontal diameter is shorter than the sagittal diameter in the segment below the orifice of the renal veins. The vena cava inferior is wider at the orifice of the renal and hepatic veins, while its phrenic portion is narrower (Fuchs 1964).

The incidence of *variations* amounts to 1·5 to 4·0 per cent (Fig. 146, Edwards 1951).

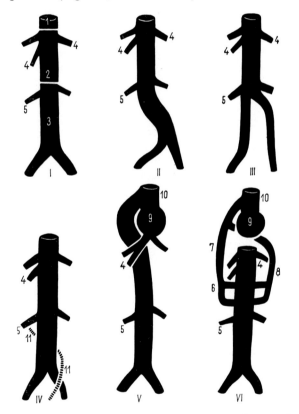

FIG. 146. Variations of the inferior vena cava. I, normal type (three segments of the inferior vena cava); II, infrarenal left inferior vena cava; III, infrarenal bilateral inferior vena cava; IV, preureteral inferior vena cava; V, partial agenesis; VI, congenital obstruction. (*1*) Hepatic part; (*2*) subcardinal part; (*3*) supracardinal part; (*4*) hepatic veins; (*5*) renal vein; (*6*) lumbar veins; (*7*) azygos vein; (*8*) hemiazygos vein; (*9*) right atrium; (*10*) superior vena cava; (*11*) right retrocaval ureter.

1. Left infrarenal inferior vena cava (Fig. 146/II). Because of the left persisting supracardinal vein the inferior vena cava runs below the orifice of the renal veins on the left side of the aorta, and after crossing the vertebral column, it passes over to its right side. The upper course is normal (Fuchs 1964, Gryska and Earthrowl 1967).

2. Bilateral infrarenal inferior vena cava (Fig. 164/III). In cases of bilaterally persisting supracardinal veins the inferior vena cava is doubled below the renal veins. The two branches unite here to follow an ascending course on the right side. The frequency of occurrence amounts to 1 per cent (Gladstone 1929, Böttger et al. 1972). Symmetrical development of the two vessels is rare (Hirsch and Chan 1963, Colborn 1964).

3. Preureteral inferior vena cava (Fig. 146/IV) is present if the right posterocardinal vein persists while the supracardinal vein diminishes. The right ureter passes from the right side of the inferior vena cava to the back, crosses it from behind and continues its path to the bladder on the left side of the vein (O'Loughlin 1961, Lemaitre et al. 1963).

4. Partial agenesis of the inferior vena cava (Fig. 146/V). The upper segment of the vein is usually missing in such cases. It continues in the azygos vein prerenally and opens into the superior vena cava. It has a frequency of 0·6 per cent. It is often accompanied by other anomalies (Petersen 1965). The hepatic veins open in such cases into the right atrium at the site of the normal orifice of the inferior vena cava, independently of the veins of the inferior segment (Stackelberg et al. 1952, Beuren 1966). Absence of the part of the inferior vena cava which develops from the middle subcardinal vein is less frequent. In such cases both renal veins empty into the persisting left cardinal vein (Bartel and Wierny 1963).

5. Congenital stenosis or obstruction of the inferior vena cava (Fig. 146/VI). The phrenic portion of the vessel is constricted or obstructed and blood flow is maintained by collateral circulation (Bücheler et al. 1966).

6. Other rare, clinically insignificant variations of the inferior vena cava have been described (Edwards 1951). Opening into the left atrium is a pathological anomaly.

Branches (parietal and viscelar). The **inferior phrenic veins** open into the inferior vena cava, either separately or together with an adjacent vessel (Rauber and Kopsch 1951).

The **lumbar veins** (Figs 169/18, 181/18, 209/5), four in number, accompany the corresponding arteries. The two upper vessels empty into the azygos vein, the lower ones into the inferior vena cava. The longitudinal anastomosis connecting them (*ascend-ing lumbar vein*, Figs 168/17, 169/17) is continuous with the azygos vein. The lumbar veins of the left side are longer than their contralateral partners. They reach the inferior vena cava after running behind the aorta.

The **testicular** (or **ovarian**) **vein** accompanies the similarly named artery. In its lower course it forms a convoluted network, called the *pampiniform plexus*. The upper segment is a single vein which opens into the renal vein on the left side, in 75 per cent of the cases laterally to the left suprarenal vein (Clegg 1970). If there are proximally two trunks on the right side, one opens into the renal vein, the other into the inferior vena cava. These vessels are provided with valves near the orifices (Rauber and Kopsch 1951). In certain cases valves are demonstrable with angiography in the entire length of the vein (Jacobs 1969).

The **renal veins** (Figs 168/15 and 16, 169/15 and 16, 171/3, 180/14 and 15, 181/15 and 16), drain the kidneys. Forming a star-shaped pattern on the surface, they accompany the arteries also outside the segment. In contrast to the renal arteries there are numerous anastomoses among the veins which were divided by Stolic and Mrvaljevic (1971) into a vertical and horizontal group. According to the same authors, the kidney can be divided into 3 to 5 segments corresponding to its veins, but the anastomoses between the veins render correct separation impossible. Uniting in the hilum they form two or three trunks which are continuous with the renal vein. The main trunk, placed in front of the renal arteries, follows a transverse course at the level of the 1st to 2nd lumbar vertebrae and opens into the inferior vena cava. The orifice of the left trunk lies usually higher than that of the right trunk. In 25 per cent of the cases their orifices are at the same level (Gillot and Gallegos 1966). The left renal vein crosses the aorta before the origins of the superior mesenteric and testicular arteries. The renal veins are sometimes provided with valves (Ahlberg et al. 1968). The length of the renal veins: left vein is 7·5 cm, the right vein is 2·5 cm (Gray 1954). Doubled renal veins (Fig. 168/16) on the right side occur in 16·3, on the left side in 3·1 per cent; triplication and quadruplication on the right side has been registered in 3·3 and 1·1 per cent, respectively (Merklin and Michels 1958). If the left renal vein is doubled it forms a ring around the aorta (Gray 1954). Ortmann (1968) observed in 12·2 per cent the existence of left retroaortal renal vein.

Branches of the left renal vein: inferior phrenic veins, left suprarenal vein, left capsular vein, left pyeloureteral veins (Fig. 171/5), left testicular vein and anastomosis with the left ascending lumbar vein. *Branches* of the right renal vein: right capsular vein, right pyeloureteral veins, and anastomosis with the right ascending lumbar vein.

Collaterals of the renal veins (Bücheler et al. 1967): 1. Subcapsular veins — ureteral veins — internal iliac vein. 2. Subcapsular veins — phrenic veins — lumbar veins. 3. Testicular vein on the left side. 4. Renal vein — lumbar veins. 5. Splenorenal anastomosis (Caron and Ribet 1964). This will be treated in context with the portal vein.

The **suprarenal veins** form a short trunk on the right side and open into the inferior vena cava about 4 cm above the orifice of the renal vein (Starer 1965). The right suprarenal vein may open into one of the hepatic veins (Reuter et al. 1967).The left suprarenal vein unites with the inferior phrenic vein before opening into the renal vein. The suprarenal veins may be double or triple (Reuter et al. 1967). There are anastomoses with the veins of the renal capsule (Anson and Cauldwell 1947), with the internal thoracic, intercostal veins, testicular and portal veins (Gagnon 1956).

The **hepatic veins** (Figs 147, 168, 169, 170, 180, 181, 182) receive blood from the hepatic artery and from the portal vein. Placed between the branches of the portal vein, they follow an ascending backward course in the grooves of the portal segments and are in close connection with the parenchyma. After reaching the posterior surface of the liver they pass obliquely into the inferior vena cava. The three principal veins measure about a little finger each, form segments which are closely correlated with the portal system (Knopp 1953, Stucke 1959, Rigaud et al. 1962, Ungváry and Faller 1963, Elias 1963). The veins of the liver, collected from the *central veins*, curve like an arch showing spiral bends. There are three segments: middle, right and left. The boundary between the middle and the left segments is between the right and left lobe of the liver, while the line separating the middle and the right segments is in the centre of the right lobe. The veins of the liver are arranged as follows (Stucke 1959, Elias 1963):

The *right hepatic vein* (Figs 147/1, 149/2, 168/6, 169/6, 170/5, 180/5, 181/6, 182/5) runs along the border of the dorsal segment and receives branches from the upper dorsal (*right superior hepatic vein*, Figs 147/2, 149/3, 168/7, 169/7, 170/6, 180/6, 181/7, 182/6) and the intermediary (*posterolateral hepatic vein*, Figs 147/3, 168/8, 169/8, 170/7, 180/7, 181/8, 182/7) segments. It may furthermore receive branches from the anterosuperior segment, the posterior and caudal parts (*hepatic vein of the caudate process*, Figs 147/5, 149/6; *posteroinferior hepatic vein*, Figs 147/10, 149/4, 168/9, 169/9, 170/9, 180/7, 181/9, 182/9). The latter vessels may open directly into the inferior vena cava. The right hepatic

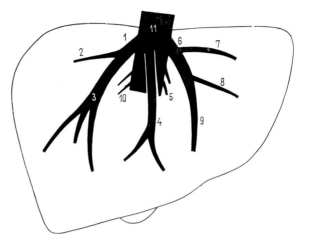

FIG. 147. Division of the hepatic veins in the liver. (*1*) Right hepatic vein; (*2*) right superior hepatic vein; (*3*) posterolateral hepatic veins; (*4*) middle hepatic vein; (*5*) inferior and superior caudate hepatic veins; (*6*) left hepatic vein; (*7*) left superior hepatic vein; (*8*) radix superior; (*9*) radix inferior; (*10*) posteroinferior hepatic veins; (*11*) inferior vena cava.

vein courses upward than backward and to the left, while it describes an arch with a right-forward convexity.

The *middle hepatic vein* (Figs 147/4, 149/5, 168/10, 169/10, 170/10, 180/9, 181/10, 182/10) runs upward from below along the main dividing line of the liver and describes a forward convex arch. It receives branches from the anterior, superior and medial aspects of the right lobe. The vein is usually formed by the union of two vessels.

The *inferior* and *superior caudate hepatic veins* (Figs 147/5, 149/6, 170/11, 182/11) are small branches from the caudate process and open separately into the inferior vena cava.

The *left hepatic vein* (Figs 147/6, 149/7, 168/11, 169/11, 170/12, 180/10, 181/11, 182/12) runs from below upward and backward along the border of the left segment. It describes an arch with a forward and left convexity. It drains the veins of the left lobe from three branches. The upper branch (*left superior hepatic vein*, Figs 147/7, 149/8, 168/12, 169/12, 170/13 180/11, 181/12, 182/13) runs horizontally, the middle and lower branches (*superior root*, Figs 147/8, 149/9, 168/13, 169/13, 170/14, 180/12, 181/13, 182/14 and *inferior root*, Figs 147/9, 149/10, 168/14, 169/14, 170/15, 180/13, 181/14, 182/15) often form a common trunk.

Rigaud and his associates (1962) distinguish three types of orifices of the principal hepatic veins. These types depend, however, also on the shape of the liver determined by constitutional factors. It is especially the right hepatic vein which displays *variations:* it may consist of one or two separately or jointly terminating major branches. The middle and left hepatic veins usually have typical orifice. The middle hepatic vein may be absent and the left hepatic vein may be rudimentary (Doehner 1968). Very rarely the trunks may be doubled (Koguerman-Lepp 1968). Banner and Bresfield (1958) made a detailed classification in this respect. The hepatic venous trunks may open directly into the right atrium. There is a valve at the orifice in such cases (Rauber and Kopsch 1951). The hepatic veins empty together and directly into the right atrium if the upper part of the inferior vena cava is agenetic (Beuren 1966). Scavo (1963) observed a thickening of the smooth muscles at the orifice of the hepatic veins, a phenomenon which, according to him, contributes to the development of "hepatic obstruction". We found a narrow shadow deficiency at the orifice of the hepatic veins. This postmortem contraction of the smooth muscles supports Scavo's histological findings.

The inferior and the superior venae cavae and the portal vein are in collateral communication. These topics are treated in detail together with the superior vena cava and the portal vein, respectively.

Contrast filling of the inferior vena cava

Dos Santos (1935) was the first to fill the inferior vena cava with radio-opaque material. Physiological research of the collateral circulation was carried out by Surrington and Jonas (1952) after the ligation of the inferior vena cava. Studies on the sacrolumbar circulation were facilitated by Helander and Lindbom's (1959) method who filled the inferior vena cava with contrast medium after its constriction by a compression balloon. Advance in anatomy and surgery also made the exploration of the hepatic veins possible. Retrograde filling is considerably more suitable for the visualization of the hepatic veins (Rappaport 1951), renal veins (Caron and Ribet 1964), suprarenal veins (Starer 1965) and the testicular vein (Gősfay 1959). Owing to condition of blood flow usually only the main trunk of the inferior vena cava can be filled in vivo with antero-grade cavography (Gansau 1955, Helander and Lindbom 1959). In such pictures the filling appears fainter at the opening of the renal veins. Side branches can be visualized only if circulation is impeded. The lumbar veins can be visualized in vivo with direct filling or retrograde azygography (Bücheler et al. 1968).

In *postmortem* **anteroposterior** *phlebograms* (Fig. 168) the projection of the lumbar segmental branches of the *inferior vena cava* (Fig. 168/5), ascending in front of the right border of the spine, as well as the projections of the *left ascending lumbar veins* (Fig. 168/17) and the vertebral venous plexuses are superimposed. The *renal veins* (Figs 168/15 and 16) and their branches can be filled in their entirety. While the *right testicular vein* is readily identifiable to the right of the inferior vena cava, its contralateral partner cannot always be easily distinguished on account of the interference of the spinal veins. Each *hepatic vein* can be followed until the minute branches. The *right hepatic* (Fig. 168/6) and the *right superior hepatic veins* (Fig. 168/7) describe a laterally convex arch upward and medially along the right border of the liver. The origin and the upper part of the *middle hepatic vein* (Fig. 168/10) fall upon the projection of the inferior vena cava. It courses to the left and upward. The initial portion of the *left hepatic vein* (Fig. 168/11) lies in front of the centre of the vertebral column. It courses steeply upward to the right. Close to the right border of the vertebrae, the *inferior root* (Fig. 168/14) ascends along an approximately straight line, the *superior root* (Fig. 168/13) runs obliquely, while the *left superior hepatic vein* (Fig. 168/12) follows a horizontal course to the right.

In the **lateral view** (Fig. 169), the *inferior vena cava* (Fig. 169/5) is seen in the projection of the anterior border of the vertebral column: its position is in accordance with the physiological lordosis. Its lumbar segment describes a forward convex curve; the further course is straight, showing a backward convex curve behind the liver. Thus, its whole course is slightly "S"-shaped. The initial part of the *right renal vein* (Fig. 169/16), in an orthoroentgenographic position, bulges backward, and the *left renal vein* (Fig. 169/15) forward from the shadow of the inferior vena cava. The transverse course of the *lumbar veins* (Fig. 169/18) and the caudocranial course of the *vertebral venous plexuses* (Fig. 169/17) are distinguishable. The *right hepatic vein* (Fig. 169/6) describes an ascending curve in front of the inferior vena cava. The *middle hepatic vein* (Fig. 169/10) lies in or somewhat behind the projection of the inferior vena cava. Occupying the highest position, the *right superior hepatic vein* (Fig. 169/7) runs horizontally, while the approximately parallel course of the *left superior hepatic vein* (Fig. 169/12) runs below its contralateral partner. Both are behind the inferior vena cava. The *left hepatic vein* (Fig. 169/11) and its branches (usually obscured by the shadow of the inferior vena cava) pursue a backward course. **Anatomical preparations of the kidney** (Fig. 171) reveal the vascular pattern of the renal vein within the kidney. The *venulae rectae* and the *interlobular veins* (Fig. 171/4), which arise from the *stellate veins*, border the cortex with a spicule-like design.

The *arcuate veins* are arched. The straight *interlobar veins* open into the *renal vein* (Fig. 171/3) in the hilum or outside it after the union of several veins. The *capsular* and the *pyeloureteral* (Fig. 171/5) *veins* and also their anastomoses can be filled.

Craniocaudal angiograms of the liver (Fig. 170) show the perpendicular course of the *central veins* to the *sublobular veins*. The triple segmentation in this third projection, complements the pictures made in the anteroposterior and lateral views.

SYSTEM OF THE PORTAL VEIN

The portal circulation occupies a peculiar position among the veins, for the afferent branches coming from the gastrointestinal tract enter the liver in the form of a common trunk, i.e., as the portal vein, where they divide into capillaries in the manner of arteries. Its ramifications follow the uniform segmental system of the arterial-venous-biliary pathways. The improving methods of postmortem angiography have considerably contributed to the exploration of the segmental system. Another characteristic feature of the portal circulation consists of the various anastomoses between the portal and the caval veins. The functional significance of these communications has long been known. They can be studied by splenoportography.

The portal vein and its branches

The portal vein (Figs 148/1, 149/11, 172/4, 173/4, 174/12, 175/4, 180/23, 181/22, 182/16, 183/4) is formed at the level of the 1st and 2nd lumbar vertebrae by the union of the superior mesenteric and splenic veins. This level may vary between the 12th thoracic and the 1st lumbar vertebrae in pyknic, and between the 1st and 3rd lumbar vertebrae in asthenic individuals (Rösch 1964). Arising, the portal vein runs to the porta hepatis at the inferior margin of the hepatoduodenal ligament between and behind the hepatic artery and the bile duct. Its initial portion is situated behind, rarely in front of the head of the pancreas and the upper horizontal segment of the duodenum (Knight 1921). The course of the vein is straight or sometimes slightly curved upward. Its projection forms an angle of 40° to 90° with the spine (Bergstrand 1964). Variations in this respect depend on constitutional factors. The vessel runs upward in asthenic and more laterally in pyknic persons. The length of the portal vein is 6 cm (3 to 9 cm) (Rousselot et al. 1953, Rösch 1964). Postmortem splenograms show the diameter to measure 2·3 cm distally and 1·9 cm proximally to the liver (Rousselot et al. 1953). In vivo values are lower: 1·39 cm (0·9 to 2·5 cm; Rösch 1964).

Variations are infrequent. If the vein is doubled, one trunk is the continuation of the splenic, the other of the superior mesenteric vein (Stauber 1965). Rarely, at the confluence of the splenic vein and superior mesenteric vein, the portal vein divides immediately into 2 to 4 branches (Ender et al. 1971). The portal vein may anomalously open into the inferior vena cava (Edwards 1951a) or it may be in communication with the pulmonary veins (*see* section on pulmonary veins). Accessory portal veins are small vessels which enter the liver from the adjacent areas, to divide there into capillaries similar to the main trunk. These vessels are classified into four groups: cystic, omental, phrenic and paraumbilical groups (Walcker 1922).

Tributaries to the portal vein are the splenic, superior mesenteric, inferior mesenteric and left gastric veins. Walcker (1922) described the following variations of these veins: 1. Splenic vein + superior mesenteric vein (the first opens into the latter; 42 per cent). 2. Splenic vein + superior mesenteric vein (the latter opens into the first; 29 per cent). 3. Splenic vein + superior and inferior mesenteric veins; 20 per cent. 4. Splenic vein + superior and inferior mesenteric veins + right gastric vein. 5. Splenic vein + superior and inferior mesenteric veins (the left gastric vein opens into the splenic or the superior mesenteric vein). Variations 4 and 5 have a combined frequency of 9 per cent.

Afferent branches of the portal vein:

The *superior mesenteric vein* (Figs 172/5, 173/5, 174/13, 180/24, 181/23) ascends on the right side of the corresponding artery in front of the inferior horizontal part of the duodenum. Its area of drainage is the same as the area supplied by the corresponding artery (*jejunal and ileal veins*, Figs 172/6, 173/6, 174/14, 178/2, 180/25, 181/24; *right gastroepiploic vein*, Figs 172/7, 173/7, 174/15, 177/3, 180/26; *pancreatic veins, ileocolic vein*, Figs 172/8, 173/6, 174/16, 179/4, 180/27; *appendicular vein, right colic vein*, Figs 172/9, 174/17, 180/28; *middle colic vein*, Figs 172/10, 174/18, 176/9, 177/5, 180/29 and *pancreaticoduodenal veins*, Fig. 174/19). The superior mesenteric vein has a diameter of 1·7 cm (Rousselot et al. 1953). Although the number of its larger branches is variable (10 to 25), the whole vessel shows a fairly constant pattern. The main trunk ascends steeply while it collects branches from both sides. The jejunal veins unite in three big trunks before emptying (50 per cent) or consist of a horizontal part with a deeper outlet and a vertical part with a higher orifice (Gillot et al. 1964). The latter opens frequently into the portal or the splenic vein. The colic veins exceed the corresponding arteries in number. Their division and arrangement into secondary arches are also different (Illarionova 1966).

The *splenic vein* (Figs 172/11, 173/9, 174/27, 176/4, 180/30, 181/25) is the other main tributary of the portal vein. It commences in the spleen with 3 to 5 branches: *superior polar vein*, V_1 (Figs 174/30, 176/11; *superior terminal branch*, V_2 (Figs 174/31, 176/12; *middle terminal branch*, V_3 (Fig. 176/13; *inferior terminal branch*, V_4 (Figs 174/32, 176/14; *inferior polar vein*, V_5 (Fig. 174/33). Each branch arises from a particular segment. No communications exist between the larger veins (Kikkawa 1966). The various segmental branches unite in a common trunk after a short course. This trunk usually describes a downward convex arch or wave behind the tail and body of the pancreas. Having reached the right border of the spine, it continues in the portal vein at the height of the 1st or 2nd lumbar vertebra. The course of the splenic vein is transverse in pyknic and obliquely descending in asthenic individuals. The length of the splenic vein is 12·8 cm (8 to 19 cm), its diameter 1·02 cm (0·6 to 1·6 cm; Rösch 1964). In addition to several small branches (*pancreatic veins*, Fig. 176/7; *short gastric veins*, Figs 172/13, 174/29, 176/6, 180/31; *left gastroepiploic vein*, Figs 172/12, 174/28, 176/8, 177/4) the vessel receives the inferior mesenteric vein. The latter opens frequently into the portal vein.

The *inferior mesenteric vein* (Figs 172/14, 173/10, 174/20, 180/32, 181/26) begins in the lesser pelvis as does the *superior rectal vein* (Figs 172/17, 173/11, 174/23, 180/35, 181/27) and, forming a left convex arch, runs toward the portal vein. It receives the *sigmoid veins* (Figs 172/16, 174/22, 180/34) and the *left colic vein* (Figs 172/15, 174/21, 180/33, 181/28). The vessel anastomoses with the system of the internal iliac vein in the lesser pelvis. The diameter of the inferior mesenteric artery is 0·6 cm (Rousselot et al. 1953).

The veins coursing along the lesser curvature of the stomach (*left and right gastric veins*, Figs 172/18, 173/8, 174/24 and 25, 180/36) unite to form a common trunk with the *prepyloric vein* which begins on the anterior aspect of the pylorus. This trunk, describing an arch upward to the left, passes in front of the spine and empties into the portal and sometimes into the splenic vein (Rauber and Kopsch 1951). They maintain important communications between the superior vena cava and the portal vein via the esophageal veins.

The *cystic vein* (Fig. 174/26), the vein of the gallbladder, according to some authors, opens into the hepatic veins (Braus and Elze 1956), but according to others it ramifies into capillaries and empties through the parenchyma of the liver into the hepatic veins (Töndury 1959) or into the portal vein (Habighorst et al. 1965). Whereas Pfuhl (1932) presumes anastomoses between the portal vein and the hepatic veins, Zielke (1962) could fill the branches of the cystic vein via the portal vein only.

The *umbilical vein* (Figs 221/31, 222/11) courses from the navel through the falciform ligament of the liver to the left sagittal groove of the liver to end in the left branch of the portal vein. From here the ductus venosus, an embryonic vessel which becomes more or less obliterated after birth, runs to the inferior vena cava. The lumen of the umbilical vein is traversable in some cases; it measures 0·2 to 0·4 cm in width (Bayly and Gonzalez 1964). The *paraumbilical veins*, connecting the portal vein to the venae cavae, empty either into the umbilical or directly into the portal vein. As a variation in orifice, the umbilical vein may, after piercing the diaphragm, open directly into the right atrium (Shryock et al. 1942).

Efferent branches of the portal vein:

Entering the liver together with the hepatic artery and the bile ducts, the portal vein divides there like the arteries (Hjorstjö 1948, Elias and Petty 1952, Healey 1954, Couinaud 1957). The portal vein may ramify in the porta hepatis in three different ways (Bergstrand 1957): 1. Division into right and left main branches is the most frequent. The right branch divides into a ventrocranial and a dorsocaudal part after the course of 1 cm. 2. The division is immediate trifurcation. 3. The right ventrocranial part arises directly from the portal vein. After that the portal vein divides into two main branches.

The *left branch* (Figs 148/2, 149/12, 172/20, 173/13, 174/35, 175/6, 180/38, 181/30, 182/18, 183/6) ascends forward and forms a bend forward and to the right at the boundary between the left and the middle lobes. It emits there a *superior branch*, V_2 (Figs 148/4, 149/14, 172/22, 173/14, 174/37, 175/8, 180/39, 182/19, 183/8) which follows a backward ascending course, further an *inferior branch*, V_3 (Figs 148/5, 149/15, 172/23, 173/15, 174/38, 175/9, 180/40, 182/20, 183/9) which runs downward and forward. The backward bending trunk (*transverse part* V_4, Figs 148/6, 149/16, 172/24, 173/16, 174/39, 175/10, 180/41, 182/21, 183/10) gives off 2 to 6 branches to the quadrate lobe. The vessels running to the caudate process spring off from the left main branch or from the bifurcation of the portal vein (*caudate branches* V_1, Figs 148/3, 149/13, 172/21, 174/36, 175/7, 182/26, 183/7).

248

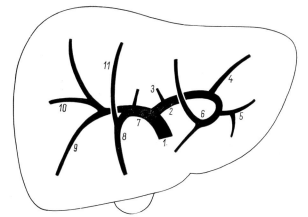

FIG. 148. Division of the portal vein in the liver. (*1*) Portal vein; (*2*) left branch; (*3*) caudate branches, V₁; (*4*) left superior branch, V₂; (*5*) left inferior branch, V₃; (*6*) transverse part, V₄; (*7*) right branch; (*8*) inferior anterior branch, V₅; (*9*) inferior posterior branch, V₆; (*10*) superior posterior branch, V₇; (*11*) superior anterior branch, V₈.

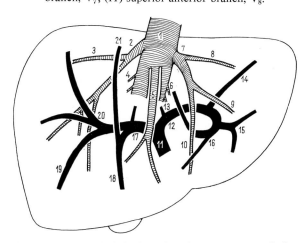

FIG. 149. Division of the hepatic veins and portal vein in the liver. (*1*) Inferior vena cava; (*2*) right hepatic vein; (*3*) right superior hepatic vein; (*4*) posteroinferior hepatic veins; (*5*) middle hepatic vein; (*6*) caudate hepatic veins; (*7*) left hepatic vein; (*8*) left superior hepatic vein; (*9*) radix superior; (*10*) radix inferior; (*11*) portal vein; (*12*) left branch; (*13*) caudate branches, V₁; (*14*) left superior branch, V₂; (*15*) left inferior branch, V₃; (*16*) transverse part, V₄; (*17*) right branch; (*18*) inferior anterior branch, V₅; (*19*) inferior posterior branch, V₆; (*20*) superior posterior branch, V₇; (*21*) superior anterior branch, V₈.

The *right branch* (Figs 148/7, 149/17, 172/19, 173/12, 174/34, 175/5, 180/37, 181/29, 182/17, 183/5), usually bifurcates. The *anterior branch* emits a descending branch (*inferior anterior branch*, V₅; Figs 148/8, 149/18, 172/25, 173/17, 174/40, 175/11, 180/42, 182/22, 183/11) and an ascending branch (*superior anterior branch*, V₈; Figs 148/11, 149/21, 172/28, 173/20, 174/43, 175/14, 180/45, 182/25, 183/14). The course of the main trunk continues backward to the right (*posterior branch*). It sends venous trunks to the inferior (*inferior posterior branch*, V₆; Figs 148/9, 149/19, 172/26, 173/18, 174/41, 175/12, 180/43,

182/23, 183/12) and to the superior part of the right border of the liver (*superior posterior branch*, V₇; Figs 148/10, 149/20, 172/27, 173/19, 174/42, 175/13, 180/44, 182/24, 183/13).

Entering the liver from above and below, the branches of the hepatic veins and of the portal vein form a characteristic pattern (Fig. 149). The two systems follow opposite courses, each in the area which — so to say — has been left free by the other.

Portocaval collateral circulation

It is by means of collateral circulation between the portal vein and the superior and inferior venae cavae that circulation is maintained if normal blood flow is anatomically impeded (Pick 1909, McIndoe 1928, Edwards 1951b, Doehner et al. 1955, Düx et al. 1962a, Maurer 1964, Hach 1971; Fig. 150). If necessary, peripheral circulation is made possible through the following anatomical communications.

1. Gastroesophageal anastomoses (Fig. 150/I). Connection of the left gastric vein, the short gastric veins and their branches with the esophageal veins ensures the possibility of collateral circulation toward the superior vena cava. The veins of the region of the cardia and fundus of the stomach may be larger without being pathological in the presence of normal esophageal veins (Parchwitz 1961).

2. Mesentericorectal anastomoses (Fig. 150/II) form a venous plexus by connecting the initial branches of the inferior mesenteric vein with the middle and inferior rectal veins.

3. Umbilicoepigastric anastomoses (Fig. 150/III) connect the left main branch of the portal vein with the epigastric vein via the umbilical vein.

4. Splenoparietal anastomoses (Fig. 150/IV) connect the veins of the surface of the spleen and of the abdominal wall (lumbar veins, hemiazygos vein, epigastric veins) with the veins of the diaphragm (phrenic and intercostal veins).

5. Retroperitoneal anastomoses (Fig. 150/V) existing between the mesenteric veins and the paravertebral venous network, ensure collateral circulation toward the inferior and the superior venae cavae.

6. Transhepatic anastomoses (Fig. 150/VI) connect the veins of the diaphragm and the abdominal wall as also the inferior vena cava with the veins of the surface of the liver (Walcker 1922).

7. Splenorenal anastomoses (Fig. 150/VII). The phrenic, peripancreatic and gastric venous networks communicate with the left renal vein via the ascending lumbar vein. The suprarenal vein opens directly into the renal vein. Direct communication between the right renal vein or the splenic and the portal

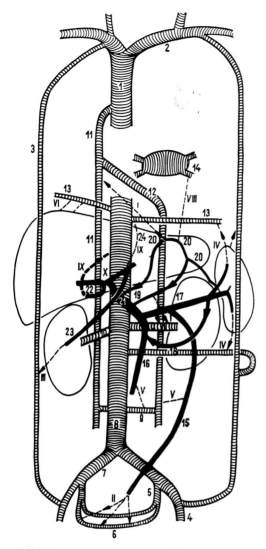

10. Intrahepatic anastomoses (Fig. 150/X) connect the right with the left branch (Guntz and Farisse 1966), or the veins of one of the lobes with each other (Myking and Halvorsen 1971).

The collateral vessels can be demonstrated by means of postmortem angiography after the ligation of the portal vein (Schoenmackers and Vieten 1964). We found that in our material where portal circulation had been normal in vivo, the contrast medium did not escape at any point when all abdominal organs were simultaneously removed at autopsy, indicating that anastomoses were closed (Fig. 174).

The portocaval anastomoses may be divided into a hepatopetal (toward the liver) and a hepatofugal (toward the inferior vena cava) group from a clinical point of view. Blood flow toward the liver is maintained by the venae ligamenti hepatoduodenales, the veins of the gall bladder, the gastroepiploic veins, the short, left and right gastric veins (Pick 1909). Hepatofugal collaterals ensure circulation via the splenoparietal, splenorenal and retroperitoneal anatomoses toward the retroperitoneal area; via the umbilicoepigastric anastomoses toward the abdominal wall; via the gastroesophageal and mesentericorectal anastomoses toward the upper and lower ends of the alimentary tract (McIndoe 1928).

Contrast filling of the portal venous system, splenoportography

Moore and Brindenbaugh (1950, cit. Zsebők 1967) were the first to fill the portal vein with radioopaque matter in vivo in order to study pathologic changes due to impeded portal circulation. They were followed by Abeatici and Campi (1951), Leger (1955), Gvozdanović and Hauptmann (1955), Bergstrand (1957), Düx et al. (1962a, b), Rösch (1964) and many others who visualized the portal vein by injecting contrast medium into the spleen (splenoportography). A more complete filling of the portal vein has been achieved recently via the umbilical vein (Piccone et al. 1967). Only the splenic vein, the portal vein and its efferent branches can be filled normally by means of splenoportography. Postmortem venography through the injection of a branch of the superior mesenteric vein permits simultaneous visualization of the entire portal system. Thus, visualization of the anastomoses is clearer than in vivo (Schoenmacker and Vieten 1953, 1954, 1964).

Postmortem venograms made in the **anteroposterior view** (Fig. 172) show the branches of the *superior mesenteric vein* (Fig. 172/5) to converge on the main trunk in front of the spine. The *inferior mesenteric*

FIG. 150. Portocaval anastomoses. I, gastroesophageal; II, mesentericorectal; III, umbilicoepigastric; IV, splenoparietal; V, retroperitoneal; VI, transhepatic; VII, splenorenal; VIII, portopulmonary; IX, direct portocaval; X, intrahepatic anastomoses. (*1*) Superior vena cava; (*2*) brachiocephalic veins; (*3*) superior and inferior epigastric veins; (*4*) external iliac vein; (*5*) internal iliac vein; (*6*) rectal veins; (*7*) common iliac vein; (*8*) inferior vena cava; (*9*) lumbar veins; (*10*) renal vein; (*11*) azygos vein; (*12*) hemiazygos vein; (*13*) inferior phrenic veins; (*14*) pulmonary veins; (*15*) inferior mesenteric vein; (*16*) superior mesen)teric vein; (*17*) splenic vein; (*18*) gastroepiploic veins; (*19* right and left gastric veins; (*20*) short gastric veins; (*21*) portal vein; (*22*) cystic vein; (*23*) umbilical vein; (*24*) ductus venosus.

veins occurs much less frequently (Grünert 1960, Düx et al. 1962b, Cronquist and Ranniger 1965).

8. Portopulmonary anastomoses (Fig. 150/VIII). The gastric veins may be connected with the pulmonary veins through the mediastinal and the pericardiac veins (Schoenmackers and Vieten 1953).

9. The portocaval rectae anastomoses (Fig. 150/IX) may maintain communication between the two systems (ductus venosus, cystic vein).

250

vein (Fig. 172/14) may terminate at various points but it follows a constant course along the left border of the vertebral column. The projections of the *left colic vein* (Fig. 172/15) and *sigmoid veins* (Fig. 172/16) and the branches of the superior mesenteric vein are superimposed. The *splenic vein* (Fig. 172/11) is seen to run transversely or obliquely from the spleen to the right border of the spine. The projections of the veins of the spleen and the fundus of the stomach are usually superimposed so that their reliable identification is often difficult. Describing an arch, the *left gastric vein* (Fig. 172/18) crosses the spine. Falling partly on the projection of the splenic vein, the *right gastric vein* cannot always be differentiated. The *portal vein* (Fig. 172/4) ascends obliquely to the right; its division determines the site of the porta hepatis with great accuracy. The intrahepatic branches offer an excellent visualization of the vascular structure.

In the **lateral view** (Fig. 173), the branches of the *superior mesenteric vein* (Fig. 173/5) are situated in front of the *inferior mesenteric vein* (Fig. 173/10). If the inferior mesenteric vein opens into the splenic vein, its orifice may be a useful aid in the recognition of the splenic vein. Occupying an oblique position, the *splenic vein* (Fig. 173/9) is mostly ortho-roentgenographic in this projection. Its branches and the spleen fall on the posterior third of the liver and are, therefore, indistinguishable. Since the *portal vein* (Fig. 173/4) pursues an obliquely ascending course forward, while the splenic vein runs obliquely backward and upward, these two vessels form a characteristic "Y" shape with the superior mesenteric vein. The degree of angle formed by the two upper limbs of the figure depends on the reciprocal position shown by the projections of the liver and the hilum of the spleen. The segmental branches can be well distinguished in the first two-third of the liver.

Anatomical preparations (Fig. 174) of the entire portal system allow the distinction of extremely fine details in respect of intraorganic ramifications. The vessels of the intestines are spread out and are projected apart. The structure of the spleen can be visualized, and the veins of the stomach followed to the minute branches.

Detailed radiograms of the rich venous network of the **stomach** (Fig. 177), the **spleen** (Fig. 176) or the **loops of the small** (Fig. 178) and the **large intestine** (Fig. 179) reveal still finer details of the small twigs and anastomoses of the portal system. Venograms of the **liver** (Fig. 175) show each efferent branch of the portal system. In addition to the usual antero-posterior pictures and the above discussed pictures in the lateral view, the branches of the portal vein are seen also in the craniocaudal projection. The poorly vascularized area of the inferior vena cava and the principal branches of the liver is striking. Beyond the various segmental branches, fine details (down to a diameter of 0·1 mm) of the interlobular and central veins can be studied in these radiograms.

With the **simultaneous filling of the portal vein and the inferior vena cava** the relative position of these two vessels can be studied. In **anteroposterior pictures** (Fig. 180), the *superior mesenteric vein* (Fig. 180/24) is seen on the left side of the inferior vena cava and usually cannot be differentiated from it. The branches of the left renal vein are intersected by the *inferior mesenteric vein* (Fig. 180/32), while the right renal vein is obliquely crossed by the *middle colic veins* (Fig. 180/29). The *splenic vein* (Fig. 180/30) and the *gastric veins* (Fig. 180/36) can be distinguished as at the simple filling of the portal vein. The *portal vein* (Fig. 180/23) crosses the projection of the inferior vena cava obliquely. Since the courses followed by the branches of the portal vein and those of the hepatic veins are intersecting in the area of the liver, they can be well differentiated. Seen **laterally** (Fig. 181), the *superior mesenteric vein* (Fig. 181/23) is situated in front of the inferior vena cava, while the *inferior mesenteric vein* (Fig. 181/26) is in the projection of the inferior vena cava. The *splenic vein* (Fig. 181/25) is obscured by the inferior vena cava and the overlapping shadows of the hepatic veins. Identification of the hepatic branches of the *portal vein* (Fig. 181/22) is difficult, since the picture is dominated by the forward and backward radiating parts of the hepatic veins. Their separation is often impossible.

Simultaneous contrast filling of the dissected liver (Fig. 182) shows in the **craniocaudal view** the two laterally running branches of the portal vein in front. The branches of the right side are crossed first by the middle hepatic then, more laterally, by the right hepatic vein. The right superior hepatic vein appears fairly isolated. On the left side, the branches of the left hepatic vein intersect peripherally the veins of the pars transversa and the branches of the lateral veins. The left superior hepatic vein is not projected upon any of the major veins.

Simultaneous contrast filling of the portal vein, the hepatic artery and the biliary paths (Fig. 183) gives a complete picture of their relative courses and segmental divisions. The triple arrangement can be observed both centrally and peripherally.

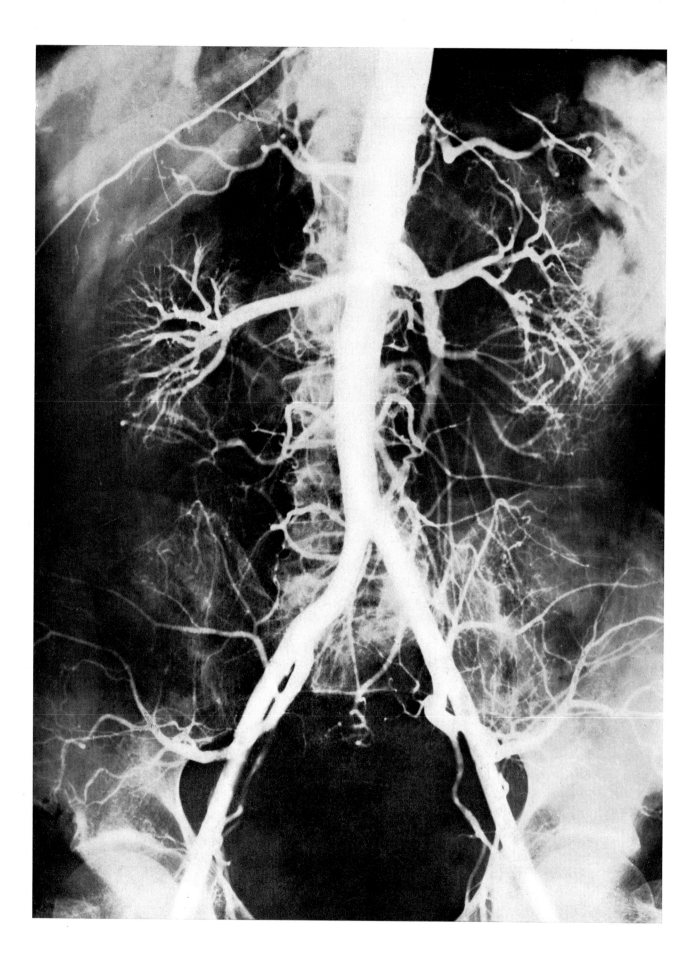

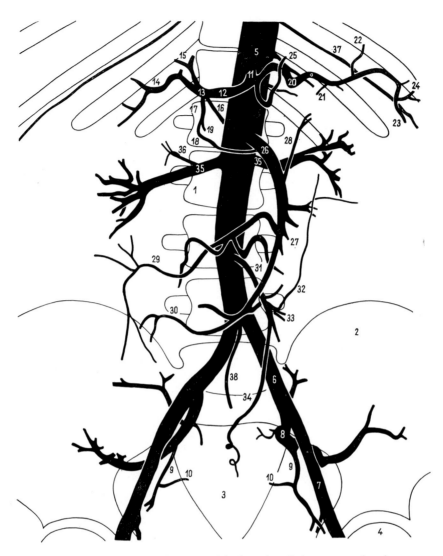

FIG. 151. The abdominal aorta and its branches, I. Anteroposterior view.

1. Lumbar vertebrae
2. Ilium
3. Sacrum
4. Head of femur
5. Abdominal aorta
6. Common iliac artery
7. External iliac artery
8. Internal iliac artery
9. Internal pudendal artery
10. Middle rectal artery
11. Celiac trunk
12. Common hepatic artery
13. Hepatic artery
14. Right branch

15. Left branch
16. Right gastric artery
17. Gastroduodenal artery
18. Anterior pancreatico-
     duodenal arch
19. Right gastroepiploic artery
20. Splenic artery
21. Pancreatic branches
22. Gastric branch
23. Left gastroepiploic artery
24. Splenic branches
25. Left gastric artery
26. Superior mesenteric
     artery

27. Jejunal and ileal arteries
28. Middle colic artery
29. Right colic artery
30. Ileocolic artery
31. Inferior mesenteric artery
32. Left colic artery
33. Sigmoid arteries
34. Superior rectal artery
35. Renal artery
36. Right inferior suprarenal
     artery
37. Posterior intercostal
     arteries
38. Median sacral artery

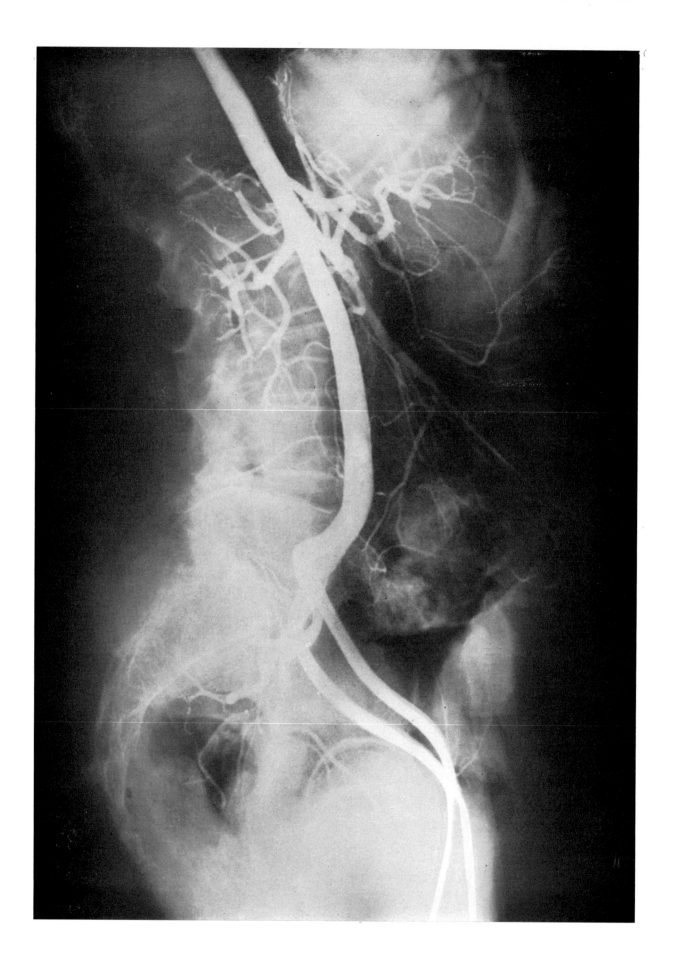

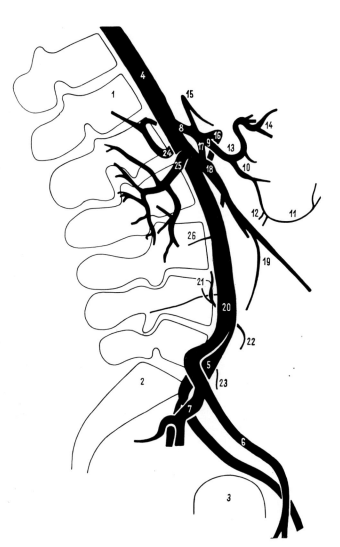

FIG. 152. The abdominal aorta and its branches, II.
Dextrosinistral view.

1. Lumbar vertebrae
2. Sacrum
3. Head of femur
4. Abdominal aorta
5. Common iliac artery
6. External iliac artery
7. Internal iliac artery
8. Celiac trunk
9. Common hepatic artery

10. Gastroduodenal artery
11. Right gastroepiploic artery
12. Supraduodenal arteries
13. Hepatic artery
14. Hepatic branches
15. Left gastric artery
16. Splenic artery
17. Anastomosis between celiac trunk and superior mesenteric artery

18. Superior mesenteric artery
19. Intestinal arteries
20. Inferior mesenteric artery
21. Left colic artery
22. Sigmoid arteries
23. Superior rectal artery
24. Left renal artery
25. Right renal artery
26. Lumbar arteries

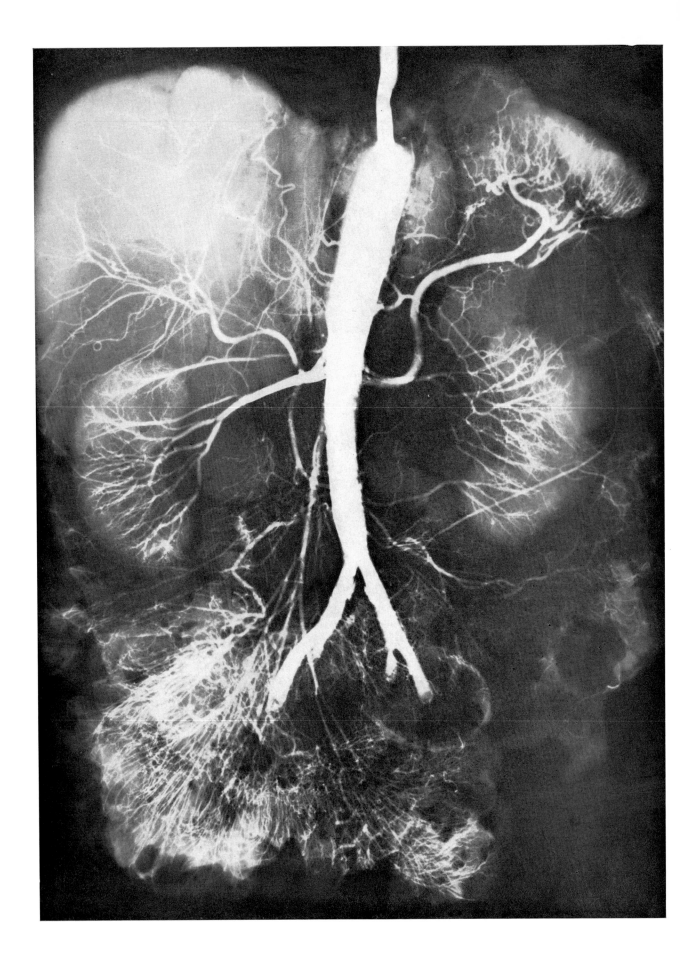

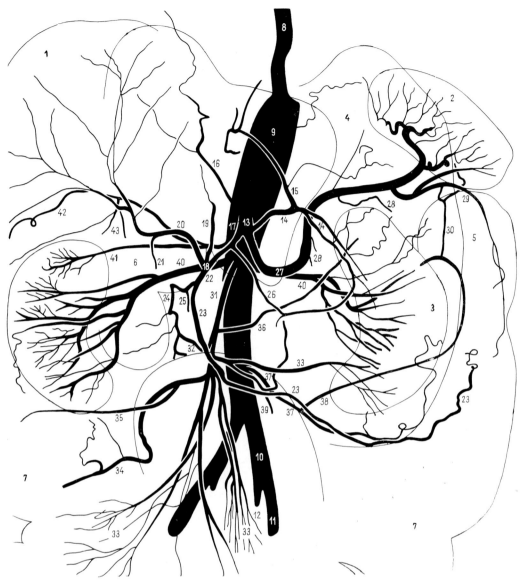

FIG. 153. The abdominal aorta and its branches, III. Anatomical preparation.
Anteroposterior view.

1. Liver
2. Spleen
3. Kidney
4. Fundus of the stomach
5. Left colic flexure
6. Gall bladder
7. Intestines
8. Cannula in aorta
9. Abdominal aorta
10. Common iliac artery
11. External iliac artery
12. Internal iliac artery
13. Celiac trunk
14. Left gastric artery
15. Left inferior phrenic artery
16. Right inferior phrenic artery

17. Common hepatic artery
18. Hepatic artery
19. Left branch
20. Right branch
21. Cystic artery
22. Gastroduodenal artery
23. Right gastroepiploic artery
24. Retroduodenal artery
25. Superior supraduodenal artery
26. Right gastric artery
27. Splenic artery
28. Pancreatic branches
29. Left gastroepiploic artery
30. Anastomosis between the splenic and the left colic artery

31. Superior mesenteric artery
32. Inferior pancreatico-duodenal artery
33. Jejunal and ileal arteries
34. Ileocolic artery
35. Right colic artery
36. Middle colic artery
37. Inferior mesenteric artery
38. Left colic artery
39. Sigmoid artery
40. Renal artery
41. Superior segmental (superior polar) artery
42. Superior capsular artery
43. Right superior suprarenal artery

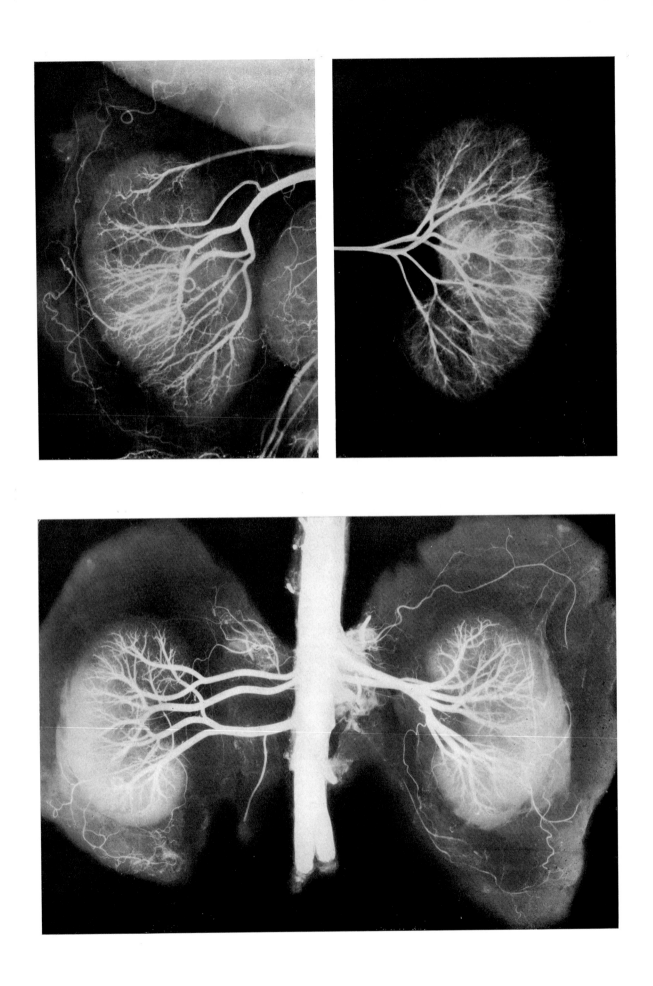

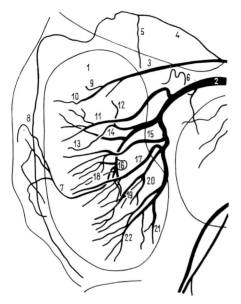

Fig. 154. The renal artery and its branches. Anatomical preparation. Anteroposterior view.

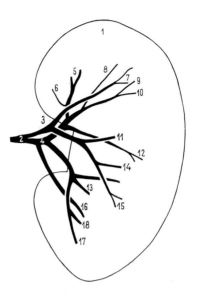

Fig. 155. Intrarenal branches of the renal artery. Anatomical preparation. Anteroposterior view.

1. Right kidney	9. 1V	17. 5V
2. Renal artery	10. 1D	18. 5D
3. Superior segmental artery	11. 2V	19. 6V
4. Superior capsular artery	12. 2D	20. 6D
5. Superior suprarenal artery	13. 3V	21. 7V
6. Inferior suprarenal artery	14. 3D	22. 7D
7. Middle capsular artery	15. 4V	
8. Perirenal arterial arch	16. 4D	

1. Left kidney	7. 2V	13. 5D
2. Renal artery	8. 2D	14. 5V
3. Anterior branch	9. 3V	15. 6V
4. Posterior branch	10. 3D	16. 6D
5. 1V	11. 4V	17. 7V
6. 1D	12. 4D	18. 7D

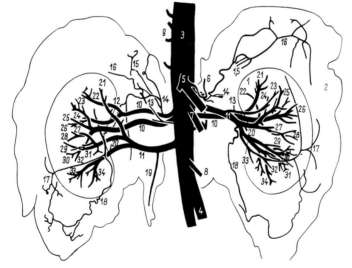

Fig. 156. Paired branches of the abdominal aorta. Anatomical preparation. Anteroposterior view.

1. Kidney	10. Renal artery (posterior branches)	17. Middle capsular artery
2. Fatty capsule of the kidney	11. Renal artery (anterior branch)	18. Inferior capsular artery
3. Abdominal aorta	12. Superior anterior segmental artery	19. Right testicular artery
4. Common iliac artery	13. Inferior suprarenal artery	20. Inferior anterior segmental artery
5. Celiac trunk	14. Middle suprarenal artery	21. 1V
6. Left gastric artery	15. Superior suprarenal artery	22. 1D
7. Superior mesenteric artery	16. Superior capsular artery	23. 2V
8. Inferior mesenteric artery		24. 2D
9. Lumbar arteries		25. 3V

26. 3D
27. 4V
28. 4D
29. 5V
30. 5D
31. 6V
32. 6D
33. 7V
34. 7D

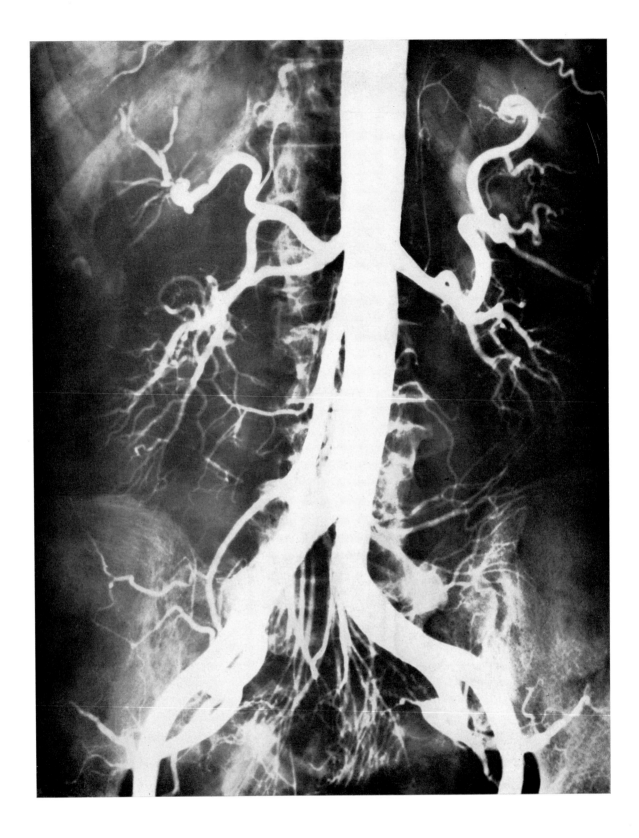

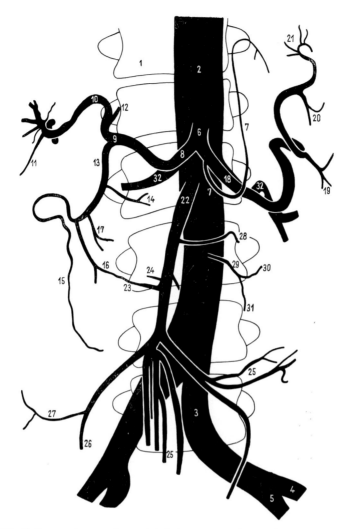

FIG. 157. Celiac trunk, superior and inferior mesenteric arteries and their branches.
Anteroposterior view.

1. Lumbar vertebrae
2. Abdominal aorta
3. Common iliac artery
4. External iliac artery
5. Internal iliac artery
6. Celiac trunk
7. Left gastric artery
8. Common hepatic artery
9. Hepatic artery
10. Right branch
11. Cystic artery
12. Left branch

13. Gastroduodenal artery
14. Right gastric artery
15. Right gastroepiploic artery
16. Retroduodenal artery
17. Superior supraduodenal artery
18. Splenic artery
19. Left gastroepiploic artery
20. Artery of the tail of the pancreas
21. Short gastric arteries
22. Superior mesenteric artery

23. Posterior inferior pancreaticoduodenal artery
24. Anterior inferior pancreaticoduodenal artery
25. Jejunal and ileal arteries
26. Ileocolic artery
27. Right colic artery
28. Middle colic artery
29. Inferior mesenteric artery
30. Left colic artery
31. Sigmoid artery
32. Renal artery

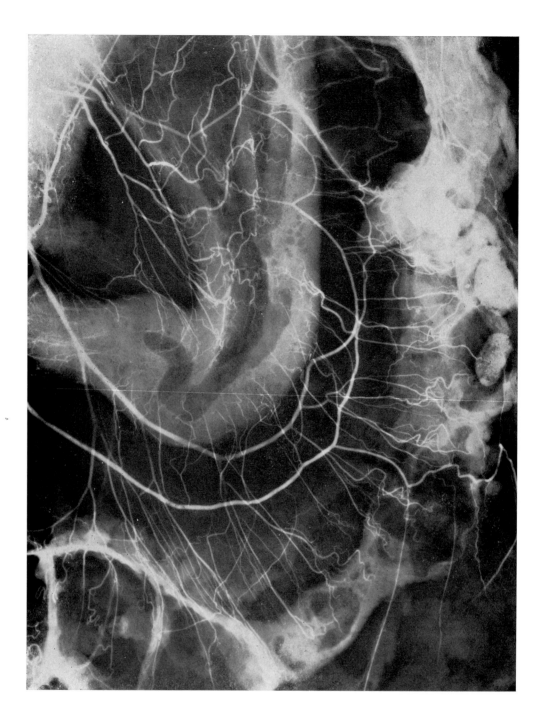

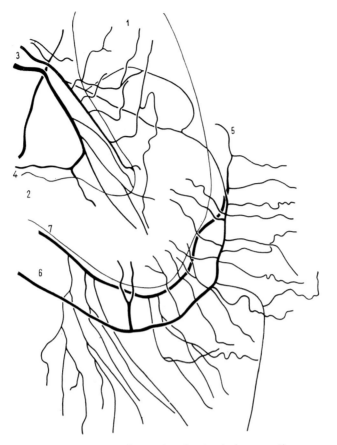

FIG. 158. The gastric arteries. Anatomical preparation.
Anteroposterior view.

1. Fundus of the stomach
2. Pyloric antrum
3. Left gastric artery
4. Right gastric artery

5. Left gastroepiploic artery
6. Right gastroepiploic
   artery
7. Middle colic artery

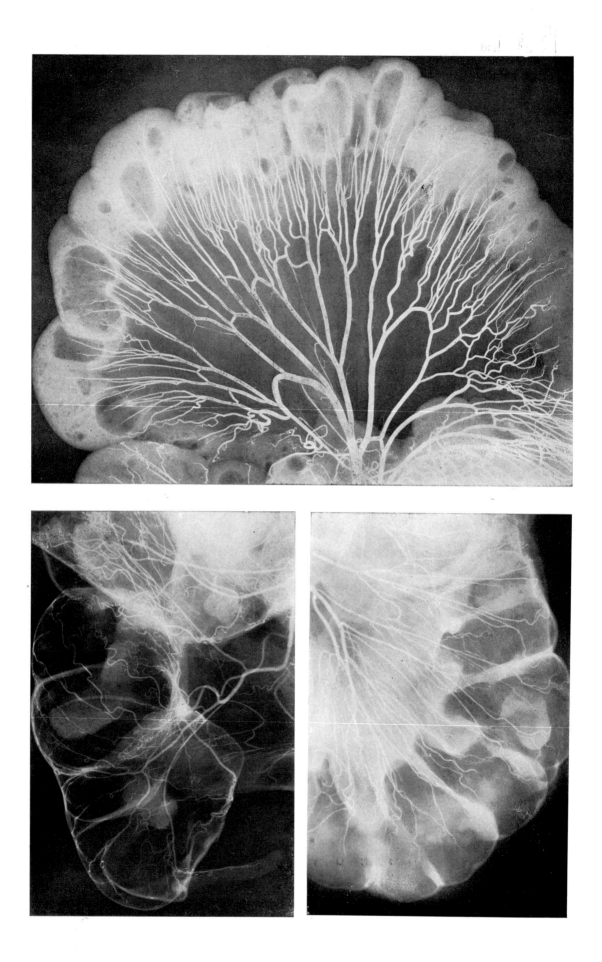

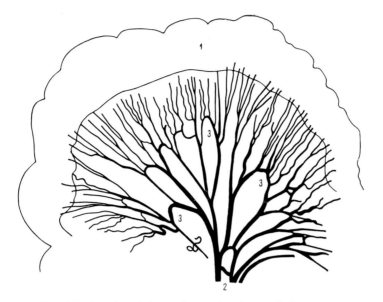

FIG. 159. Arteries of the small intestine. Anatomical preparation.
Anteroposterior view.

1. Jejunum
2. Jejunal arteries
3. Arterial arches

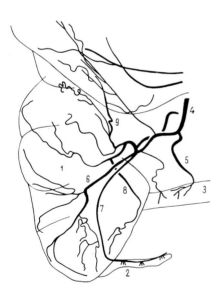

FIG. 160. Arteries of the cecum.
Anatomical preparation. Anteroposterior view.

1. Cecum   *6.* Anterior cecal artery
2. Vermiform appendix   *7.* Appendicular artery
3. Ileum   *8.* Posterior cecal artery
4. Ileocolic artery   *9.* Ascending artery
5. Iliac branch

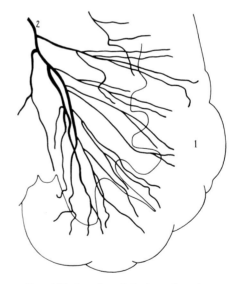

FIG. 161. Arteries of the large intestine.
Anatomical preparation. Anteroposterior view.

1. Descending colon
2. Left colic artery

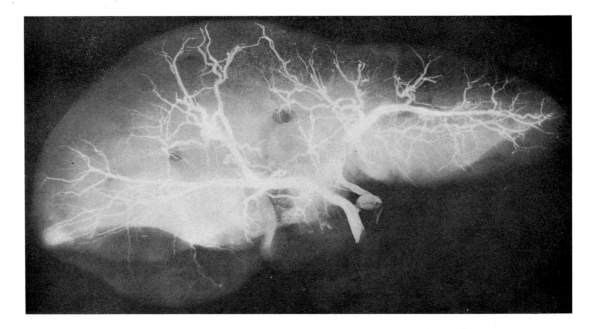

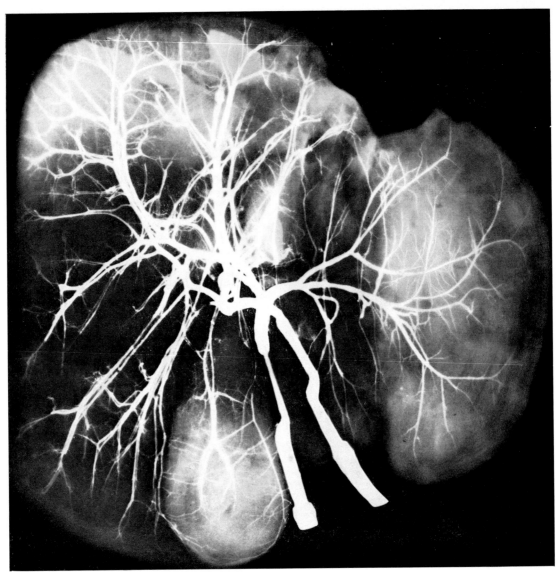

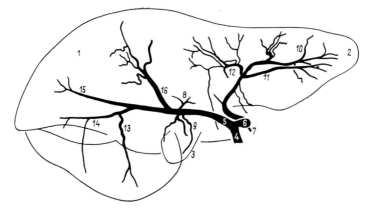

FIG. 162. The hepatic artery and its branches, I. Anatomical preparation.
Anteroposterior view.

1. Right lobe of liver
2. Left lobe
3. Gall bladder
4. Hepatic artery
5. Right branch
6. Left branch
7. Left accessory hepatic artery

8. Artery of caudate lobe, A_1
9. Cystic artery
10. Superior lateral segmental artery, A_2
11. Inferior lateral segmental artery, A_3
12. Medial segmental artery, A_4

13. Inferior anterior segmental artery, A_5
14. Inferior posterior segmental artery, A_6
15. Superior posterior segmental artery, A_7
16. Superior anterior segmental artery, A_8

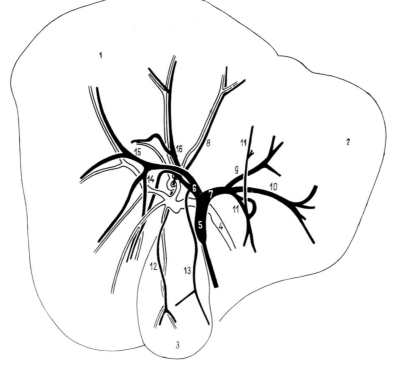

FIG. 163. The hepatic artery, the right hepatic duct and their branches.
Anatomical preparation. Craniocaudal view.

1. Right lobe of liver
2. Left lobe
3. Gall bladder
4. Right hepatic duct
5. Hepatic artery
6. Right branch
7. Left branch

8. Artery of caudate lobe, A_1
9. Superior lateral segmental artery, A_2
10. Inferior lateral segmental artery, A_3
11. Medial segmental artery, A_4
12. Inferior anterior segmental artery, A_5

13. Cystic artery
14. Inferior posterior segmental artery, A_6
15. Superior posterior segmental artery, A_7
16. Superior anterior segmental artery, A_8

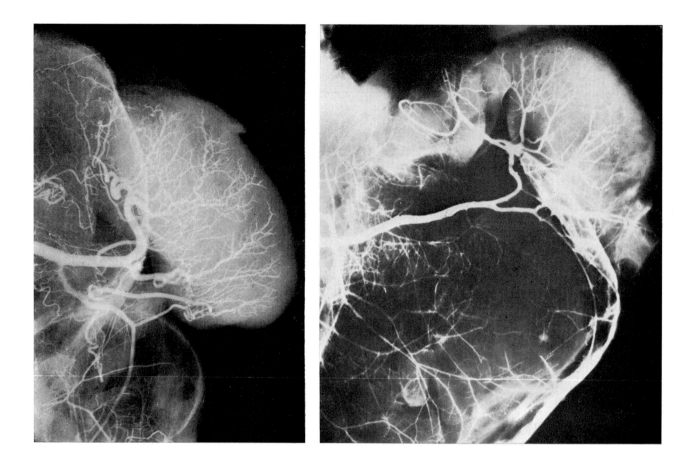

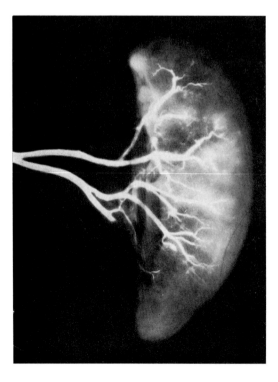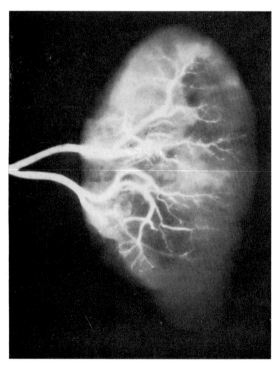

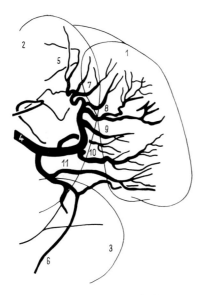

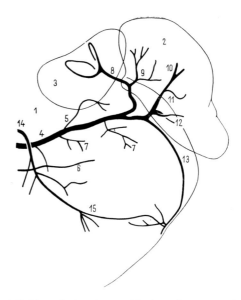

FIG. 164. The splenic artery and its branches. Anatomical preparation. Anteroposterior view.

FIG. 165. The splenic artery and its branches; succenturiate spleen. Anatomical preparation. Anteroposterior view.

1. Spleen
2. Fundus of stomach
3. Left colic flexure
4. Splenic artery
5. Short gastric arteries
6. Left gastroepiploic artery
7. Superior polar artery, A_1

8. Superior terminal artery, A_2
9. Middle terminal artery, A_3
10. Inferior terminal artery, A_4
11. Inferior polar artery, A_5

1. Fundus of stomach
2. Spleen
3. Succenturiate spleen
4. Splenic artery
5. Short gastric arteries
6. Dorsal pancreatic artery
7. Arteries of the tail of pancreas
8. Succenturiate branch of splenic artery

9. Superior polar artery, A_1
10. Superior terminal artery, A_2
11. Inferior terminal artery, A_4
12. Inferior polar artery, A_5
13. Left gastroepiploic artery
14. Left gastric artery
15. Anastomosis between left gastric and left gastro-epiploic arteries

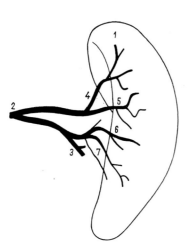

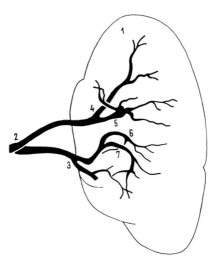

FIGS 166 and 167. Terminal branches of the splenic artery. Anatomical preparation. Anteroposterior view (Fig. 166) and dextrosinistral view (Fig. 167).

1. Spleen
2. Splenic artery
3. Left gastroepiploic artery

4. Superior polar artery, A_1
5. Superior terminal artery, A_2
6. Inferior terminal artery, A_4
7. Inferior polar artery, A_5

269

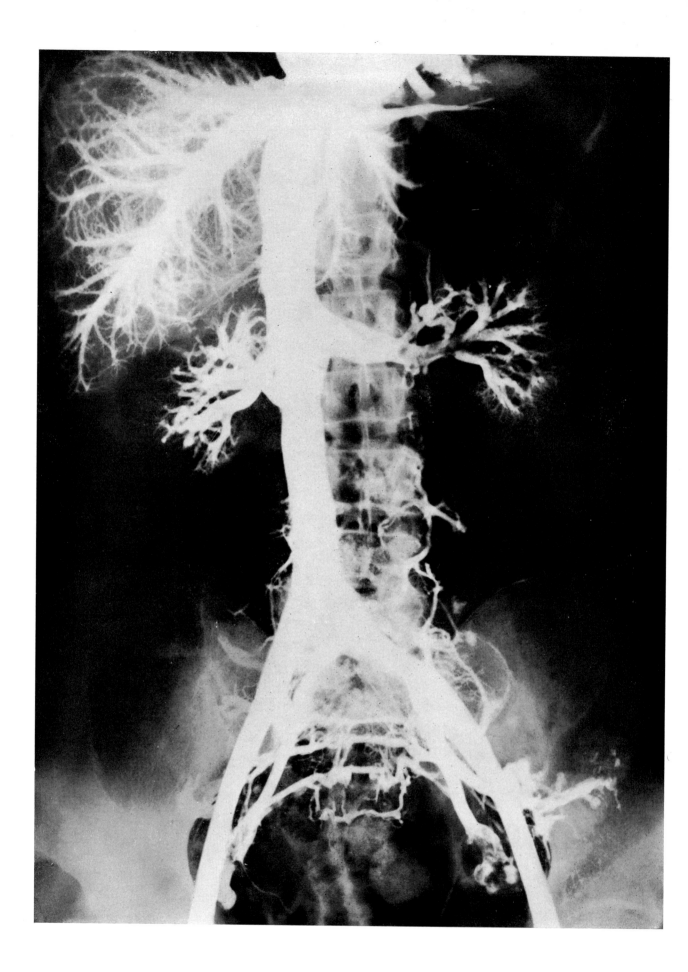

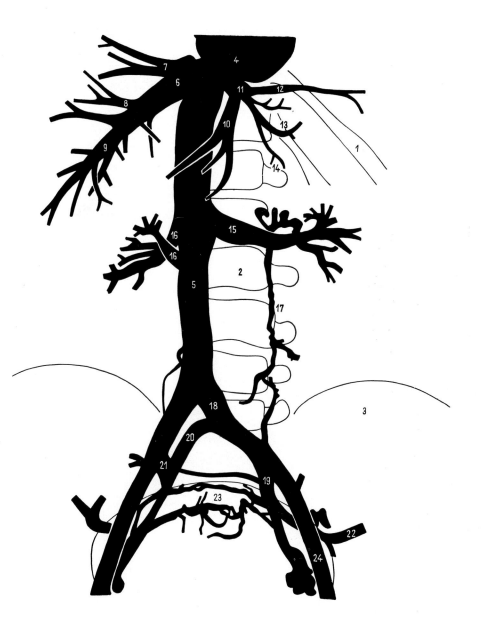

Fig. 168. The inferior vena cava and its branches, I.
Anteroposterior view.

1. Ribs
2. Lumbar vertebrae
3. Ilium
4. Right atrium
5. Inferior vena cava
6. Right hepatic vein
7. Right superior hepatic vein
8. Posterolateral hepatic vein
9. Posteroinferior hepatic vein

10. Middle hepatic vein
11. Left hepatic vein
12. Left superior hepatic vein
13. Superior root
14. Inferior root
15. Left renal vein
16. Right renal veins
17. Ascending lumbar vein

18. Common iliac vein
19. Left internal iliac vein
20. Right internal iliac vein (left branch)
21. Right internal iliac vein (right branch)
22. Superior gluteal vein
23. Sacral venous plexus
24. External iliac vein

271

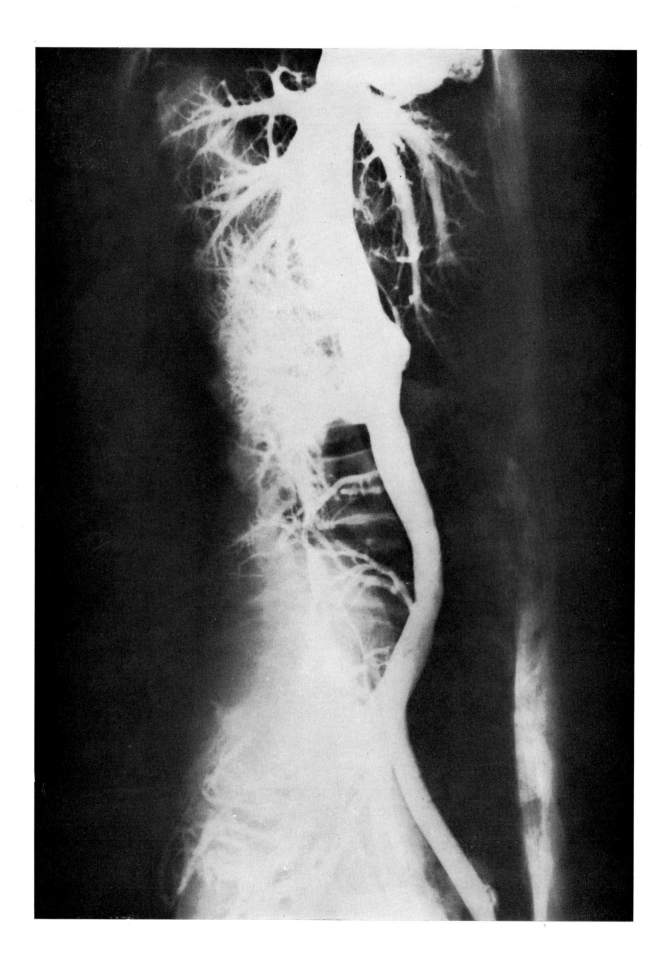

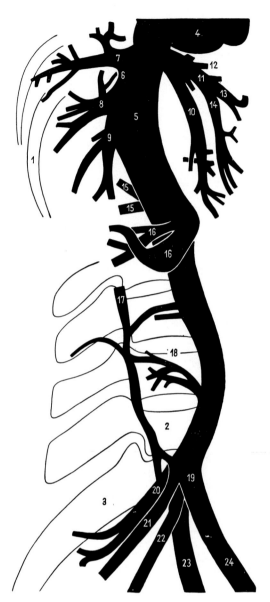

FIG. 169. The inferior vena cava and its branches, II.
Dextrosinistral view.

1. Ribs
2. Lumbar vertebrae
3. Sacrum
4. Right atrium
5. Inferior vena cava
6. Right hepatic vein
7. Right superior hepatic vein
8. Posterolateral hepatic vein
9. Posteroinferior hepatic vein

10. Middle hepatic vein
11. Left hepatic vein
12. Left superior hepatic vein
13. Superior root
14. Inferior root
15. Left renal vein
16. Right renal veins
17. Vertebral venous plexuses
   and ascending lumbar vein

18. Lumbar veins
19. Common iliac veins
20. Left internal iliac vein
21. Right internal iliac vein
   (right branch)
22. Right internal iliac vein
   (left branch)
23. Left external iliac vein
24. Right external iliac vein

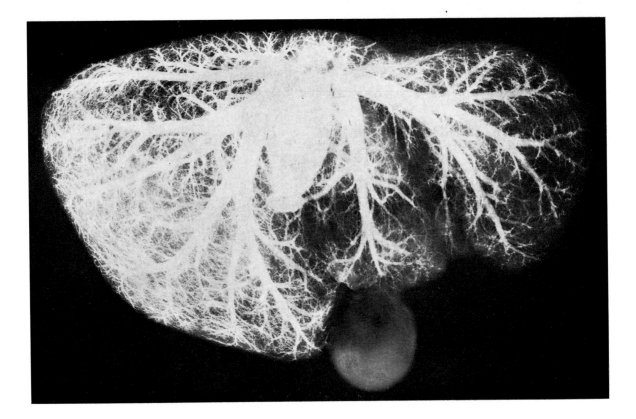

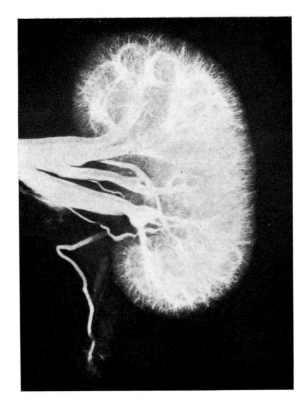

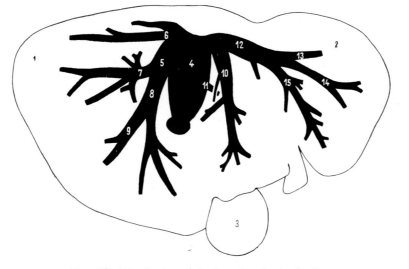

FIG. 170. Distribution of the hepatic veins in the liver.
Anatomical preparation. Craniocaudal view.

1. Right lobe of liver
2. Left lobe
3. Gall bladder
4. Inferior vena cava
5. Right hepatic vein

6. Right superior hepatic vein
7. Posterolateral hepatic vein
8. Posterointermediary hepatic vein
9. Posteroinferior hepatic vein
10. Middle hepatic vein

11. Caudate hepatic veins
12. Left hepatic vein
13. Left superior hepatic vein
14. Superior root
15. Inferior root

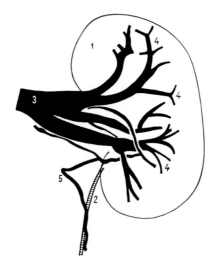

FIG. 171. The renal vein and its branches.
Anteroposterior view.

1. Left kidney
2. Ureter
3. Renal vein
4. Interlobular veins
5. Left pyeloureteral vein

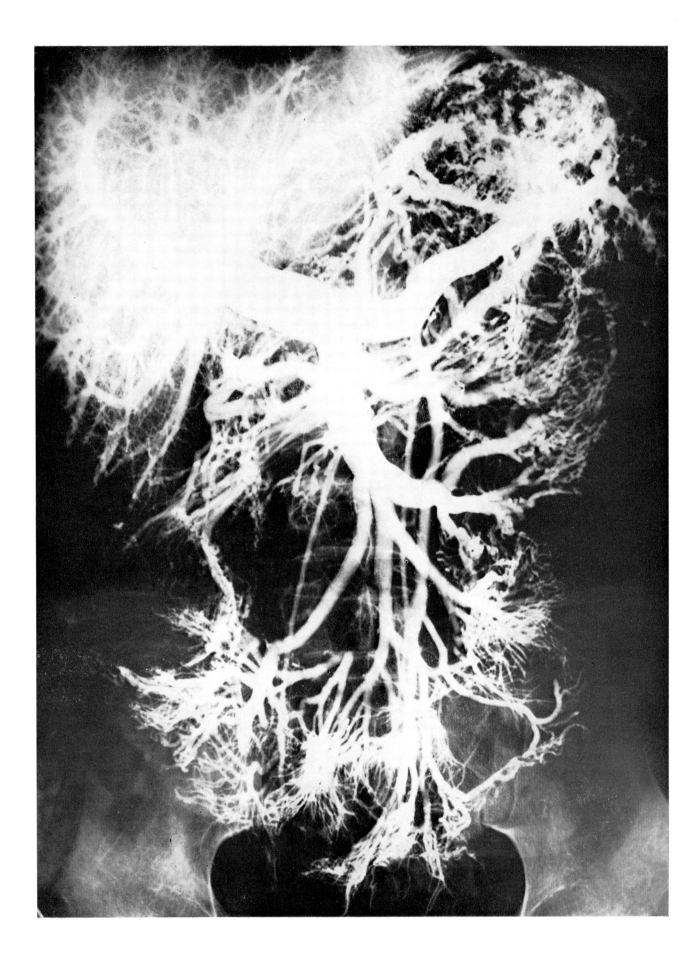

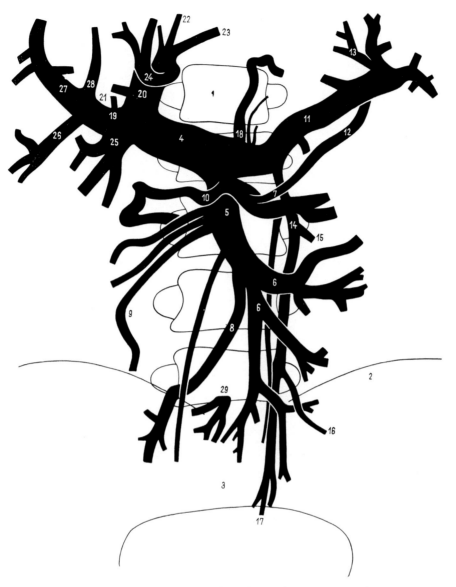

FIG. 172. The portal vein and its branches, I. Anteroposterior view.

1. Lumbar vertebrae
2. Wing of the ilium
3. Sacrum
4. Portal vein
5. Superior mesenteric vein
6. Jejunal and ileal veins
7. Right gastroepiploic vein
8. Ileocolic vein
9. Right colic vein
10. Middle colic vein
11. Splenic vein

12. Left gastroepiploic vein
13. Short gastric veins
14. Inferior mesenteric vein
15. Left colic vein
16. Sigmoid veins
17. Superior rectal veins
18. Left gastric vein
19. Right branch of portal vein
20. Left branch of portal vein
21. Caudate branches, V_1

22. Left superior branch, V_2
23. Left inferior branch, V_3
24. Transverse part, V_4
25. Inferior anterior branch, V_5
26. Inferior posterior branch, V_6
27. Superior posterior branch, V_7
28. Superior anterior branch, V_8
29. Cannula in jejunal vein

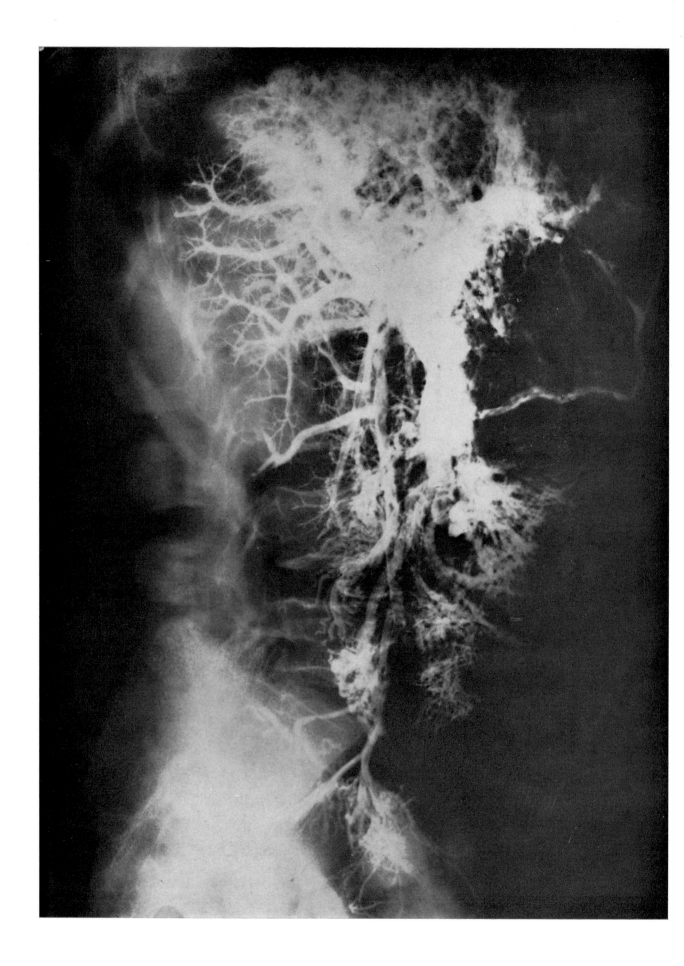

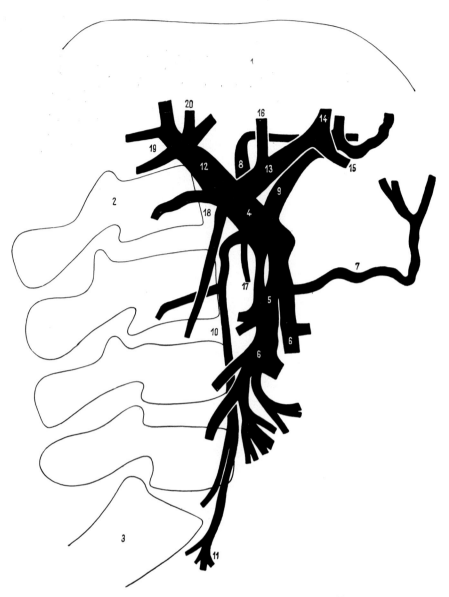

FIG. 173. The portal vein and its branches, II.
Dextrosinistral view.

1. Diaphragm
2. Lumbar vertebrae
3. Sacrum
4. Postal vein
5. Superior mesenteric vein
6. Jejunal, ileal, ileocolic, right and middle colic veins
7. Right gastroepiploic vein
8. Left gastric vein
9. Splenic vein
10. Inferior mesenteric vein
11. Superior rectal vein
12. Right branch of portal vein
13. Left branch of portal vein
14. Left superior branch, V_2
15. Left inferior branch, V_3
16. Transverse part, V_4
17. Inferior anterior branch, V_5
18. Inferior posterior branch, V_6
19. Superior posterior branch, V_7
20. Superior anterior branch, V_8

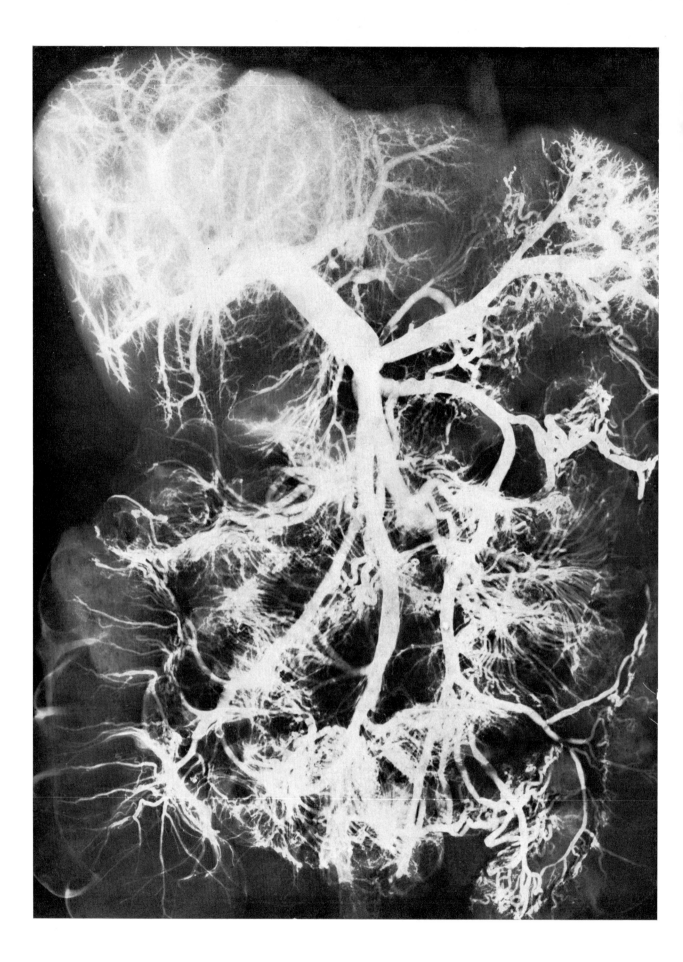

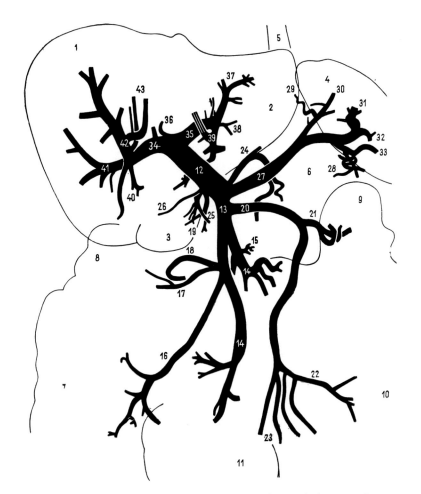

FIG. 174. The portal vein and its branches, III. Anatomical preparation.
Anteroposterior view.

1. Right lobe of liver	*17*. Right colic vein	*32*. Inferior terminal branch, V_4
2. Left lobe	*18*. Middle colic vein	*33*. Inferior polar vein, V_5
3. Gall bladder	*19*. Pancreaticoduodenal veins	*34*. Right branch of portal vein
4. Spleen	*20*. Inferior mesenteric vein	*35*. Left branch of portal vein
5. Esophagus	*21*. Left colic vein	
6. Stomach	*22*. Sigmoid veins	*36*. Caudate branches, V_1
7. Cecum	*23*. Superior rectal veins	*37*. Superior branch, V_2
8. Right colic flexure	*24*. Left gastric veins	*38*. Inferior branch, V_3
9. Left colic flexure	*25*. Right gastric vein	*39*. Transverse part, V_4
10. Sigmoid colon	*26*. Cystic vein	*40*. Inferior anterior branch, V_5
11. Rectum	*27*. Splenic vein	*41*. Inferior posterior branch, V_6
12. Portal vein	*28*. Left gastroepiploic vein	
13. Superior mesenteric vein	*29*. Short gastric veins	*42*. Superior posterior branch, V_7
14. Jejunal and ileal veins	*30*. Superior polar vein, V_1	
15. Right gastroepiploic vein	*31*. Superior terminal branch, V_2	*43*. Superior anterior branch, V_8
16. Ileocolic vein		

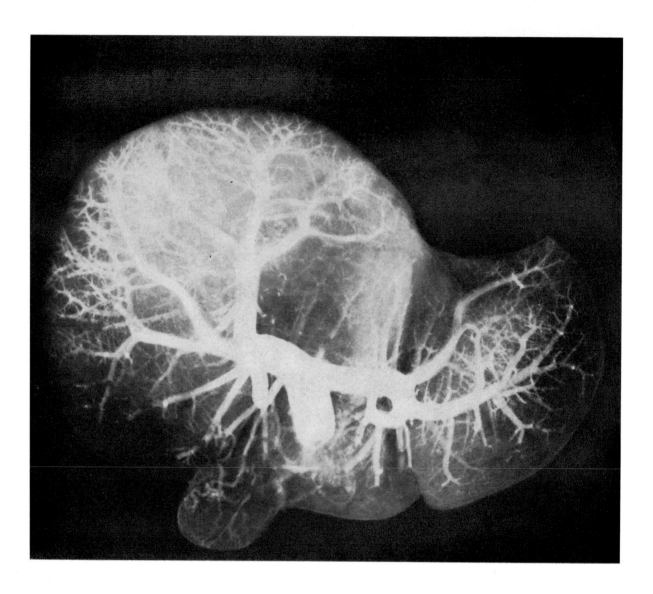

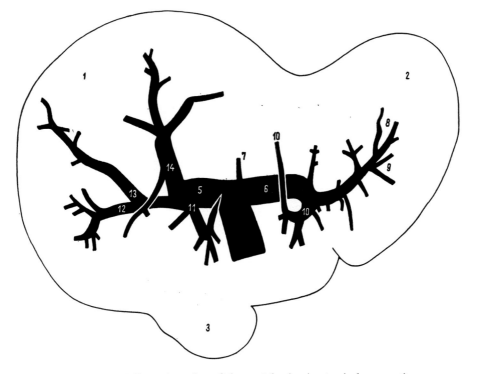

FIG. 175. Efferent branches of the portal vein. Anatomical preparation.
Craniocaudal view.

1. Right lobe of the liver
2. Left lobe
3. Gall bladder
4. Portal vein
5. Right branch
6. Left branch

7. Caudate branches, V_1
8. Superior branch, V_2
9. Inferior branch, V_3
10. Transverse part V_4
11. Inferior anterior branch, V_5

12. Inferior posterior branch, V_6
13. Superior posterior branch, V_7
14. Superior anterior branch, V_8

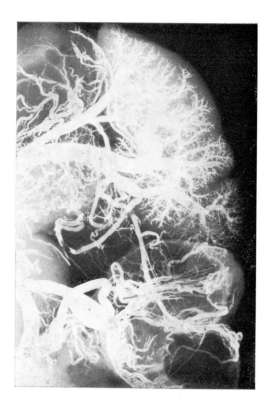

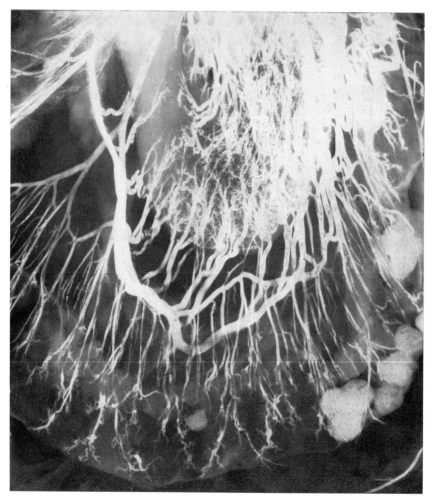

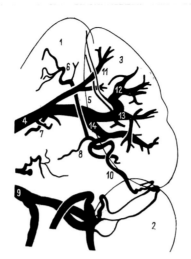

FIG. 176. The splenic vein and its branches. Anatomical preparation.
Anteroposterior view.

1. Stomach
2. Left colic flexure
3. Spleen
4. Splenic vein
5. Perilienal vein
6. Short gastric veins

7. Pancreatic veins
8. Left gastroepiploic vein
9. Middle colic vein
10. Anastomosis between splenic and middle colic veins
11. Superior polar vein, V_1

12. Superior terminal branch, V_2
13. Middle terminal branch, V_3
14. Inferior terminal branch, V_4

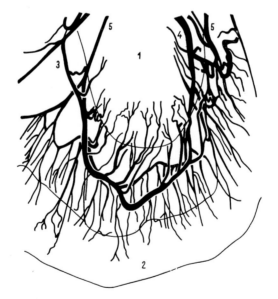

FIG. 177. Veins of the stomach and the transverse colon.
Anatomical preparation. Anteroposterior view.

1. Stomach
2. Transverse colon
3. Right gastroepiploic vein
4. Left gastroepiploic vein
5. Middle colic vein

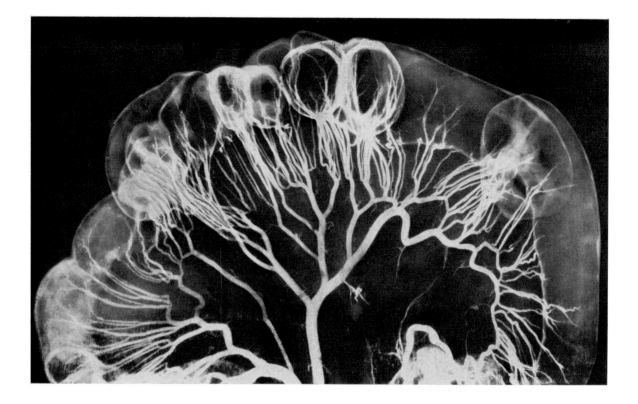

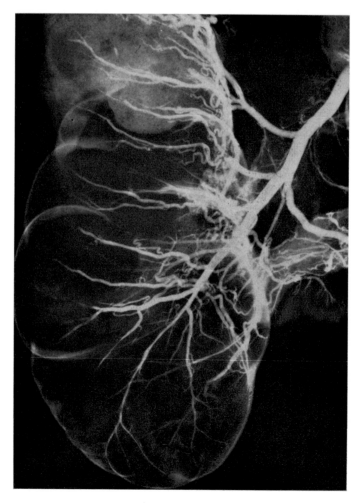

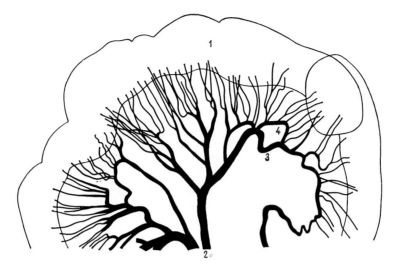

FIG. 178. Veins of the small intestine.
Anatomical preparation. Anteroposterior view.

1. Jejunum   *3.* Venous arch I
2. Jejunal veins   *4.* Venous arch II

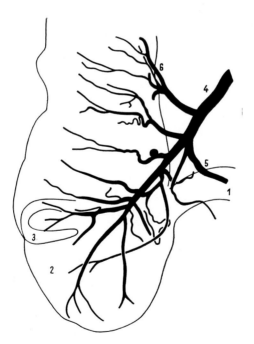

FIG. 179. Veins of the cecum. Anatomical preparation.
Anteroposterior view.

1. Ileum   *5.* Anastomosis between ileo-
2. Cecum   colic vein and ileal veins
3. Vermiform appendix   *6.* Anastomosis between ileo-
4. Ileocolic vein   colic and right colic veins

287

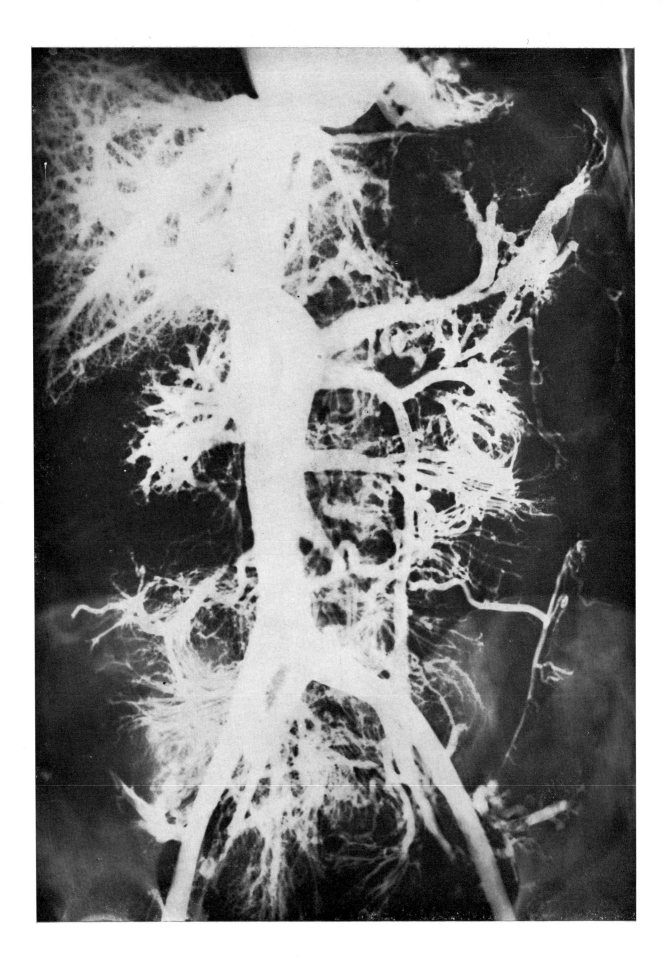

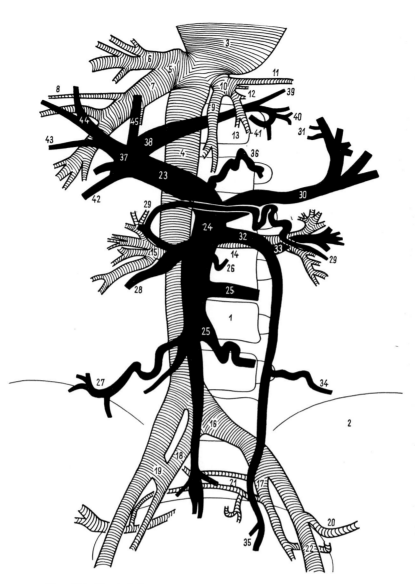

FIG. 180. The inferior vena cava, portal vein and their branches, I.
Anteroposterior view.

1. Lumbar vertebrae
2. Wing of the ilium
3. Right atrium
4. Inferior vena cava
5. Right hepatic vein
6. Right superior hepatic vein
7. Posterolateral hepatic vein
8. Posterointermediary hepatic vein
9. Middle hepatic vein
10. Left hepatic vein
11. Left superior hepatic vein
12. Superior root
13. Inferior root
14. Left renal vein
15. Right renal vein
16. Common iliac vein

17. Left internal iliac vein
18. Right internal iliac vein (left branch)
19. Right internal iliac vein (right branch)
20. Superior gluteal vein
21. Sacral venous plexus
22. External iliac vein
23. Portal vein
24. Superior mesenteric vein
25. Jejunal and ileal veins
26. Right gastroepiploic vein
27. Ileocolic vein
28. Right colic vein
29. Middle colic vein
30. Splenic vein
31. Short gastric veins

32. Inferior mesenteric vein
33. Left colic vein
34. Sigmoid vein
35. Superior rectal veins
36. Left gastric vein
37. Right branch of portal vein
38. Left branch of portal vein
39. Superior branch, V_2
40. Inferior branch, V_3
41. Transverse part, V_4
42. Inferior anterior branch, V_5
43. Inferior posterior branch, V_6
44. Superior posterior branch, V_7
45. Superior anterior branch, V_8

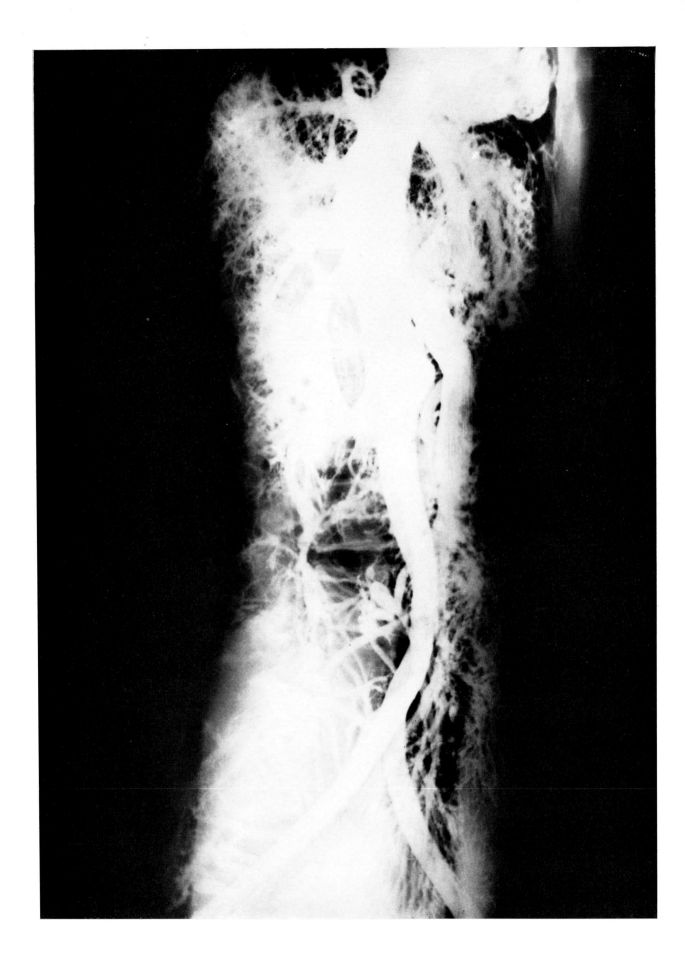

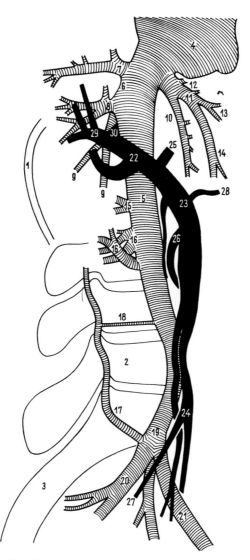

FIG. 181. The inferior vena cava, portal vein and their branches, II.
Dextrosinistral view.

1. Ribs
2. Lumbar vertebrae
3. Sacrum
4. Right atrium
5. Inferior vena cava
6. Right hepatic vein
7. Right superior hepatic vein
8. Posterolateral hepatic vein
9. Posteroinferior hepatic vein
10. Middle hepatic vein

11. Left hepatic vein
12. Left superior hepatic vein
13. Superior root
14. Inferior root
15. Left renal vein
16. Right renal veins
17. Vertebral venous plexus
18. Lumbar veins
19. Common iliac veins
20. Internal iliac veins

21. External iliac veins
22. Portal vein
23. Superior mesenteric vein
24. Jejunal and ileal veins
25. Splenic vein
26. Inferior mesenteric vein
27. Superior rectal veins
28. Left colic vein
29. Right branch of portal vein
30. Left branch of portal vein

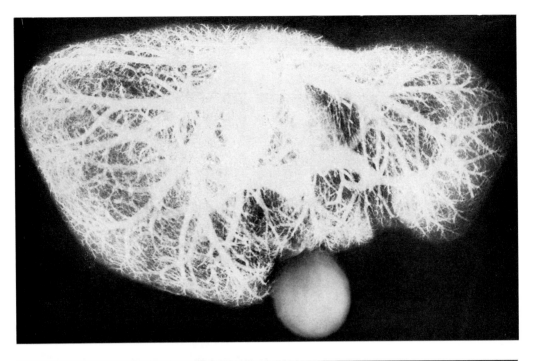

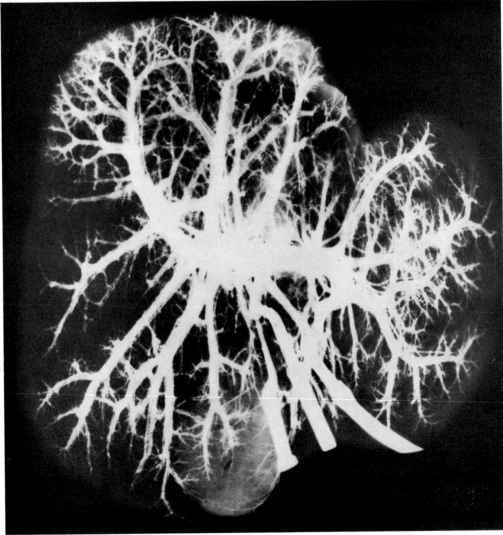

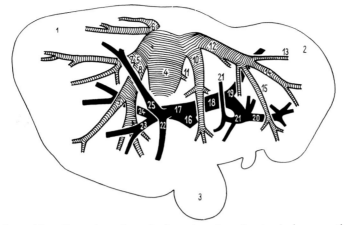

FIG. 182. The portal vein and its efferent branches; the hepatic veins. Anatomical preparation. Craniocaudal view.

1. Right lobe of liver
2. Left lobe
3. Gall bladder
4. Inferior vena cava
5. Right hepatic vein
6. Right superior hepatic vein
7. Posterolateral hepatic vein

8. Posterointermediary hepatic vein
9. Posteroinferior hepatic vein
10. Middle hepatic vein
11. Caudate hepatic veins
12. Left hepatic vein
13. Left superior hepatic vein

14. Superior root
15. Inferior root
16. Portal vein
17. Right branch
18. Left branch
19. Superior branch, V_2
20. Inferior branch, V_3

21. Transverse part, V
22. Inferior anterior branch, V_5
23. Inferior posterior branch, V_6
24. Superior posterior branch, V_7
25. Superior anterior branch, V_8
26. Caudate branches, V_1

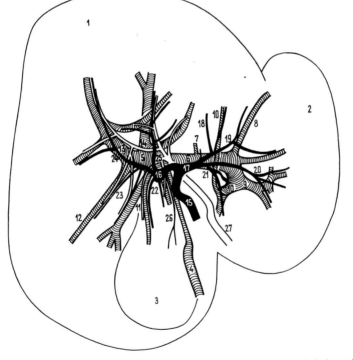

FIG. 183. The portal vein, hepatic artery, right hepatic duct and their branches.
Anatomical preparation. Craniocaudal view.

1. Right lobe of liver
2. Left lobe of liver
3. Gall bladder
4. Cannula in portal vein
5. Right branch of the portal vein
6. Left branch of the portal vein
7. Caudate branches, V_1
8. Superior branch, V_2
9. Inferior branch, V_3

10. Pars transversa, V_4
11. Inferior anterior branch, V_5
12. Inferior posterior branch, V_6
13. Superior posterior branch, V_7
14. Superior anterior branch, V_8
15. Cannula in hepatic artery

16. Right branch of the hepatic artery
17. Left branch of the hepatic artery
18. Artery of caudate lobe, A_1
19. Superior lateral segmental artery, A_2
20. Inferior lateral segmental artery, A_3
21. Middle segmental artery, A_4

22. Inferior anterior segmental artery, A_5
23. Inferior posterior segmental artery, A_6
24. Superior posterior segmental artery, A_7
25. Superior anterior segmental artery, A_8
26. Cystic artery
27. Cannula in right hepatic duct

293

BLOOD VESSELS OF THE PELVIS AND THE LOWER EXTREMITIES

THE COMMON ILIAC ARTERY AND ITS BRANCHES

Blood pressure in the pelvis and the lower extremities is 40 to 60 mm Hg higher than that in the upper limbs, a fact which determines their susceptibility to vascular disorders. The collateral circulation is less developed so that clinical symptoms of vascular insufficiency are more frequent. The arteries of the lesser pelvis play a significant part in the collateral circulation of the aorta and of the urogenital apparatus.

The common iliac artery

The common iliac artery (Figs 151/6, 152/5, 153/10, 157/3, 184/1, 192/9, 193/3, 194/6, 195/5) is a large vessel formed by the bifurcation of the abdominal aorta. It is distributed to the pelvic organs and the lower limbs. Its origin is most frequently at the level of the 4th lumbar vertebra (81 per cent) and sometimes between the 3rd lumbar and 1st sacral vertebrae in the midline (De Luca and De Serio 1961). From its origin the common iliac artery pursues a forward-lateral-downward course and bifurcates in front of the sacroiliac joint. Its initial portion rests on the lumbar spine, its lower part on the psoas major muscle. The beginning of the inferior vena cava lies behind the right artery. The right common iliac artery is crossed from behind by the right common iliac vein. The division of the inferior mesenteric artery lies to the left of the left common iliac artery. Both arteries are in their last segment crossed frontally by the ureter in an oblique direction. The angle of division of the aorta is 65° in males, 75° in females (40° to 80°). The right artery has a length of 6·5 cm, the left 6·3 cm (3·5 to 12 cm) (De Luca and De Serio 1961). Reich and Nechtow (1964) found that the left artery was longer than its contralateral partner in 72 per cent of the cases. The diameter measures 0·89 cm on the right side, 0·83 cm on the left (0·5 to 1·2 cm; De Luca and De Serio 1961). Reich and Nechtow (1964) found further that the bifurcation of the right artery was 1·5 cm, the left 2·0 cm below the line connecting the two anterior superior iliac spines. The surface projection of the common iliac arteries beginning

1 cm below the umbilicus, corresponds to a straight line to the point midway between the anterior superior iliac spine and the symphysis pubis (Gray 1954).

Variations are rare. The internal and the external iliac arteries may emerge directly from the aorta if the common iliac is too short (Adachi 1928).

Branches. Some minor branches are distributed to the peritoneum, the ureter and the psoas major muscle. The median sacral, aberrant renal and iliolumbar arteries may constitute its supernumerary branches (Rauber and Kopsch 1951, Gray 1954).

The internal iliac artery and its branches

The internal iliac artery (Figs 151/8, 152/7, 153/12, 157/5, 184/3, 192/10, 193/4, 194/7, 195/6), a short and bulky vessel, secures the blood supply to the pelvic organs. Arising at the bifurcation of the common iliac artery, it runs to the greater sciatic foramen while it divides into branches. In front of the vessel are the ovary and the ureter; behind it are the internal iliac vein, the lumbosacral plexus and the sacroiliac joint; laterally, near its origin, the external iliac vein; medially, the peritoneum. It describes either an outward concave (39 per cent) or straight line (31 per cent), or an inward concave (22 per cent) or tortuous line (8 per cent). The internal iliac artery on the right side has a length of 3·9 cm, on the left side 4 cm (2 to 7 cm); the diameter measures 0·5 cm (0·3 to 0·7 cm) (De Luca and De Serio 1962a, b). The internal is smaller than the external iliac artery in adults, and larger in the newborn.

Variations are rare. If the internal iliac artery is absent, the common iliac artery arches into the pelvis to continue as the external iliac artery. The arteries of the pelvic organs arise from this arch (Rauber and Kopsch 1951). The numerous variations in division can hardly be classified (Fig. 184). In general, it divides into an anterior and a posterior trunk from which the side branches arise. Roberts and Krishingner (1967) described five types of origin: 1. The superior gluteal artery forms a common trunk with the umbilical artery, and the inferior gluteal with the internal pudendal artery forms another common trunk (51 per cent). 2. The superior and inferior gluteal form one, the internal pudendal artery and the umbilical arteries another trunk (26·8 per cent). 3. Each of the four vessels has a separate origin (14·4 per cent). 4. The superior and inferior gluteal and the internal pudendal arteries arise together, the umbilical artery originates separately (7·2 per cent). 5. Exceptionally a common trunk is formed by the superior gluteal and the internal pudendal, another by the inferior gluteal and the umbilical arteries.

The uterine artery frequently arises together with the umbilical artery on the anterior aspect of the internal iliac artery. *Branches:*

The *iliolumbar artery* (Figs 184/4, 192/11, 193/5, 194/8) has two side branches, namely the *lumbar branch* (the 5th lumbar artery) and the *iliac branch;* the latter communicates with the deep circumflex iliac artery in the muscles of the ilium. The *lateral sacral arteries* (Figs 192/12, 193/6, 194/9) originate as a rule from the iliolumbar and sometimes from the superior gluteal artery. They give off branches to the vertebral canal.

The *obturator artery* (Figs 184/5, 185/6, 192/13, 193/7, 194/10, 195/9, 200/5) arises in typical cases from the internal iliac artery but may originate also from the inferior epigastric (28·5 per cent), the external iliac (1·2 per cent), or the femoral artery (0·4 per cent; Jaschtschinski 1891). Anomalous origin in women is more frequent on the right side (Rauber and Kopsch 1951). The obturator artery has a diameter of 0·2 to 0·3 cm (De Luca and De Serio 1962a, b). Its lateral course is below the terminal line of the pelvis toward the obturator canal and, passing through it, the obturator artery divides into an *anterior* (Fig. 194/26) and a *posterior branch* (Fig. 194/25) between the adductors of the thigh. It distributes a branch through the acetabular notch to the head of the femur (*acetabular branch*, Figs 193/8, 194/12) and another branch in the pelvic cavity which runs to the symphysis pubis (*pubic branch*, Figs 193/9, 194/11, 200/8). The terminal branches of the obturator artery anastomose with the inferior epigastric artery and with the medial circumflex femoral artery (Müssbichler 1971). If the inferior epigastric artery is strongly developed the obturator artery may arise from it.

The *superior gluteal artery* (Figs 184/6, 192/14, 193/10, 194/13, 195/7) is the largest branch of the internal iliac artery. Its main trunk passes through the greater sciatic foramen above the piriformis between the gluteal muscles supplying them by way of its *superficial* and *deep branches*. Sometimes the iliolumbar or the lateral sacral artery originates

from the superior gluteal artery (Rauber and Kopsch 1951).

The *inferior gluteal artery* (Figs 184/7, 192/15, 193/11, 194/14, 195/8, 200/6) passes through the greater sciatic foramen below the piriformis to gain

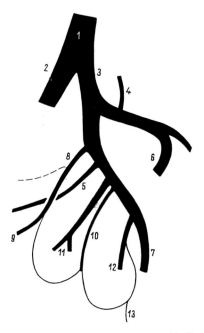

Fig. 184. Branches of the internal iliac artery. (*1*) Common iliac artery; (*2*) external iliac artery; (*3*) internal iliac artery; (*4*) iliolumbar artery; (*5*) obturator artery; (*6*) superior gluteal artery; (*7*) inferior gluteal artery; (*8*) umbilical artery; (*9*) superior vesical artery; (*10*) inferior vesical artery; (*11*) uterine artery; (*12*) internal pudendal artery; (*13*) middle rectal artery.

the gluteus maximus muscle. It arises from the pelvis in a line connecting the posterior superior iliac spine and the sciatic tuberosity (Gray 1954). The accompanying artery of the sciatic nerve, a long thin vessel, accompanies the sciatic nerve. If, exceptionally, this vessel is very strong, it may constitute the main artery of the lower extremity instead of the femoral artery. In these cases it continues distally in the popliteal artery (Rauber and Kopsch 1951). The accompanying artery of the sciatic nerve may also occur on both sides (Martinez et al. 1968).

The *umbilical artery* (Figs 184/8, 220/25, 222/10), the largest branch of the internal iliac artery in the fetus and in the newborn, runs in the median umbilical ligament to the umbilicus. After birth it atrophies. Its unilateral aplasia has a frequency of 0·4 to 1·0 per cent (Carrier et al. 1966, Dehalleux et al. 1966). The *artery of the ductus deferens* usually originates from the vestigial remnant of this vessel or from the vesical arteries. Arising from the umbilical artery the branches of the *superior vesical arteries* (Figs 184/9, 185/2, 192/16, 193/12, 194/15) communicate with the inferior epigastric artery (Shehata 1964).

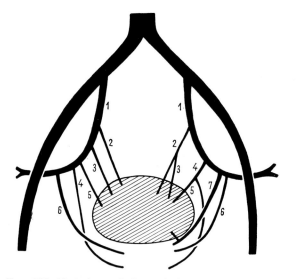

Fig. 185. Variations of the vesical arteries. (*1*) Internal iliac artery; (*2*) superior vesical artery; (*3*) middle vesical artery; (*4*) internal pudendal artery; (*5*) middle rectal artery; (*6*) obturator artery; (*7*) inferior vesical artery.

The *inferior vesical artery* (Figs 184/10, 185/7, 192/17, 193/13, 194/16) is usually a direct branch of the internal iliac artery. It is often doubled (*middle vesical artery*, Fig. 185/3). In addition to these vessels the middle rectal artery also contributes to the blood supply of the bladder. Converging from two sides, these vessels form an arterial network (Maranta et al. 1964). The internal pudendal artery may also distribute a branch to the anterior wall.

The *uterine artery* (Figs 184/11, 192/18, 194/17, 199/5) is the largest branch of the anterior root of the internal iliac artery; in men it corresponds to the artery of the ductus deferens. The uterine artery follows a tortuous course in the lower border of the broad ligament, crosses the ureter in front, and reaches the cervix of the uterus. The length of the uterine artery is 15 cm, its diameter 0·3 cm (Paturet 1958). From the cervix the uterine artery gives off the *vaginal artery* (Fig. 194/19) which supplies the wall of that organ and anastomoses with the vessel of the opposite side as also with the branches of the internal pudendal artery. The tortuous main trunk runs along the uterus to the angle of the tube giving off a branch there which courses in the mesosalpinx parallel to the tube (*tubal branch*, Figs 194/18, 199/7). The other part of the uterine artery, i.e., the *ovarian branch* (Fig. 199/6), runs in the mesovarium

to the ovary. Both vessels communicate with the ovarian artery and form an arterial arch with it. The course of the uterine artery is more tortuous along the body of the uterus than at the cervix of the uterus. The blood supply of the posterior wall of the uterus is more abundant than that of the anterior wall. Converging, the cervical branches run toward the orifice of the uterus. The branches of the vessels of the body of the uterus form, with transverse stout trunks, a network which connects the opposite sides (Fernström 1955). The branch to the ovary divides in the mesovarium, and gives off parallel branches to the substance of the ovary. The main trunk gives off a small vessel in the round ligament of the uterus.

The *middle rectal artery* (Figs 151/10, 184/13, 185/5, 192/17, 193/14, 194/24) is an independent branch of the internal iliac artery. It may sometimes arise together with the internal pudendal artery or the inferior vesical artery (Rauber and Kopsch 1951). It forms important anastomoses with the inferior mesenteric artery upward and with the internal pudendal artery downward. The middle rectal artery has a diameter of 0·1 to 0·25 cm. It is multiple in 50 per cent of the cases (Michels et al. 1965).

The *internal pudendal artery* (Figs 151/9, 184/12, 185/4, 192/19, 193/15, 194/20, 195/10), supplying the perineum and the external genitalia, arises from the pelvis through the greater sciatic foramen below the piriformis, runs forward on the lateral side of the ischiorectal fossa, passes through the urogenital diaphragm and divides into terminal branches between the cavernous bodies. The *inferior rectal artery* (Figs 193/16, 194/21) anastomoses with the other rectal arteries. The *perineal artery* (Figs 193/17, 194/22), another branch of the internal pudendal artery, courses along the perineum to the external genitalia and divides in the scrotum or at the posterior end of the labium majus, respectively (*scrotal or posterior labial branches*, Fig. 194/23). The *artery to the bulb of the penis* (Fig. 193/18) or *artery to the bulb of the vestibulum* enters the bulb. From it originates the *urethral artery* (Figs 196 and 197/5) which runs to the urethra and reaches the glans of the penis where it anastomoses with the deep and the dorsal arteries of the penis. The vessel arises sometimes directly from the internal pudendal artery (Kiss 1963). The deep arteries which, distributed to the cavernous bodies (*deep artery of the penis*, Figs 193/19, 196 and 197/3) or the *deep artery of the clitoris*, are larger than the *dorsal artery of the penis* (Figs 193/20, 196 and 197/4) or the *dorsal artery of the clitoris*. The unpaired dorsal vein of the penis (clitoris) is situated in the midline between the bilateral dorsal arteries of the penis.

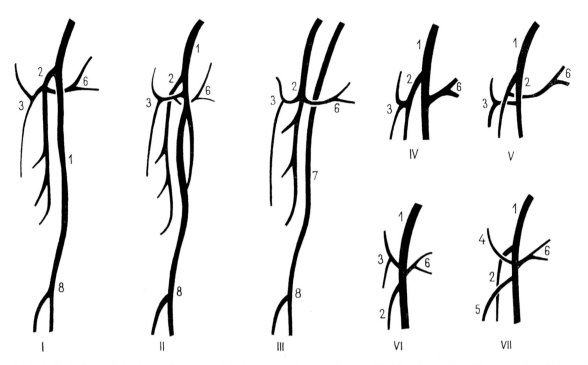

FIG. 186. Variations of the femoral artery and its branches. I, normal type; II, islet formation (the medial and lateral circumflex femoral arteries arise together from the femoral artery); III, accompanying artery of the sciatic nerve; IV, the medial circumflex femoral artery arises from the femoral artery; V, the lateral circumflex femoral artery arises from the femoral artery; VI, both the medial and the lateral circumflex femoral arteries arise from the main trunk; VII, the one branch of the lateral circumflex femoral artery arises separately, the branches of the medial circumflex femoral artery arise together from the femoral artery. (*1*) Femoral artery; (*2*) deep femoral artery; (*3*) lateral circumflex femoral artery; (*4*) ascending branch; (*5*) descending branch; (*6*) medial circumflex femoral artery; (*7*) accompanying artery of the sciatic nerve; (*8*) popliteal artery.

The external iliac artery, the femoral artery and their branches

The **external iliac artery** (Figs 151/7, 152/6, 153/11, 157/4, 192/20, 193/21, 194/28, 195/11) supplies the lower extremity. It is the larger branch of the common iliac artery which descends from the sacroiliac joint forward and laterally to the inguinal ligament and, passing below it, it reaches the thigh and is continous with the femoral artery. It runs along the psoas major muscle. In front, the beginning of the artery is crossed by the ureter; its end, by the testicular vessels. The internal iliac artery lies on the medial side of the external iliac artery. Its course may be straight (57 per cent), curved (29 per cent) or tortuous (14 per cent). The length of the vessel is 9 cm on the right, 8·8 cm on the left side (6 to 12 cm). The diameter is 0·68 cm (0·4 to 1·0 cm; De Luca and De Serio 1962a, b). Noteworthy variations have not been observed. It has the following *branches:*

The *inferior epigastric artery* (Figs 192/21, 195/13) originates 0·5 cm above the inguinal ligament. Quain (1884) found it to arise from the femoral artery in exceptional cases. The vessel follows a medial and then an ascending course. It runs on the dorsal surface of the rectus abdominis muscle and communicates with the terminal branches of the internal thoracic artery. Its position falls in the line of the anterior inferior iliac spine in 80 per cent of the cases (Harsányi 1951). Its *pubic branch* runs toward the symphysis and anastomoses with the obturator artery. The latter may sometimes arise from here (Jaschtschinski 1891). Another branch, the *cremasteric artery*, enters the inguinal canal and divides in the skin of the scrotum.

The *deep circumflex iliac artery* (Figs 192/22, 193/22, 195/12) describes an ascending curve along the crest of the ilium and communicates with the iliolumbar artery; then its *ascending branch* forms anastomoses with the lumbar arteries and the inferior epigastric artery. A bridge, important for collateral circulation, is thus formed between the external iliac artery and the abdominal aorta (Gray 1954).

The **femoral artery** (Figs 186, 192/23, 193/24, 195/14, 200 and 201/9, 202 and 203/4) is continuous with the external iliac artery. It begins at the inguinal ligament and extends to the popliteal fossa to become the popliteal artery. The upper third of the vessel is placed in the middle of the subinguinal triangle between the femoral vein and the femoral nerve below the fascia lata. Its middle third is covered by the sartorius muscle. The upper two-third of the artery lie in front of the femoral vein. In the adductor canal the femoral vein runs in front and medial to the femoral artery. The course of the artery corresponds to a line between the midpoint of the inguinal ligament and the medial condyle of the femur. The length of the femoral artery is 15 to 30 cm, its diameter 0.8 to 0.9 cm (Paturet 1958).

Variations. The femoral artery is rarely absent; when it is, it is replaced by the accompanying artery of the sciatic nerve (Pernkopf 1922, Pirker and Schmidberger 1972, Fig. 186/III). The vascular area of the thigh is sometimes supplied by the deep femoral artery (Braedel 1961). A doubling of the artery may be due to islet formation below the origin of the deep femoral artery, while the lower segment of the vessel consists again of a single trunk (Fig. 186/II, Müller 1967). Complete doubling may also occur (Krasemann 1972). The saphenous artery, a small supernumerary branch, accompanies the saphenous vein (Manners-Smith 1912).

Branches of the femoral artery:

The *superficial epigastric artery* (Figs 192/24, 195/15, 200 and 201/10) passes superficially to the umbilicus and communicates with the cutaneous branches of the internal thoracic artery.

The *superficial circumflex iliac* artery (Figs 192/25, 200/11) runs to the anterior superior iliac spine. It often arises together with the superficial epigastric artery (Adachi 1928).

The *external pudendal arteries* (Figs 192/26, 200/12) consist of two or three trunks distributed to the groin (*inguinal branches*, Fig. 200/14), the scrotum or the labium majus (*anterior scrotal* or *labial branches*, Fig. 200/13).

The *deep femoral artery* (Figs 186/2, 192/27, 193/25, 195/16, 200 and 201/15) is the largest branch. It usually arises 3 to 4 cm (0 to 8 cm) below the inguinal ligament from the lateral border of the dorsal side, but it may sometimes originate from the medial side (Lanz and Wachsmuth 1938). The vessel passes below the adductor longus muscle and lies against the bone on the posterior side of the thigh. The diameter of the deep femoral artery is 3.18 to 6.68 mm (Gyurkó and Szabó 1968). In half of the cases, it gives off medial and lateral branches from its initial segment (*medial*, Figs 186/6, 192/28, 193/23, 200 and 201/16 and *lateral*, Figs 186/3, 192/31, 200 and 201/18 *circumflex femoral arteries*). These branches may originate separately (Figs 186/IV—VI) or together (Figs 186/II, VII) so that the number of arteries arising from the femoral artery in the subinguinal triangle totals one to four. The medial artery divides between the superficial and the deep muscles (*ascending branch*, Figs 192/29, 200 and 201/17 and *deep branch*, Fig. 192/30) as also

in the hip joint (*acetabular branch*) and communicates with the lateral vessel in the trochanteric fossa (*transverse branch*). The medial circumflex femoral artery together with the obturator artery participates with several branches in the blood supply of the head of the femur (Müssbichler 1971). The lateral circumflex femoral artery gives off an *ascending* (Figs 192/31, 200/19) and a *descending branch* (Figs 186/5, 200 and 201/20) as also a branch connecting it with the medial circumflex artery. The *perforating arteries* (Figs 200 and 201/21) i.e., those branches of the deep femoral artery which penetrate the dorsal muscles, form anastomoses with each other and the adjacent vessels. There are 3 to 4 perforating arteries. They maintain collateral circulation between the proximal portion of the femoral artery and the popliteal artery.

The *descending genicular artery* (Figs 201/22, 202 and 203/5) arises in the adductor canal and distributes a branch to the arterial network of the knee (*articular branches*, Fig. 201/24) and a branch to accompany the great saphenous vein (*saphenous branch*, Fig. 201/23).

The popliteal, anterior and posterior tibial arteries and their branches

The **popliteal artery** (Figs 187, 200 and 201/25, 202 and 203/6, 204 and 205/5) extends from the inferior border of the adductor canal to that of the popliteus muscle and divides there into terminal branches. This area is 6 cm below the knee joint in adults (Morris et al. 1960). The entire course of the artery runs in the deeper layers; it rests first on the femur, then on the capsule of the joint, and finally on the popliteus muscle. The popliteal vein is in front of and somewhat lateral to the artery. The tibial nerve occupies the most superficial position. The initial portion of the popliteal artery passes from the medial side to the midline in an oblique direction and descends thereafter vertically. The length of the popliteal artery is 18 cm, its diameter 0.7 cm (Paturet 1958).

Variations. Islet formation is rare (Adachi 1928). Pässler and Pässler (1963) distinguish the following types of division: Normal type (94.62 per cent; Fig. 187/I). High division of the anterior tibial artery (2.22 per cent; Fig. 187/II). High division of the posterior tibial artery; the peroneal artery originates from the anterior tibial artery (1.2 per cent). Trifurcation at the normal site (1.26 per cent; Fig. 187/III). Normal division; the peroneal artery originates from the anterior tibial artery (0.6 per cent; Fig. 187/IV). The peroneal artery arises from the popliteal artery at a high point (0.1 per cent).

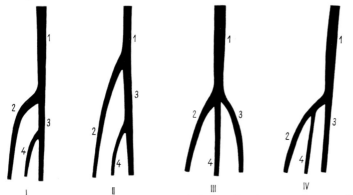

FIG. 187. Variations in the division of the popliteal artery. I, normal type; II, high division; III, trifurcation; IV, the peroneal artery arises from the anterior tibial artery. (*1*) Popliteal artery; (*2*) anterior tibial artery; (*3*) posterior tibial artery; (*4*) peroneal artery.

The popliteal artery has the following *branches:*

The *medial and lateral superior genicular arteries* (Figs 202 and 203/8 and 7, 204/6 and 7) wind around the lower end of the femur and divide in the arterial network of the knee. They communicate with the descending genicular artery.

The *middle genicular artery* (Figs 202 and 203/9) pierces the capsule of the knee joint from behind.

The *medial and lateral inferior genicular arteries* (Figs 202 and 203/11 and 12, 204 and 205/9 and 10) surround the condyles of the tibia and contribute to the formation of the arterial network. They are in communication with the anterior tibial recurrent artery.

The *sural arteries* (Figs 202 and 203/10, 204 and 205/8) begin between the upper and middle articular branches and distribute branches to the gastrocnemius muscle and to the skin.

The **anterior tibial artery** (Figs 188/1, 202 and 203/13, 204 and 205/11, 206/11, 207/11) is one of the terminal branches of the popliteal artery and courses at the lower bordre of the popliteus muscle. Passing through the interosseous membrane it runs between the extensor muscles of the leg from where it descends steeply. The course of its projection extends from the midpoint of the line between the head of the fibula and the tuberosity of the tibia to the line midway between the two malleoli. The vessel is continued on the dorsum of the foot as the dorsalis pedis artery. The diameter of the anterior tibial artery is 1·19 to 3·5 mm (Gyurkó and Szabó 1968).

Variations are due to the superficial or the lateral position of the vessel. Sometimes it is rudimentary when it is replaced by the perforating branches of the posterior tibial artery (Rauber and Kopsch 1951). A rare supernumerary branch accompanies the peroneal nerve (arteria nervi peronei superficialis; Adachi 1928). Further variations depend on those of the posterior tibial artery. Pässler and Pässler (1963) distinguished the following combinations in the configuration of the arteries around the ankle joint (Fig. 188): Normal type (98·16 per cent; Fig. 188/I). Rudimentary posterior tibial artery; the plantar arteries originate from the peroneal artery (1·21 per cent; Fig. 188/II). Rudimentary anterior tibial artery; the dorsalis pedis artery arises from the peroneal artery (0·5 per cent; Fig. 188/III). Both the anterior and the posterior tibial arteries are absent; the foot is supplied by the peroneal artery (0·13 per cent; Fig. 188/IV).

The *branches* of the anterior tibial artery are as follows:

The *posterior tibial recurrent artery* (Figs 202 and 203/14, 204 and 205/12) curves back to the knee joint.

The *anterior tibial recurrent artery* (Figs 202 and 203/15, 204 and 205/13) arising from the frontal aspect of the interosseous membrane, runs to the arterial network of the knee.

The *muscular branches* are distributed to the muscles on either side of the vessel.

The *anterior (medial and lateral) malleolar arteries* run to the ankles and participate in the formation of the arterial network.

The *dorsalis pedis artery* (Figs 206/12, 207/12) follows a straight course from the midpoint of the

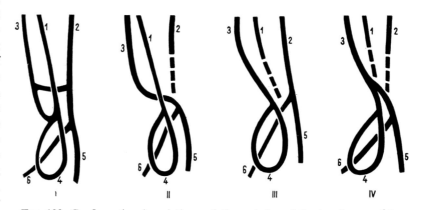

FIG. 188. Configurational variations of the arteries of the leg. I, normal type; II, rudimentary posterior tibial artery; III, rudimentary anterior tibial artery; IV, both principal vessels are rudimentary. (*1*) Anterior tibial artery; (*2*) posterior tibial artery; (*3*) peroneal artery; (*4*) arcuate artery; (*5*) medial plantar artery; (*6*) lateral plantar artery.

ankle joint to the first interosseous space. The vessel is rarely absent (Garusi 1968). In addition to the branches which run to the dorsum pedis (*lateral and medial tarsal arteries*, Figs 206/13, 207/13), the vessel gives off a branch (*arcuate artery*, Figs 188/4, 206/14, 207/14) which describes a bend in the tarsometatarsal line. The five *dorsal metatarsal arteries* (Fig. 207/21) arise from the arcuate artery; they communicate with the plantar vessels via the perforating branches and, bifurcating in the clefts between the toes, continue as the *dorsal digital arteries*. Penetrating to the plantar side, the terminal branch of the dorsalis pedis artery assists in the formation of the plantar arch (*deep plantar branch*, Figs 206/15, 207/15).

The **posterior tibial artery** (Figs 188/2, 202 and 203/16, 204 and 205/14, 206/16, 207/16), the other terminal branch of the popliteal artery, passes between the superficial and the deep muscles in a straight downward line from the middle of the popliteal space to midway between the medial malleolus and the medial tubercle of the calcaneus to divide into end branches on the sole. The diameter of the posterior tibial artery is 2·23 to 4·15 mm (Gyurkó and Szabó 1968). The formation of *variations* is chiefly due to the full development of the peroneal artery (Gray 1954) in which case the posterior tibial artery is rudimentary or absent (Ferrante et al. 1967). *Branches:*

The *circumflex fibular branch* (Figs 202 and 203/17, 204 and 205/15) passes round the neck of the fibula.

The *(fibular) peroneal artery* (Figs 188/3, 202/18, 204 and 205/18), arising 2·3 cm (0 to 5·6 cm) below the origin of the posterior tibial artery, passes obliquely toward the fibula and runs along it to the lateral malleolus (Adachi 1928). Its absence is rare. If both tibial arteries are rudimentary, the peroneal artery alone supplies the leg (Ferrante et al. 1967). Besides muscular branches, the vessel gives off a branch which pierces the interosseous membrane 4 to 6 cm above the ankle (*perforating branch*); through these, communications are formed with the network of the dorsum pedis, while, somewhat lower, anastomosis is formed with the posterior tibial artery (*communicating branch*, Fig. 205/19). The *lateral* and *medial malleolar branches* (Fig. 207/17) communicate with the arterial *network of the calcaneus* (Fig. 207/18).

The *medial and lateral plantar arteries* (Figs 188/5 and 6, 206/17 and 18, 207/19 and 20), arising behind the medial malleolus, run distally in the plantar grooves. The lateral artery is larger; it passes in an arched course medially at the base of the metatarsal bones (*plantar arch*, Fig. 206/19) and anastomoses with the terminal branch of the dorsalis pedis artery as also with the deep portion of the medial artery (*deep branch*, Figs 206/15, 207/15). The *superficial branch* of the medial artery continues its course along the medial border of the first metatarsal bone and supplies the medial surface of the 1st toe and the proximal surfaces of the 1st and 2nd toes. The surfaces between the 2nd to 4th toes are supplied by the branches from the plantar arch (*plantar metatarsal arteries*, Figs 206/20, 207/22) which, dividing, form the *common and proper plantar digital arteries* (Figs 206/21, 207/23). The lateral side of the 5th toe is usually supplied by a vessel which arises directly from the lateral plantar artery. The common plantar digital arteries communicate with the vessels of the dorsum pedis. The numerous variations of the arteries of the foot arise from the shifting of the compensating equilibrium. The plantar arch may be replaced by the dorsalis pedis artery (Rauber and Kopsch 1951). The variability of the metatarsal and digital arteries is of no practical importance.

Collateral circulation of the pelvis and the lower extremities

Anatomically, the collateral circulation of the pelvis and the lower extremities is ensured by three groups of anastomoses (Fig. 189; Brantigan 1963).

1. The system of iliac anastomoses is not as good as that of the scapular region. Connections between the aorta (lumbar, median sacral, testicular, superior and inferior mesenteric arteries, Figs 189/3, 2 and 1), the internal iliac artery (superior and inferior gluteal, internal pudendal, obturator, iliolumbar arteries, Figs 189/5, 6, 9, 8 and 7), external iliac artery (inferior epigastric, deep circumflex iliac arteries, Figs 189/12 and 13) and the femoral artery (superficial epigastric, superficial circumflex iliac, external pudendal, deep femoral, medial and lateral circumflex femoral arteries, Figs 189/15, 16 and 19) are able to compensate for the insufficiency of the iliac arteries (Lériche 1940). No adequate circulation in the extremity can develop if the proximal part of the femoral artery is obstructed because the deep femoral artery ceases to function in such cases (Bellmann and Herwig 1964), whereas sufficient collateral circulation in the lower third can be maintained through the anastomoses between the femoral and popliteal arteries.

2. Genicular anastomoses are formed among the femoral artery (descending genicular artery, Fig. 189/22), the deep femoral artery (third perforating artery, descending branch of the lateral circumflex femoral artery, Fig. 189/21), the popliteal artery (superior, middle and inferior genicular arteries, Figs 189/24 and 25) and the anterior tibial artery

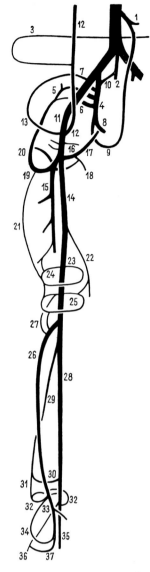

FIG. 189. Collateral circulation in the arteries of the pelvis and the lower extremities. (*1*) Inferior mesenteric artery; (*2*) median sacral artery; (*3*) lumbar arteries; (*4*) internal iliac artery; (*5*) superior gluteal artery; (*6*) inferior gluteal artery; (*7*) iliolumbar artery; (*8*) obturator artery; (*9*) internal pudendal artery; (*10*) lateral sacral artery; (*11*) external iliac artery; (*12*) inferior epigastric artery; (*13*) deep circumflex iliac artery; (*14*) femoral artery; (*15*) deep femoral artery; (*16*) medial circumflex femoral artery; (*17*) deep branch; (*18*) transverse branch; (*19*) lateral circumflex femoral artery; (*20*) ascending branch; (*21*) descending branch; (*22*) descending genicular artery; (*23*) popliteal artery; (*24*) superior genicular arteries; (*25*) inferior genicular arteries; (*26*) anterior tibial artery; (*27*) anterior and posterior tibial recurrent arteries; (*28*) posterior tibial artery; (*29*) peroneal artery; (*30*) communicating branch; (*31*) perforating branch; (*32*) medial and lateral malleolar arteries; (*33*) dorsalis pedis artery; (*34*) arcuate artery; (*35*) medial plantar artery; (*36*) lateral plantar artery; (*37*) plantar arch.

(anterior and posterior tibial recurrent arteries, Fig. 189/27). This communication is not always adequate. Collateral circulation is functionally sufficient only if the arterial network of the knee can compensate satisfactorily (Bellmann and Herwig 1964).

3. Anastomoses in the legs and feet between the three arteries of the leg are formed in the region of the ankles (malleolar, arteries, Fig. 189/32) and in that of the heels (calcanean arteries) through the connections of the peroneal artery (communicating branch, perforating branch, Figs 189/30 and 31) and by way of the vessels which compose the plantar arch (dorsalis pedis and plantar arteries, Figs 189/33, 35 and 36). The initial segment of the posterior tibial artery (Fig. 189/28) is of primary importance in this connection. Its deficiency can be compensated only by the sural arteries. The anterior tibial artery (Fig. 189/26) may be replaced by its communication with the peroneal artery and the arterial network of the knee. The peroneal artery (Fig. 189/29) has so many anastomoses that its elimination elicits no clinical manifestation.

Arteriography of the pelvis and the lower extremities

Brooks (1924) made the first arteriogram of the leg using sodium iodide. Lumbar aortography, introduced by Dos Santos et al. (1929), made the visualization of the pelvic arteries possible. Following the pioneer works (Sgalitzer et al. 1930, Lériche 1935, Fontaine 1937, Ratschow 1937, Dimtza and Jäger 1938), anatomic aspects and pathologic anomalies have been studied intensively on the basis of a large material (Lindbom 1952, Wellauer 1957, Malchiodi and Ruberti, 1957, Pässler 1958, Ratschow 1959, Abrams 1961).

Olovson (1941) carried out preliminary studies regarding the radiographic examination of pelvic vessels by post-mortem filling of the collaterals. Gesenius (1949) and subsequently Loose (1953, 1957) and Pässler (1952, 1957) reported on a larger material of arteriography in vivo, as well as Orlandi et al. (1968). Introduction of selective methods (Ödman 1956, Gollmann 1957) has facilitated the isolated filling of separate vessels. Visualization of the arteries of the uterus (Fernström 1955) and of the urinary bladder (Boijsen and Nilsson 1962, Bücheler and Thurn 1964, Kelemen et al. 1965) are clinically the most significant.

While arteriograms of the extremity reveal even vessels with diameters of 0·1 mm, the thickness of the layers in the pelvis makes it impossible to visualize vessels with a diameter less than 0·3 mm in anteroposterior pictures and in the lateral view those of less than 0·5 mm. Malchiodi and Ruberti (1957) registered variations in 10 per cent of the examined cases, while Pässler and Pässler (1963) studying arteriograms of the leg, observed variations formed by branches of the popliteal artery in 5·38 and those of the malleolar vessels in 1·84 per cent. Anatomical examinations revealed, on the other hand, variations in 20 to 40 per cent

(Quain 1884, Adachi 1928, Lanz and Wachsmuth 1938). The differences are partly due to a more accurate registration of anatomical observations and partly to the fact that deviations from the normal are not always traceable to angiographic demonstration.

Postmortem **anteroposterior** *angiograms* **of the pelvis** (Figs 192, 193, 194) show the two branches of the aorta formed by its bifurcation at the level of the 4th lumbar vertebra (*common iliac arteries*, Figs 192/9, 193/3, 194/6) to lie in the projection of the sacroiliac joints. Superposition of the projections of the external and internal iliac arteries at their beginning makes it sometimes impossible to locate their site of division with accuracy. The *internal iliac artery* (Figs 192/10, 193/4, 194/7) describes a medially convex arch and winds to the lateral side. The *superior and inferior gluteal arteries* (Figs 192/14 and 15, 193/10 and 11, 194/13 and 14), arch-shaped continuations of the main trunk, run to the gluteal muscles and cross the external iliac artery; their further course lies in the projection of the ilium. In the upper half of the ilium a well developed anastomosis often exists between the *iliolumbar artery* (Figs 192/11, 193/5, 194/8) and the deep circumflex iliac artery. Placed in front of the sacrum, the *lateral sacral arteries* (Figs 192/12, 193/6, 194/9) communicate with the median sacral artery. The terminal portion of the latter can be followed as far as the apex of the coccyx. Of the numerous vessels projected on one another on the two borders of the lesser pelvis, the *internal pudendal artery* (Figs 192/19, 193/15, 194/20) passes through the greater sciatic foramen below the piriformis, describes a laterally convex arch, runs toward the pubic bones and, after crossing the projection of the obturator foramen, extends below the symphysis. The vessel is larger in males than in females. The *dorsal artery of the penis* (Fig. 193/20) describes a slight upward curve to the medial side and, reaching the midline, turns downward and courses parallel with the contralateral vessel along the longitudinal axis of the penis. The *deep artery of the penis* (Fig. 193/19) represents the smaller branch. It usually arises in the projection of the lower border of the ischium and runs obliquely and medially downward. The deep artery of the penis is always more laterally placed than the dorsal artery of the penis. From its origin the *obturator artery* (Figs 192/13, 193/7, 194/10) crosses obliquely the upper limb of the pubic bone and passes into the projection of the obturator foramen so that its branches cannot easily be distinguished from the internal pudendal artery. Its anastomosis with the medial circumflex femoral artery usually fills easily. The *artery of the ductus deferens* cannot be differentiated from the vesical arteries. The *uterine artery* (Figs 192/18, 194/17) passes obliquely across the approximate centre of the lesser pelvis. Its course depends to a great extent on the actual position of the uterus. Reaching the cervix of the uterus, the upward curving tortuous main trunk of the artery emits perpendicular corkscrew-like side branches that meet in the midline. The smaller branches surround the fundus in an arch. The *tubal branch* and the *ovarian branch* can best be studied in preparations of the removed organs (Fig. 199). This way their connection with the ovarian artery and also with the small vessels of the ovary can be observed. The *vesical arteries* (Figs 192/16 and 17, 193/12 and 13, 194/15 and 16) consist of several small branches; arising at the border of the pelvis, they form multiple anastomoses around the bladder. The *middle rectal artery* (Figs 192/17, 193/14, 194/24) usually arises together with the inferior vesical artery so that the two vessels are mostly indistinguishable. The *vaginal artery* (Fig. 194/19) is likewise situated below or within the area of the inferior vesical arteries and cannot always be filled. The *pelvic arteries* differ in development *in males and females:* the internal pudendal artery is larger in men and the obturator artery in women. The uterine artery and its branches can be best studied on *preparations of the removed organ* (Fig. 199), the arteries of the penis can be visualized in *two-directional pictures of the penis* (Figs 196, 197). The testicular artery and the epididymal artery can be best visualized in *isolated pictures showing the testicle dissected out of the scrotum* (Fig. 198). Describing a lateral slightly convex arch at the border of the pelvis, the *external iliac artery* (Figs 192/20, 193/21, 194/28) runs to the head of the femur. In this projection it is already continuous with the femoral artery. The *inferior epigastric artery* (Fig. 192/21), describing mild curves, ascends steeply in the projection of the ilium. The *deep circumflex iliac artery* (Figs 192/22, 193/22) describes a wide arch at the lateral border of the wing of the ilium.

Only large branches are distinguishable on **lateral roentgenograms** (Fig. 195). The *common iliac artery* (Fig. 195/5) descends slightly backward in front of the sacrum. Superposition of the bilateral projections makes a reliable location of the origin of the *internal iliac artery* (Fig. 195/6) difficult also in this view. Of the branches given off by the internal iliac artery, the *superior and inferior gluteal arteries* (Figs 195/7 and 8) are distributed chiefly to the gluteal muscles and follow a descending backward course, while the *internal pudendal artery* (Fig. 195/10) describes a forward curve. The *obturator artery* (Fig. 195/9) runs obliquely forward and downward. Owing to their small size and orthoroentgenographic course, the other arteries of the lesser pelvis cannot be identified in this view. The *external iliac artery* (Fig. 195/11) describes in its forward descending course an "S" with a backward convex line in its upper and a forward convex line in its lower part. The bilateral vessels pass across the middle of the pelvic projection. Emerging from the pelvis, they descend in front of the head of the femur.

In **anteroposterior pictures of the thigh** (Fig. 200), the *femoral artery* (Fig. 200/9) crosses the head of the femur obliquely and descends steeply, sometimes describing a medially mild curve; when arriving at the level of the adductor canal it turns laterally and intersects the projection of the femur. Arising immediately below the border of the neck of the femur, the *deep femoral artery* (Fig. 200/15) pursues a slightly lateral descending course. That branch of the *medial circumflex femoral artery* (Fig. 200/16) which is connected with the obturator artery, runs medially, while its *deep branch* bends back to the neck of the femur. The medial circumflex femoral artery communicates with the *ascending branch* (Fig. 200/19) of the *lateral circumflex femoral artery* (Fig. 200/18). The *descending branch* (Fig. 200/20) describes a laterally convex arch in its downward course. Running laterally, the *perforating arteries* (Fig. 200/21) cross the projection of the femur. The *descending genicular artery* (Fig. 200/22) winds medially or laterally toward the knee joint.

The **lateral picture** (Fig. 201) shows the *femoral artery* (Fig. 201/9) to cross the projection of the bone in an anteroposterior direction at the boundary between its middle and lower third, meanwhile the vessel is continuous with the popliteal artery in the popliteal fossa. The descending branches of the *deep femoral artery* (Fig. 201/15) pursue a similar course. The medial branches of the femoral artery (superficial epigastric artery, superficial circumflex iliac artery, external pudendal arteries) run partly to the ischium and the pubic bone and partly to the ilium; they can be studied on the roentgenograms of the pelvis.

Anteroposterior pictures of the knee (Fig. 202) show the upper and lower arched branches (*superior and inferior genicular arteries*, Fig. 202/7, 8, 11 and 12) of the *popliteal artery* (Fig. 202/6), which passes from the medial aspect of the thigh to the midline, to surround the femoral and tibial condyles. The *middle genicular artery* (Fig. 202/9) is placed at the height of the joint space. The *sural arteries* (Fig. 202/10) follow an oblique descending path. The division of the popliteal artery is usually about 6 cm below the space of the knee joint.

In the **lateral view** (Fig. 203), the *popliteal artery* (Fig. 203/6) is seen behind the knee joint near the bone. The branches surrounding the articulation

from below and above can be well identified also in this view. The *sural arteries* (Fig. 203/10) course backward and downward in the soft tissues. The division of the popliteal artery appears below the neck of the fibula.

Anteroposterior pictures of the arteries of the leg (Fig. 204) show the following arrangement. The *anterior tibial artery* (Fig. 204/11), after describing a lateral curve, pursues a medial downward course in front of the projection of the fibula. At the height of the ankle, the vessel can be found midway between the two malleoli. The *posterior tibial artery* (Fig. 204/14), a straight continuation of the popliteal artery, runs downward and slightly medially in the projection of the tibia. Reaching the ankle, the vessel is seen behind the medial malleolus. Arising as a rule from the trunk of the posterior tibial artery, the *peroneal artery* (Fig. 204/18) courses between the two major vessels and traverses the projection of the anterior tibial artery in its lower course.

In the **lateral view** (Fig. 205), the initial portion of the *anterior tibial artery* (Fig. 205/11) runs forward to turn downward in the projection of the posterior border of the tibia. In its lower third, the vessel crosses the tibia in an oblique direction and lies in front of the bones at the height of the ankle. The *posterior tibial artery* (Fig. 205/14) follows a straight descending course in the projection of the fibula. Its lower part lies behind the medial malleolus. The *peroneal artery* (Fig. 205/18) courses behind the two vessels, crosses the posterior tibial artery obliquely and runs forward.

Dorsoplantar pictures of the malleolar region and the foot (Fig. 206) show the *lateral plantar artery* (Fig. 206/18) to follow an oblique lateral course from the medial malleolus and to cross the projections of the tarsal bones and the dorsalis pedis artery. The *medial plantar artery* (Fig. 206/17) passes in a straight line toward the first metatarsal bone. The *plantar arch* (Fig. 206/19) pursues a transverse path at the base of the metatarsal bones. The *common and proper plantar digital arteries* (Fig. 206/21) follow a distal course between the metatarsal bones and at the two sides of the toes. The *dorsalis pedis artery* (Fig. 206/12) extends from the midpoint of the line connecting the malleoli to the first intermetatarsal space and gives off in its course branches which run bilaterally to the tarsal bones and wind to the dorsum pedis.

In the **lateral view** (Fig. 207), the *dorsalis pedis artery* (Fig. 207/12), a continuation of the anterior tibial artery, lies in front of the tibia in the malleolar region and is seen at the dorsal border of the tarsal bones in the projection of the soft tissues. Then it winds over to the plantar side in the projection of the first metatarsal bone. The *posterior* *tibial artery* (Fig. 207/16), emerging from behind the medial malleolus, traverses the projection of the calcaneus in an oblique direction and descends to the sole. The *calcaneal branches* (Fig. 207/18) usually form a rich network in the projection of the calcaneus and the heel. The main trunk divides in the projection of the calcaneus. Passing below the tarsal bones, the *lateral plantar artery* (Fig. 207/20) descends along their inferior border and joins the dorsalis pedis artery in the plantar arch. Coursing forward from the projection of the calcaneus, the *medial plantar artery* (Fig. 207/19) ramifies in the area of the tarsal bones. The projections of the arteries lying between the metatarsi and the toes are mostly overlapping in this view which makes their identification difficult. This projection is suitable for the study of the plantar arch formed by the dorsalis pedis and plantar vessels.

THE COMMON ILIAC VEIN AND ITS BRANCHES

Intercommunicating plexuses and a close connection with the portal circulation are the characteristic features of the pelvic veins. The intricate haemodynamic conditions of the venous circulation of the lower extremities can only be understood by the correct visualization of the communications between the superficial and deep veins.

The common, internal and external iliac veins and their branches

The **common iliac veins** (Figs 168/18, 169/19, 180/16, 181/19, 208/9, 209/7), arising in front of the sacroiliac joint, run to the right side of the 4th and 5th lumbar vertebrae; they unite in the inferior vena cava. They drain the veins of the pelvis and the lower extremity. The left common iliac vein ascends obliquely on the medial side of the common iliac artery. The right common iliac vein ascends more steeply behind and to the right of its artery and reaches the inferior vena cava. The length of the common iliac vein is 7·5 cm on the left, 5·5 cm on the right side; the diameter measures 1·6 to 1·8 cm (Paturet 1958). The posterior wall of the veins shows the impression which corresponds to the inclination of the angle of the promontory (Liechti 1948). This occurs in 15 to 22 per cent in adult persons (May and Nissl 1959).

Variations are rare. If the left common iliac vein does not join its contralateral partner, it ascends along the left side of the aorta. The lower portion of the inferior vena cava is doubled in such cases (*see* Variations of the inferior vena cava). Agenesis is associated with the simultaneous absence of the inferior vena cava (Bétoulières et al. 1959).

Branches: The *median sacral vein* (Fig. 208/8) opens into the left common iliac vein; the *iliolumbar* vein empties either into this vessel or into the internal iliac vein.

Internal iliac vein (Figs 168/19, 20 and 21, 169/20, 21 and 22, 180/17, 18 and 19, 181/20, 208/10, 209/8).

The bilateral internal iliac veins ascend behind and slightly medial to the corresponding artery in front of the sacroiliac joint and open into the common iliac vein. They return blood from the pelvic veins. They have no valves. Length of the internal iliac vein is 4 to 5 cm, diameter 1·2 to 1·3 cm. The diameter may vary according to whether the vessel is single, double or plexiform (Paturet 1958). As a *variation*, the vein may arise with two trunks one of which empties into the common iliac vein of the opposite side (Figs 168/20 and 21, 169/21 and 22). A similar case was reported by May and Nissl as well (1973).

Its *branches* accompany the corresponding arteries in pairs. The so-called venous plexuses are constitute a special feature.

The parietal branches, converging from the gluteal region (*superior and inferior gluteal veins*, Figs 208/11, 209/9 and 10) are in connection with the *obturator veins* (Figs 208/13, 209/11). The latter form anastomoses with the external iliac vein. The *lateral sacral veins* (Fig. 208/12) form the *sacral venous plexus* (Fig. 208/14) and are in communication with the median sacral vein.

The visceral branches form numerous anastomoses at the floor of the pelvis. The dorsal vein of the penis or clitoris is an exception in this respect (Rauber and Kopsch 1951). The *internal pudendal vein* (Figs 210 and 211/7) receives the veins from the scrotum or the labium majus (*scrotal* or *posterior labial veins*) and receives moreover the *deep vein of the penis* or *clitoris* (Figs 210 and 211/6) which accompanies the similarly named artery. The internal pudendal vein anastomoses with the rectal venous plexus. The *vesical veins* (Fig. 208/15) form a rich network around the bladder (*vesical venous plexus*, Fig. 208/16) that communicates with the prostatic and rectal veins. The *prostatic venous plexus* (Figs 208/16, 210 and 211/7), situated behind the symphysis, receives the *dorsal vein of the penis*. The latter is formed by the union of two veins at the crown of the glans penis (Abeshouse and Ruben

1952). The *rectal venous plexus*, developed around the similarly named arteries, forms an important anastomosis with the inferior mesenteric vein. The *uterine and vaginal venous plexus*, the largest of the pelvic plexuses in women, consists of a network surrounding the body and neck of the uterus as well as the upper part of the vagina. It is drained into the internal iliac vein by the *uterine veins* that course laterally between the membranes of the broad ligament.

The **external iliac vein** (Figs 168/24, 169/23 and 24, 180/22, 181/21, 208/17, 209/12, 212/5) returns venous blood of the lower extremity from the region of the inguinal ligament toward the sacroiliac joint and opens in front of it into the common iliac vein. It lies on both sides medial to the accompanying artery. The course of the left vein is more curved. It has a valve at the initial portion in 1 to 7 per cent of the cases (Basmajian 1952). The vessel is in communication with the obturator vein. The diameter of the external iliac vein measures 1·3 to 1·4 cm (Paturet 1958).

The external iliac vein has two constant *branches*, namely the *inferior epigastric vein* and the *deep circumflex iliac vein*. The former communicates with the internal thoracic, the latter with the iliolumbar vein. Thus, they are important collaterals of the inferior vena cava.

Peculiarities of the veins of the lower extremities

The veins of the lower limb are divided into deep and superficial veins. The *deep veins* lie in a common sheath with the arteries and they are doubled distally to the popliteal vein. Via anastomoses between the two trunks they form a plexus around the arteries. Despite their variability, the deep veins display a certain constant arrangement. Of the *muscle veins* which open into the deeper veins, those of the soleus and the gastrocnemius have a particular haemodynamic function. Their normal typically arcade-shaped course (Charpy and Hovelacque 1920) is demonstrable only up to age 25 (Gullmo 1957). These vessels fill with blood on muscle relaxation, and eject the blood centripetally on a muscle contraction (Almén and Nylander 1962).

Forming loops and plexuses, the *subcutaneous veins* are embedded in loose adipose tissue. They have valves only at the divisions. They communicate with the deep veins. These vessels are drained by the small and great saphenous veins which follow straight courses and have stronger walls than the deep veins. They have less valves.

The superficial and the deep veins are connected by the *communicating* and *perforating veins* (Figs 212 and 213/9, 214 and 215/8, 216 and 217/11, 218/12 and 13). They follow transverse courses (Raivio 1948). About ten communicating veins belong to each paired trunk. Linton (1938) termed the vessels running directly to the deep veins communicating veins and those linked to the muscle veins, perforating veins. Their differentiation in practice is not possible. Only those exposed to the greatest haemodynamic stresses attain clinical significance. The valves are such as to direct the flow of blood from the surface to the deeper layers (Pirner 1956). Gullmo (1959) described orificial loops in them that are hardly 0·1 cm wide. These loops make circulation possible without angulation of the perforating veins even if the fasciae are displaced.

The *valves* are of primary importance for the maintenance of circulation. They can be found even in postcapillaries over a size of 20 μ (Staubesand 1959). The valves are mainly situated distally to the orifices. Longer veins have valves not only at their orifices but elsewhere, too. The free margin of the cusps of the valves parallels the long axis of the body (Braus and Elze 1956). The valve of the subinguinal femoral vein (0·5 to 1·0 cm below the inguinal ligament) and the valve of the popliteal vein below the knee joint are of particular importance (Basmajian 1952). These valves produce a pumping-pressing regulation when the limb is flexed (Kügelen 1951). The femoral vein has 1 to 6 valves of which the one situated above the orifice of the saphenous vein and the other valve situated below the opening of the deep vein of the thigh are the most constant (Basmajian 1952). Valves in the deep veins are placed at 2·2, in the superficial veins at 4 cm intervals. There are 10 (7 to 15) valves in the great, and 8 in the small saphenous vein (Raivio 1948). Valves may be missing in the popliteal, femoral or iliac veins (Luke 1951) and even in the whole leg (Lodin 1958/9, cit. May and Nissl 1959). Total absence of all deep veins has also been described (Tonitza et al. 1967).

The femoral vein and its branches

The femoral vein (Figs 190, 208/18, 212 and 213/6, 214 and 215/5) is the continuation of the popliteal vein. It courses along the femoral artery to the inguinal ligament and passes into the external iliac vein. In addition to the veins which accompany the corresponding arteries it receives the great (and possibly the accessory) saphenous vein. The femoral vein has a diameter of 0·9 to 1·0 cm (Paturet 1958).

Four *variations* have been described by May and Nissl (1966). Normal type (Fig. 190/I; 62·34 per

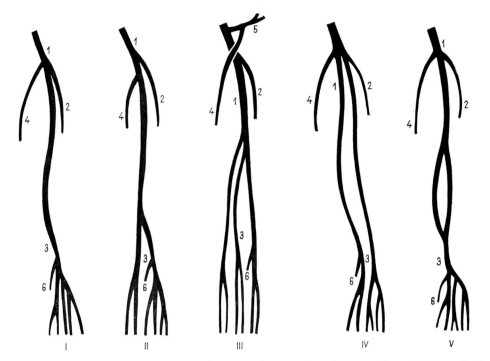

FIG. 190. Variations of the femoral, popliteal and great saphenous veins. I, normal type; II, femoral vein divided in the lower segment; duplication of popliteal vein; distal orifice of great saphenous vein; III, triple femoral and popliteal veins; great saphenous vein opens into superficial epigastric vein; IV, femoral vein divided along its entire course; V, islet formation on the femoral vein. (*1*) Femoral vein; (*2*) deep femoral vein; (*3*) popliteal vein; (*4*) great saphenous vein; (*5*) superficial epigastric vein; (*6*) small saphenous vein.

cent). Two femoral veins in the lower segment subsequently uniting (Fig. 190/II; 21·16 per cent). Multiple femoral veins (Fig. 190/III; 13·72 per cent). Division of the vein in its entire course (Fig. 190/IV; 2·78 per cent). In cases of agenesis of the femoral vein it is replaced by the accompanying vein of the sciatic nerve or by a superficial collateral (Olivier 1957, May and Nissl 1971). Formation of islets has also been observed (Fig. 190/V).

The **popliteal vein** (Figs 190, 212 and 213/10, 216 and 217/5) runs dorsally to the corresponding artery in the popliteal fossa. Its diameter measures 0·8 cm (Paturet 1958). In addition to the veins accompanying the arteries it receives the small saphenous vein. Since the confluence of the veins of the lower limb is fairly variable, the length of the popliteal vein varies accordingly. It begins below the line of the knee joint in only half of the cases. The vein may be single (55·85 per cent), double (39·15 per cent), double with two femoral veins (2·78 per cent) and triple (2·22 per cent; May and Nissl 1966). Agenesis is rare (Servelle 1952).

Posterior and anterior tibial veins, peroneal veins. The three veins of the leg accompany the corresponding arteries in pairs. They divide sometimes into three or four segments which unite in the proximal segment. Their orifice is sometimes situated below the knee joint (47·5 per cent), sometimes at

the level of the joint (8·35 per cent) and in other cases above it (44·15 per cent; May and Nissl 1966). The *anterior tibial veins* (Figs 216 and 217/8) drain the dorsum pedis. They lie medial to the peroneal veins. The *posterior tibial veins* (Figs 216 and 217/6, 218/11) course from behind the medial malleolus along the back of the leg toward the popliteal fossa. The *peroneal veins* (Figs 216 and 217/7) lie first on the medial side of the anterior tibial veins and then lateral to them (Netzer 1958). Agenesis of the veins of the leg is very rare (Gullmo 1964).

Veins of the foot (Fig. 218). The deep veins accompany the corresponding arteries. The plantar veins are connected with the superficial venous plexus of the dorsum of the foot via the communicating vein of the 1st interosseous space. Limborgh (1963), in addition to the interdigital communications, distinguishes 15 *plantar*, 14 *marginal* and 20 *dorsal communicating veins of the foot* (Figs 218/12 and 13).

Superficial veins. The *great saphenous vein* (Figs 208/21, 212 and 213/11, 214 and 215/7, 216 and 217/9, 218/15) begins in the medial margin of the foot, ascends in front of the medial malleolus and runs up the leg. It passes on the medial side to the thigh and crosses the medial condyle of the femur from behind. The entire course of the vessel

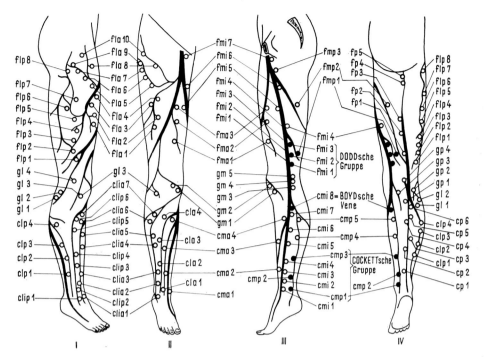

FIG. 191. Diagram showing the communicating veins of the lower extremities (after May, R. and Nissl, R. from Limborgh, J. et al.: De venae communicantes van het been. *Ned. T. Geneesk* 106, 1962, 415). I, leg seen from the lateral side; II, leg seen from the front; III, leg seen from the medial side; IV, leg seen from behind: *cma*, anterior medial communicating veins of the leg, *cmi*, intermediary medial communicating veins of the leg, *cmp*, posterior medial communicating veins of the leg, *cla*, anterior lateral communicating veins of the leg, *clia*, anterior intermediary lateral communicating veins of the leg, *clip*, posterior intermediary lateral communicating veins of the leg, *clp*, posterior lateral communicating veins of the leg, *cp*, posterior communicating veins of the leg, *gm*, medial genicular communicating veins, *gl*, lateral genicular communicating veins, *gp*, posterior genicular communicating veins, *fma*, anterior medial femoral communicating veins, *fmi*, intermediary medial femoral communicating veins, *fmp*, posterior medial femoral communicating veins, *fla*, anterior lateral femoral communicating veins, *flp*, posterior lateral femoral communicating veins, *fp*, posterior femoral communicating veins.

lies in the subcutaneous connective tissue. It passes through the saphenous opening into the deeper layers and ends in the femoral vein. The orifice of the vessel is on a level with the orifice of the deep vein of the thigh about 9 cm below the groin (May and Nissl 1959). The great saphenous vein usually receives an anterior and a larger posterior branch on both the leg and the thigh in the genicular region and a few cm before its orifice, respectively. The latter are termed *medial and lateral accessory saphenous veins* (Limborgh 1963). The *external pudendal veins*, the *superficial epigastric vein* and the *superficial circumflex iliac vein* empty into its upper end. The orifice of the great saphenous vein may be a few cm more distal than typically or, it may open into one of the veins of the abdominal wall after crossing the femoral vein. The great shapenous vein has a diameter of 0·4 to 0·5 cm at the beginning and 0·7 to 0·8 cm at the upper end (Paturet 1958).

The *small saphenous vein* (Figs 216 and 217/10, 218/16) begins at the lateral border of the dorsum of the foot, runs behind the lateral malleolus and

reaches the dorsal aspect of the leg. Piercing the fascia it passes to the deeper layers between the two heads of the gastrocnemius muscle and opens into the popliteal vein. The vein may open in common with the femoropopliteal vein, occasionally present on the dorsal side of the thigh, or it may have a separate orifice (May and Nissl 1966). The orifice of the small saphenous vein lies at the approximate height of the knee joint, sometimes slightly above and very rarely below it (May and Nissl 1968).

Communicating (and perforating) veins (Fig. 191). Linton (1938), Cockett (1955) and Limborgh (1963) gave precise anatomical descriptions of the communicating veins. Their number and arrangement are presented here according to Limborgh's description.

Communicating veins of the leg. Medial veins: These form three groups (consisting of 1 to 6, 5 to 10 and 3 to 6 branches, respectively) between the great saphenous vein and the posterior tibial veins. Lateral veins: Two groups (consisting of 2 to 5 and 5 to 10 branches, respectively) link the great saphenous vein with the anterior tibial veins; another group of 4 to 10 branches forms communications between the great saphenous and the peroneal veins; a fourth group of 2 to 5 members connects the great saphenous with the veins of the gastrocnemius muscle. Posterior veins consist of 2 to 6 branches between the small saphenous vein and the veins of the gastrocnemius muscle.

Communicating veins of the knee. Medial veins: 2 to 6 branches running from the great saphenous to the popliteal vein. Lateral veins: 2 to 6 branches running from the lateral veins to the popliteal vein. Posterior veins: 2 to 7 branches running from the small saphenous to the popliteal vein.

Femoral communicating veins. Medial veins: Arranged in three groups (consisting of 1 to 4, 4 to 8 and 1 to 5 branches, respectively), run from the accessory saphenous vein to the muscle veins and from the great saphenous to the femoral vein. Lateral veins: Arranged in two groups (6 to 12 and 3 to 9 branches, respectively), these vessels connect the subcutaneous and the muscle veins. Posterior veins: 4 to 7 branches running from the femoro-popliteal to the femoral vein or to one of the perforating veins.

Collateral venous circulation of the pelvis and the lower limbs

Abundant bilateral anastomoses guarantee the collateral circulation of pelvic veins. The sacral, prostatic, rectal, uterine and vaginal plexuses, between the internal iliac veins, are in close communication within the lesser pelvis. The scrotal (labial) veins form collateral paths with each other as also with the medial circumflex femoral vein and the rectal venous plexus. Thus there are communications here between the femoral and the internal iliac vein. In case of insufficient circulation communication between the external and internal veins is maintained partly by the homolateral and partly by the contralateral veins (Thomas et al. 1967).

Collateral circulation in the lower limbs is maintained via the communicating veins connecting the superficial with the deep vessels. The deep veins are also linked. Anastomoses between the deep vein of the thigh and the popliteal vein as also between the venae comitantes femorales and popliteales are able to maintain circulation if necessary. Even the terminal branches of the venae comitantes femorales maintain significant peripheral communications (Mavor and Galloway 1967). Anastomoses between the deep veins of the leg are ensured mainly via the muscle veins and indirectly through the superficial vessels.

Phlebography of the pelvis and the lower limbs

After animal experiments, Berberich and Hirsch (1923) were the first to fill the veins of the lower limbs of men with contrast material. The valves could be visualized on phlebograms obtained with strontium bromide injections. It took a long time until the technical and anatomical problems were solved (Ratschow 1930, Barber and Orley 1932, Dos Santos 1938, Lindblom 1941, Fine et al. 1942) that made the routine application of phlebography possible. The clinical importance of phlebography consists of the correct evaluation of the deep and superficial veins and their anastomoses (Linton 1938, Cockett 1955, Gullmo 1957, 1964, Limborgh 1963, May and Nissl 1959, 1966, 1968). Radiographic examination of the pelvic veins yielded significant anatomical results (Liechti 1948, Abeshouse and Ruben 1952, Basmajian 1952, De La Pena 1956). Presently selective filling of the deep vein of the penis (De La Pena 1956), the vein of the clitoris (Petković 1953), the cavernous body of the penis (Molnár and Hajós 1960) as well as the uterine (Schlüssler et al. 1966) and ovarian veins (Delorme et al. 1968), can be carried out. Although there are numerous variations, the phlebographies of the lower extremities may be divided into the retrograde (Martineti 1959) and the anterograde group (Greitz 1955, May and Nissl 1959). Intraosseous venography (Drasnar 1946, Leger and Masse 1951, Vas and Kerpel 1954, Olivier 1957, Zsebők et al. 1957, Luzsa 1959/60, Arnoldi 1961) is essentially a version of the anterograde procedure.

In *postmortem phlebography* we could visualize the veins of the pelvis and the lower limbs by anterograde percutaneous filling. The side branches, commencing from the trunks, were thus filled through the anastomoses only. The valves impede retrograde filling.

Lateral pictures of the ankle and foot (Fig. 218) show a good filling of both the superficial veins of the dorsum pedis and the deep veins of the sole. Their anastomoses and the perimalleolar venous plexus can be visualized only in this view. The shadow of the *posterior tibial veins* (Fig. 218/11), originating from *the plantar veins*, further that of the *great saphenous vein* (Fig. 218/15) appear at the posterior and the anterior border of the tibia, respectively. The *small saphenous vein* (Fig. 218/16) casts its shadow on the soft tissues slightly behind the posterior tibial veins.

Anteroposterior roentgenograms of the leg (Fig. 216) show the following pattern. The branches of the popliteal vein which ramifies below the knee, i.e., the *deep veins*, pass along the arteries in the projections of the tibia and the fibula. The *great* *saphenous vein* (Fig. 216/9) runs along the medial border of the leg; its numerous communications with the deep veins are clearly visible. Being projected together with the deep veins, the *small saphenous vein* (Fig. 216/10) is usually hardly identifiable.

Lateral pictures (Fig. 217) show the *deep veins* mostly as a common bundle in or behind the projection of the fibula. Only certain segments of the *great saphenous vein* (Fig. 217/9) can be differentiated before *the deep veins*. The *small saphenous vein* (Fig. 217/10) appears under the skin on the leg behind and then in the muscles. Its orifice is at various sites. Both its course and anastomoses are clearly visible.

Anteroposterior phlebograms of the thigh (Fig. 212) show the *femoral vein* (Fig. 212/6) as it follows the corresponding artery. It is most often situated in the shape of an "S". Its side branches can hardly be visualized. The course of the *great saphenous vein* (Fig. 212/11) lies medial to the femoral vein; the height of its orifice is variable.

Lateral pictures (Fig. 213) show the *femoral vein* (Fig. 213/6) to follow the course of its artery and to cross the femur. It appears to be placed somewhat higher than the femoral artery. The projection of the *great saphenous vein* (Fig. 213/11) appears first behind the femoral vein and then, after crossing the bone in its upper third, it is seen to lie against the femoral vein.

By ligating the deep veins and simultaneously filling the superficial veins it is possible to visualize the anastomoses between the superficial and the deep veins too. **Two-directional pictures** of the thigh, with the application of this technique (Figs 214, 215), show the filled *great saphenous vein* and its *communicating veins* (Figs 214 and 215/7 and 8) as

also the *muscle veins* and the *vena profunda femoris* (Figs 214 and 215/6).

Anteroposterior roentgenograms of the pelvis (Fig. 208) reveal the *common iliac veins* (Fig. 208/9) to course in front of the sacroiliac joint toward the right border of the vertebral column. Of the branches of the *internal iliac vein* (Fig. 208/10), only the *superior* and *inferior gluteal veins* (Fig. 208/11) can be seen, and even these only in their initial portion. The *obturator vein* (Fig. 208/13) can usually be filled only via the anastomosis of the medial circumflex femoral vein. It is through the *internal pudendal vein* that the roots of the *rectal venous plexus*, the *deep veins of the penis*, the *dorsal vein of the penis*, further the *prostatic venous plexus* (Fig. 208/16) open into the internal iliac vein. The *sacral venous plexus* (Fig. 208/14) can always be identified.

Owing to the formation of abundant plexuses it is usually impossible to differentiate the side branches on **lateral pictures** (Fig. 209) because the iliac veins in view also have the characteristic "S" shape like the corresponding arteries.

By filling the cavernous body of the penis (cavernosography), the **anteroposterior view of the penis** (Fig. 210) presents a clear visualization of the septum between the corpora cavernosa. The crura penis, projected orthoroentgenographically cast, each, an apricot stone-sized confluent shadow between the rami of the ischium.

Phlebograms made in the **oblique view** (Fig. 211) present the entire course of the cavernous bodies. Their projections are superposed in this view. The septa between them are obscured from view in this projection by the intensive contrast medium. The efferent *dorsal and deep veins of the penis* (Figs 210 and 211/6) as well as the *internal pudendal vein* (Figs 210 and 211/7) are invariably filled.

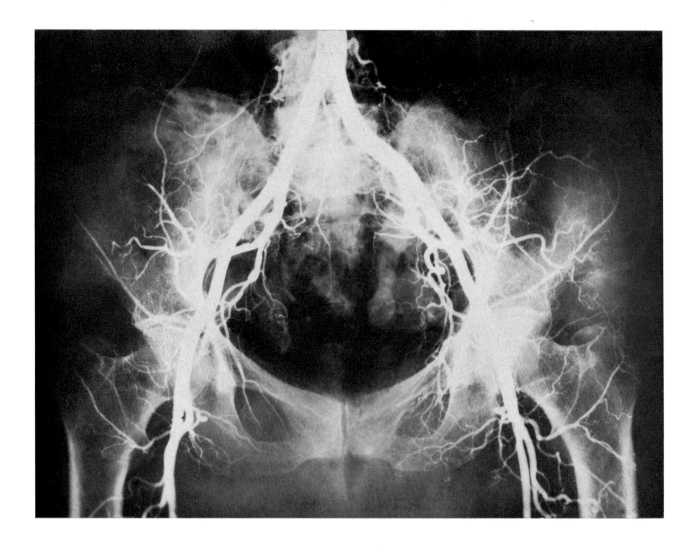

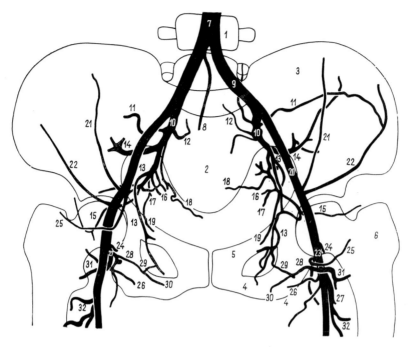

Fig. 192. The common iliac artery and its branches, I.
Anteroposterior view.

1. 4th lumbar vertebra
2. Sacrum
3. Ilium
4. Ischium
5. Pubic bone
6. Femur
7. Abdominal aorta
8. Median sacral artery
9. Common iliac artery
10. Internal iliac artery
11. Iliolumbar artery
12. Lateral sacral arteries

13. Obturator artery
14. Superior gluteal artery
15. Inferior gluteal artery
16. Superior vesical artery
17. Inferior vesical and middle
rectal arteries
18. Uterine artery
19. Internal pudendal artery
20. External iliac artery
21. Inferior epigastric artery
22. Deep circumflex iliac artery
23. Femoral artery

24. Superficial epigastric artery
25. Superficial circumflex iliac
artery
26. External pudendal artery
27. Deep femoral artery
28. Medial circumflex femoral
artery
29. Ascending branch
30. Deep branch
31. Ascending branch of lateral
circumflex femoral artery
32. Descending branch

311

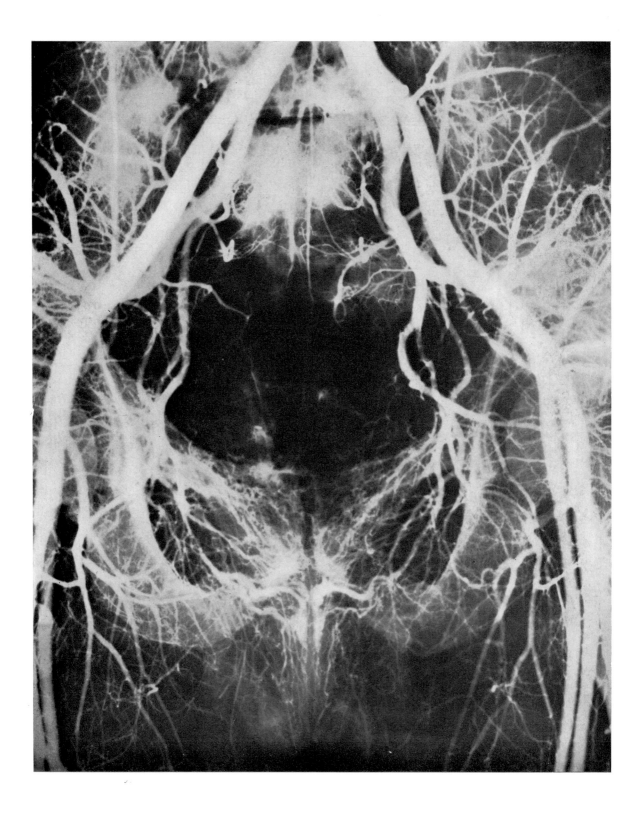

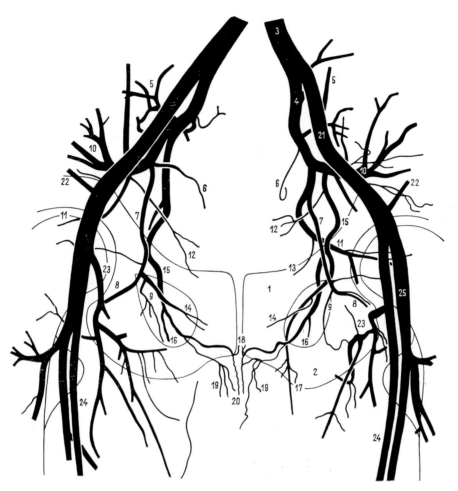

FIG. 193. The common iliac artery and its branches, II.
Arteries of the male genital organs. Anteroposterior view.

1. Pubic bone
2. Ischium
3. Common iliac artery
4. Internal iliac artery
5. Iliolumbar artery
6. Lateral sacral artery
7. Obturator artery
8. Acetabular branch
9. Pubic branch

10. Superior gluteal artery
11. Inferior gluteal artery
12. Superior vesical artery
13. Inferior vesical artery
14. Middle rectal artery
15. Internal pudendal artery
16. Inferior rectal artery
17. Perineal artery
18. Artery to the bulb of the penis

19. Deep artery of the penis
20. Dorsal artery of the penis
21. External iliac artery
22. Deep circumflex iliac
artery
23. Medial circumflex femoral
artery
24. Femoral artery
25. Deep femoral artery

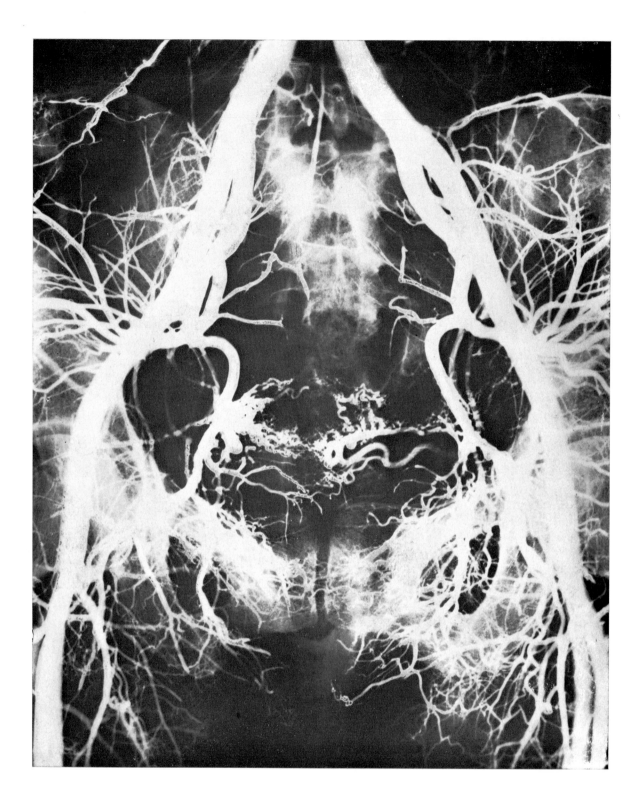

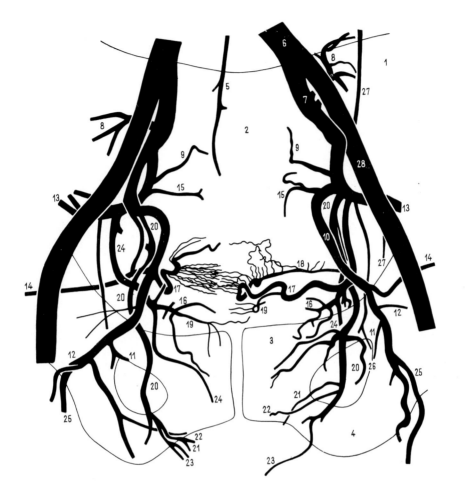

FIG. 194. The common iliac artery and its branches, III.
Arteries of the female genital organs. Anteroposterior view.

1. Ilium
2. Sacrum
3. Pubic bone
4. Ischium
5. Median sacral artery
6. Common iliac artery
7. Internal iliac artery
8. Iliolumbar artery
9. Lateral sacral arteries
10. Obturator artery

11. Pubic branch
12. Acetabular branch
13. Superior gluteal artery
14. Inferior gluteal artery
15. Superior vesical artery
16. Inferior vesical artery
17. Uterine artery
18. Tubal branch
19. Vaginal artery
20. Internal pudendal artery

21. Inferior rectal artery
22. Perineal artery
23. Posterior labial branches
24. Middle rectal artery
25. Posterior branch of obturator artery
26. Anterior branch
27. Ovarian artery
28. External iliac artery

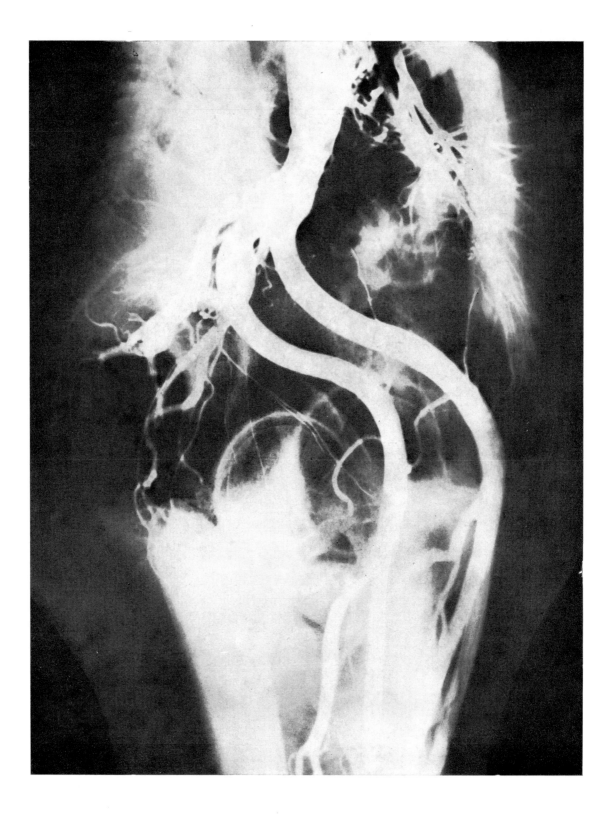

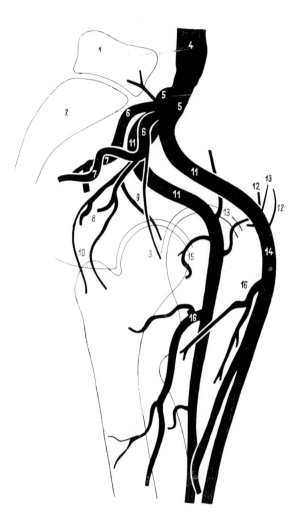

FIG. 195. The common iliac artery and its branches, IV.
Dextrosinistral view.

1. 5th lumbar vertebra
2. Sacrum
3. Femur
4. Abdominal aorta
5. Common iliac artery

6. Internal iliac artery
7. Superior gluteal artery
8. Inferior gluteal artery
9. Obturator artery
10. Internal pudendal artery
11. External iliac artery

12. Deep circumflex iliac artery
13. Inferior epigastric artery
14. Femoral artery
15. Superficial epigastric artery
16. Deep femoral artery

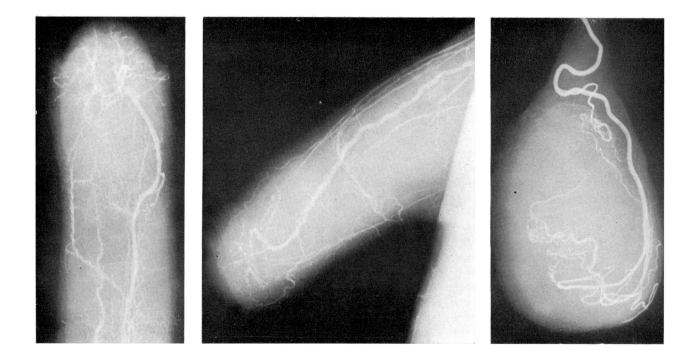
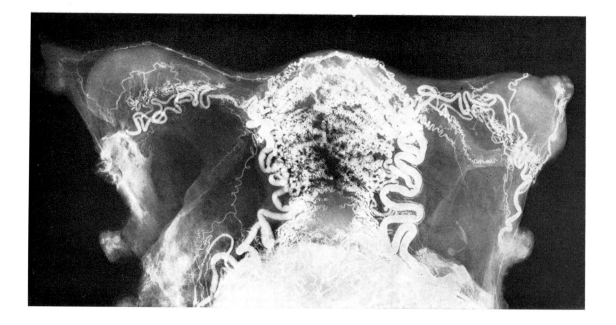

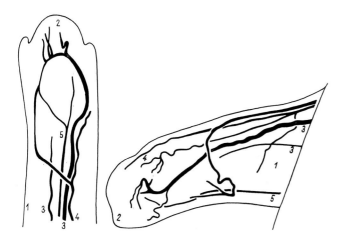

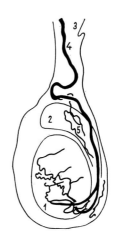

FIGS 196 and 197. Arteries of the penis. Anteroposterior
view (Fig. 196) and laterolateral view (Fig. 197).

1. Body of penis
2. Glans of penis
3. Deep artery of penis
4. Dorsal artery of penis
5. Urethral artery

FIG. 198. Arteries of the testicle and epididymis.
Anatomical preparation. Laterolateral view.

1. Testicle
2. Epididymis
3. Spermatic cord
4. Testicular artery
5. Epididymal artery

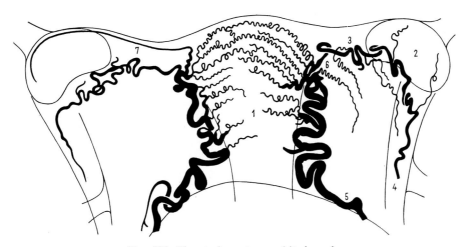

FIG. 199. The uterine artery and its branches.
Anatomical preparation. Anteroposterior view.

1. Uterus
2. Ovary
3. Uterine tube

4. Ligament of ovary
5. Uterine artery

6. Ovarian branch
7. Tubal branch
8. Ovarian artery

319

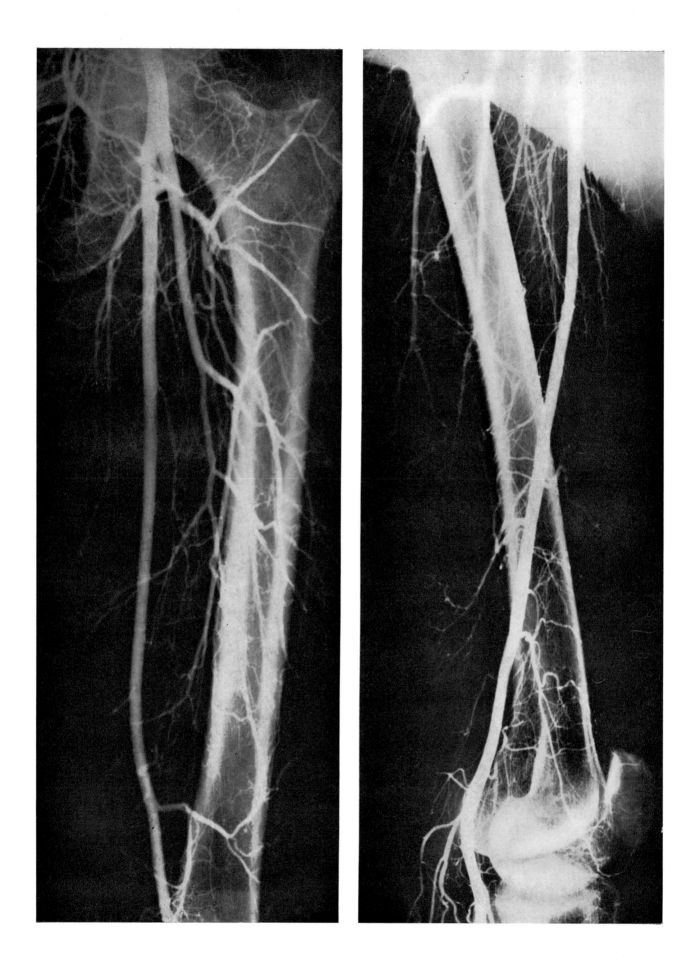

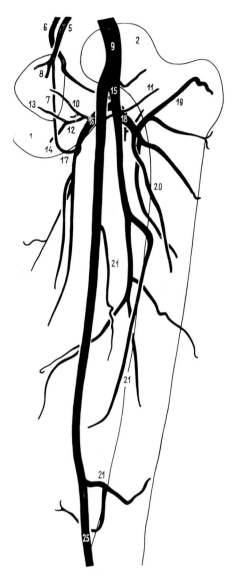
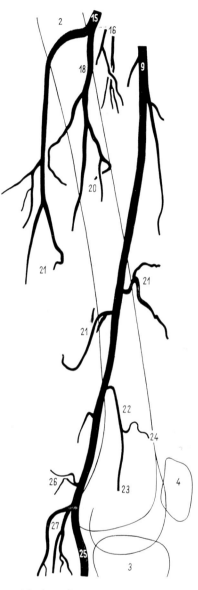

Figs 200 and 201. The femoral artery and its branches.
Anteroposterior view (Fig. 200) and dextrosinistral view (Fig. 201).

1. Ischium
2. Femur
3. Tibia
4. Patella
5. Obturator artery
6. Inferior gluteal artery
7. Anastomosis between obturator and deep femoral arteries
8. Pubic branch
9. Femoral artery
10. Superficial epigastric artery
11. Superficial circumflex iliac artery
12. External pudendal artery
13. Anterior labial branches
14. Inguinal branches
15. Deep femoral artery
16. Medial circumflex femoral artery
17. Ascending branch
18. Lateral circumflex femoral artery
19. Ascending branch
20. Descending branch
21. Perforating arteries
22. Descending genicular artery
23. Saphenous branch
24. Articular branches
25. Popliteal artery
26. Superior genicular arteries
27. Sural arteries

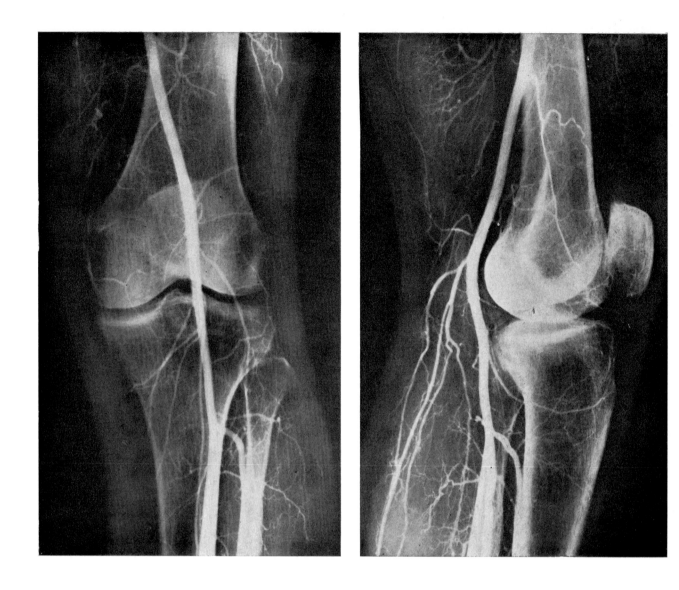

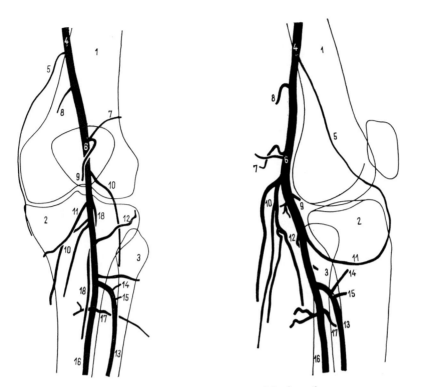

FIGS 202 and 203. Popliteal artery and its branches.
Anteroposterior view (Fig. 202) and dextrosinistral view (Fig. 203).

1. Femur
2. Tibia
3. Fibula
4. Femoral artery
5. Descending genicular artery
6. Popliteal artery
7. Lateral superior genicular artery

8. Medial superior genicular artery
9. Middle genicular artery
10. Sural arteries
11. Medial inferior genicular artery
12. Lateral inferior genicular artery

13. Anterior tibial artery
14. Posterior tibial recurrent artery
15. Anterior tibial recurrent artery
16. Posterior tibial artery
17. Circumflex fibular branch
18. Peroneal artery

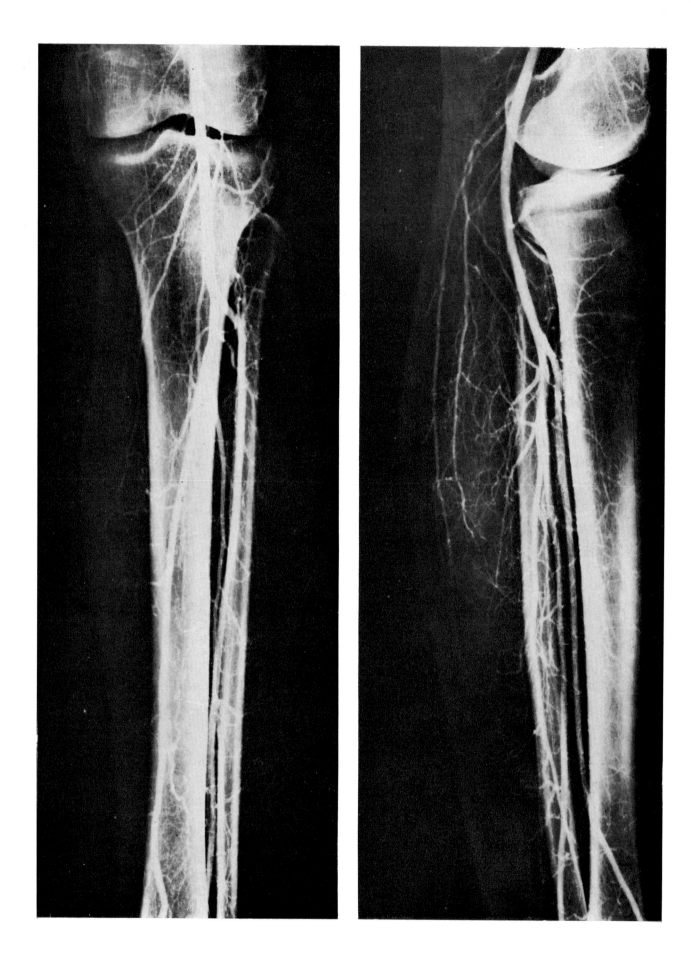

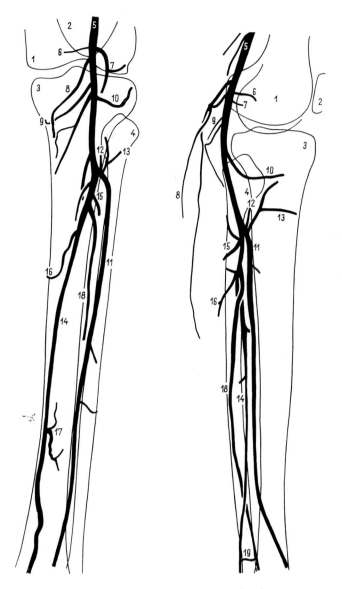

FIGS 204 and 205. Branches of the popliteal artery.
Anteroposterior view (Fig. 204) and dextrosinistral view (Fig. 205).

1. Femur
2. Patella
3. Tibia
4. Fibula
5. Popliteal artery
6. Medial superior genicular artery
7. Lateral superior genicular artery

8. Sural arteries
9. Medial inferior genicular artery
10. Lateral inferior genicular artery
11. Anterior tibial artery
12. Posterior tibial recurrent artery

13. Anterior tibial recurrent artery
14. Posterior tibial artery
15. Circumflex fibular branch
16. Muscular branch
17. Nutrient fibular artery
18. Peroneal artery
19. Communicating branch

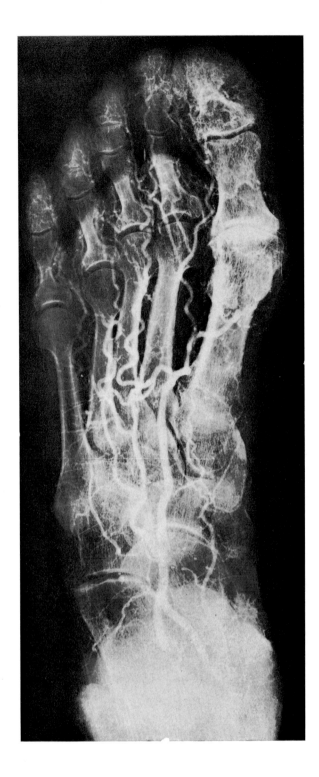

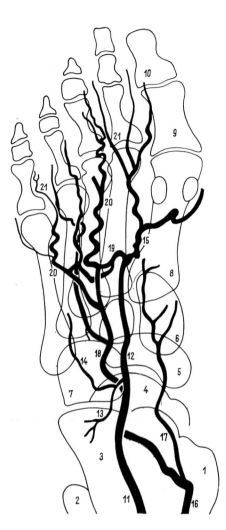

Fig. 206. The anterior and posterior tibial arteries and their branches, I.
Dorsoplantar view.

1. Tibia	*8*. Metatarsal bones	*15*. Deep plantar branch
2. Fibula	*9*. Proximal phalanges	*16*. Posterior tibial artery
3. Calcaneus	*10*. Distal phalanges	*17*. Medial plantar artery
4. Talus	*11*. Anterior tibial artery	*18*. Lateral plantar artery
5. Navicular bone	*12*. Dorsalis pedis artery	*19*. Plantar arch
6. Cuneiform bones	*13*. Lateral tarsal artery	*20*. Plantar metatarsal artery
7. Cuboid bone	*14*. Arcuate artery	*21*. Plantar digital arteries

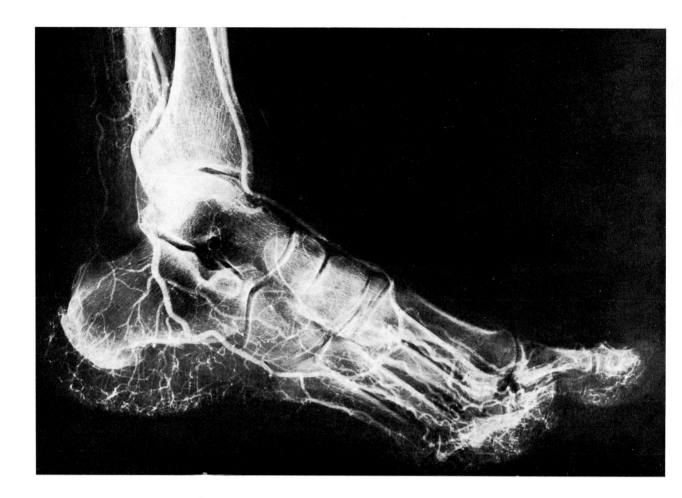

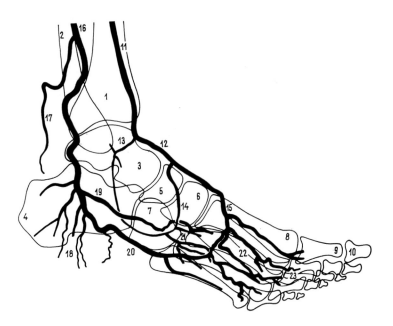

FIG. 207. The anterior and posterior tibial arteries and their branches, II.
Dextrosinistral view.

1. Tibia	*9.* Proximal phalanges	*17.* Medial malleolar branch
2. Fibula	*10.* Distal phalanges	*18.* Calcaneal branches
3. Talus	*11.* Anterior tibial artery	*19.* Medial plantar artery
4. Calcaneus	*12.* Dorsalis pedis artery	*20.* Lateral plantar artery
5. Navicular bone	*13.* Lateral tarsal artery	*21.* Dorsal metatarsal arteries
6. Cuneiform bones	*14.* Arcuate artery	*22.* Plantar metatarsal
7. Cuboid bone	*15.* Deep plantar branch	arteries
8. Metatarsal bones	*16.* Posterior tibial artery	*23.* Plantar digital arteries

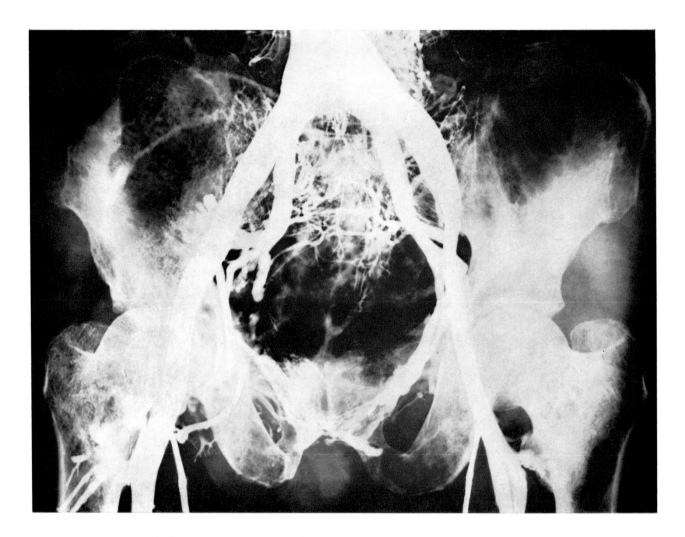

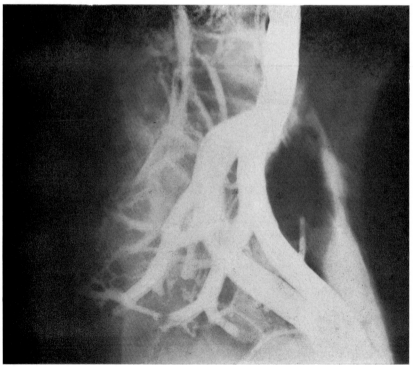

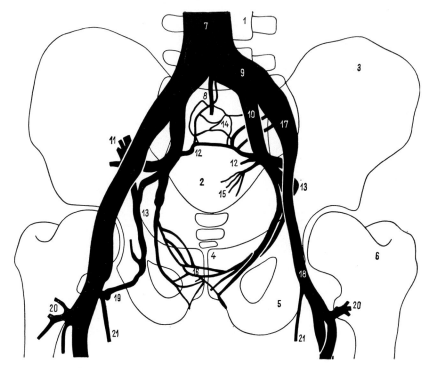

FIG. 208. The common iliac vein and its branches, I.
Anteroposterior view.

1. 4th lumbar vertebra
2. Sacrum
3. Ilium
4. Pubic bone
5. Ischium
6. Femur
7. Inferior vena cava
8. Median sacral vein

9. Common iliac vein
10. Internal iliac vein
11. Superior gluteal vein
12. Lateral sacral veins
13. Obturator vein
14. Sacral venous plexus
15. Vesical veins

16. Vesical and prostatic
    venous plexus
17. External iliac vein
18. Femoral vein
19. Medial circumflex femoral vein
20. Lateral circumflex femoral vein
21. Great saphenous vein

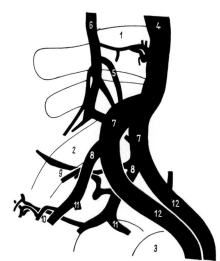

FIG. 209. The common iliac vein and its branches, II.
Dextrosinistral view.

1. 4th lumbar vertebra
2. Sacrum
3. Hip joints
4. Inferior vena cava

5. Lumbar veins
6. Vertebral venous plexus
7. Common iliac vein
8. Internal iliac vein

9. Superior gluteal vein
10. Inferior gluteal vein
11. Obturator vein
12. External iliac vein

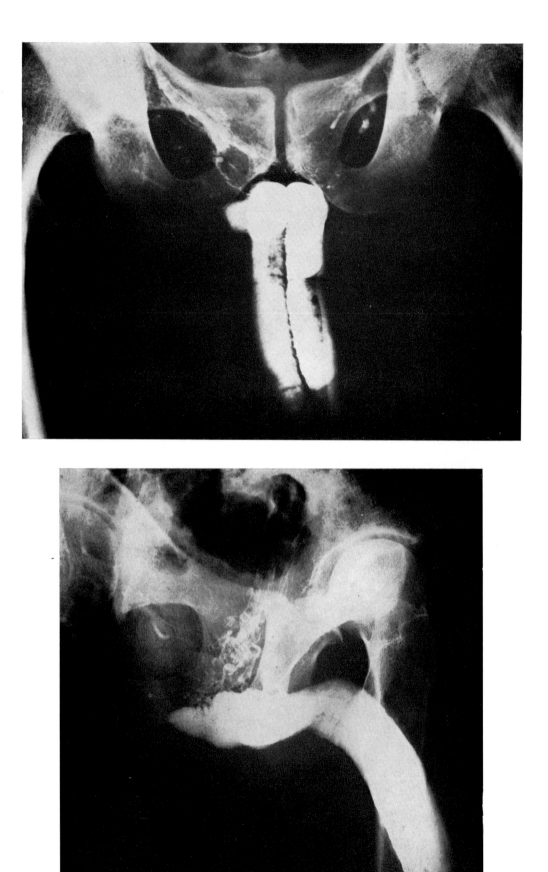

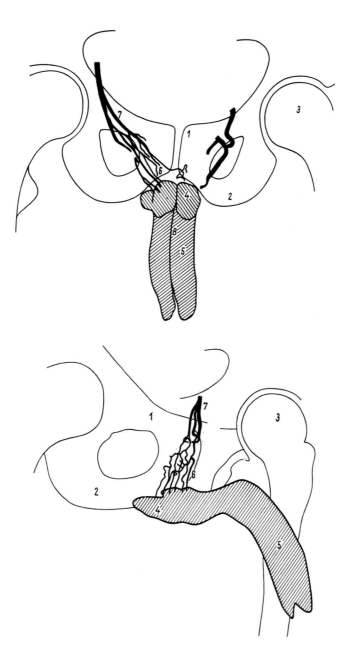

FIGS 210 and 211. Contrast filling of the cavernous body of the penis (cavernosography). Anteroposterior view (Fig. 210) and first oblique view (Fig. 211).

1. Pubic bone	*4.* Crura of penis	*7.* Prostatic venous plexus and
2. Ischium	*5.* Cavernous body of penis	internal pudendal vein
3. Femur	*6.* Deep veins of penis	*8.* Septum of the penis

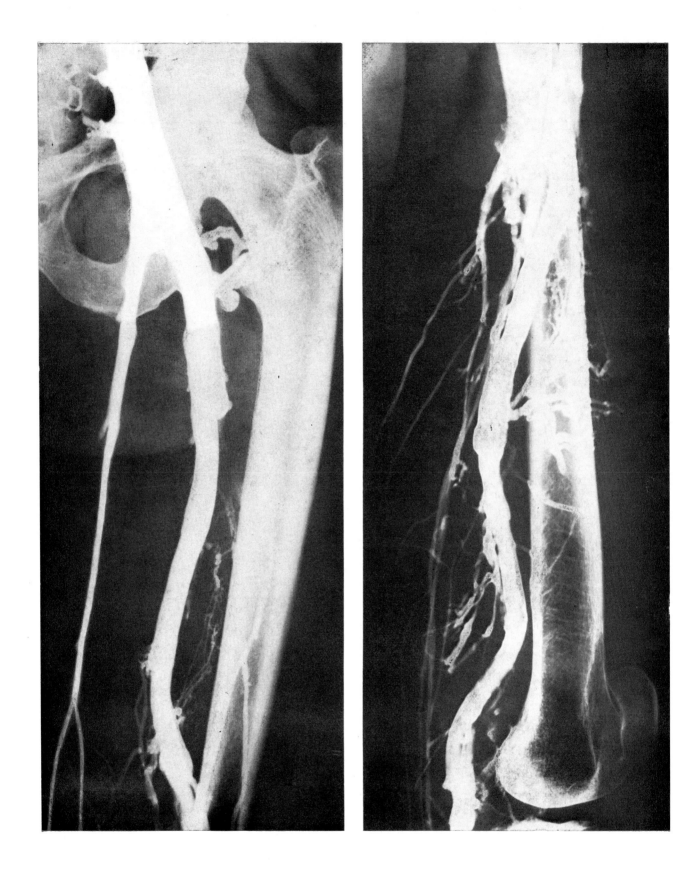

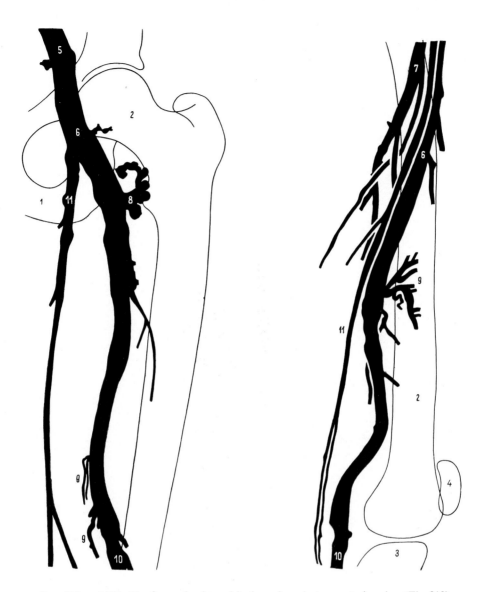

Figs 212 and 213. The femoral vein and its branches. Anteroposterior view (Fig. 212)
and dextrosinistral view (Fig. 213).

1. Ischium	*5.* External iliac vein	*9.* Perforating veins
2. Femur	*6.* Femoral vein	*10.* Popliteal vein
3. Tibia	*7.* Deep femoral vein	*11.* Great saphenous vein
4. Patella	*8.* Lateral circumflex femoral vein	

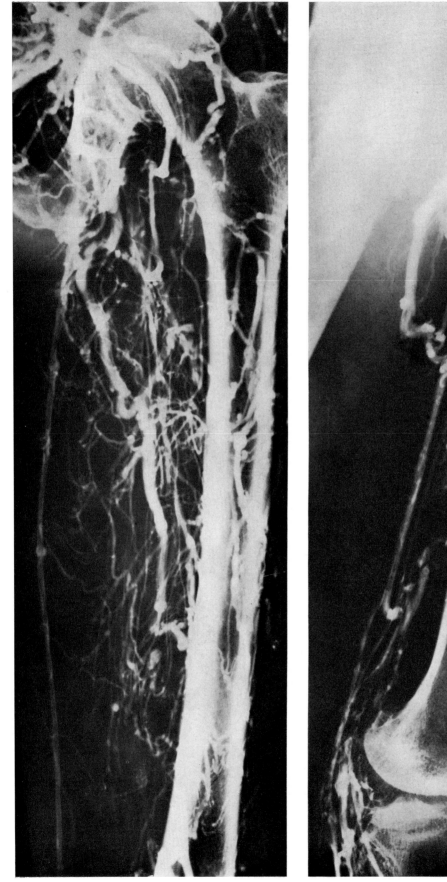
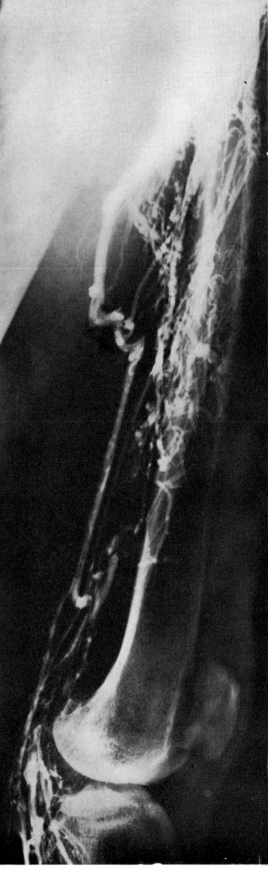

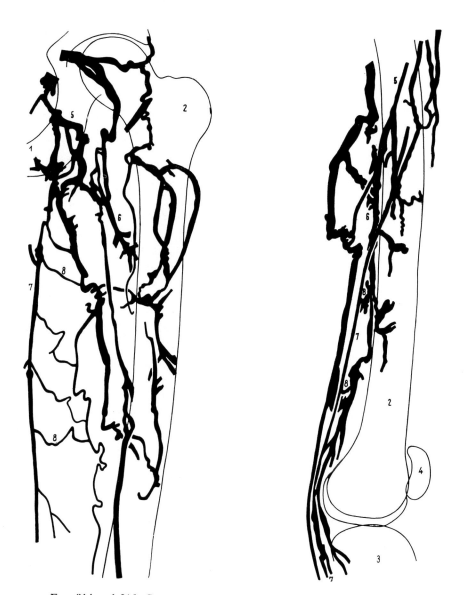

FIGS 214 and 215. Communicating branches of the great saphenous vein.
Anteroposterior view (Fig. 214) and dextrosinistral view (Fig. 215).

1. Ischium

2. Femur

3. Tibia

4. Patella

5. Femoral vein

6. Deep femoral vein

7. Great saphenous vein

8. Communicating veins

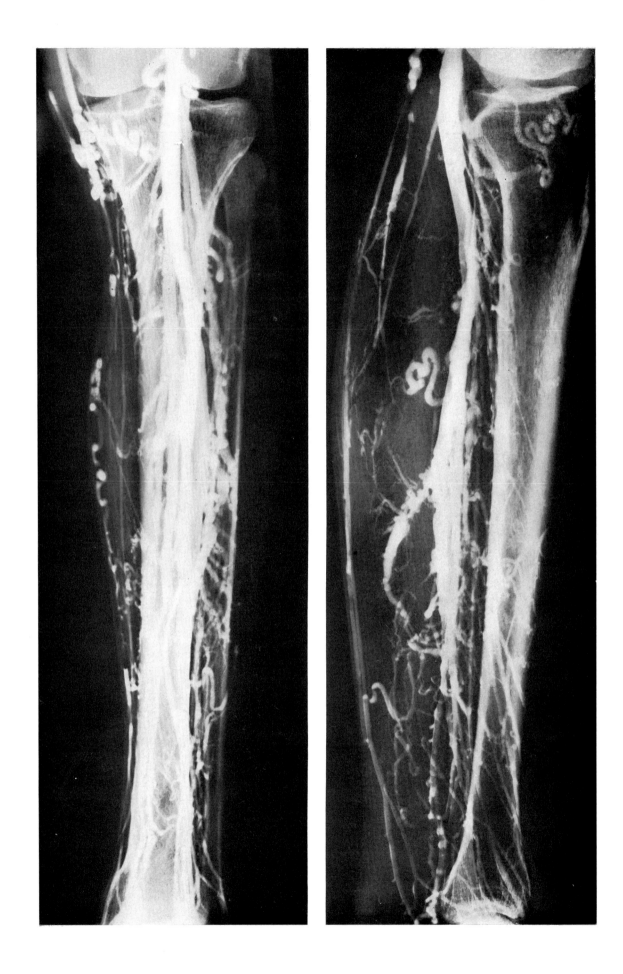

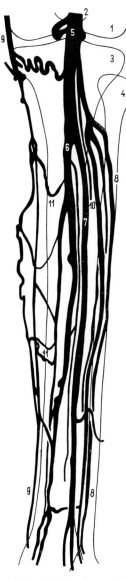
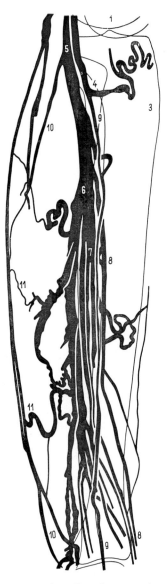

FIGS 216 and 217. The popliteal vein and its branches; great and small saphenous veins.
Anteroposterior view (Fig. 216) and dextrosinistral view (Fig. 217).

1. Femur	*5*. Popliteal vein	*8*. Anterior tibial veins
2. Patella	*6*. Posterior tibial veins	*9*. Great saphenous vein
3. Tibia	*7*. Peroneal veins	*10*. Small saphenous vein
4. Fibula		*11*. Communicating veins

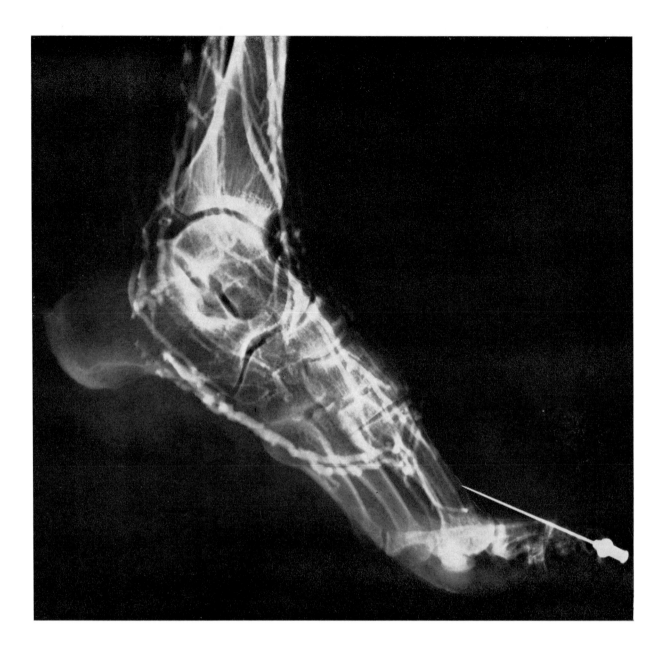

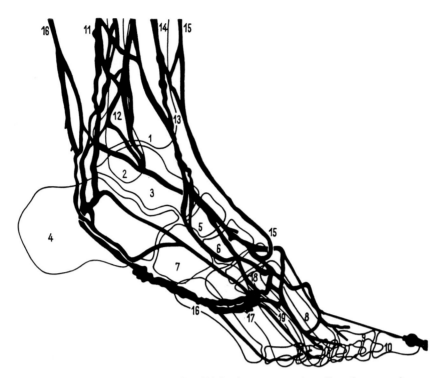

FIG. 218. Anterior and posterior tibial veins; great and small saphenous veins. Dextrosinistral view.

1. Tibia
2. Fibula
3. Talus
4. Calcaneus
5. Navicular bone
6. Cuneiform bones
7. Cuboid bone
8. Metatarsal bones

9. Proximal phalanges
10. Distal phalanges
11. Posterior tibial veins
12. Communicating veins
   (small saphenous vein —
   posterior tibial veins)
13. Communicating veins
   (great saphenous vein —
   anterior tibial veins)

14. Anterior tibial veins
15. Great saphenous vein
16. Small saphenous vein
17. Dorsal venous arch of
   the foot
18. Dorsal venous network
   of the foot
19. Dorsal metatarsal veins

APPENDIX

RADIOGRAPHIC MORPHOLOGY OF NEONATAL CIRCULATION

Circulation of the newborn differs essentially in several aspects from that of the adult (Fig. 219). Fresh blood is supplied to the embryo from the placenta by the *umbilical vein* (Figs 219/8, 221/31, 222/11) which runs in the ligamentum teres of the liver to the porta hepatis and divides there into two branches. One of them (*left umbilical vein,* Fig. 221/29) empties into the left branch of the portal vein, the other (*ductus venosus,* Figs 219/10, 221/30, 222/18) opens directly into the inferior vena cava.

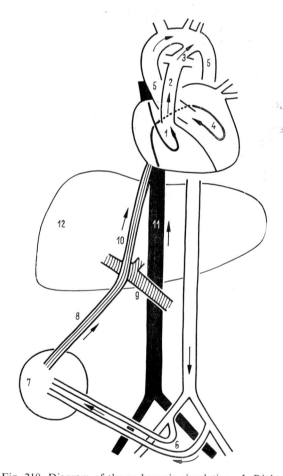

Fig. 219. Diagram of the embryonic circulation. *1.* Right atrium and ventricle; *2.* pulmonary trunk; *3.* ductus arteriosus; *4.* left atrium and ventricle; *5.* aorta; *6.* umbilical arteries; *7.* placenta; *8.* umbilical vein; *9.* portal vein; *10.* ductus venosus; *11.* inferior vena cava; *12.* liver.

Fresh oxygenated blood, mixed with the venous blood of the lower half of the body, passes from the right atrium through the foramen ovale to the left atrium, while most of the blood of the superior vena cava gains access to the pulmonary trunk. A mingling of the blood of the two systems is prevented by the valve situated at the orifice of the inferior vena cava (valvula venae cavae inferioris) which directs the flow of blood to the foramen ovale. Blood flowing from the superior vena cava is directed by the intervenous tubercle of the right ventricle. The *ductus arteriosus* (Fig. 219/3), extending from the division of the pulmonary trunk to the aortic arch, practically eliminates the lung from the circulation. The *umbilical arteries* (Figs 219/6, 220/25, 222/10), branches of the internal iliac artery, return the utilized embryonic blood to the maternal organism. These characteristic phenomena of embryonic circulation persist some time after the partition of the umbilical cord. Shunts existing between the arterial and the venous system of the newborn create circulatory conditions that are essentially different from those in adults. Differences of this kind may persist for a while without significance, while their persistence gives rise to anomalies with serious disturbances in certain cases.

The *umbilical vein* is usually not completely obliterated and can, therefore, be used for direct portography in adults (Bayly and Gonzalez 1964). The vein attains significance when the necessity of collateral portal circulation arises.

According to postmortem statistics, the *foramen ovale* remains open in 25 per cent of the adults (Haranghy 1966). This has no clinical significance as long as pressure in the left atrium is higher then in the right atrium since the aperture is closed by the valve of the foramen.

The unclosed *ductus arteriosus,* due to admixture of the systemic and the pulmonary circulation, gives rise to circulatory disturbances.

The *umbilical artery* atrophies in all cases. According to Dehalleux et al. (1966), this vessel is solitary in 0·7 to 1·1 per cent of the newborns.

Radiography. Conditions of neonatal circulation in vivo have been studied on the umbilical vein

(Hirvonen et al. 1961) and the umbilical artery alike (Kauffmann and Weisser 1963, Emmanouilides and Rein 1964). Postmortem angiograms by Schoenmackers and Vieten (1954), showed the cerebral, cardiac and renal vessels to be more developed than those of the other organs.

In *postmortem angiography*, contrast medium injected into the aorta (after the ligation of its proximal segment, Fig. 220), fills the embryonic arteries and, via the ductus arteriosus, also the branches of the pulmonary trunk. The pulmonary vascular apparatus is very little developed as long as the lungs are still airless. The embryonic brain and abdominal cavity are, on the other hand, well vascularized. Chiefly the physiological collaterals can be filled in the extremities. Even the palmar and plantar arterial arches can be visualized in full. The *umbilical arteries* (Fig. 229/25) are nearly as large as the common iliac artery. They turn over an angle of 180° about 1 cm after their origin and run to the navel.

In *venography* (Fig. 221), the veins of the trunk and the head, and the pulmonary veins can be filled after the ligation of the pulmonary trunk and the aorta. In the region of the pelvis and the shoulder girdle, retrograde filling of the veins of the extremities is prevented by the valves. The heart chambers fill entirely through the open foramen ovale. The right half of the heart is larger than the left. The pulmonary veins can be followed down to the minutest branches. The projection of the hepatic part of the inferior vena cava and that of the *ductus venosus* (Fig. 221/30) are superimposed. Both the portal and the caval system of vessels can be visualized in the liver. Running first medially, the *umbilical vein* (Fig. 221/31) describes an elbow-shaped downward bend and projected on the branches of the portal vessels, is lost in the umbilicus.

If the *entire embryonic vascular system* is filled (Fig. 222), the relative positions of the arteries and veins can be well followed. The inferior vena cava shows in the right upper part of the abdominal cavity, the *ductus venosus* (Fig. 222/18) appears in the middle, while the aorta is seen on the left side. The inferior vena cava lies in the right lower part of the abdominal cavity, while, to the left of it in the midline, the *umbilical vein* is (Fig. 222/11) projected on the summated shadows of the aorta and the portal vessels.

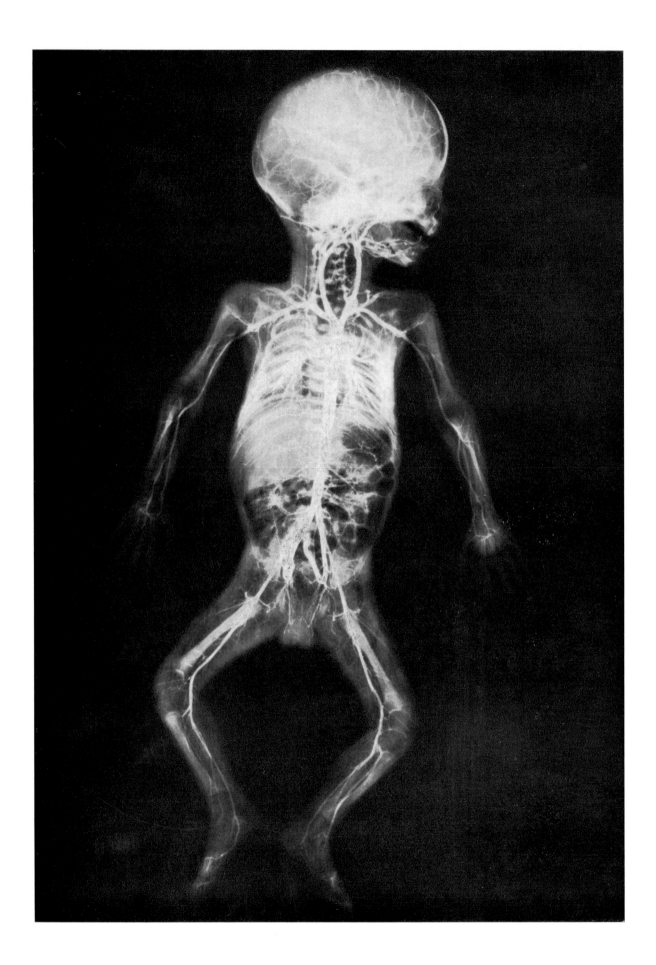

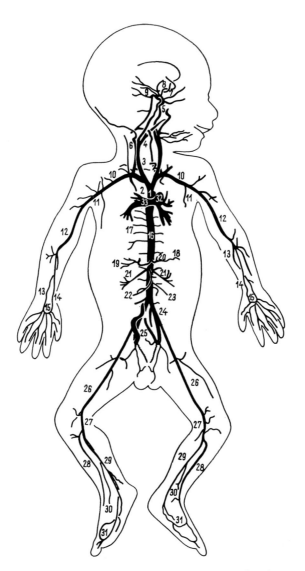

FIG. 220. Arteries of the newborn. Anteroposterior view.

1. Aorta
2. Brachiocephalic trunk
3. Common carotid artery
4. External carotid artery
5. Internal carotid artery
6. Vertebral artery
7. Anterior cerebral artery
8. Middle cerebral artery
9. Posterior cerebral artery
10. Subclavian artery
11. Axillary artery

12. Brachial artery
13. Ulnar artery
14. Radial artery
15. Deep palmar arch
16. Descending aorta
17. Posterior intercostal arteries
18. Splenic artery
19. Hepatic artery
20. Left gastric artery
21. Renal artery
22. Superior mesenteric artery

23. Inferior mesenteric artery
24. Common iliac artery
25. Umbilical artery
26. Femoral artery
27. Popliteal artery
28. Anterior tibial artery
29. Posterior tibial artery
30. Peroneal artery
31. Plantar arch
32. Left pulmonary artery
33. Right pulmonary artery

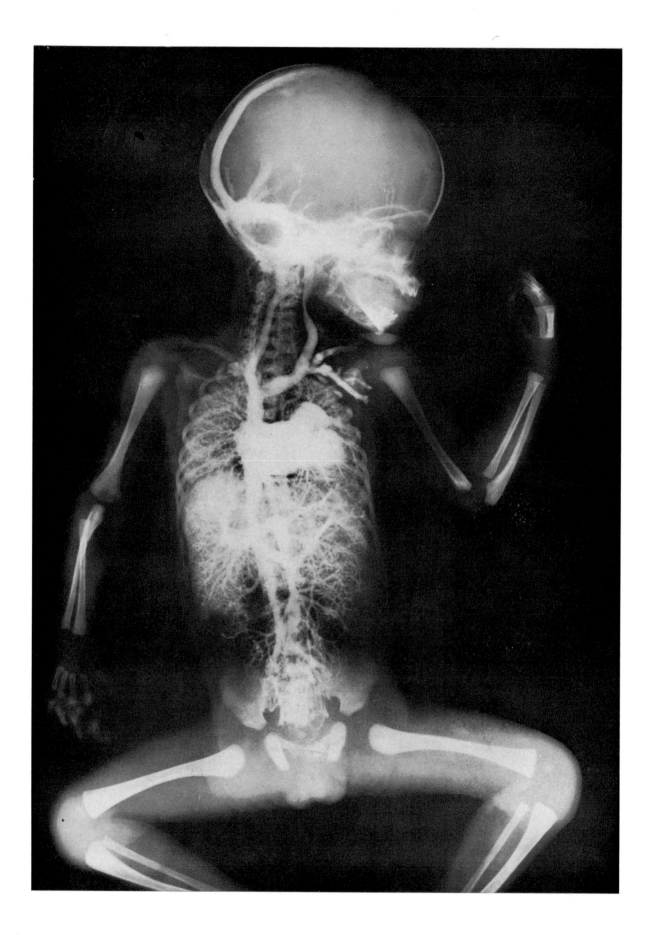

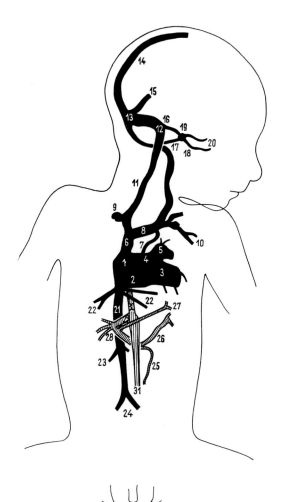

FIG. 221. Veins of the newborn. Anteroposterior view.

1. Right atrium	*11.* Internal jugular vein	*22.* Hepatic veins
2. Right ventricle	*12.* Sigmoid sinus	*23.* Renal vein
3. Left ventricle	*13.* Confluence of sinuses	*24.* Common iliac vein
4. Left atrium	*14.* Superior sagittal sinus	*25.* Inferior mesenteric vein
5. Pulmonary trunk	*15.* Straight sinus	*26.* Splenic vein
6. Superior vena cava	*16.* Superior petrosal sinus	*27.* Left branch of portal
7. Persistent left superior vena	*17.* Inferior petrosal sinus	vein
cava	*18.* Sphenoparietal sinus	*28.* Portal vein
8. Brachiocephalic vein	*19.* Cavernous sinus	*29.* Left umbilical vein
9. Subclavian vein	*20.* Ophthalmic vein	*30.* Ductus venosus
10. Axillary vein	*21.* Inferior vena cava	*31.* Umbilical vein

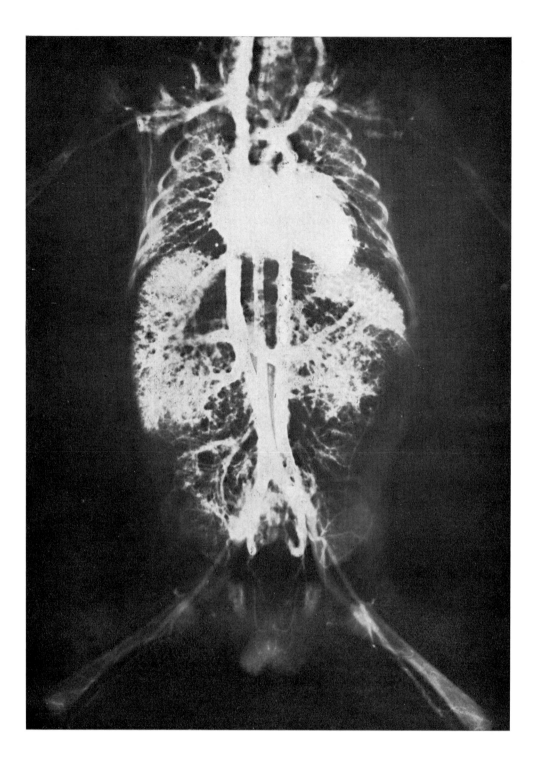

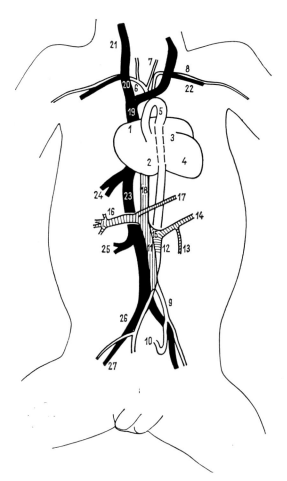

FIG. 222. Arteries and veins of the newborn. Anteroposterior view.

1. Right atrium	*10.* Umbilical artery	*19.* Superior vena cava
2. Right ventricle	*11.* Umbilical vein	*20.* Brachiocephalic vein
3. Left atrium	*12.* Superior mesenteric vein	*21.* Internal jugular vein
4. Left ventricle	*13.* Inferior mesenteric vein	*22.* Subclavian vein
5. Aorta	*14.* Splenic vein	*23.* Inferior vena cava
6. Brachiocephalic trunk	*15.* Portal vein	*24.* Hepatic veins
7. Common carotid artery	*16.* Right branch	*25.* Renal vein
8. Subclavian artery	*17.* Left branch	*26.* Common iliac vein
9. Common iliac artery	*18.* Ductus venosus	*27.* External iliac vein

REFERENCES

Generally used handbooks, monographs and anatomical atlases

ABRAMS, H. L. (1961) *Angiography*, vol. 2. Little, Brown & Co., Boston.

ADACHI, B. (1928) *Das Arteriensystem der Japaner*. Kenkyu-Sha, Kyoto.

ADACHI, B. (1933) *Das Venensystem der Japaner*. Kenkyu-Sha, Tokio.

ANSON, B. J. (1951) *An Atlas of Human Anatomy*. Saunders, Philadelphia—London.

BENNINGHOFF, A. (1930) Blutgefäße und Herz (in: *Handbuch der mikroskopischen Anatomie des Menschen*, 6. vol. Ed. by Möllendorff, W.). Springer, Berlin.

BRANTIGAN, O. (1963) *Clinical Anatomy*. McGraw-Hill Book Co., New York—Toronto—London.

GRAY's (1954) *Anatomy Descriptive and Applied*. (Ed. by Johnston, T. B. and Whillis, J.). Longmans, Green and Co., London—New York—Toronto.

HAYEK, H. (1958) Normale Anatomie (in: *Handbuch der Thoraxchirurgie*, vol. 1. Ed. by Derra, E.). Springer, Berlin—Göttingen—Heidelberg.

KISS, F. (1963) *Rendszeres bonctan* (Systematic Anatomy). Medicina Könyvkiadó, Budapest.

KISS, F. and SZENTÁGOTHAI, J. (1968) *Anatomischer Atlas des menschlichen Körpers*, vols 2—3. 35rd ed. Akadémiai Kiadó—Medicina Könyvkiadó, Budapest.

KOVÁTS, F. jr. and ZSEBŐK, Z. (1961) *The Thorax: A Radiographical and Anatomical Atlas*. 1st English ed. Akadémiai Kiadó, Budapest.

NAGY, D. (1965) *Radiological Anatomy*. Akadémiai Kiadó, Budapest.

NAGY, D. (1962) *Chirurgische Anatomie. Thorax*. Akadémiai Kiadó, Budapest.

PATURET, G. (1958) *Traité d'anatomie humaine*, vols 2—3. Masson, Paris.

PERNKOPF, E. (1937) *Topographische Anatomie des Menschen*, vols 1—4. Urban and Schwarzenberg, Berlin—Wien.

QUAIN, R. (1884) *Anatomy of the Arteries of Human Body*. Taylor and Walston, London.

RAUBER, A. and KOPSCH, FR. (1951) *Lehrbuch und Atlas der Anatomie des Menschen*. (Ed. by Kopsch, Fr.) vol. 2. Thieme, Leipzig.

SCHINZ, H. R., BAENSCH, W. E., FRIEDL, E. and UEHLINGER, E. (1952) *Lehrbuch der Röntgendiagnostik*, vols 3—4. Thieme, Stuttgart.

SCHOENMACKERS, J. and VIETEN, H. (1954) *Atlas postmortaler Angiogramme*. Thieme, Stuttgart.

SOBOTTA, J. (1911) *Az ember anatómiájának atlasza* (Atlas of Human Anatomy), vol. 3. Franklin-Társulat, Budapest.

TÖNDURY, G. (1959) *Angewandte und topographische Anatomie*. Thieme, Stuttgart.

TÖRŐ, I. and CSABA, GY. (1964) *Az ember normális és pathológiás fejlődése* (The Normal and Pathological development of Man). Akadémiai Kiadó, Budapest.

ZDANSKY, E. (1962) *Röntgendiagnostik des Herzens und der großen Gefäße*. Springer, Wien.

ZSEBŐK, Z. B. (1969) *Technic of Roentgenologic Investigations*. Akadémiai Kiadó, Budapest.

Introduction

BERBERICH, J. and HIRSCH, S. (1923) Die röntgenologische Darstellung der Arterien und Venen am lebenden Menschen. *Klin. Wschr.* **2**, 2226.

CASTELLANOS, A., PEREIAS, R. and GARCIA, A. (1937) La angiocardiografia radioopaca. *Arch. Soc. Estud. clin. Habana* **31**, 523.

CRAINICIANU, A. (1922) Anatomische Studien über die Coronararterien und experimentelle Untersuchungen über ihre Durchgängigkeit. *Virchows Arch. path. Anat.* **238**, 1.

CZMÓR, S. and URBÁNYI, E. (1939) Arteriographische Beobachtungen an den Herzgefäßen. *Röfo* **60**, 57.

DOS SANTOS, R. (1935) Phlébographie d'une veine cave inférieure suturée. *J. Urol. méd. chir.* **39**, 586.

FRIK, W. and PERSCH, W. F. (1969) Der Einfluß des Kontrastmitteltyps auf das Arterienkaliber. *Röfo* **111**, 620.

HASCHEK, E. and LINDENTHAL, O. TH. (1896) Ein Beitrag zur praktischen Verwertung der Photographie nach Röntgen. *Wien. klin. Wschr.* **9**, 63.

HEINZ, E. R. (1968) Stereoangiography. *Amer. J. Roentgenol.* **104**, 220.

JAMIN, F. and MERKEL, H. (1907) *Stereoskopische Röntgenbilder des Herzens*. Fischer, Jena.

LAUBRY, CH., COTTENOT, P., ROUTIER, D. and HEIM DE BALSAC, R. (1939) *Radiologie clinique du cœur et des gros vaisseaux*. Masson, Paris.

MONIZ, E. (1940) *Die zerebrale Arteriographie und Phlebographie*. Springer, Berlin.

MONIZ, E. and LIMA, P. A. (1927) L'encéphalographie artérielle: son importance dans la localisation des tumeurs cérébrales. *Rev. neurol.* **34**, 72.

RÁNKY, L. (1962) A collateralis háiózat kialakulása és jelentősége az elzáródásos verőérbetegségekben (Development and importance of the collateral network in obliterating arterial diseases). Thesis. Budapest.

ROBB, G. P. and STEINBERG, I. (1940) Visualization of chambers of the heart, pulmonary circulation and great vessels. Summary of methods and results. *J. Amer. med. Ass.* **114**, 474.

SCHOENMACKERS, J. (1960) Technik der postmortalen Angiographie mit Berücksichtigung verwandter Methoden postmortaler Gefäßdarstellung. *Ergebn. allg. Path. path. Anat.* **39**, 53.

SICARD, J. A. and FORESTIER, G. (1923) Injections intra-vasculaires d'huile iodée sous contrôle radiologique. *C. R. Soc. Biol. (Paris)* **88**, 1200.

SUTTON, D. (1962) *Arteriography.* Livingstone, Edinburgh—London.

TUCKER, J. L. and KREMENTZ, E. T. (1957) Anatomical corrosion specimen I. Heart-lung models prepared from dogs. *Anat. Rec.* **127**, 655.

VASTESAEGER, M. M., VAN DER STRAETEN, P. P. and BERNARD, R. M. (1955) La coronarographie hyper-stéréoscopique, méthode d'examen post mortem de la vascularisation myocardique et des anastomoses inter-coronariennes. *Acta cardiol. (Brux.)* **10**, 495.

The heart

ASSMANN, H. (1934) *Die klinische Röntgendiagnostik der inneren Krankheit.* Vogel, Berlin.

AYRES, S. M. and STEINBERG, I. (1963) Dextrorotation of heart: Angiocardiographic study of forty-one cases. *Circulation* **27**, 268.

BARGMANN, W. and DOERR, W. (1963) *Das Herz des Menschen,* vol. 1. Thieme, Stuttgart.

BAUER, D. F. DE (1944) *Heterotoxity. A bibliography of visceral transposition (s.i.v.c.) in man.* Duke Univ. School of Med., Michigan.

BELOU, P. (1934) *Revision anat. del sistema arterial.* Ateneo, Buenos Aires.

BENSON, P. A. and LACK, A. R. (1968) Anomalous aortic origin of left coronary artery. *Arch. Path.* **86**, 214.

BEUREN, A. J. (1966) *Die angiokardiographische Darstellung kongenitaler Herzfehler.* W. de Gruyter, Berlin.

BJÖRK, L. (1966) Angiographic demonstration of extra-cardial anastomoses to the coronary arteries. *Radiology* **87**, 274.

BLAND, E. F., WHITE, P. D. and GARLAND, J. (1933) Congenital anomalies of the coronary arteries: Report of an unusual case associated with cardiac hyperthrophy. *Amer. Heart J.* **8**, 787.

BOEREMA, I. and BLICKMAN, J. R. (1955) Reduced intra-thoracic circulation as an aid in angiocardiography. *J. thorac. Surg.* **30**, 129.

BOPP, F. (1947) *Über den Situs inversus.* Inaug. speech. Heidelberg.

BROOKS, H. ST. J. (1886) Two cases of an abnormal coronary artery of the heart arising from the pulmonary artery; with some remarks upon the effect of this anomaly in producing cirsoid dilatation of the vessels. *J. Anat. Physiol.* **20**, 26.

BRÜCKE, E. (1885) *Vorlesungen über Physiologie,* vol. 1.

CAMPBELL, M. and FORGÁCS, P. (1953) Laevocardia with transposition of the abdominal viscera. *Brit. Heart J.* **15**, 401.

CASTELLANOS, A. et al. (1953) Arterias coronarias super-numerias. *Rev. Cubana Cardiol.* (cit. by Hayek, H. 1958).

CASTELLANOS, A., PEREIAS, R. and GARCIA, A. (1937) La angiocardiografia radioopaca. *Arch. Soc. Estud. clin Habana* **31**, 523.

CEBALLOS, R. (1970) Unusually large communication between the coronary sinus and the left atrium without associated anomalies. Presentation of a case and review of the literature. *Ala. J. med. Sci.* **7**, 291.

CHENG, T. O. (1972) Arteriographic demonstration of intercoronary arterial anastomosis in living man with coronary artery disease. *Angiology* **23**, 76.

CHRISTIAENS, L., DUPUIS, C. and AVINÉE, J. C. (1964) Les dextroversions cardiaques. *Arch. Malad. Cœur* **57**, 809.

CORDIER, G. and HEFFEZ, A. (1952) Anatomie chirurgicale du sinus veineux coronaire du cœur. *C. R. Ass. Anat.* **39**, 817.

CORREIA, M. (1939) Les anastomoses entre les artères coronaires du cœur. *Presse méd.* **47**, 1542.

CRAINICIANU, A. (1922) Anatomische Studien über die Coronararterien und experimentelle Untersuchungen über ihre Durchgängigkeit. *Virchows Arch. path. Anat.* **1**, 238.

CZMÓR, S. and URBÁNYI, E. (1939) Arteriographische Beobachtungen an den Herzgefäßen. *Röfo* **60**, 57.

DAVIS, P. L. and COMPTON, V. (1962) Congenital absence of the left coronary artery. *Med. Tms (Lond.)* **90**, 293.

DEBIEC, B. (1967) Studies concerning the children extra-coronary blood supply of the atria. *Aggiorn. pediat.* **18**, 138.

DEBIERRE, C. (1908) La projection des orifices du cœur. *J. Anat. (Paris)* **34**, 1.

DIETLEN, H. (1909) Klinische Bedeutung der Verände-rungen am Zirkulationsapparat, insbesondere der wechselnden Herzgröße, bei verschiedenen Körper-stellungen (Liegen und Stehen). *Dtsch. Arch. klin. Med.* **97**, 132.

DIETLEN, H. (1910) Ergebnisse des medizinischen Röntgen-verfahrens für die Physiologie. *Ergebn. Physiol.* **10**, 598.

DIETLEN, H. (1923) *Herz und Gefäße im Röntgenbild.* Barth, Leipzig.

DI GIORGI, S. and GENSINI, G. G. (1965) The coronary venous pressure. *Cardiologia (Basel)* **46**, 337.

DI GUGLIELMO, L. and GUTTADAURO, M. (1954) Anatomic variations in the coronary arteries. *Acta radiol. (Stockh.)* **41**, 393.

DOERR, W. (1955) Die Mißbildungen des Herzens und der großen Gefäße (in: *Lehrbuch der spezielle pathologi-schen Anatomie.* Ed. by Kaufmann, E. and Staemmler, M.). W. de Gruyter, Berlin.

DUTRA, F. R. (1950) *Arch. intern. Med.* **85**, 955 (cit. by Doerr, W. 1955).

DÜX, A. (1967) *Koronarographie.* Thieme, Stuttgart.

DÜX, A., HASPER, M., HILGER, H. H., SCHAEDE, A. and THURN, P. (1964) Die Koronarsklerose im intravitalen Koronarogramm. *Röfo* **100**, 9.

DÜX, A., HILGER, H. H., SCHAEDE, A. and THURN, P. (1961) Zur Koronarographie. Koronararterienbefunde im se-lektiven Aorto- und Lävokardiogramm bei angebore-nen und erworbenen Herzfehlern. *Röfo* **95**, 1.

EDWARDS, J. E. (1958) Anomalous coronary arteries with special reference to arterio-venous-like communica-tions. *Circulation* **17**, 1001.

ESTES, E. H., jr., ENTMAN, M. L., DIXON II, H. B. and HACKEL, D. B. (1966) The vascular supply of the left ventricular wall. Anatomic observations, plus a hypo-thesis regarding acute events in coronary artery disease. *Amer. Heart J.* **71**, 58.

EVANS W. (1933) Congenital stenosis (coarctation), atresia, and interruption of the aortic arch. *Quart. J. Med.* **26**, 11.

FELDT, R. H., ONGLEY, P. A. and TITUS, J. L. (1965) Total coronary arterial circulation from pulmonary artery with survival to age seven. *Mayo Clin. Proc.* **40**, 539.

FORSSMANN, W. (1931) Über Kontrastdarstellung der Höh-len des lebenden rechten Herzens und der Lungen-schlagader. *Münch. med. Wschr.* **78**, 489.

GÄBERT, E. (1924) Die Lagebeziehungen des Oesophagus zur hinteren Herzfläche und ihre veränderungen durch Erweiterung des linken Vorhofes im Röntgenbild. *Röfo* **32**, 410.

GENSINI, G. G., BUONANNO, C. and PALACIO, A. (1967) Anatomy of the coronary circulation in living man. *Dis. Chest* **52**, 125.

GENSINI, G. G., DI GIORGI, S., COSKUN, O., PALACIO, A. and KELLY, A. E. (1965) Anatomy of the coronary circulation in living man. *Circulation* **31**, 778.

GENSINI, G. G., DI GIORGI, S. and MURAD-NETTO, S. (1963) Coronary venous occluded pressure. *Arch. Surg.* **86**, 72.

GOBEL, F. L., ANDERSON, C. F., BALTAXE, H. A., AMPLATZ, K. and WANG, Y. (1970) Shunts between the coronary and pulmonary arteries with normal origin of the coronary arteries. *Amer. J. Cardiol.* **25**, 655.

GROSS, L. (1921) *The Blood Supply to the Heart in its Anatomical and Clinical Aspects.* Hoeber, New York.

HACKENSELLNER, H. A. (1955a) Über akzessorische, von der Arteria pulmonalis abgehende Herzgefäße und ihre Bedeutung für das Verständnis der formalen Genese des Ursprungs einer oder beider Koronararterien von der Lungenschlagader. *Frankf. Z. Path.* **66**, 463.

HACKENSELLNER, H. A. (1955b) Koronaranomalien unter 1000 Herzen. *Anat. Anz.* **101**, 123.

HALLMAN, G. L., COOLEY, D. A. and SINGER, D. B. (1966) Congenital anomalies of the coronary arteries: anatomy, pathology and surgical treatment. *Surgery* **59**, 133.

HALPERN, M. H. (1954) Extracardiac anastomoses of the coronary arteries in the human newborn. *Anat. Rec.* **118**, 2.

HELLWING, E. (1967) Untersuchungen über die Variabilität der Länge der Arteria coronaria sinistra. *Thoraxchirurgie* **15**, 218.

HETTLER, M. G. (1965) Die semiselektive, bilaterale Koronarographie. Eine neue klinische Untersuchungsmethode der Herzkranzarterien. *Röfo* **103**, 3.

HETTLER, M. G. (1966) Zur normalen und pathologischen Anatomie der Koronararterienversorgung des Herzens im intravitalen Angiogramm. *Röfo* **105**, 480.

HILLESTAD, L. and EIE, H. (1971) Single coronary artery. *Acta med. scand.* **189**, 409.

HOLZMANN, M. (1952) Erkrankungen des Herzens und der Gefäße (in: *Lehrbuch der Röntgendiagnostik.* Ed. by Schinz, H. R., Baensch, W. E., Friedl, E. and Uehlinger, E.). Thieme, Stuttgart.

JAMES, TH. N. (1970) The delivery and distribution of coronary collateral circulation. *Dis. Chest* **58**, 183.

JAMESON, A. G., ELLIS, K. and LEVINE, O. R. (1963) Anomalous left coronary artery arising from pulmonary artery. *Brit. Heart J.* **25**, 251.

JANKER, R. (1936) Roentgen cinematography. *Amer. J. Roentgenol.* **36**, 384.

JANKER, R. (1950) Ein röntgenkinematographischer Film über die Kontrastdarstellung der Herzinnenräume und der großen Gefäße bei angeborenen Herzfehlern. *Langenbecks Arch. klin. Chir.* **226**, 322.

JOESSEL, G. (1889) *Lehrbuch der topographisch-chirurgischen Anatomie,* vol. 2/1. Cohen, Bonn.

JÖNSSON, G. (1948) Visualization of the coronary arteries: Preliminary report. *Radiology* **29**, 536.

KÁDÁR, F. (1956) Topographische Beziehungen zwischen arteriellen und venösen Kranzgefäße des Herzens. *Anat. Anz.* **103**, 113.

KÁDÁR, F. (1963) Die topographischen Verhältnisse zwischen Gefäßen und Muskelfasern des Herzens. *Anat. Anz.* **113**, 381.

KIRSCH, O. (1929) *Grundlagen der orthodiagraphischen Herzgröße und Thoraxbreitenbeurteilung im Kindesalter.* Karger, Berlin.

KLAFTEN, E. and PALUGYAY, J. (1927) Vergleichende Untersuchungen über Lage und Ausdehnung von Herz und Lunge in der Schwangerschaft und im Wochenbett. *Arch. Gynäk.* **131**, 347.

KNESE, K. H. (1963) Topographie des Herzens (in: *Das Herz des Menschen.* Ed. by Bargmann, W. and Doerr, W.). Thieme, Stuttgart.

KÖNIG, K. and BICHMANN, R. (1967) Vergleichende Untersuchungen zur röntgenologischen Herzvolumenbestimmung in Rücken- und Bauchlage. *Röfo* **107**, 38.

KREUZFUCHS, S. (1936) Aortenverlauf und Meßbarkeit im Kindesalter. *Röfo* **54**, 396.

LAUBRY, C., COTTENOT, P., ROUTIER, D. and HEIM DE BALSAC, R. (1935a) Étude anatomoradiologique du cœur et des gros vaisseaux par opafication. *J. Radiol. Électrol.* **19**, 195.

LAUBRY, C., COTTENOT, P., ROUTIER, D. and HEIM DE BALSAC, R. (1935b) Étude anatomoradiologique du cœur et des gros vaisseaux par opafication. *J. Radiol. Électrol.* **19**, 561.

LAUBRY, C., COTTENOT, P., ROUTIER, D. and HEIM DE BALSAC, R. (1935c) Étude anatomoradiologique du cœur et des gros vaisseaux par opafication. *J. Radiol. Électrol.* **19**, 700.

LAUBRY, C., COTTENOT, P., ROUTIER, D. and HAIM DE BALSAC, R. (1936) Étude anatomoradiologique du cœur et des gros vaisseaux par opafication. *J. Radiol. Électrol.* **20**, 65.

LAUX, G. and MARCHAL, G. (1948) Contribution à l'étude de la morphologie et de la topographie des veines du cœur. *Arch. Anat. (Strasbourg)* **31**, 179.

LILJESTRAND, G., LYSHOLM, E., NYLIN, G. and ZACHRISSON, C. (1939) The normal heart volume in man. *Amer. Heart J.* **17**, 406.

LIND, J. and WEGELIUS, C. (1952) Angiographic studies in children III (in: *Advances in Pediatrics,* vol. 5). Academic Press, New York.

LONGENECKER, C. G., REEMTSMA, K. and CREECH, O. (1961) Surgical implications of single coronary artery. *Amer. Heart J.* **61**, 382.

LUDWIG, H. (1939) Röntgenologische Beurteilung der Herzgröße. *Röfo* **59**, 139.

LUDWIG, H. (1941) Die röntgenologische Beurteilung der Herzgröße bei der Frau. *Röfo* **63**, 311.

LUSCHKA, H. (1858) Die fibrösen Bänder des menschlichen Herzbeutels. *Z. nation. Med.* **3**, 4.

MASON, D. G. and HUNTER, W. C. (1937) *Amer. J. Path.* **13**, 835 (cit. by Doerr, W. 1955).

MOBERG, A. (1967) Anastomoses between extracardiac vessels and coronary arteries via bronchial arteries. *Acta radiol. (Stockh.)* **6**, 177.

MOCHIZUKI, S. (1933) Vv. cordis (in: *Das Venensystem der Japaner.* Ed. by Adachi, B.). Kenkyu-Sha, Tokio.

MORITZ, F. (1931) Über die Norm der Größe und Form des Herzens beim Manne. *Dtsch. Arch. klin. Med.* **171**, 431.

MORITZ, F. (1932) Über die Norm der Größe und Form des Herzens beim Manne. *Dtsch. Arch. klin. Med.* **172**, 462.

MORITZ, F. (1934) Über die Norm der Größe und Form des Herzens beim Manne. *Dtsch. Arch. klin. Med.* **174**, 330.

MURRAY, R. M. (1963) Single coronary artery with fistulous communication. *Circulation* **28**, 437.

NAGY, D. (1949) Adatok a coronariák anatómiájához (Data to the anatomy of the coronary arteries). *Orv. Hetil.* **90**, 181.

NEIL, C. and MOUNSEY, P. (1958) Auscultation in patent ductus arteriosus. With a description of two fistulae simulating patent ductus. *Brit. Heart J.* **20**, 61.

NEUFELD, H. N., LESTER, R. G., ADAMS, P., jr., ANDERSON, R. C., LILLEHEI, C. W. and EDWARDS, J. E. (1961) Congenital communication of a coronary artery with a cardiac chamber of the pulmonary trunk (coronary artery, fistula). *Circulation* **24**, 171.

NORDENSTRÖM, B., OVENFORS, C. O. and TÖRNELL, G. (1962a) Coronary angiography in 100 cases of ischaemic heart disease. *Radiology* **78**, 714.

NORDENSTRÖM, B., OVENFORS, C. O. and TÖRNELL, G. (1962b) Myocardiography of the cardiac veins in coronary angiography. *Acta radiol. (Stockh.)* **57**, 11.

OGDEN, J. A. (1970) Congenital anomalies of the coronary arteries. *Amer. J. Cardiol.* **25**, 474.

OGDEN, J. A. and STANSEL, H. C., JR (1971) Roentgenographic manifestation of congenital coronary artery disease. *Amer. J. Roentgenol.* **113**, 538.

PALTAUF, R. (1901) Dextrocardie und Dextroversio cordis. *Wien. klin. Wschr.* **13**, 120.

PARSONNET, V. (1952) The anatomy of the veins of the human heart with special reference to normal anastomotic channels. *J. med. Soc. N. J.* **50**, 446.

PAULIN, S. (1964) Coronary Angiography. A technical, anatomic and clinical study. *Acta radiol. (Stockh.) Suppl.* **233.**

PETELENZ, T. (1965) Radiological picture of extracoronary arteries of myocardium in man. *Cardiologia (Basel)* **46**, 65.

PRIBBLE, R. H. (1961) Anatomic variations of the coronary arteries and their clinical significance. The third reported case of an unusual anomaly. *J. Indiana med. Ass.* **54**, 329.

RADNER, S. (1945) An attempt at the roentgenologic visualization of coronary blood vessels in man. *Acta radiol. (Stockh.)* **26**, 497.

RAGHIB, G., RUTTENBERG, H. D., ANDERSON, R. C., AMPLATZ, K., ADAMS, P., jr. and EDWARDS, J. E. (1965) Termination of left superior vena cava in left atrium, atrial septal defect, and absence of coronary sinus. *Circulation* **31**, 906.

RANNINGER, K., THILENIUS, O. G. and CASSELS, D. E. (1967) Angiographic diagnosis of an anomalous right coronary artery arising from the pulmonary artery. *Radiology* **88**, 29.

RAUTMANN, H. (1951) *Untersuchung und Beurteilung der röntgenologischen Herzgröße.* Kreislaufbücherei Bd. 9, Darmstadt.

ROBB, G. P. and STEINBERG, I. (1938) Visualization of the chambers of the heart. *Amer. J. Roentgenol.* **41**, 1.

ROBERTSON, H. F. (1930) Vascularization of the epicardial and periaortic fat pads. *Amer. J. Path.* **6**, 209.

ROBICSEK, F., SANGER, P. W., DAUGHERTY, H. K. and GALLUCCI, V. (1967) Origin of the anterior interventricular (descending) coronary artery and vein from the left mammary vessels. *J. thorac. cardiovasc. Surg.* **53**, 602.

ROESLER, H. (1934) The relation of the shape of the heart to the shape of the chest. *Amer. J. Roentgenol.* **32**, 464.

ROHRER, F. (1916) Volumenbestimmung von Körperhöhlen und Organen auf orthodiagraphischem Wege. *Röfo* **24**, 285.

ROHRER, F. (1929) Volumenbestimmung von Körperhöhlen bei Herzschlagverlangsamung. *Röfo* **40**, 519.

RUBLI, H. (1933/34) *Anat. Anz.* **77**, 169 (cit. by Doerr, W. 1955).

SABISTON, D. C., jr., PELLARGONIO, S. and TAUSSIG, H. B.

(1960) Myocardial infarction in infancy; surgical management of complication of congenital origin of left coronary artery from pulmonary artery. *J. thorac. cardiovasc. Surg.* **40**, 321.

SANDERS, W. J. and POORMAN, D. H. (1968) Complete situs inversus with anomalous right carotid artery. *Arch. Surg.* **96**, 86.

SARRAZIN, R. (1965) A propos des valvules du sinus coronaire. *Arch. Anat. path.* **13**, 124.

SCHAEDE, A. (1963) Die Bedeutung des Koronarogrammes bei den Koronarerkrankungen. *Verh. dtsch. Ges. inn. Med.* **69**, 624.

SCHLESINGER, M. J., ZOLE, P. M. and WESSLER, S. (1949) The conus artery: a third coronary artery. *Amer. Heart J.* **38**, 823.

SCHOENMACKERS, J. and VIETEN, H. (1954) Postmortale Angiogramme der Koronararterien bei angeborenen und erworbenen Herzfehlern. *Dtsch. med. Wschr.* **79**, 671.

SICK, C. (1885) Einige Untersuchungen über den Verlauf der Pleurablätter am Sternum, die Lage der arteriellen Herzklappen zur Brustwand und den Stand der rechten Herzfellkuppe. *Arch. Anat.* 324.

SMITH, J. C. (1950) Review of single coronary artery with report of 2 cases. *Circulation* **1**, 1168.

SMITH, S. C., ADAMS, D. F., HERMAN, M. V. and PAULIN, S. (1972) Coronary to bronchial anastomoses: An in vivo demonstration by selective coronary arteriography. *Radiology* **104**, 289.

SOLOFF, L. (1942) Anomalous coronary arteries from the pulmonary artery; report of a case in which left coronary artery arose from pulmonary artery. *Amer. Heart J.* **24**, 118.

SONES, F. M., jr. and SHIREY, E. K. (1962) Cine coronary arteriography. *Mod. Conc. cardiov. Dis.* **31**, 735.

SPALTEHOLZ, W. (1924) *Die Arterien der Herzwand.* Hirzel, Leipzig.

SPRER, F. (1959) Über quantitative formgerechte Darstellung der Herzhöhlen im Ausgußverfahren. *Z. Kreisl.-Forsch.* **408**, 501.

STEIN, H. L., HAGSTROM, J. W. C., EHLERS, K. H. and STEINBERG, I. (1965) Anomalous origin of the left coronary artery from the pulmonary artery. *Amer. J. Roentgenol.* **93**, 320.

STUMPF, P. (1928) Die Gestaltänderung des schlagenden Herzens im Röntgenbild. *Röfo* **38**, 1055.

SYMMERS, W. and CLAIR, ST. (1907) Note on accessory coronary arteries. *Inl Anat. & Physiology* **61**, 141.

SZEDERKÉNYI, GY. and STECZIK, A. (1964) Arteria pulmonalisból eredő coronariák (Coronary arteries arising from the pulmonary artery). *Morph. igazságü. Orv. Szle* **4**, 134.

TESCHENDORF, W. (1952) *Lehrbuch der röntgenologischen Differentialdiagnose der Erkrankungen der Brustorgane.* Thieme, Stuttgart.

TESTUT, L. and JACOB, O. (1921) *Traité d'anatomie topographique,* vol. 1. Doinet Cie, Paris.

THURN, P. (1958) Diagnose und Differentialdiagnose der Herzerkrankungen im Röntgenbild (in: *Lehrbuch der röntgenologischen Differentialdiagnostik,* vol. 1. Ed. by Teschendorf, W.). Thieme, Stuttgart.

THURN, P. and DÜX, A. (1963) Zur Methodik der Koronarographie. *Röntgen-Bl.* **16**, 97.

THURN, P., DÜX, A. and HILGER, H. H. (1963) Zur Physiologie und Morphologie des Koronarkreislaufes im Koronarogramm. *Röfo* **98**, 381.

TORI, G. (1952) Radiological visualization of the coronary sinus and coronary veins. *Acta radiol. (Stockh.)* **36**, 405.

VAN PRAAGH, R., VAN PRAAGH, S., VLAD, P. and KEITH,

354

J. D. (1964) Anatomic types of congenital dextrocardia. *Amer. J. Cardiol.* **13**, 510.

VESTERMARK, S. (1965) Single coronary artery. *Cardiologia (Basel)* **46**, 79.

VIRCHOW, H. (1913) Ein nach Form zusammengesetztes Thoraxskelett. *Arch. Anat. Entwickl.-Gesch.* 157.

VOSS, R. (1856) Cyanosis congenita. *Norsk. mag. f. laegevidensk.* **10**, 670.

WEGELIUS, C. and LIND, J. (1950) New trends in angiocardiography. *Med. Illust.* **4**, 135.

WHITE, N. K. and EDWARDS, J. E. (1948) Anomalies of the coronary arteries. Report of 4 cases. *Arch. Path.* **45**, 766.

WIGGERS, C. J. (1952) *Circulation* **5**, 609 (cit. by Thurn, P. 1958).

WILDER, R. J. and PERLMAN, A. (1964) Roentgenographic demonstration of anomalous left coronary artery arising from the pulmonary artery. *Amer. J. Roentgenol.* **91**, 511.

WILSON, P. (1965) An unusual variation of the coronary arteries. *Anat. Anz.* **116**, 299.

ZDANSKY, E. (1951) Zur Röntgenologie der Dynamik des Herzens. *Röfo* **75**, Special issue 179.

The thoracic arteries
(arteries of the greater circulation)

ALEKSANDROWICZ, R. (1967) Dwa przypadki braku pnia ramienno-głowowego. *Fol. Morph.* **16**, 235.

ÁLMOS, S. and LÓNYAI, T. (1962) A felső mediastinum verőér rendellenességei (Anomalies of the arteries of the upper mediastinum). *Magy. Radiol.* **15**, 92.

ARKIN, A. (1936) Double aortic arch with total persistence of the right and isthmus stenosis of the left arch: a new clinical and X-ray picture. *Amer. Heart J.* **11**, 44.

ASSMANN, H. (1934) *Die klinische Röntgendiagnostik der inneren Krankheiten.* Vogel, Berlin.

BAYFORD, D. (1789) An account of a singular case of obstructive deglutition. *Mem. med. Soc. Lond. Ed.* **2**, 27.

BEDFORD, D. E. and PARKINSON, J. (1936) Right-sided aortic arch (situs inversus aortae). *Brit. J. Radiol.* **9**, 776.

BENDER, F., MENGES, G. and SCHULZE, W. (1964) Seltene Verlaufsanomalie des Aortenbogens mit rechtsthoracaler Schleifenbildung. *Röfo* **100**, 203.

CASTELLANOS, A., PEREIAS, R. and GARCIA, A. (1937) La angiocardiografia radioopaca. *Arch. Soc. Estud. clin. Habana* **31**, 523.

DEFFRENNE, P. and VERNEY, R. (1968) L'aorte cervicale. *Ann. Radiol.* **11**, 525.

EDWARDS, J. E. (1948) Retro-esophageal segment of the left aortic arch, right ligamentum arteriosum and right descending aorta causing a congenital vascular ring about the trachea and esophagus. *Proc. Mayo Clin.* **108**, 23.

ENNABLI, E. (1967) Les artères intercostales. Thesis. Paris.

EXALTO, J., DICKE, W. K. and AALSMEER, W. C. (1950) Congenital stricture of trachea and esophagus by double aortic arch. *Arch. chir. neerl.* **2**, 170.

FLEISCHNER, F. (1926) Korrigierte Kreuzfuchssche Messung. *Röfo* **34**, 426.

FRANKE, H. (1950) Über Entwicklungs- und Lageanomalien der Aorta. *Röfo* **73**, 267.

FRAY, W. W. (1936) Right aortic arch. *Radiology* **26**, 27.

GROB, M. (1949) Über Anomalien des Aortenbogens und ihre entwicklungsgeschichtliche Genese. *Helv. paediat. Acta* **4**, 274.

GROLLMAN, J. H., BEDYNEK, J. L., HENDERSON, H. S. and HALL, R. J. (1968) Right aortic arch with an aberrant retro-esophageal innominate artery: Angiographic diagnosis. *Radiology* **90**, 782.

GROSSE-BROCKHOFF, F., LOTZKE, H., SCHAEDE, A. and THURN, P. (1954) Verlaufsanomalien des Aortenbogens und der Arcusgefäße. *Röfo* **80**, 314.

HEWITT, R. L. and BREWER, P. L. (1970) Aortic arch anomalies. *J. thorax. cardiovasc. Surg.* **60**, 746.

HOLZAPFEL, G. (1899) Ungewöhnlicher Ursprung und Verlauf der Arteria subclavia dextra. *Anat. Hefte* **12**, 369.

HOLZMANN, M. (1952) Erkrankungen des Herzens und der Gefäße (in: *Lehrbuch der Röntgendiagnostik.* Ed. by Schinz, H. R., Baensch, W. E., Friedel, E. and Uehlinger, E.). Thieme, Stuttgart.

JANKER, R. (1955) *Die Röntgenuntersuchung des Herzens und der großen Gefäße.* Girardet, Wuppertal—Elberfeld.

JÖNSSON, G., BRODEN, B. and KARNELL, J. (1951) Thoracic aortography. *Acta radiol. (Stockh.) Suppl.* **89**.

JUNGBLUT, R. (1966) Ursprungsvarietäten der großen Gefäße der Aortenbogens. *Röntgen-Bl.* **19**, 472.

KEATS, T. E. and MARTT, J. M. (1962) Tracheo-esophageal constriction produced by unusual combination of anomalies of great vessels: Case report. *Amer. Heart J.* **63**, 265.

KIS-VÁRDAY, GY. (1963) Érgyűrűt képező aortaív (Aortic arch forming a vessel ring). *Orv. Hetil.* **104**, 1953.

KRAUSE, W. (1880) *Anatomische Varietäten.* (cit. by Adachi, B. 1928).

KREUZFUCHS, S. (1936) Aortométrie précise. *Presse méd.* **44**, 2013.

LIECHTY, J. D., SHIELDS, T. W. and ANSON, B. J. (1957) Variations pertaining to aortic arches and their branches; with comments on surgically important types. *Quart. Bull. Northw. Univ. med. Sch.* **31**, 136.

(MAKRASHOV, A. M.) Макрашов, А. М. (1970) Функциональная анатомия колларатеральцых связей между венами позвоночника и прилежамних органов (Functional anatomy of the collateral circulation of the spinal cord and adjacent organs). *Arkh. Anat. Gistol. Embriol.* **59**, 104.

MURRAY, G. and BARON, M. G. (1971) Right aortic arch. *Circulation* **44**, 1137.

NEUHAUSER, E. B. D. (1946) The roentgendiagnosis of double aortic arch and other anomalies of the great vessels. *Amer. J. Roentgenol.* **56**, 1.

PÓKA, L. and NAGY, D. (1952) A nyelőcső artériái (Arteries of the oesophagus). *Sebész Nagygyűlés*, Eü. Kiadó, Budapest.

PONTES, A. P. DE (1963) Artérias supra-aorticas. Thesis. Rio de Janeiro.

REUTERWALL, O. (1922) Zur Frage der Arterienelastizität. *Virchows Arch. path. Anat.* **239**, 363.

SCHMIDT, J. (1957) Röntgendiagnostische Besonderheiten der Arteria lusoria. *Röfo* **86**, 188.

SHAPIRO, A. and ROBILLARD, G. (1950) The esophageal arteries (their configurational anatomy and variations in relation to surgery). *Ann. Surg.* **130**, 2.

SIMAY, A., VEZENDI, S. and DAYKA, Á. (1967) Pseudocoarctatio aortae. *Magy. Radiol.* **19**, 355.

SNELLING, C. E. and ERB, J. H. (1933) Double aortic arch. *Arch. Dis. Child.* **8**, 401.

SONDERS, C. R., PEARSON, C. M. and ADAMS, H. D. (1951) Aortic deformity simulating mediastinal tumor: subclinical form of coarctation. *Dis. Chest* **20**, 35.

STEINBERG, I. (1962) Anomalies (pseudocoarctation) of the arch of the aorta. *Amer. J. Roentgenol.* **88**, 73.

THURNER, B. (1951) Die angeborenen Anomalien der Aorta thoracica im Röntgenbild. *Wien. Z. inn. Med.* **32**, 132.

VAQUEZ, H. and BORDET, E. (1928) *Radiologie du cœur et des vaisseaux de la base.* Baillière, Paris.

WHEELER, P. C. and KEATS, T. E. (1963) The left aortic diverticulum as a component of a constricting vascular ring: Report of two neonatal cases. *Amer. J. Roentgenol.* **89**, 989.

ZDANSKY, E. (1932) Zur Kritik der Kreuzfuchsschen Aortenmessung. *Röfo* **45**, 40.

(ZGRIVETS, S. G.) Згивеч, С. Г. (1970) Клапаны непарной вены человека (Valves in the azygos vein in man). *Arkh. Anat. Gistol. Embriol.* **58**, 79.

The thoracic veins
(veins of the greater circulation)

ABRAMS, H. L. (1957) Vertebral and azygos systems and some variations in systematic venous return. *Radiology* **69**, 508.

BEUREN, A. J. (1966) *Die angiokardiographische Darstellung kongenitaler Herzfehler.* W. de Gruyter, Berlin.

BOZSÓ, G. (1966) Zur Röntgenanatomie der Vena azygos. *Röntgen-Bl.* **19**, 215.

CAMPBELL, M. and DEUCHAR, D. C. (1954) The left-sided superior vena cava. *Brit. Heart J.* **16**, 423.

CARLSON, H. A. (1934) Obstruction of superior venacava; experimental study. *Arch. Surg.* **29**, 669.

CHEVREL, J. P., HUREAU, J., ALEXANDRE, J. H. and LASSAU, J. P. (1965) Deux nouvelles voies de drainage veineux du corps thyroïde. *Arch. Anat. path.* **13**, 97.

CHLYVITCH, B. (1932) Cas de veine supérieure gauche avec persistance du segment transverse et de la corne gauche du sinus réumiens. Embouchure de la veine sushépatique gauche dans l'oreillette droite. *Ann. Anat. path.* **9**, 1053.

DERRA, E., LOOGEN, F. and SATTER, P. (1965) Anomalien der unteren Hohlvene. *Dtsch. med. Wschr.* **90**, 689.

DOERR, W. (1955) Die Mißbildungen des Herzens und der großen Gefäße (in: *Lehrbuch der speziellen pathologischen Anatomie.* Ed. by Kaufmann, E. and Staemmler, M.). W. de Gruyter, Berlin.

DREWES, J. (1963) *Die Phlebographie der oberen Körperhälfte.* Springer, Berlin—Göttingen—Heidelberg.

DREWES, J. and SELING, A. (1966) Persistieren der linken oberen Hohlvene mit Doppelung der linken Vena subclavia. *Röfo* **104**, 677.

DÜNNER, L. and CALM, A. (1923) Die Röntgenologie der Gefäße, insbesondere Lungengefäße am lebenden Menschen. *Röfo* **31**, 635.

DÜX, A., BÜCHELER, E., DOHMEN, M. and FELIX, R. (1967) Die direkte retrograde Azygographie. *Röfo* **107**, 310.

ERDÉLYI, M. (1944) *Röntgenrétegvizsgálatok* (Tomographic examinations). Egyetemi Nyomda, Budapest.

FRIEDRICH, A., BING, R. J. and BLOUNT, S. G., jr. (1950) Physiological studies in congenital heart disease. IX. Circulatory dynamics in the anomalies of venous return to the heart including pulmonary arteriovenous fistula. *Bull. Johns Hopk. Hosp.* **86**, 20.

GARDNER, F. and ORAM, S. (1953) Persistent left superior vena draining pulmonary veins. *Brit. Heart J.* **15**, 305.

GENSINI, G. G., CALDINI, P., CASACCIO, F. and BLOUNT, S. G. (1959) Persistent left superior vena cava. *Amer. J. Cardiol.* **4**, 677.

GLASGOW, E. F. (1963) Persistent left superior vena cava with bilateral azygos system in adult. *Brit. Heart J.* **25**, 264.

GOERTTLER, KL. (1958) Normale und pathologische Entwicklung des menschlichen Herzens. Thesis. Kiel 1957 (in: *Zwanglose Abhandlungen auf dem Gebiete der normalen und pathologischen Anatomie).* Thieme, Stuttgart.

GROSSE-BROCKHOFF, F., LOOGEN, F. and SCHAEDE, A. (1960) Angeborene Herz- und Gefäßmißbildungen (in: *Handbuch der inneren Medizin*, vol. 9/3. Ed. by Bergmann, G., Frey, F. and Schiegk, H.). Springer, Berlin—Göttingen—Heidelberg.

HAGEDORN, A. (1954) *Venenanomalie und Mißbildung des Vorhofes bei einem 15jährigen Jungen.* Inaug. speech. Berlin.

HALPERT, B. and COMAN, F. D. (1930) Complete situs inversus of the vena cava superior. *Amer. J. Path.* **6**, 191.

HOLZMANN, M. (1952) Erkrankungen des Herzens und der Gefäße (in: *Lehrbuch der Röntgendiagnostik.* Ed. by Schinz, H. R., Baensch, W. E., Friedl, E. and Uehlinger, E.). Thieme, Stuttgart.

JAKUBCZIK, I. (1963) Seltene Anomalien der großen intrathoracalen Blut- und Lymphgefäßstämme. *Anat. Anz.* **112**, 257.

JONNESCO, T. (1914) Appareil digestif (in: *Anatomie humaine*, vol. 4/1. Ed. by Poirier, P. and Charpy, A.). Masson, Paris.

KNAPPE, J., HASCHE, E., EGER, H., FIEHRING, H., ERBSTÖSSER, H. and GIEGLER, I. (1968) Seltene Verlaufsanomalien intrathoracaler Körpervenen und Lungenvenen. *Röfo* **109**, 309.

KUBIK, ST. and MÜNTENER, M. (1971) Bronchusanomalien: tracheale, eparterielle und präeparterielle Bronchi. *Röfo* **114**, 147.

LAND, R. E., (1972) The relationship of the left subclavian vein to the clavicle. *J. thorac. cardiovasc. Surg.* **63**, 564.

(MAKRASHOV, A. M.) Макрашов, А. М. (1970) Функциональная анатомия коллатеральцых связей между венами позвоночника и прилежамних органов Functional anatomy of the collateral circulation ot the spinal cord and adjacent organs). *Arkh. Anat. Gistol. Embriol.* **59**, 104.

NAKAYAMA, T. and KITAGAWA, T. (1965) Pri la vejnoj de la ezofago. *Okajimas Folia anat. jap.* **40**, 807.

REED, A. F. (1938) A left superior vena cava draining the blood from a closed coronary sinus. *J. Anat.* **73**, 195.

ROMINGER, C. J. (1958) The normal axillary venogram. *Amer. J. Roentgenol.* **80**, 217.

SAXENA, S. K. (1965) A case of bilateral superior vena cava with bilateral azygos vein. *J. anat. Soc. India* **14**, 37.

SCHOBINGER, R. A. (1960) *Intraosseous Venography.* Grune and Stratton, New York.

SGALITZER, M., KOLLERT, V. and DEMEL, R. (1931) Kontrastdarstellung der Venen im Röntgenbilde. *Klin. Wschr.* **10**, 1659.

SICARD, J. A. and FORESTIER, G. (1922) Méthode générale d'exploration radiologique par l'huile iodée (lipidol). *Bull. Soc. méd. Hôp.* **46**, 463.

STEINBERG, I. (1962) Dilatation of the hemiazygos veins in superior venae cavae occlusion simulating mediastinal tumour. *Amer. J. Roentgenol.* **87**, 248.

SÜSSE, H. J. and AURIG, G. (1954) Das transosseale Venogramm der Venae intercostales, der Vena azygos und der Vena thoracica interna. *Röfo* **81**, 335.

SWART, B. (1959) Die Breite der Vena azygos als röntgendiagnostisches Kriterium. *Röfo* **91**, 416.

SZABÓ, I. and SIMAI, A. (1972) A kis- és nagyvérkör közötti anastomozisok post mortem angiogrammon (Anastomoses between the lesser and greater circulation in postmortem angiograms). *Tuberk. és Tüdőbetegs.* **25**, 16. (In Hungarian).

SZÜCS, S. (1964) Mellkasi intraossealis venographia (Thoracic intraosseals venography). Thesis. Budapest.

SZÜCS, S., MISKOVITS, G. and GAÁL, J. (1960) Durch Azygographie verifizierter lobus venae azygos. *Radiol. diagn. (Berl.)* **1**, 120.

Tarkiainen, E. (1967) Intercostal vein meningorachidography. A technical, anatomical and clinical study. *Acta radiol. (Stockh.) Suppl.* **271.**

Tori, G. (1954) The radiological demonstration of the azygos and other thoraco-abdominal veins in the living. *Brit. Heart J.* **27,** 16.

Winter, F. S. (1954) Persistent left superior vena cava. *Angiology* **5,** 90.

Wishart, D. L. (1972) Normal azygos vein in children. *Radiology* **104,** 115.

Zágreanu, D., Rádulescu, D. and Vlaicu, R. (1964) Contribution au diagnostique des anomalies veineuses supérieures. *Cor et vasa (Praha)* **6,** 49.

Blood vessels of the lung

Abesi, E. J. (1966) Abnormaler Ursprung einer Bronchialarterie. *Anat. Anz.* **119,** 104.

Abrams, H. L. (1957) Vertebral and azygos venous systems, and some variations in systematic venous return. *Radiology* **69,** 508.

Anderson, R. C., Adams, P. and Burke, B. (1961) Anomalous inferior vena cava with azygos continuation (infrahepatic interruption of the inferior vena cava). *J. Pediat.* **59,** 370.

Appleton, A. B. (1944) Segments and blood vessels of the lung. *Lancet* **2,** 592.

Appleton, A. B. (1945) The arteries and veins of the lungs. *J. Anat.* **79,** 97.

Assmann, H. (1911) Das anatomische Substrat der normalen Lungenzeichnung im Röntgenbild. *Röfo* **17,** 141.

Aviado, D. M. (1965) *The Lung Circulation.* Pergamon Press, Oxford—London—Edinburgh—New York—Paris—Frankfurt.

Aviado, D. M., Daly, M., B. Lee, C. Y. De and Schmidt, C. F. (1961) The contribution of the bronchial circulation to the venous admixture in pulmonary venous blood. *J. Physiol. (Lond)* **155,** 602.

Bell, A. L. L., jr., Shimomura, S., Guthrie, W. J., Hempel, H. F., Fritzportrick, H. F. and Begg, Ch. F. (1959) Wedge pulmonary arteriography, its application in congenital and acquired heart disease. *Radiology* **73,** 566.

Bhagvant, R. K., Carlson, R. G., Ferlic, R. M., Sellers, R. D. and Lillehei, C. W. (1967) Partial anomalous pulmonary venous connections. *Amer. J. Cardiol.* **20,** 91.

Bikfalvi, A., Scheifer, D., Becker, H. and Arold, R. (1967) Untersuchungen zur arteriellen Versorgung der Trachea. *Med. Welt* **18,** 693.

Björk, L. (1966) Anastomoses between the coronary and bronchial arteries. *Acta radiol. (Stockh.)* **4,** 93.

Blake, Hu. A., Hall, R. J. and Manion, W. C. (1965) Anomalous pulmonary venous return. *Circulation* **32,** 406.

Bland, E. F., White, P. D. and Garland, J. (1933) Congenital anomalies of coronary arteries: Report of an unusual case associated with cardiac hypertrophy. *Amer. Heart J.* **8,** 787.

Bogsch, A. (1958) Beiträge zu den Röntgen-Darstellungsmöglichkeiten der Pulmonalarterien. *Röfo* **88,** 401.

Bolt, W., Forssmann, W. and Rink, H. (1957) *Selektive Angiographie in der praeoperativen Diagnostik und in der inneren Klinik.* Thieme, Stuttgart.

Botenga, A. S. J. (1968) Selectieve arteriografie van arteria bronchialis en intercostalis. *Ned. T. Geneesk.* **112,** 1119.

Boyden, E. A. (1955) *Segmental Anatomy of the Lungs.* McGraw-Hill, New York.

Boyden, E. A. and Hartmann, J. (1946) *Amer. J. Anat.* **79,** 321 (cit. by Hornykiewytsch, Th. and Stender, H. St. 1954).

Boyden, E. A. and Scannel, J. G. (1946) An analysis of variations in the bronchovascular pattern of the right upper lobe of fifty lungs. *Amer. J. Anat.* **79,** 321.

Brantigan, O. C. (1952) Anomalies of the pulmonary veins. Their surgical significance. *Dis. Chest* **21,** 174.

Brooks, H. St. J. (1886) Two cases of abnormal coronary artery of heart arising from pulmonary artery with some remarks upon effect of this anomaly in producing cirsoid dilatation of vessels. *J. Anat. Physiol.* **20,** 26.

Brown, S., McCarthy, J. E. and Eine, A. (1939) The pulmonary artery. A roentgenographic and roentgenkymographic study. *Radiology* **32,** 175.

Bruwer, A., Clagett, O. Th. and McDonald, J. R. (1950) *J. thoracic. Surg.* **19,** 957 (cit. by Doerr, W. 1955).

Campbell, M. and Deuchar, D. C. (1954) Left-sided superior vena cava. *Brit. Heart J.* **16,** 423.

Castellanos, A. and Garcia, O. (1951) Classification des anomalies de l'artère pulmonaire et de ses branches. *Arch. Mal. Cœur* **44,** 193.

Cauldwell, E. W., Siekert, R. G., Lininger, R. E. and Anson, B. J. (1948) The bronchial arteries. An anatomic study of 150 human cadavers. *Surg. Gynec. Obstet.* **86,** 395.

Chang, C. H. J. (1965) The normal x-ray measurement of the right descending pulmonary artery in 1085 cases and its clinical application. *Nagoya J. med. Sci.* **28,** 67.

Cohnheim, J. and Litten, M. (1875) Über die Folgen der Embolie der Lungenarterien. *Virchows Arch. path. Anat.* **65,** 99.

Cory, R. A. S. and Valentini, E. J. (1959) Varying patterns of the lobar branches of the pulmonary artery. *Thorax* **14,** 267.

Csákány, Gy. (1965) Újabb szempontok a tüdő röntgenvizsgálatában (Recent aspects in the X-ray examination of the lung). Thesis. Budapest.

Csákány, Gy. and Varga, L. (1966) A partialis vena pulmonalis transpositio röntgen-diagnosisának lehetőségéről (On the possibilities concerning the X-ray diagnosis of the partial transposition of the pulmonary vein). *Tuberk. és Tüdőbetegs.* **19,** 193.

Cudkowicz, L. and Armstrong, J. B. (1951) Observations on the normal anatomy of the bronchial arteries. *Thorax* **6,** 343.

Delarue, J., Abelauet, R., Chomette, G. and Levame, M. (1960) Recherches sur les interdépendances entre les réseaux artériels coronariens et médiastinaux chez l'homme: Mise en évidence d'anastomoses coronaro-bronchiques par angiographie post mortem du système artériel bronchique. *C. R. Soc. Biol. (Paris)* **154,** 937.

Delmas, A. E. (1954) Projection de l'artère pulmonaire sur la paroi thoracique. *C. R. Ass. Anat.* **80,** 658.

Diaz, W. H., Jordan, F. R. and Snymau, H. W. (1959) Persistent left superior vena cava draining into left atrium, as isolated anomaly. *Amer. Heart J.* **57,** 616.

Didion, H. (1942) *Virchows Arch. path. Anat.* 1309 (cit. by Doerr, W. 1955).

Doerr, W. (1955) Die Mißbildungen des Herzens und der großen Gefäße (in: *Lehrbuch der speziellen pathologischen Anatomie.* Ed. by Kaufmann, E. and Staemmler, M.). W. de Gruyter, Berlin.

Dotter, Ch. T., Hardisty, N. M. and Steinberg, I. (1949) Anomalous right pulmonary vein entering the inferior vena cava. Two cases diagnosed during life by angiocardiography and cardiac catheterization. *Amer. J. med. Sci.* **31,** 218.

DOTTER, CH. T. and STEINBERG, I. (1949) Angiographic study of the pulmonary artery. *J. Amer. med. Ass.* **139**, 566.

DOWNING, D. F. (1953) Absence of inferior vena cava. *Pediatrics* **12**, 675.

ELLIS, F. H., GRINDLAY, J. H. and EDWARDS, J. E. (1952) The bronchial arteries. II. Their role in pulmonary embolism and infarction. *Surgery* **31**, 167.

FELIX, W. (1928) Topographische Anatomie des Brustkorbes, der Lunge und der Pleura (in: *Die Chirurgie der Brustorgane*, vol. 1. Ed. by Sauerbruch, F.). Springer, Berlin

FERRY, R. M. and BOYDEN, E. A. (1951) Variations in the bronchovascular patterns of the right lower lobe of 50 lungs. *J. thorac. Surg.* **22**, 188.

FIANDRA, O., BARCIA, A., CORTES, R. and STANHOM, J. (1962) Partial anomalous pulmonary venous drainage into the inferior vena cava. *Acta radiol. (Stockh.)* **57**, 301.

FISHMAN, A. P. (1961) Respiratory gases in the regulation of the pulmonary circulation. *Physiol. Rev.* **41**, 214.

FLORANCE, W. (1960) Anatomie und Pathologie der Arteria bronchialis. *Ergebn. allg. Path. path. Anat.* **39**, 152.

FOGEL, M., SOMOGYI, ZS. and GÁCS, J. (1959) Transposition der Pulmonalvenen. *Röfo* **90**, 32.

FONÓ, R. (1968) Az arteria pulmonalis jobb ágának hiányáról (About the absence of the right pulmonary artery). *Magy. Radiol.* **20**, 7.

FORSSMANN, W. (1931) Über die Kontrastdarstellung der Höhlen des lebenden rechten Herzens und der Lungenschlagader. *Münch. med. Wschr.* **78**, 489.

FRANCESCHI, E. (1927) Le vena polmonari nella stasi di vizio mitralico. *Anat. Berichte* **9**, 511.

GIESE, W. (1957) Über die Endstrombahn der Lunge. *Zbl. allg. Path. path. Anat.* **97**, 233.

GREMMEL, H. (1962) Die Transversalschichtuntersuchung des Herzens und der großen Gefäße. *Röfo* **96**, 3.

GROEN, A. S., ZIEDSES DES PLANTES, B. G., DE JONG, J. and WESTRA, D. (1966) Angiografie van de bronchiale arterien met toepassing van de subtractiemethode. *Ned. T. Geneesk.* **110**, 2201.

HALMÁGYI, D. F. J. (1957) *Die klinische Physiologie des kleinen Kreislaufs*. Fischer, Jena.

HARLEY, H. R. S. (1958) Sinus venosus type of interatrial septal defect. *Thorax* **13**, 12.

HAYEK, H. (1940) Über einen Kurzschlußkreislauf. *Z. Anat. Entwickl.-Gesch.* **110**, 412.

HAYEK, H. (1942) Kurz- und Nebenschlüsse in der Pleura. *Z. Anat. Entwickl.-Gesch.* **112**, 221.

HAYEK, H. (1953) *Die menschliche Lunge*. Springer, Berlin — Göttingen — Heidelberg.

HEALEY, J. E., jr. (1952) An anatomic survey of anomalous pulmonary veins; their clinical significance. *J. thorac. Surg.* **23**, 433.

HERRNHEISER, G. and KUBAT, A. (1936) Systematische Anatomie der Lungengefäße. *Z. Anat. Entwickl.-Gesch.* **105**, 570.

HERRNHEISER, G. and KUBAT, A. (1951) Systematische Anatomie der Lunge. *Röfo* **74**, 623.

HORNYKIEWYTSCH, TH. and STENDER, H. ST. (1953a) Normale und pathologisch veränderte Lungengefäße im Schichtbild. *Röfo* **79**, 44.

HORNYKIEWYTSCH, TH. and STENDER, H. ST. (1953b) Normale und pathologisch veränderte Lungengefäße im Schichtbild. *Röfo* **79**, 639.

HORNYKIEWYTSCH, TH. and STENDER, H. ST. (1953c) Normale und pathologisch veränderte Lungengefäße im Schichtbild. *Röfo* **79**, 704.

HORNYKIEWYTSCH, TH. and STENDER, H. ST. (1954a) Normale und pathologisch veränderte Lungengefäße im Schichtbild. *Röfo* **80**, 458.

HORNYKIEWYTSCH, TH. and STENDER, H. ST. (1954b) Normale und pathologisch veränderte Lungengefäße im Schichtbild. *Röfo* **81**, 36.

HORNYKIEWYTSCH, TH. and STENDER, H. ST. (1954c) Normale und pathologisch veränderte Lungengefäße im Schichtbild. *Röfo* **81**, 134.

HORNYKIEWYTSCH, TH. and STENDER, H. ST. (1954d) Normale und pathologisch veränderte Lungengefäße im Schichtbild. *Röfo* **81**, 455.

HORNYKIEWYTSCH, TH. and STENDER, H. ST. (1954e) Normale und pathologisch veränderte Lungengefäße im Schichtbild, *Röfo* **81**, 642.

HORNYKIEWYTSCH, TH. and STENDER, H. ST. (1955a) Normale und pathologisch veränderte Lungengefäße im Schichtbild. *Röfo* **82**, 228.

HORNYKIEWYTSCH, TH. and STENDER, H. ST. (1955b) Normale und pathologisch veränderte Lungengefäße im Schichtbild. *Röfo* **82**, 331.

HORNYKIEWYTSCH, TH. and STENDER, H. ST. (1955c) Normale und pathologisch veränderte Lungengefäße im Schichtbild. *Röfo* **82**, 642.

HOWALD, E. (1949) *Helv. paediat. Acta* **4**, 322 (cit. by Doerr, W. 1955).

JAMESON, A. G., ELLIS, K. and LEVINE, O. R. (1963) Anomalous left coronary artery from pulmonary artery. *Brit. Heart J.* **25**, 251.

JANKER, R. (1954) *Röntgenologische Funktionsdiagnostik*. Girardet, Wuppertal — Elberfeld.

JOVANOVIC, M. S., BERNIER, R. and TURNEL, N. (1967) Agénésie isolée de l'artère pulmonaire gauche. *Laval Méd.* **38**, 668.

JUNGHANS, W. (1958) Die Endstrombahn der Lunge im postmortalen Angiogramm. *Virchows Arch. path. Anat.* **331**, 263.

KÁRPÁTI, A. (1957) Über das röntgenmorphologische und röntgenkinetische Bild der Stamm- und Lungengefäße. *Med. Mschr.* **11**, 784.

KASSAI, D. (1950) *A tüdő segmentumai* (Segments of the lung). Akadémiai Kiadó, Budapest.

KASSAI, T. and KUROTAKI, M. (1967) Anomalous origin of the left pulmonary artery. A case report and review. *Okajimas Folia Anat. Jap.* **44**, 29.

KENT, E. M. and BLADES, B. (1942) The surgical anatomy of the pulmonary lobes. *J. thorac. Surg.* **12**, 18.

KOVÁCS, G. (1965) A bronchopulmonalis kollateralis keringés vizsgálata és klinikai jelentősége (Examination and clinical importance of the bronchopulmonary collateral circulation). Thesis. Szeged.

KREUZFUCHS, S. (1937) *Röfo* **56**, 756 (cit. by Richter, K. 1963).

KUBIK, ST. and MÜNTENER, M. (1971) Bronchusanomalien: tracheale, eparterielle und präeparterielle Bronchi. *Röfo* **114**, 147.

LATARJET, M. and JUTTIN, P. (1951) Données nouvelles sur la circulation des artères bronchiques. *Poumon* **7**, 35.

LINDSKOG, G. E. (1949) Bilobectomy. Surgery and consideration in resection of right, middle and lower lobes. *J. thorac. Surg.* **18**, 619.

LÖHR, H. H., GRILL, W., SCHOLTZE, H. and SCHÖLMERICH, P. (1964) *Beiträge zur Angiocardiographie chirurgischer Lungenerkrankungen*. Springer, Berlin — Göttingen — Heidelberg.

LÖHR, H., SCHOLTZE, H. and GRILL, W. (1959) Normale und pathologische Lungensegmente im selektiven Angiogramm. *Acta radiol. (Stockh.)* **51**, 33.

LÜDIN, M. (1952) *Beitr. path. Anat.* **112**, 380 (cit. by Doerr, W. 1955).

MANHOFF, L. J., jr. and HOWE, J. S. (1949) Absence of the pulmonary artery: a new classification for pulmonary arteries of anomalous origin. Report of a case of absence of the pulmonary artery with hypertrophied bronchial arteries. *Arch. Path.* **48**, 155.

MARCHAND, P., GILROY, J. C. and WILSON, V. H. (1950) Anatomical study of the bronchial vascular system and its variations in disease. *Thorax* **5**, 207.

MASSUMI, R. A., RIOS, J. C. and DONOHOE, R. R. (1965) The pathogenesis of angiographic nonvisualization or attenuation of a patent pulmonary artery and the role of bronchial artery-pulmonary artery anastomosis. *J. thorac. cardiovasc. Surg.* **49**, 772.

MEHN, W. H. and HIRSCH, F. E. (1947) *Amer. J. Path.* **23**, 125 (cit. by Doerr, W. 1955).

MELNIKOW, A. (1924) Die Varietäten der intrapulmonalen Gefäße. *Z. Anat. Entwickl.-Gesch.* **71**, 185.

MILLER, W. S. (1906a) The arrangement of the bronchial blood vessels. *Anat. Anz.* **28**, 432.

MILLER, W. S. (1906b) The vascular supply of pleura pulmonalis. *Anat. Rec.* **1**, 73.

MILLER, W. S. (1925) The vascular supply of the bronchial tree. *Amer. Rev. Tuberc.* **12**, 87.

MILLER, W. S. (1947) *The Lung.* Thomas, Springfield/Ill.

MOBERG, A. (1967) Anastomoses between extracardiac vessels and coronary arteries — via bronchial arteries. *Acta radiol. (Stockh.)* **6**, 177.

MOORE, C. B., KRAUS, W. Z., DOCK, D. S., WOODWARD, E. and DEXLER, L. (1959) The relationship between pulmonary arterial pressure and roentgenographic appearance in mitral stenosis. *Amer. Heart J.* **58**, 576.

NARATH, A. (1901) *Der Bronchialbaum der Säugetiere und des Menschen.* Bibl. med. Abt. A, Stuttgart.

NORDENSTRÖM, B. (1967) Selective catheterization and angiography of bronchial and mediastinal arteries in man. *Acta radiol. (Stockh.)* **6**, 13.

OLIVEROS, G. L. (1951) Arterias y venas pulmonarias. Anatomia segmentaria. *Arch. esp. Morfol. Suppl.* **3**.

O'RAHILLY, R., DEBSON, H. and KING, T. S. (1950) Subclavian origin of bronchial arteries. *Anat. Rec.* **108**, 227.

PRINZMETAL, M., jr., ORNITZ, E. M., SIMKIN, D. and BERGMANN, H. C. (1948) Arterio-venous anastomoses in liver, spleen and lungs. *Amer. J. Physiol.* **152**, 48.

RÉMY, J., VOISON, C. and GOGUILLON, P. (1972) Les collatérales des artères bronchiques. *Ann. Radiol.* **15**, 471.

RICHTER, K. (1963) *Die zentrale Lungenschlagader im Röntgenbild.* Akademie-Verlag, Berlin.

RICHTER, K. and BÖCK, G. (1967) Die anomalie der epibronchialen rechten Pulmonalarterie als Leitsymptom eines pulmokardiovasculären Syndroms. *Röfo* **107**, 31.

ROBB, G. P. and STEINBERG, I. (1938) A practical method of visualization of the chambers of the heart, the pulmonary circulation and the great blood vessels in man. *J. clin. Invest.* **17**, 507.

ROMANKEVITCH, V. (1931) Topographisch-anatomische Untersuchungen über den Lungenabschnitt des Vagus und die Bronchialgeflechte. *Dtsch. Z. Chir.* **231**, 593.

ROMODA, T., ISTVÁNFFY, M. and ZÁBORSZKY, B. (1963) A v. pulmonalis transpositio diagnosticus nehézségeiről (About the diagnostic difficulties in case of transposition of the pulmonary vein). *Orv. Hetil.* **49**, 2325.

RUYSCH, F. (1696) *Epistola anatomica, problematica secta.* Amsterdam.

SABISTON, D. C., jr., NEILL, C. A. and TAUSSIG, H. B. (1960) Direction of blood flow in anomalous coronary artery arising from pulmonary artery. *Circulation* **22**, 591.

SANISH, R. and GESSNER, J. (1958) *Atlas der selektiven. Lungenangiographie.* Fischer, Jena.

SCHOBER, R. (1964) Selektive Bronchialisarteriographie. *Röfo* **101**, 337.

SCHOEDEL, W. (1964) Über broncho-pulmonale Gefäßverbindungen. *Ann. Acad. Sci. fenn.* A **102**.

SCHOENMACKERS, J. (1960a) Über Bronchialvenen und ihre Stellung zwischen großem und kleinem Kreislauf. *Arch. Kreisl.-Forsch.* **32**, 1.

SCHOENMACKERS, J. (1960b) Technik der postmortalen Angiographie mit Berücksichtigung verwandter Methoden postmortaler Gefäßdarstellung. *Ergebn. allg. Path. path. Anat.* **39**, 53.

SCHOENMACKERS, J. and VIETEN, H. (1953) Porto-cavale und porto-pulmonale Anastomosen im postmortalen Angiogramm. *Röfo* **79**, 488.

SCHOENMACKERS, J. and VIETEN, H. (1954) Porto-cavale Anastomosen. *Zbl. Chir.* **76**, 1236.

SCHWARTZ, G. (1910) Röntgenoskopische Beobachtungen von Eigenpulsation der Hilusschatten und ihrer Verzweigungen. *Wien. klin. Wsch.* **23**, 892.

SHEDD, D. P., ALLEY, R. D. and LINDSKOG, G. E. (1951) Observations on the hemodynamics of bronchial-pulmonary vascular communications. *J. thorac. Surg.* **22**, 537.

SIELAFF, H. J. (1964) Lungenarterien und Lungenvenen (in: *Handbuch der medizinischen Radiologie*, vol. 10/3. Ed. by Diethelm, L., Olsson, O., Strnad, F. and Zuppinger, A.). Springer, Berlin.

SILVER, C. P. (1952) The radiological pattern of injected pulmonary and bronchial arteries. *Brit. J. Radiol.* **25**, 617.

STEIN, H. L., HAGSTROM, J. W. C., EHLERS, K. H. and STEINBERG, I. (1965) Anomalous origin of the left coronary artery from the pulmonary artery. *Amer. J. Roentgenol.* **93**, 320.

STEINBACH, H. L., KEATS, TH. E. and SHELINE, G. E. (1955) The roentgen appearance of the pulmonary veins in heart disease. *Radiology* **65**, 157.

SWAN, H. J. C., BURCHELL, H. B. and WOOD, E. H. (1953) Differential diagnosis at cardiac catheterization of anomalous pulmonary venous drainage related to an atrial septal defect or abnormal venous connection. *Proc. Mayo Clin.* **25**, 452.

SZABÓ, I. and SIMAI, A. (1972) A kis- és nagyvérkör közötti anastomosisok post mortem angiogrammon (Anastomoses between the lesser and greater circulation in postmortem angiograms). *Tuberk. és Tüdőbetegs.* **25**. 16.

SZEDERKÉNYI, GY. and STECZIK, A. (1964) Arteria pulmonalisból eredő coronariák (Coronaries arising from the pulmonary artery). *Morph. igazságü. Orv. Szle.* **4**, 134.

TAN, P. M., LOH, T. F., YONG, N. K. and SUGAI, K. (1968) Aberrant left pulmonary artery. *Brit. Heart J.* **30**, 110.

TÖNDURY, G. and WEIBEL, E. (1956) Über das Vorkommen von Blutkreislaufanastomosen in der menschlichen Lunge. *Schweiz. med. Wschr.* **86**, 265.

TÖNDURY, G. and WEIBEL, E. (1958) Anatomie der Lungengefäße (in: *Ergebnisse der gesamten Tuberkulose- und Lungenforschung*, vol. 14. Ed. by Engel, S. T., Heilmeyer, L., Hein, J. and Uehlinger, E.). Thieme, Stuttgart.

VERLOOP, M. C. (1948) The arteriae bronchiales and their anastomoses with the arteriae pulmonales. *Acta anat. (Basel)* **5**, 171.

VIAMONTE, Mc., jr., PARKS, R. E. and SMOAK, W. M. (1965) Guided catheterization of the bronchial arteries. *Radiology* **85**, 205.

VIAMONTE, MC., jr. (1967) Intrathoracic extracardiac shunts. *Sem. Roentgenol.* **2**, 342.

WALDHAUSEN, J. A., FRIEDMAN, S., TYERS, G. F. O., RASHKIND, W. J., PETRY, E. and MILLER, W. W. (1968) Ascending aorta-right pulmonary artery anastomosis. *Circulation* **38**, 463.

WATZKA, M. (1936) Über Gefäßsperren und arterio-venose Anastomosen. *Z. mikr.-anat. Forsch.* **39**, 521.

WEIBEL, E. (1958) Die Entstehung der Längsmuskulatur in den Ästen der A. bronchialis. *Z. Zellforsch.* **47**, 440.

WEIBEL, E. (1959) Die Blutgefäßanastomosen in der menschlichen Lunge. *Z. Zellforsch.* **50**, 653.

WEINTRAUB, R. A. (1966) Ectopic origin of one pulmonary artery from the ascending aorta. *Radiology* **86**, 666.

WINTER, F. S. (1954) Persistent left superior vena cava. Survey of world literature and report of 30 additional cases. *Angiology* **5**, 90.

ZDANSKY, E. (1951) Zur Röntgenologie der Dynamik des Herzens. *Röfo* **75**, Special issue 179.

ZENKER, R., HEBERER, G. and LÖHR, H. H. (1954) *Die Lungenresectionen.* Springer, Berlin—Göttingen—Heidelberg.

ZUCKERKANDL, E. (1882) Über die Anastomosen der Venae pulmonales mit den Bronchialvenen und mit dem mediastinalen Venennetze. *S.-B. Akad. Wiss. Wien. math.-nat. Kl.* **84**, 110.

ZUCKERKANDL, E. (1883) Über die Verbindungen zwischen den arteriellen Gefäßen der menschlichen Lunge. *S. B. Akad. Wiss. Wien, math.-nat. Kl.* **87**, 171.

Vascular system of the common carotid and subclavian arteries

AARON, C. and CHAWAF, A.-R. (1967) Variations de la carotide externe et de ses branches. *Bull. Ass. Anat. (Nancy)* **52**, 125.

AARON, C., DOYON, D. and RICHARD, J. (1966) Morphologie de la carotide externe et de ses branches à la lumière de l'artèriographie. *Bull. Ass. Anat. (Nancy)* **51**, 79.

ALEXANDER, L. (1942) The vascular supply of the strio-pallidum. *Assoc. Res. Nerv. Dis. Proc.* **21**, 77.

ALTMANN, F. (1947) Anomalies of the internal carotid artery. *Laryngoscope* **57**, 313.

AMISTANI, B. (1950) Minute vascularisation of the thyroid in various types of goiter. *Arch. ital. Anat. Istol. pat.* **23**, 365.

ANGERMAYER, S. (1907) Ein Fall von getrenntem Ursprung der Carotis interna sinistra und der Carotis externa sinistra aus dem Aortenbogen. *Anat. Hefte* **32**, 213.

ARNOULD, G., TRIDON, P. and LAXENAIRE, M. (1968) L'artère hypoglosse primitive. Étude anatomique et radio-clinique. *Rev. neurol.* **118**, 372.

ATKINSON, W. J. (1949) The anterior inferior cerebellar artery. *J. Neurol. Neurosurg. Psychiat.* **12**, 137.

BATUJEFF, N. (1889) Eine seltene Arterienanomalie. *Anat. Anz.* **4**, 282.

BEAN, R. B. (1905) Observations on a study of the subclavian artery in man. *Amer. J. Anat.* **4**, 303.

BEKÉNY, GY. and FÉNYES, GY. (1955) Az arteria carotis interna elsődleges thrombosisáról 7 angiographiával kórismézett eset kapcsán (Primary thrombosis of the internal carotid artery on the basis of 7 cases diagnosed with angiography). *Ideggyógy. Szle* **8**, 78.

BENEDEK, L. and HÜTTL, TH. (1938) *Über den diagnostischen Wert der zerebralen Stereoangiographie, hauptsächlich bei intrakraniellen Tumoren.* Karger, Basel—Leipzig.

BERRY, R. J. A. and ANDERSON, J. H. (1910) A case of nonunion of the vertebrales with consequent abnormal origin of the basilaris. *Anat. Anz.* **35**, 54.

BINSWANGER, O. (1879) Anatomische Untersuchungen über die Ursprungstelle und den Anfangsteil der Carotis interna. *Arch. Psychiat.* **9**, 351.

BLACKBURN, J. W. (1907) Anomalies of the encephalic arteries among the insane. *J. Comp. Neurol. Physiol.* **17**, 493.

BLADT, A. (1903) *Die Arterien des menschlichen Kehlkopfes.* Inaug. speech. Königsberg.

BOERI, R. and PASSERINI, A. (1964) The megadolichobasilar anomaly. *J. neurol. Sci.* **1**, 475.

BONNAL, J. and LEGRÉ, J. (1958) *L'angiographie cérébrale.* Masson et Cie, Paris.

BOSTRÖM, K. and GREITZ, T. (1967) Kinking of the internal carotid artery. *Acta radiol. (Stockh.)* **6**, 105.

BROWN, ST. J. and TATLOW, W. F. F. (1963) Radiographic studies of the vertebral arteries in cadavers. *Radiology* **81**, 80.

BULLEN, F. and JOHN, ST. 1890) Absence of one anterior cerebral with both coming from opposite carotid. *J. ment. Sci.* **36**, 32.

BUSSE, O. (1921) Aneurysmen und Bildungsfehler der A. communicans anterior. *Virchows Arch. path. Anat.* **228**, 178.

CARPENTER, M. B., NOBACK, C. R. and MOSS, M. L. (1954) The anterior chorioideal artery. *Arch. Neurol. Psychiat.* **71**, 714.

CAVATORTI, P. (1907) Di una rara variazione delle arterie della base dell'encefalo nell'uomo. *Monit. Zool. Ital.* **18**, 294.

CHAKRAVORTY, B. G. (1971) Arterial supply of the cervical spinal cord (with special reference to the radicular arteries). *Anat. Rec.* **170**, 311.

CHANMUGAM, P. K. (1936) Note on an unusual ophthalmic artery associated with other abnormalities. *J. Anat.* **70**, 580.

CHASE, N. E. and TAVERAS, J. M. (1963) Temporal tumours studied by serial angiography. *Acta radiol. (Stockh.)* **1**, 225.

CLARA, M. (1953) *Das Nervensystem des Menschen.* Barth, Leipzig.

CRITCHLEY, M. and SCHUSTER, P. (1933) Beiträge zur Anatomie und Pathologie der A. cerebellaris superior. *Z. ges. Neurol. Psychiat.* **144**, 681.

CROMPTON, M. P. (1962) The pathology of ruptured middle cerebral aneurysms. *Lancet* **2**, 421.

CURRY, R. W. and CULBERTH, G. G. (1951) The normal cerebral angiogram. *Amer. J. Roentgenol.* **65**, 345.

DALL'AQUA, U. (1900) L'arteria temporale superficiale dell'uomo. *Schwalbe's Jahresberichte* **6**, 201.

DANDY, W. E. (1947) *Intracranial arterial aneurysms.* Comstock Co., Ithaca/N. Y.

DANIEL, P. M. and PRICHARD, M. M. L. (1966) Observations on the vascular anatomy of the pituitary gland and its importance in pituitary function. *Amer. Heart J.* **72**, 147.

DE ALMEIDA, F. (1931) Note sur les collatérales de l'artère communicante cérébrale antérieure. *Arch. Anat. Antrop. Lisboa* **13**, 551.

DE VRIESE, B. (1905) Sur la signification morphologique des artères cérébrales. *Arch. Biol. (Liège)* **21**, 357.

DILENGE, D. (1962) *L'angiographie de l'artère carotide interne.* Masson et Cie, Paris.

DILENGE, D. and CONSTANS, J. P. (1963) Sémiologie angiographique de l'artère cérébrale antérieure. *Acta radiol. (Stockh.)* **1**, 248.

DILENGE, D. and DAVID, M. (1965) La branche méningée de l'artère vertébrale. *Neuro-chirurgie* **8**, 121.

DILENGE, D., DAVID, M. and METZGER, J. (1966) L'angiographie de l'artère ophtalmique (in: *L'exploration neuroradiologique en ophtalmologie*. Ed. by Guillot, R., Saraux, H. and Sedan, R.). Masson, Paris.

DILENGE, D., FISCHGOLD, H. and DAVID, M. (1961) L'artère ophtalmique. Aspects angiographiques. *Neuro-chirurgie* 4, 249.

DJINDJIAN, R., FAURÉ, C. and DEBRUN, G. (1964) L'artériographie du corps thyroïde. *Ann. Radiol.* 7, 6.

DJINDJIAN, R. and HURTH, M. (1970) L'artériographie de la moelle épinière. *Rev. Prat. (Paris)* 20, 1901.

DOPPMAN, J. and DI CHIRO, G. (1968) The arteria radicularis magna: Radiographic anatomy in the adult. *Brit. J. Radiol.* 41, 40.

DOYON, D. (1966) Modalités de l'artériographie de la carotide externe. Thésis. Paris.

DURET, H. (1874) Recherches anatomiques sur la circulation de l'encéphale. *Arch. Physiol.*

ECKER, A. D. (1951) *The Normal Cerebral Angiogram*. Thomas, Springfield/Ill.

EDINGTON, G. H. (1901) Tortuosity of both internal carotid arteries. *Brit. med. J.* 1, 1526.

ELLIOT, H. C. (1963) *Textbook of Neuroanatomy*. Lippincott, Philadelphia — Montreal.

FALCONER, H. cit. by Finkemeyer, H. (1956) Der Kollateraliskreislauf zwischen Arteria carotis externa und interna im Arteriogramm. *Zbl. Neurochir.* 16, 342.

FAWCETT, E. and BLACKFORD, J. V. (1905/06) The circle of Willis: An examination of 700 specimens. *J. Anat. Physiol.* 40, 63.

FELDMAN, F., HABIF, D. V., FLEMING, R. J., KANTER, I. E. and SEAMAN, W. B. (1967) Arteriography of the breast. *Radiology* 89, 1053.

FESANI, F. and PELLEGRINO, F. (1968) Il circolo collaterale attraverso le mammarie interne nella obliterazione dell'arteria succlavia all'origine. *Minerva Cardioangiol.* 16, 1249.

FIEBACH, O. and AGNOLI, A. (1973) Betrachtungen zu Strömungsdynamik bei der A. trigemina primitiva im Angiogram. *Röfo* 118, 293.

FIEGEL, A. and NADJMI, M. (1971) Variationen der Arterien und ihre topometrischen Verhältnisse im retrograden Brachialisangiogramm. *Röntgen-Bl.* 24, 73.

FIELDS, W. S., BRUETMAN, M. E. and WEIBEL, J. (1965) Collateral circulation of the brain. *Monogr. Surg. Sci.* 2, 183.

FIFE, C. D. (1921) Absence of common carotid. *Anat. Rec.* 22, 115.

FISCHER-BRÜGGE, E. (1938) Lage — Abweichungen der vorderen Hirnarterie im Gefäßbild. *Zbl. Neurochir.* 3, 300.

FISHER, M. (1954) Occlusion of the carotid artery. *Arch. Neurol. Psychiat. (Chic.)* 72, 187.

FLEMMING, E. E. (1895) Absence of the left internal carotid. *J. Anat. Phys.* 29, 23.

GABRIELE, O. F. and BELL, D. (1967) Ophthalmic origin of the middle meningeal artery. *Radiology* 89, 841.

GABRIELSEN, T. O. and AMUDSEN, P. (1969) The pontine arteries in vertebral angiography. *Amer. J. Roentgenol.* 106, 296.

GADO, M. and MARSHALL, J. (1971) Clinico-radiological study of collateral circulation after internal carotid and middle cerebral occlusion. *J. Neurol. Neurosurg. Psychiat.* 34, 163.

GALLIGIONI, F., ANDRIOLI, G. C., MARIN, G., BRIANI, S. and IRACI, G. (1971) Hypoplasia of the internal carotid artery associated with cerebral pseudoangiomatosis. *Amer. J. Roentgenol.* 112, 251.

GALLOWAY, J. R., GREITZ, T. and SJÖRGEN, S. E. (1964) Vertebral angiography in the diagnosis of ventricular dilatation. *Acta radiol. (Stockh.)* 2, 321.

GERLACH, J. and VIEHWEGER, G. (1955) Die Abhängigkeit des Angiogramms der Hirngefäße von der Strahlen-Projection. *Acta Neurochir. (Wien) Suppl.* 3, 211.

GIUFFRIDA-RUGGERI, V. (1913) Über die endocranischen Furchen der Arteria meningea media beim Menschen. *Z. Morph. Anthr.* 16, 15.

GORDON-SCHAW, G. (1910) Two cases of reduplication of the art. cerebri post. *J. Anat. Physiol.* 44, 249.

GREITZ, T. (1956) Radiologic study of brain circulation by rapid serial angiography of carotid artery. *Acta radiol. (Stockh.) Suppl.* 140.

GREITZ, T. and LAURÉN, T. (1968) Anterior meningeal branch of the vertebral artery. *Acta radiol. (Stockh.)* 7, 219.

GREITZ, T. and SJÖRGEN, S. E. (1963) The posterior inferior cerebellar artery. *Acta radiol. (Stockh.)* 1, 284.

GRISOLI, J., RICHELME, H., SALAMON, G. and GUERINEL, G. (1969) Les anastomoses artérielles entre les systèmes circulatoires carotidiens interne et externe vertébral par des branches méningées intracraniennes. *C. R. Ass. Anat.* 142, 961.

GRÖNROSS, H. (1902) Eine seltene Anordnung der Arteria maxillaris externa bei einem Erwachsenen. *Anat. Anz.* 20, 9.

GROTE, G. (1901) Die Varietäten der Arteria temporalis superficialis. *Z. Morph. Antrop.* 3, 1.

GUND, A. (1960) Die Bedeutung der zerebralen Serienangiographie. *Wien. klin. Wschr.* 72, 28.

GYURKÓ, GY. and SZABÓ, M. (1968) Adatok az emberi artériás rendszer nagyobb értörzseinek méreteire vonatkozóan (Data concerning the dimensions of the larger vessel trunks of the human arterial system). *Magy. Sebész.* 21, 276.

HACKER, H. and ALONSO, A. (1968) Über die angiographische Darstellung eines kapillaren Gefäßnetzes am Dorsum sellae und seine Deutung als Neurohypophyse. *Röfo* 108, 141.

HANDA, H., HANDA, J. and TAZUMI, M. (1966) Tentorial branch of the internal carotid artery (arteria tentorii). *Amer. J. Roentgenol.* 98, 595.

HANDA, J., KIKUCHI, H. and HANDA, H. (1967) Persistierende karotido-basiläre Anastomose. Die A. primitiva hypoglossica. *Röfo* 107, 421.

HANDA, J., SETA, K. and HANDA, H. (1968) Die akzessorische Arteria cerebri media. *Röfo* 108, 539.

HANDA, J. MATSUDA, M. and HANDA, H. (1972) Lateral position of the external carotid artery. *Radiology* 102, 361.

HANDA, J., WAGA, S. and HANDA, H. (1971) Dural cortical anastomosis as a collateral channel in carotid occlusive disease. *Clin. Radiol.* 22, 302.

HARRISON, C. R. and LUTTRELI, G. (1953) Persistent carotid-basilar anastomosis. *J. Neurosurg.* 10, 205.

HARVEY, J. C. and HOWARD, L. M. (1945) A rare type of anomalous ophthalmic artery in a negro. *Anat. Rec.* 92, 87.

HARZER, K. and TÖNDURY, G. (1966) Zum Verhalten der Arteria vertebralis in der alternden Halswirbelsäule. *Röfo* 104, 687.

HASEBE, K. (1928) Arterien der Hirnbasis (in: *Das Arteriensystem der Japaner*, vol. 1. Ed. by Adachi, B.). Kenkyu-Sha, Kyoto.

HAWKINS, T. D. (1966) The collateral anastomoses in cerebrovascular occlusion. *Clin. Radiol.* 17, 203.

HAWKINS, T. D. and MELCHER, D. H. (1966) A meningeal artery in the falx cerebelli. *Clin. Radiol.* 17, 377.

HAYREK, S. S. and DASS, R. (1962) The ophthalmic artery. I. Origin and intracranial and intracanalicular course. *Brit. J. Ophthal.* **46,** 65.

HERMAN, E. H., OSTROWSKI, A. Z. and GURDJIAN, E. S. (1963) Perforating branches of the middle cerebral artery. *Arch. Neurol.* **8,** 32.

HEUBNER, A. (1872) Zur Topographie der Ernährungsgebiete der einzelnen Hirnarterien. *Zbl. med. Wiss.* **52,** 817.

HINCK, V. C. (1964) Persistent primitive trigeminal artery. *Radiology* **83,** 41.

HOCHSTETTER, A. (1963) Eine einzigartig abnorme Anordnung der Arterien des Gesichtes. *Anat. Anz.* **113,** 221.

HOCHSTETTER, F. R. (1937) Über einige Fälle einer bisher anscheinend noch nicht beobachteten Varietät der Arteria cerebralis posterior des Menschen. *Z. Anat. Entwickl.-Gesch.* **107,** 633.

HORÁNYI, B. and KÁRPÁTI, M. (1959) Az arteria cerebri media lefutásbeli variátióinak diagnosztikus jelentőségéről (Diagnostic significance of variations in the course of the middle cerebral artery). *Ideggyógy. Szle* **12,** 193.

HROMODA, J. (1957) Anatomische Bemerkungen über die A. chorioidea anterior in bezug auf die Cooper'sche Operation bei der Behandlung des Parkinsonismus. *Zbl. Neurochir.* **17,** 209.

HUBER, P. (1966) Die prognostische Bedeutung des angiographisch sichtbaren Kollateralkreislaufs bei Verschlüssen der Arteria cerebri media. *Röfo* **104,** 82.

HYRTL, J. (1836) Beiträge zur pathologischen Anatomie des Gehörorganes. *Med. Jb. öst. Staates* **11,** 421.

HYRTL, J. (1887) *Lehrbuch der Anatomie des Menschen.* Braumüller, Wien.

JAIN, K. K. (1964) Some observations of the anatomy of the middle cerebral artery. *Canad. J. Surg.* **7,** 134.

JENNY, H. (1910) Abnorme einseitige Verdoppelung der Arteria thyreoidea inferior. *Anat. Anz.* **40,** 623.

KAPLAN, H. A. and FORD, D. H. (1966) *The Brain Vascular System.* Elsevier, Amsterdam—London—New York.

KAPLAN, H. A., RABINER, A. M. and BROWDER, J. (1954) Anatomical study of blood vessels of the brain: The perforating arteries of the base of the forebrain. *Trans. Amer. neurol. Ass.* **79,** 38.

KAUTZKY, R. and ZÜLCH, K. J. (1955) *Neurologisch-neurochirurgische Röntgendiagnostik und andere Methoden zur Erkennung intracranieller Erkrankungen.* Springer, Berlin.

KELLER, H. L. and WEISS, D. (1973) Ursprung einer des Vertebralisgebiet versorgenden Arterie aus dem Halsabschnitt der rechten Arteria carotis interna. *Röfo* **118,** 473.

KEMMETMÜLLER, H. (1911) Über eine seltene Varietät der Arteria vertebralis. *Anat. Hefte* **44,** 305.

KETTUNEN, K. (1965) Arteriographic visualisation of the alveolar (inferior dental) artery of the mandible. *Brit. J. Radiol.* **38,** 599.

KIMMERLE, A. (1930) Mitteilung über einen eigenartigen Befund am Atlas. *Röntgenpraxis* **2,** 479.

KIRGIS, H. D. and PEEBLES, E. MC. C. (1961) Sympathetic control of the activity of the cerebral arteries of the cat. *Anat. Rec.* **139,** 246.

KISS, F. (1949) A szem vérkeringése (Blood circulation of the eye). *Szemészet* **86,** 1.

KRAUSE, W. (1880) *Anatomische Varietäten.* (cit. by Adachi, B. 1928).

KRAYENBÜHL, H. and RICHTER, R. (1952) *Die zerebrale Angiographie.* Thieme, Suttgart.

KRAYENBÜHL, H. and YASARGIL, M. G. (1957) *Die vaskulären Erkrankungen im Gebiet der Arteria vertebralis und Arteria basilaris.* Thieme, Stuttgart.

KRAYENBÜHL, H. and YASARGIL, M. G. (1958) Der zerebrale kollaterale Blutkreislauf im angiographischen Bild. *Acta neurochir. (Wien)* **6,** 30.

KRAYENBÜHL, H. and YASARGIL, M. G. (1965) *Die zerebrale Angiographie.* 2nd ed. Thieme, Stuttgart.

KUHN, R. A. (1961) Normal roentgenographic anatomy of the human circle of Willis. *Amer. J. Roentgenol.* **86,** 1040.

KUHN, R. A. (1962) Speed of cerebral circulation. *New Engl. J. Med.* **267,** 689.

KUKWA, A. and ZBRODOWSKI, A. (1966) Rzadki pozypadek odejecia tetnicy tarczowej górnej od tetnicy szyjnej wspólnej lewej. *Folia morph. (Warszawa)* **25,** 641.

LAHL, R. (1966) Carotido-basiläre Anastomose (A. primitiva trigemina) in Kombination mit Anomalien des Circulus arteriosus cerebri. *Psychiatr. Neurol.* **151,** 365.

LANG, E. K., HANN, E. C. and LUROS, TH. J. (1964) Arteriographic demonstration of external-internal carotid anastomoses and their correlation to RISA circulation studies. *Radiology* **83,** 632.

LANGE, H. (1939) Die zweiwurzelige Arteria vertebralis. *Anat. Ber.* **39,** 40.

LANGE-COSACK, H., NORLÉN, G., TÖNNIS, W. and WALTER, W. (1966) Klinik und Behandlung der raumbeengenden intrakraniellen Prozesse (in: *Handbuch der Neurochirurgie.* Ed. by Olivecrona, H. and Tönnis, W.). Springer, Berlin—Göttingen—Neidelberg—New York.

LAUBER, H. (1901) Über einige Varietäten im Verlauf der Arteria maxillaris interna. *Anat. Anz.* **19,** 444.

LAZORTHES, G. (1961) *Vascularisation et circulation cérébrales.* Masson, Paris.

LECHI, A. and NIZZOLI, V. (1964) Contributo angiografico allo studio del settore posteriore del circolo di Willis. *Sist. nerv.* **4,** 224.

LEEDS, N. E. and GOLDBERG, H. I. (1970) Lenticulostriate artery abnormalities. *Radiology* **97,** 377.

LEHRER, H. Z. (1968) Relative calibre of the cervical internal carotid artery. *Brain* **91,** 339.

LELLI, G. F. (1939) Comportamento dell'arteria uditiva interna e dei suoi rami labirintici nell'uomo. *Z. Anat. Entwickl.-Gesch.* **110,** 48.

LEMAY, M. and GOODING, CH. A. (1966) The clinical significance of the azygos anterior cerebral artery (A.C.A.). *Amer. J. Roentgenol.* **98,** 602.

LENHOSSÉK, M. (1922) *Az ember anatómiája* (Atlas of Human Anatomy). Budapest.

LINDGREN, E. (1950) Percutaneous angiography of vertebral artery. *Acta radiol. (Stockh.)* **33,** 289.

LINDGREN, E. (1954) Röntgenologie einschließlich Kontrastmethoden (in: *Handbuch der Neurochirurgie,* vol. 2. Ed. by Olivecrona, H. and Tönnis, W.). Springer, Berlin—Göttingen—Heidelberg.

LINDGREN, E. (1957) Radiologic examination of the brain and spinal cord. *Acta radiol. (Stockh.) Suppl.* **151.**

LIVINI, F. (1900) Studio morfologico delle arterie tiroidee. *Schwalbe's Jahresberichte* **6,** 201.

LOMAN, J. and MYERSON, A. (1936) Visualization of cerebral vessels by direct intracarotid injection of thoriumdioxide. *Amer. J. Roentgenol.* **35,** 188.

LONGO, L. (1905) Le anomalie del poligono di Willis nell'uomo studiate comparativamente in alcuni mammiferi ed uccelli. *Anat. Anz.* **27,** 170.

MANI, R. L., NEWTON, TH. H. and GLICKMAN, M. G. (1968) The superior cerebellar artery: An anatomic-roentgenographic correlation. *Radiology* **91,** 1102.

MATUSHIMA, T. (1970) Study on the radiological anatomy of the ophthalmic artery. *Tokyo Jikeikai Med. J.* **85,** 691.

MINNE, J. DEPREUX, R. and FRANCKE, J. P. (1970) Les artères periodontoidiennes. *C. R. Ass. Anat.* **149**, 914.

MITTERWALLNER, FR. (1955) Variationsstatistische Untersuchungen an den basalen Hirngefäßen. *Acta anat. (Basel)* **24**, 51.

MOFFAT, D. B. (1967) A case of persistence of the primitive olfactory artery. *Anat. Anz.* **121**, 477.

MONIZ, E. (1927) L'encéphalographie artérielle, son importance dans la localisation des tumeurs cérébrales. *Rev. neurol.* **34**, 72.

MONIZ, E. (1934) *L'angiographie cérébrale.* Masson et Cie, Paris.

MONIZ, E. (1940) *Die zerebrale Arteriographie und Phlebographie.* Springer, Berlin.

MONIZ, E., LIMA, P. A. and CALDAS, P. (1933) A filmogen da cirçulacao cerebral. *A medic. contemp.* **3**.

MOREAU, F. (1965) *L'angiographie thyroïdienne.* Impr. Delteil, Bordeaux.

MORRIS, L. (1962) Non-union of the vertebral arteries. *Brit. J. Radiol.* **35**, 415.

MOUNT, L. A. and TAVERAS, J. M. (1957) Arteriographic demonstration of the collateral circulation of the cerebral hemispheres. *Arch. Neurol. Psychiat. (Chic.)* **78**, 235.

MRACEK, Z., ULC, M. and KOHUTEK, V. (1971) Aplazie nitrolebniho useku vnitrni kravice s krvacejicim aneurysmatem na arteria communicans anterior. *Čs. Neurol.* **34**, 289.

MULTANOVSKY, J. M. (1928) Variation der Arteria vertebralis. *Anat. Anz.* **13**, 362.

NAGY, D. (1948) Az arteria meningea media anastomosisairól (Anastomoses of the middle meningeal artery). *Orv. Hetil.* **89**, 348.

NEUMÄRKER, K. J. and NEUMÄRKER, M. (1971) Ein atypischer Abgang der Arteria cerebralis anterior im Karotisangiogramm. *Röfo* **114**, 852.

NEWTON, TH. H. and YOUNG, D. A. (1968) Anomalous origin of the occipital artery from the internal carotid artery. *Radiology* **90**, 550.

NIERLING, D. A., WOLLSCHLAEGER, P. B. and WOLLSCHLAEGER, G. (1966) Ascending pharyngeal-vertebral anastomosis. *Amer. J. Roentgenol.* **98**, 599.

NISHIMOTO, A. and TAKEUCHI, S. (1968) Abnormal cerebrovascular network related to the internal carotid arteries. *J. Neurosurg.* **29**, 255.

OBLORCA, F. (1940) Seltene Varietäten der linken Arteria vertebralis. *Anat. Ber.* **40**, 2.

OERTEL, O. (1922) Über die Persistenz embrionaler Verbindungen zwischen der A. carotis interna und der A. vertebralis cerebralis. *Anat. Anz.* **55**, 281.

OLIVECRONA, H. (1934) *Die parasagittalen Meningeome.* Thieme, Leipzig.

ORMAI, S. and SZY, S. (1962) Über die arteriographische Untersuchung des Gefäßnetzes der Schilddrüse. *Röfo* **96**, 411.

PADGET, D. H. (1947) The circle of Willis. Its embryology and anatomy (in: *Intracranial Arterial Aneurysms*. Ed. by Dandy, W. E.). Comstock, Ithaca/N. Y.

PADGET, D. H. (1948) The development of the cranial arteries in human embryo. *Contr. Embryol. Carneg. Instn.* **32**, 205.

PAILLAS, J. E., SEDAN, R., PELLET, W. and LAVIEILLE, J. (1966) Valeur de la suppléance circulatoire par l'anastomose artérielle maxillo-ophtalmique au cours de la thrombose carotidienne. *Press Méd.* **74**, 1631.

PARAICZ, E. (1965) *A központi idegrendszer röntgen-kontrasztvizsgálatainak új útjai csecsemő- és gyermekkorban* (New procedures in the X-ray contrast examination in infancy and childhood). Thesis, Budapest.

PARAICZ, E. and SZÉNÁSSY, J. (1966) *Neurologisch-klinische Untersuchungen im Säuglings- und Kindesalter.* Akadémiai Kiadó, Budapest.

PEETERS, F. L. M. (1968) Die Arteriae tentorii. *Röfo* **109**, 65.

PELLEGRINI, A. (1904) Il tipo normale e le variazioni delle Arteriae subclavia e axillaris. *Monit. Zool. Ital.* **15**, 232.

PLATZER, W. (1956) Der Carotissiphon und seine anatomische Grundlage. *Röfo* **84**, 200.

POLLOCK, J. A. and NEWTON, TH. H. (1968) The anterior falx artery: Normal and pathologic anatomy. *Radiology* **91**, 1089.

PONTES, A. P. DE (1963) *Artérias supra-aorticas.* Thesis, Rio de Janeiro.

QUANDT, J. (1959) *Die zerebralen Durchblutungsstörungen des Erwachsenenalters.* Volk und Gesundheit, Berlin.

RAAD, R. (1964) An angiographic study of the course of the ophthalmic artery in normal and pathological conditions. *Brit. J. Radiol.* **37**, 826.

RABE, W. (1970) Ein seltener Kollateralkreislauf zwischen der Arteria maxillaris und der Arteria carotis interna. *Z. Neurol.* **198**, 342.

RABISCHONG, P., PALEIRAC, R., TEMPLE, J. P., OLIVIER, J. and ZOURGANE, M. (1962) Étude anatomo-radiologique de la portion prétransversaire de l'artère vertébrale. *Bull. Ass. Anat. (Nancy)* **48**, 1137.

RADNER, S. (1955) Intracranial angiography via the vertebral artery. *J. Neurosurg.* **12**, 369.

REIVICH, M., HOLLING, H. E., ROBERTS, B. and TOOLE, J. F. (1961) Reversal of blood flow through vertebral artery and its effect on cerebral circulation. *New Engl. J. Med.* **265**, 878.

RICKENBACHER, J. (1964) Der suboccipitale und der intracraniale Abschnitt der Arteria vertebralis. *Z. Anat. Entwickl.-Gesch.* **124**, 171.

RIGGS, H. E. and RUPP, C. (1963) Variation in form of the circle of Willis. The relation of the variations to collateral circulation: Anatomic analysis. *Arch. Neurol. (Chic.)* **8**, 24.

RING, B. A. and WADDINGTON, M. (1967a) Ascending frontal branch of middle cerebral artery. *Acta radiol. (Stockh.)* **6**, 209.

RING, B. A. and WADDINGTON, M. (1967b) Intraluminal diameters of the intracranial arteries. *Vasc. Surg.* **1**, 137.

RING, B. A. and WADDINGTON, M. (1968) Roentgenographic anatomy of the pericallosal arteries. *Amer. J. Roentgenol.* **104**, 109.

ROSSI, P., TRACHT, D. G. and RUZICKA, F. F., JR. (1971) Thyroid angiography techniques, anatomy and indications. *Brit. J. Radiol.* **44**, 911.

ROWLANDS, R. P. and SWAN, R. H. J. (1902) Tortuosity of both internal carotid arteries. *Brit. med. J.* **1**, 76.

RUGGIERO, G., CALABRO, A., METZGER, J. and SIMON, J. (1963) Arteriography of the external carotid artery. *Acta radiol. (Stockh.)* **1**, 395.

RUGGIERO, G. and CONSTANS, J. P. (1954) L'artériographie vertébrale. Analyse de 42 cas. *Rev. neurol.* **5**, 467.

SACHS, E., jr. (1954) Arteriographic demonstration of collateral circulation through the ophthalmic artery in internal carotid artery thrombosis. *J. Neurosurg.* **11**, 405.

SALAMON, G., GRISOLI, J., PAILLAS, J. E., FAURE, J. and GIUDICELLI, G. (1967) Étude artériographique des artères méningées. *Neuro-chirurgie* **10**, 1.

SALAN, A. and ASTENGO, A. (1964) L'arteria basilare. Studio anatomico radiologico del puncto di vista angiografico in relazione a sesso, età e stato morboso. *Min. Radiol.* **9**, 28.

SCHÄFER (1878) Über die aneurysmatische Erweiterung der Carotis interna an ihrem Ursprung. *Allg. Z. Psychiat.* **34**, 438.

SCHECHTER, M. M. (1964) The occipital vertebral anastomosis. *J. Neurosurg.* **21**, 758.

SCHECHTER, M. M. and ZINGESSER, L. H. (1965) The anterior spinal artery. *Acta radiol. (Stockh.)* **3**, 489.

SCHIEFER, W. and VETTER, K. (1957) Das cerebrale Angiogramm in verschiedenen Altersstufen. *Zbl. Neurochir.* **17**, 218.

SCHIEFER, W. and WALTER, W. (1959) Die Persistenz embryonaler Gefäße als Ursache von Blutungen des Hirns und seine Häute. *Acta Neurochir. (Wien)* **7**, 53.

SCHLESINGER, B. (1953) The insulo-opercular arteries of the brain, with special reference to angiography of striothalamic tumors. *Amer. J. Roentgenol.* **70**, 555.

SCHMIEDEL, G. (1933) Die Entwicklung der Arteria vertebralis des Menschen. *Morph. Jb.* **71**, 315.

SCHOENMACKERS, J. and SCHEUNEMANN, H. (1956) Angiographische Untersuchungen der A. carotis externa. *Dtsch. Zahn-, Mund- u. Kieferheilk.* **23**, 346.

SCHÜRMANN, K. (1954) Darstellung der A. vertebralis und ihrer Äste im Angiogramm von der A. carotis externa aus. *Zbl. Neurochir.* **6**, 362.

SCHWALBE, G. (1878) Über Wachstumverschiebungen und ihr Einfluß auf die Gestaltung des Arteriensystems. *J. Z. Naturwiss.* **12**, 267.

SCOTT, H. (1963) Carotid basilar anastomosis-persistent hypoglossal artery. *Brit. J. Radiol.* **36**, 431.

SEIDEL, K. (1965) Arteriographische Beobachtungen einer seltenen Carotisanomalie. *Röfo* **103**, 390.

SINDERMANN, F. (1967) Angiographische und klinische Bedeutung der Kollateralen bei Verschluß der Arteria carotis interna. *Arch. Psychiat. Nervenkr.* **209**, 207.

SIQUEIRA, E. B. and AMADOR, L. V. (1964) Normal angiographic configuration of the carotid siphon in the pediatric patient. *J. Neurology* **21**, 215.

SJÖRGEN, S. E. (1953) Percutaneous vertebral angiography. *Acta radiol. (Stockh.)* **40**, 113.

SMALTINO, F., BERNINI, F. P. and ELEFANTE, R. (1971) Normal and pathological findings of the angiographic examination of the internal auditory artery. *Neuroradiology* **2**, 216.

STAFFORD, F. and GONZALEZ, A. A. (1957) Branches of the anterior communicating artery in man. *Anat. Rec.* **127**, 449.

STOPFORD, J. S. B. (1916) The arteries of the pons and medulla oblongata. *J. Anat. Physiol.* **50**, 132.

STRONG, O. S. and ELWYN, A. (1948) *Human Neuroanatomy.* Williams and Wilkins, Baltimore.

SUNDERLAND, S. (1948) Neurovascular relations and anomalies of the base of the brain. *J. Neurol. Neurosurg. Psychiat.* **11**, 243.

SUZUKI, B. (1894) Ein Fall der Varietät der Arteria subclavia dextra. *Tokyo Igaku Zasshi* **8**, 1031.

SZENTÁGOTHAI, J., ROZSOS, I. and KUTAS, J. (1957) A hypophysis hátsó lebenyének szerepe a mellső lebeny vérkeringésében (Role of the posterior lobe of the hypophysis in the blood circulation of the inferior lobe). *Magy. Tud. Akad. Biol. orv. Tud. Oszt. Közl.* **8**, 104.

TAKAHASHI, K. (1940) Die perkutane Arteriographie der Arteria vertebralis und ihrer Versorgungsgebiete. *Arch. Psychiat.* **111**, 373.

TAPTAS, J. N. (1948) Les dilatations et allongements de l'artère carotide interne; états fonctionnées et organiques. *Rev. neurol.* **80**, 338.

TARTARINI, E., DAVINI, V. and GUIGNI, L. (1955) Studio arteriografico del sifone carotideo in condizioni normali e patologiche. *Sist. nerv.* **3**, 3.

TÖNDURY, G. (1934) Einseitiges Fehlen der Arteria carotis interna. *Morph. Jb.* **74**, 625.

VIETEN, H. (1964) Röntgendiagnostik des Herzens und der Gefäße (in: *Handbuch der medizinischen Radiologie*, vol. 10/3. Ed. by Diethelm, L., Olsson, O., Strnad, F., Vieten, H. and Zuppinger, A.). Springer, Berlin.

VIGNAUD, J., CLAY, C. and AUBIN, M. L. (1972) Orbital arteriography. *Radiol. Clin. North America* **10**, 39.

VOGELSANG, H. (1968) Angiographisch selten nachweisbarer Kollateralkreislauf bei Arteria-carotis-interna-Verschluß. *Röfo* **108**, 794.

VOIGT, K., BRANDT, T. and SAUER, M. (1972) Röntgenanatomische Variationsstatistik zur topographischen Beziehung zwischen A. basilaris und schädelbasisstrukturen: Neuroradiologische Untersuchungen an Vertebralis und Brachialisangiographien. *Arch. Psychiat. Nervenkr.* **215**, 376.

WEIBEL, J. and FIELDS, W. S. (1965) Tortuosity, coiling and kinking of the internal carotid artery. *Neurology* **15**, 7.

WESTBERG, G. (1963) The recurrent artery of Heubner and the arteries of the central ganglia. *Acta radiol. (Stockh.)* **1**. 949.

WHEELER, E. C. (1964) The ophthalmic arterial complex in angiographic diagnosis. *Radiology* **83**, 26.

WILLIS, T. (1684) *Two Discourses Concerning the Soul of Brutes.* (cit. by Lang, E. K., Hann, E. C. and Luros, Th. J. 1964).

WOLF, B. S., NEWMAN, CH. M. and KHILNANI, M. T. (1962) The posterior inferior cerebellar artery on vertebral angiography. *Amer. J. Roentgenol.* **87**, 322.

WOLLSCHLAEGER, G. and WOLLSCHLAEGER, P. B. (1964a) The primitive trigeminal artery as seen angiographically and post-mortem examination. *Amer. J. Roentgenol.* **92**, 761.

WOLLSCHLAEGER, P. B. and WOLLSCHLAEGER, G. (1964b) Arterial anastomoses of the human brain (a radiographic-anatomical study). In: *VII. Symp. Neurol.*, New York.

ZAPPE, L., JUHÁSZ, J. and VIDOVSZKY, T. (1965) Collaterális keringés és prognózis összefüggései agyi artériás elzáródások esetén (Correlation between the collateral circulation and prognosis in cases of cerebral arterial obstruction). *Magy. Radiol.* **17**, 138.

ZOLNAI, B. (1960) Topography of the vertebral artery and the system of vertebral veins. *Acta morph. Acad. Sci. hung. Suppl.* **9**, 37.

ZUCKERKANDL, E. (1873) Über die Arteria stapedia des Menschen. *Mschr. Ohrenheilk.* 5.

YASUSADA, F. (1964) The X-ray findings of the thalamoperforate artery. *Nipp. Acta Radiol.* **24**, 60.

The internal jugular vein and its area of drainage

ARON-ROSA, D., RAMÉE, A., FISCHGOLD, H. and OFFRET, C. (1966a) Opafication du sinus caverneux par injection de produit opaque dans la veine ophtalmique. *Arch. Ophtal.* **26**, 737.

ARON-ROSA, D., RAMÉE, A. and METZGER, J. (1966b) La phlébographie orbitaire (in: *L'exploration neuroradiologique en ophtalmologie.* Ed. by Guillot, P., Saraux, H. and Sedan, R.). Masson et Cie, Paris.

BARGMAN, B. (1957) *Angiographie im Zahn-, Mund- und Kieferbereich.* Inaug. speech, München.

BAUMGARTNER, J., WORINGER, E., BRAUN, J. P. and ABADA, M. (1963) Phlébogramme cérébral profond de face et ses variations en cas de processus expansifs de l'espace intra-cranien sus-tentoriel. *Acta radiol. (Stockh.)* **1**, 182.

BEN AMOR, M., MARION, CH. and HELDT, N. (1971) Normal and pathological radioanatomy of the superior choroid vein. *Neuroradiology* **3**, 16.

CHEVREL, J. P., HUREAU, J., ALEXANDRE, J.-M. and LASSAU, J.-P. (1965) Deux nouvelles voies de drainage veineux du corps thyroïde. *Arch. Anat. path.* **97**, 13.

CHIRAIC, V., FRASIN, CH. and CHIRAIC, R. (1972) Varietät des Sinus durae matris des oberen aboralen Gruppe. *Anat. Anz.* **130**, 526.

CLARA, M. (1953) *Das Nervensystem des Menschen.* Barth, Leipzig.

CURRY, R. W. and CULBERTH, G. G. (1951) The normal cerebral angiogram. *Amer. J. Roentgenol.* **65**, 341.

DAS, A. C. and HASAN, M. (1970) The occipital sinus. *J. Neurosurg.* **33**, 307.

DE DOMINICIS, R. BUFALINI, G. N. and RAGAGLINI, G. (1964) Il flebogramma cerebrale nei suoi aspetti morfologici e funzionali. *Nunt. radiol. (Roma)* **30**, 1.

DÉJEAN, CH. and BOUDET, CH. (1951) Du diagnostic des varices de l'orbite et de leurs complications par la phlébographie. *Bull. Soc. Ophtal. Paris* **64**, 374.

DELMAS, A., PERTUISET, B. and BERTRAND, G. (1951) Les veines du lobe temporal. *Rev. Oto-neuro-ophtal.* **23**, 224.

DILENGE, D. (1962) *L'angiographie de l'artère carotide interne chez le sujet normal.* Masson, Paris.

DREWES, J. (1963) *Die Phlebographie der oberen Körperhälfte unter besonderer Berücksichtigung anatomischer Varietäten und hämodynamisch bedinger Phänomene im Venenkontrastbild.* Springer, Berlin—Göttingen—Heidelberg.

ELLIOTT, H. C. (1963) *Textbook of Neuroanatomy.* Lippincott, Philadelphia—Montreal.

ELMOHAMED, A. and HEMPEL, K. J. (1966) Über die Typenhäufigkeit des Confluens sinuum beim Menschen. *Frankf. Z. Path.* **75**, 321.

ELMOHAMED, A. and HEMPEL, K. J. (1966) Über einen Parasinus transversus durae matris. *Acta Neurochir. (Wien)* **15**, 120.

FISCHGOLD, H., ADAM, H., ÉCOIFFIER, L. and PIEQUET, J. (1952) Opafication des plexus rachidiennes et des veines azygos par voie osseuse. *J. Radiol. Électrol.* **33**, 37.

GEJROT, T. and LAUREN, T. (1964) Retrograde venography of the internal jugular veins and transverse sinuses. *Acta otolaryng. (Stockh.)* **57**, 1.

GVOZDANOVIĆ, V. (1952) Some observations about the normal cerebral phlebogram and its variations. *Rad. jug. Akad. Znan. Umj. Od. med. Nauke* **291**, 33.

HEMPEL, K. J. and ELMOHAMED, A. (1971) Anatomie, Formvarianten und Typisierungen des venösen intrakraniellen System beim Menschen. *Radiologe* **11**, 451.

JOHANSON, C. (1954) The cerebral veins and deep dural sinuses of the brain. *Acta radiol. (Stockh.) Suppl.* **107**.

KÁDÁR, F. and KOCSIS, A. G. (1959) Beiträge zur Anatomie und zu den klinischen Beziehungen des Plexus venosus pterygoideus. *Schweiz. Mschr. Zahnheilk.* **69**, 618.

KESSEL, F. (1928) Verlauf des Nervus accessorius durch eine Insel der Vena jugularis interna. *Anat. Anz.* **65**, 162.

KISS, F. (1949) A szem vérkeringése (Blood circulation of the eye). *Szemészet* **86**, 1.

KISS, F. (1957) Az agy vér és liquor keringése (Blood and CSF circulation of the brain). *Orv. Szle* **3**, 14.

KRAYENBÜHL, H. and RICHTER, H. R. (1952) *Die zerebrale Angiographie.* Thieme, Stuttgart.

KRAYENBÜHL, H. and YASARGIL, M. G. (1965) *Die zerebrale Angiographie*, 2nd ed. Thieme, Stuttgart.

LINDGREN, E. (1954) Röntgenologie, einschließlich Kontrastmethoden (in: *Handbuch der Neurochirurgie*, vol. 2. Ed. by Olivecrona, H. and Tönnis, W.). Springer, Berlin—Göttingen—Heidelberg.

LOMBARDI, G. and PASSERINI, A. (1968) Venography of the orbit: Technique and anatomy. *Brit. J. Radiol.* **41**, 282.

MINE, T. (1971) The medial inferior cerebellar vein. *Brain Nerve (Tokyo)* **23**, 129.

MOREAU, F. (1965) *L'angiographie thyreoïdéenne.* Imp. Delteil, Bordeaux.

NEBAUER, H. and SÜSSE, H. J. (1966) Die Phlebographie der Orbita über die Vena frontalis. *Klin. Mbl. Augenheilk.* **148**, 202.

PORTELA-GOMES, F. (1964) Seio longitudinal superior. *Gaz. méd. port.* **17**, 354.

RABINOV, K. R. (1964) The postvertebral neck veins in cerebral angiography. *Radiology* **83**, 626.

RODRIGUEZ, I. and ADRIAO, M. (1931) Variation de la veine jugulaire interne. Absence de jugulaire externe. Rameau nerveux traversant une veine. *Folia anat. Coimbra* **6**, 1.

SCHEUNEMANN, H. and SCHRUDDE, J. (1964) Angiographische Untersuchungen der A. carotis externa (in: *Handbuch der medizinischen Radiologie*, vol. 10/3. Ed. by Diethelm, L., Olsson, O., Strnad, F., Vieten, H. and Zuppinger, A.). Springer, Berlin.

SCHMIDT-WITTKAMP, E. and ROSCHER, M. (1966) Zur Lagebestimmung des "Angulus venosus" im seitlichen Phlebogramm. *Röfo* **105**, 92.

SHIU, PH. C., HANAFEE, W. N., WILSON, G. H. and RAND, R. W. (1968) Cavernous sinus venography. *Amer. J. Roentgenol.* **104**, 57.

SÜSSE, H. J. and KUNITS, G. (1966) Die Phlebographie der extrakraniellen Kopfvenen über die Vena frontalis. *Röfo* **104**, 184.

TENCHINI L. (1900) Sul bulbo giugulare inferiore dell'uomo. *Ric. Lab. Anat. Roma e altri Lab. Biol. V*, VII (1899) (ref. Anat. Jb. 5/1900/189).

TÖNNIS, W. and SCHIEFER, W. (1959) *Zirkulationsstörungen des Gehirns im Serienangiogramm.* Springer, Berlin—Göttingen—Heidelberg.

WACKENHEIM, A., HELDT, N. and BEN AMOR, M. (1971) Variations in the drainage of the lateral mesencephalic vein. *Neuroradiology* **2**, 154.

WENDE, S. and CIBA, K. (1968) Der Wert der Jugularis-Venographie für die Darstellung des Sinus cavernosus. *Röfo* **109**, 56.

WOLF, B. S. and HUANG, Y. P. (1964) The subependymal veins of the lateral ventricles. *Amer. J. Roentgenol.* **91**, 406.

WOLF, B. S., HUANG, Y. P. and NEWMAN, C. M. (1963) The lateral anastomotic mesencephalic vein and other variations in drainage of the basal cerebral vein. *Amer. J. Roentgenol.* **89**, 411.

WOODHALL, V. (1939) Anatomy of the cranial blood sinuses with particular reference to the lateral. *Laryngoscope (St. Louis)* **49**, 966.

ZOLNAI, B. (1960) Topography of the vertebral artery and the system of vertebral veins. *Acta morph. Acad. Sci. hung. Suppl.* **9**, 37.

The axillary artery and its branches

BERBERICH, J. and HIRSCH, S. (1923) Die röntgenologische Darstellung der Arterien und Venen am lebenden Menschen. *Klin. Wschr.* **2**, 2226.

EDWARDS, E. A. (1960) Organization of the small arteries of the hand and digits. *Amer. J. Surg.* **99**, 837.

FLINT, M. H. (1955) *Brit. J. plast. Surg.* **8**, 186 (cit. by Strickland, B. and Urquhart, W. 1963).

HASCHEK, E. and LINDENTHAL, O. TH. (1896) Ein Beitrag zur praktischen Verwertung der Photographie nach Röntgen. *Wien. Klin. Wschr.* **9**, 63.

JASCHTSCHINSKI, S. N. (1897) Morphologie und Topographie des Arcus volaris sublimis und profundus des Menschen. *Anat. Hefte* **7**, 161.

KADANOFF, D. and BALKANSKY, G. (1966) Zwei Fälle mit seltenen Varietäten der Arterien der oberen Extremität. *Anat. Anz.* **118**, 289.

KENESI, C. and HONNART, F. (1969) Les artères interosseuses à l'avant-bras. *C. R. Ass. Anat.* **142**, 1057.

LOETZKE, H. H. and KLEINAU, W. (1968) Gleichzeitiges Vorkommen der Aa. brachialis superficialis, radialis und antebrachialis dorsalis superficialis, sowie deren Aufzweigungen. *Anat. Anz.* **122**, 137.

MCCORMACK, L. J., CAULDWELL, E. W. and ANSON, B. J. (1953) Brachial and antibrachial arterial patterns. *Surg. Gynec. Obstet.* **96**, 43.

NEIHARDT, J. H. and SPANTA, A. D. (1969) Aspect anatomique de la vascularization de l'extrémité supérieure de l'humerus. *Lyon méd.* **222**, 689.

RATSCHOW, M. (1959) *Angiologie.* Thieme, Stuttgart.

SOILA, P., WEGELIUS, U. and VIITANEN, S. M. (1963) Notes on the technique of angiography of the upper extremity. *Angiology* **14**, 297.

STRICKLAND, B. and URQUHART, W. (1963) Digital arteriography, with reference to nail dystrophy. *Brit. J. Radiol.* **36**, 427.

WEATHERBY, H. T. (1955) *Anat. Rec.* **122**, 57 (cit. by Strickland, B. and Urquhart, W. 1963).

WELLAUER, J. (1957) Arteriographie der Extremitäten (in: *Lehrbuch der Röntgendiagnostik, Ergebnisse der medizinischen Trahlenforschung* 1952–1956. Ed. by Schinz, H. R., Glauner, R. and Uehlinger, F. E.). Thieme, Stuttgart.

The axillary vein and its area of drainage

BILE, S. (1935) Ostacoli e pericoli che si possono incontrare durante la ligatura dell'arteria ascellare in alto, per la presenza di un aderente e cospicuo "anelo venoso" interno all'arteria. *Monit. Zool. ital.* **46**, 259.

BRECHER, G. A. (1956) *A Venous Return.* Grune and Stratton, New York – London.

DREWES, J. (1963) *Die Phlebographie der oberen Körperhälfte unter besonderer Berücksichtigung anatomischer Varietäten und hämodynamisch bedingter Phänomene im Venenkontrastbild.* Springer, Berlin – Göttingen – Heidelberg.

DREWES, J. (1964) Varietäten der Vena cephalica im Phlebogramm. *Röfo* **100**, 490.

DREWES, J. (1965) Veneninseln im Phlebogramm der oberen Extremität. *Röfo* **102**, 667.

FISCHER, F. K. (1951) Die Phlebographie von Schulter und Hals und Mediastinum. *Schweiz. med. Wschr.* **81**, 1198.

GARUSI, G. F. and MORETTI, S. (1963) Aspetti morfo-funzionali del tronco axillo-succlavio e dell'apparato valvolare della vena succlavia. *Radiol. med. (Torino)* **49**, 757.

KADANOFF, D., ČUČKOV, CHR. and ZRINOV, B. (1966) Die Unterschiede im Typ der Hauptanastomose zwischen den großen Hautvenen der oberen Extremität beim Menschen. *Morph. Jb.* **109**, 340.

KALDYI, H. (1877) Einiges über die Vena basilica und die Venen des Oberarmes. *Arch. Anat.* **2**.

LAVIZZARI, E. and OTTOLINI, V. (1955) La dimostrazione radiologica del tronco axillo-succlavio. *Atti Soc. lombarda Sci. med.-biol.* **10**, 134.

MOBERG, E. (1960) The shoulder-hand-finger syndrome. *Surg. Clin. N. Amer.* **40**, 376.

ROMINGER, C. J. (1958) The normal axillary venogram. *Amer. J. Roentgenol.* **80**, 217.

SAÏFI, Y. (1967) *Études sur la face dorsale de la main.* Mem. Lab. Anat., Paris.

SGALITZER, M., KOLLERT, V. and DEMEL, R. (1931) Kontrastdarstellung der Venen im Röntgenbilde. *Klin. Wschr.* **10**, 1659.

SZÜCS, S. (1964) Mellkasi intraossealis venographia (Thoracic intraosseal venography). Thesis. Budapest.

TAGARIELLO, P. (1952) Value of phlebography in the diagnosis of intermittent obstruction of the subclavian vein. *J. int. Coll. Surg.* **17**, 789.

The abdominal aorta and its branches

ALFIDI, R. J., RASTOGI, H., BUONOCORE, E. and BROWN, CH. H. (1968) Hepatic arteriography. *Radiology* **90**, 1136.

ALKEN, C. F. and SOMMER, F. (1950) Die Renovasographie. *Z. Urol.* **43**, 420.

ANSON, B. J., CAULDWELL, E. W., PICK, J. W. and BEATON, L. E. (1947) The blood supply of the kidney, suprarenal gland and associated structures. *Surg. Gynec. Obstet.* **84**, 313.

ANSON, B. J. and KURTH, L. E. (1955) Common variations in the renal blood supply. *Surg. Gynec. Obstet.* **100**, 156.

AUGIER, M. A. (1923) Appareil urinaire (in: *Traité d'anatomie humaine.* Ed. by Poirier, P. and Charpy, A.). Masson, Paris.

BABICS, A. (1945) Kóros vesék verőérelváltozásai (Arterial changes in pathological kidneys). *Orv. Lapja* **1**, 264.

BÁLINT, J. and PALKOVICH, I. (1952) Rendellenes vesearteriák intrarenalis viszonya az art. renalishoz (Intrarenal relation of the anomalous renal arteries to the renal artery). *Magy. Sebész* **5**, 130.

BARBACCIA, F. and POMPILI, G. (1960) I circoli collaterali nelle ostruzioni dell'aorta abdominale e dei suoi rami terminali. *Radiol. med. (Torino)* **46**, 129.

BASMAJIAN, J. V. (1954) The marginal anastomoses of the arteries to the large intestine. *Surg. Gynec. Obstet.* **99**, 614.

BAYLIN, G. J. (1939) Collateral circulation following an obstruction of the abdominal aorta. *Anat. Rec.* **75**, 405.

BELLMANN, G. and HERWIG, H. (1964) *Die Aortographie in der angiologischen Diagnostik.* Thieme, Leipzig.

BERNARDI, R., FRASSON, F. and PISTOLESI, G. F. (1971) Normal angiographic patterns of the inferior mesenteric artery. *Radiol. Clin. Biol.* **40**, 153.

BOATMAN, D. L., CORNELL, S. H. and KÖLLN, C. P. (1971) The arterial supply of horseshoe kidneys. *Amer. J. Roentgenol.* **113**,, 447.

BOIJSEN, E. (1959) Angiographic studies of the anatomy of single and multiple renal arteries. *Acta radiol. (Stockh.) Suppl.* **183**.

BOIJSEN, E. and OLIN, T. (1964) Zöliakographie und Angiographie der Arteria mesenterica superior (in: *Ergebnisse der medizinischen Strahlenforschung.* Ed. by Schinz, H., Glauner, R. and Rüttmann, A.). Thieme, Stuttgart.

BROWNE, E. Z. (1940) Variations in origin and course of the hepatic artery and its branches. *Surgery* **8**, 424.

BÜCHELER, E., DÜX, A. and THURN, P. (1966) Die Stenose der abdominellen Aorta. *Röfo* **104**, 22.

CAMERINI, F. and SCAGNOL, A. (1967) Mesenterialer Kollateralkreislauf bei Verschluß der Nierenarterie. *Röfo* **107**, 290.

CARUCCI, J. J. (1963) Mesenteric vascular occlusion. *Amer. J. Surg.* **85**, 47.

CHÉRIGIÉ, E., MELLIÈRE, D. amd BENNET, J. (1967) Anatomie radiologique de la vascularisation du pancréas. *J. Radiol. Électrol.* **48**, 316.

COUINAUD, C. (1954a) Distribution de l'artère hépatique dans le foie. *Acta anat. (Basel)* **22**, 17.

COUINAUD, C. (1954b) Lobes et segments hépatiques. *Presse méd.* **62**, 709.

DASELER, T. C. and CUTTER, W. W. (1948) Arterial blood supply of the common bile duct. *Arch. Surg.* **57**, 599.

DEBRAY, CH., MARTIN, ET. and LEYMARIOS, J. (1961) Les lésions dégénératives du tronc et de l'artère mésentérique supérieure. *Sem. Hôp. Paris* **37**, 3561.

DELANNOY, E. (1923) Artère mésentérique supérieure double. *Bull. Soc. Anat. Paris* **93**, 346.

DE LUCA, C. and DE SERIO, N. (1959) Studi di anatomia radiologica angiographica sul vivente. *Radiol. med. (Torino)* **45**, 972.

DE LUCA, C. and DE SERIO, N. (1960a) Studi di anatomia radiologica angiographica sul vivente. *Radiol. med. (Torino)* **46**, 120.

DE LUCA, C. and DE SERIO, N. (1960b) Studi di anatomia radiologica angiographica sul vivente. *Radiol. med. (Torino)* **46**, 355.

DE LUCA, C. and DE SERIO, N. (1960c) Studi di anatomia radiologica angiographica sul vivente. *Radiol. med. (Torino)* **46**, 435.

DE LUCA, C .and DE SERIO, N. (1960d) Studi di anatomia radiologica angiographica sul vivente. *Radiol. med. (Torino)* **46**, 1074.

DE LUCA, C. and DE SERIO, N. (1961) Studi di anatomia radiologica angiographica sul vivente. *Radiol. med. (Torino)* **47**, 322.

DEUTSCH, V. (1967) Cholecysto-angiography. *Amer. J. Roentgenol.* **101**, 608.

DIEMEL, H., RAU, G. and SCHMITZ-DRÄGER, H. G. (1964) Die Riolanische Kollaterale. *Röfo* **101**, 253.

DIEMEL, H. and SCHMITZ-DRÄGER, H. G. (1965) Intraabdominelle Kollateralbahnen bei Verschlußkrankheiten der Eingeweidearterien. *Röfo* **103**, 652.

DOS SANTOS, R., LAMAS, A. C. and CALDAS, J. (1931) *Artériographie des membres et de l'aorte abdominale.* Masson, Paris.

DOUIVILLE, E. and HOLLINSHEAD, W. H. (1955) The blood supply of the normal renal pelvis. *J. Urol.* **73**, 906.

DREYFUSS, J. R., NEBESAR, R. A. and POLLARD, J. J. (1967) Hepatic angiography (in: *Progress in Radiology.* Symposium and invital papers of the 11th International Congress of Radiology, Rom, 22.—28. Sept. 1965. Ed. by Turano, L., Ratti, A. and Biagnini, C.). Excerpta Medica Foundation, Amsterdam—New York—London.

DRUMMOND, H. (1913) Some points relating to the surgical anatomy of the arterial supply of the large intestine. *Proc. roy. Soc. Med.* **7**, 185.

DÜX, A., BÜCHELER, E. and THURN, P. (1966) Der arterielle Kollateralkreislauf der Leber. *Röfo* **105**, 1.

DWIGHT, T. (1903) The branches of the superior mesenteric artery of the jejunum and ileum. *Anat. Anz.* **23**, 184.

EATON, P. B. (1917) The coeliac axis. *Anat. Rec.* **13**, 369.

EDSMAN, G. (1957) Angionephrography and suprarenal angiography. *Acta radiol.(Stockh.) Suppl.* **155**.

EDWARDS, E. A. and LEMAY, M. (1955) Occlusion patterns and collaterals in arteriosclerosis of the abdominal aorta and iliac arteries. *Surgery* **38**, 950.

ELISKA, O. (1968) The perforating arteries and their role in the collateral circulation of the kidneys. *Acta anat. (Basel)* **70**, 184.

FALCONER, C. W. A. and GRIFFITHS, E. (1950) The anatomy of the blood vessels in the region of the pancreas. *Brit. J. Surg.* **37**, 334.

FALLER, J. and UNGVÁRI, GY. (1962) Die arterielle Segmentation der Niere. *Zbl. Chir.* **87**, 23.

FINE, H. and KEEN, D. N. (1966) The arteries of the human kidney. *J. Anat. (Lond.)* **100**, 881.

FRY, W. J. and KRAFT, R. O. (1963) *Surg. Gynec. Obstet.* **117**, 417 (cit. by Schmidt, H. and Schimanski, K. 1967).

GAGNON, R. (1957) The arterial supply of the human adrenal gland. *Rev. canad. Biol.* **16**, 421.

GAGNON, R. (1964) Middle suprarenal arteries in man: "A statistical study of two hundred human adrenal glands". *Rev. canad. Biol.* **23**, 461.

GAGNON, R. (1966) Les artères surrénales inférieures chez l'homme. *Rev. canad. Biol.* **25**, 135.

GEYER, J. R. and POUTASSE, E. F. (1962) Incidence of multiple renal arteries on aortography. *J. Amer. Med. Ass.* **182**, 120.

GILLOT, CLAUD, DELMAS (1959) cit. in: *Handbook of circulation.* Ed. by Dittmer, D. S. and Grebe, R. M. Saunders, Philadelphia—London.

GÖBBELER, TH. and LÖHR, E. (1968) Abdominelle Aortenverschlüsse und deren Umgebungkreisläufe, unter besonderer Berücksichtigung angiographischer Untersuchungstechnik. *Röfo* **109**, 471.

GÖMÖRI, P., NAGY, Z., ZOLNAY, B., JAKAB, I. and MÉSZÁROS, A. (1965) The problem of the arterio-venous anastomoses of the kidney. *Acta med. Acad. Sci. hung.* **21**, 197.

GOTTLOB, R. (1956) *Angiographie und Klinik.* Maudrich, Wien—Bonn.

GRAVES, F. T. (1954) The anatomy of the intrarenal arteries and its application to segmental resection of the kidney. *Brit. J. Surg.* **42**, 132.

GRAVES, F. T. (1956) The aberrant renal artery. *J. Anat.* **90**, 553.

GWYN, D. G. and SKILTON, I. S. (1966) A rare variation of the inferior mesenteric artery in man. *Anat. Rec.* **156**, 235.

GYURKÓ, GY. and SZABÓ, M. (1966) A lép érszerkezetének vizsgálata sebészeti anatómiai szempontból (Study of the angioarchitecture of the spleen from a surgical anatomical aspect). *Morph. igazságü. orv. Szle* **6**, 1.

HAAGE, H. and REHM, A. (1964) Zum Kollateralkreislauf der Niere. *Röfo* **100**, 736.

HABERER, H. (1901) Lien succenturiatus und Lien accessorius. *Arch. J. Anat. Entwickl.-Gesch.* 47.

HABIGHORST, L. V., ALBERS, P. and ZEITLER, E. (1965) Die Gefäße der Gallenblase im postmortalen Angiogramm. *Röfo* **103**, 63.

HABIGHORST, L. V., KÖSSLING, F. K. and ALBERS, P. (1966) Die perirenalen Arterien und der Kollateralkreislauf der Niere im postmortalen Angiogramm. *Röfo* **105**, 35.

HALLER (1759) *First Lines of Physiology.* (cit. by Diemel, H., Rau, G. and Schmitz-Dräger, H. G. 1964).

HAYEK, H. (1935) Bau und Funktion der Arterien als Stütz- und Halteorgane. *Z. Anat. Entwickl.-Gesch.* **104**, 359.

HEALEY, J. E., SCHROY, P. C. and SORENSEN, R. J. (1953) The intrahepatic distribution of the hepatic artery in man. *J. int. Coll. Surg.* **20**, 133.

HEIDSIECK, E. (1928) Zur Skeletotopie der großen Äste der Bauchaorta. *Anat. Anz.* **66**, 6.

HELLSTRÖM, J. (1928) Über die Varianten der Nierengefäße. *Z. urol. Chir.* **24**, 253.

HENSCHEN, C. (1928) Die chirurgische Anatomie der Milzgefäße. *Schweiz. med. Wschr.* **58**, 164.

HESS, W. (1961) *Die Erkrankungen der Gallenwege und des Pankreas.* Thieme, Stuttgart.

INAMURA, H. (1923) Blutgefäße des Processus vermiformis. *Kyoto Igakkai Zasshi* **20**.

JACKSON, B. B. (1963) *Occlusion of the superior mesenteric artery.* Thomas, Springfield, Ill.

KÁDÁR, F. (1950) A lép vérkeringése korróziós készítmények alapján (Blood circulation of the spleen on the basis of corrosion preparations). *Kísérl. Orvostud.* **4**, 1.

KÁDÁR, F. and BÁLINT, J. (1953) Adatok az epehólyag vérellátásához (Data to the blood supply of the gallbladder). *Magy. Sebész.* **6**, 106.

KAHN, P. C. (1967) Selective angiography of the inferior phrenic arteries. *Radiology* **88**, 1.

KAHN, P. C. and ABRAMS, H. L. (1964) Inferior mesenteric arterial patterns. *Radiology* **82**, 429.

KÁPOLNÁSI, J. and VÉGH, E. (1972) Csecsemőn észlelt solitaer arteria renalis (Solitary renal artery observed in infant). *Gyermekgyógyászat* **23**, 96.

KIKKAWA, F. (1966a) The segmental arrangement of the trabecular arteries of the spleen in the human. *Acta Anat. Nippon* **41**, 105.

KIKKAWA, F. (1966b) Über die extralienale Verästelung der Arteria lienalis und die Ansatzfigur des Hilus. *Okajimas Folia anat. jap.* **42**, 1.

KISS, F. (1926) Über einige Varietäten der Arteria hepatica und Arteria cystica. *Z. Anat. Entwickl.-Gesch.* **81**, 601.

KÖHLER, R. (1963) Incomplete angiogram in selective renal angiography. *Acta radiol. (Stockh.)* **1**, 1011.

KOKAS, F. and KUBIK, I. (1954) Adatok a duodenum vérellátásához (Data to the blood supply of the duodenum). *Magy. Sebész.* **7**, 99.

KOURIAS, B. G. and PEVERETOS, P. (1972) Variations et anomalies artères hépatobiliaires. *J. Chirurg.* **103**, 221.

KUPIC, E. A., MARSHALL, W. H. and ABRAMS, H. L. (1967) Splenic arterial patterns. Angiographic analysis and review. *Invest. Radiol.* **2**, 70.

KYAW, M. M. and NEWMAN, H. (1971) Renal pseudotumors due to ectopic accessory renal arteries: The angiographic diagnosis. *Amer. J. Roentgenol.* **113**, 443.

LANG, H. (1947) Die arterielle Blutversorgung der tiefen Gallenwege. *Chirurg* **17/18**, 67.

LARDENNOIS, G. and OKINCZYC, J. (1910) La véritable terminaison de l'artère mésentérique supérieure. *Bull. Soc. Anat. Paris* **85**, 13.

LEVASSEUR, J. C. and COUINAUD, C. (1968) Étude de la distribution des artères gastriques. *J. Chir.* **95**, 57.

LIBSHITZ, H., BEN-MENACHEM, Y. and KURODA, K. (1972) Unusual renal vascular supply. *Brit. J. Radiol.* **45**, 536.

LÖFGREN, F. (1949) *Das topographische System der Malpigischen Pyramiden der Menschenniere.* Gleerupska Univ.-bokhandeln, Lund.

LUDIN, H. (1963) Angiographische Nebennierendarstellung. *Röfo* **99**, 654.

LUZSA, GY. (1963) Hasi szervek postmortalis angiographiája (Postmortem angiography of the abdominal viscera). *Magy. Radiol.* **15**, 361.

LUZSA, GY. (1965) Posmrtná angiografie břišnich orgánů (Postmortem angiography of the abdominal viscera). *Čs. Rentgenol.* **19**, 2.

MÁTYUS, E. (1965) A veseerek fejlődési rendellenességei, segmentum ischaemia és a vese megbetegedései (Congenital anomalies and segmental ischaemia of the renal vessels and renal diseases). Thesis. Budapest.

MERCIER, R. and VANNEUVILLE, G. (1968) *Anatomie radiologique de l'aorta abdominale et de ses branches terminales et collatérales.* Brosch, Paris.

MERKLIN, R. J. and MICHELS, N. A. (1958) Variant renal and suprarenal blood supply with data on inferior phrenic, ureteral and gonadal arteries: Statistical analysis based on 185 dissections and review of literature. *J. int. Coll. Surg.* **29**, 41.

MEYERS, M. A., FRIEDENBERG, R. M. and KING, M. C. (1967) The significance of the renal capsular arteries. *Brit. J. Radiol.* **401**, 949.

MICHELS, N. A. (1953) Collateral arterial pathways to the liver after ligation of the hepatic artery and removal of the celiac axis. *Cancer* **6**, 708.

MICHELS, N. A. (1955) *Blood Supply and Anatomy of the Upper Abdominal Organs.* Lippincott, Philadelphia.

MICHELS, N. A. (1957) The ever varied blood supply of the liver and its collateral circulation. *J. int. Coll. Surg.* **27**, 1.

MICHELS, N. A., SIDDHARTH, P., KORNBLITH, P. L. and PARKE, W. W. (1965) The variant blood supply to the descending colon, rectosigmoid and rectum, based on 400 dissections. *Dis. Colon Rect.* **8**, 251.

MICHELS, N. A., SIDDHARTH, P., KORNBLITH, P. L. and PARKE, W. W. (1968) Routes of collateral circulation of the gastrointestinal tract as ascertained in a dissection of 500 bodies. *Int. J. Surg.* **49**, 8.

MLYNARCZYK, L., WOZNIAK, W. and KIERSZ, A. (1966) Varianten in der Anzahl und im Verlauf der Nierenarterien. *Anat Anz.* **118**, 67.

MORETTI, S. (1965) Le arterie della testa del pancreas. *Ann. Radiol. diagn. (Bologna)* **38**, 569.

MÖRIKE, K. D. (1965) Der Verlauf der Nierenarterien und ihr möglicher Einfluß auf die Lage der Nieren. *Anat. Anz.* **116**, 485.

MORINO, F. (1959) Die Arteriographie der Arteria hepatica (in: *Röntgendiagnostik der Leber.* Ed. by Anecker, H., Morino, F., Rösch, J., Schumacher, W. and Zuppinger, A.). Springer, Berlin—Göttingen—Heidelberg.

MULLER, R. F. and FIGLEY, M. M. (1957) The arteries of the abdomen, pelvis and thigh. *Amer. J. Roentgenol.* **77**, 296.

NARATH, P. A. (1951) *Renal Pelvis and Ureter.* Grune and Stratton, New York.

ÖDMAN, P. (1958) Percutaneous selective angiography of the coeliac artery. *Acta radiol. (Stockh.) Suppl.* **159**.

ÖDMAN, P. (1959) Percutaneous selective angiography of the superior mesenteric artery. *Acta radiol. (Stockh.)* **51**, 25.

OLSSON, O. (1964) Selektive Nierenangiographie (in: *Ergebnisse der medizinischen Strahlenforschung* vol. 1. Ed. by Schinz, H. R., Glauner, R. and Rüttmann, A.). Thieme, Stuttgart.

OLSSON, O. and JÖNSSON, G. (1962) Roentgen examination of the kidney and ureter (in: *Handbuch der Urologie.* Ed. by Alken, C. E., Dix, V. W., Weirauch, H. M. and Wildbolz, E.). Springer, Berlin—Göttingen—Heidelberg.

PALUBINSKAS, A. J. (1964) "Stretching" of the arteries in renal arteriography. *Radiology* **82**, 40.

PICK, J. W. and ANSON, B. J. (1940) Inferior phrenic artery: Origin and suprarenal branches. *Anat. Rec.* **78**, 413.

PIERSON, J. M. (1943) The arterial blood supply of the pancreas. *Surg. Gynec. Obstet.* **77**, 426.

PIQUAND, G. (1910) Recherches sur l'anatomie du tronc cœliaque et ses branches. *Bibl. anat. (Basel)* **19**, 159.

PIRLET, FR. and DELVIGNE, J. (1965) L'artériographie rénale. *Acta urol. belg.* **33**, 161.

RATSCHOW, M. (1937) Leistung und Bedeutung der Vasographie als Funktionsprüfung der peripheren Blutgefäße. *Röfo* **55**, 253.

RATSCHOW, M. (1959) *Angiologie.* Thieme, Stuttgart.

REUTER, S. R. and OLIN, T. (1965) *Radiology* **85**, 617 (cit. by Schmidt, H. and Schimanski, K. 1967).

RIO BRANCO, P. (1912) Essai sur l'anatomie et la médecine opératoire du tronc cœliaque et de ses branches et de l'artère hépatique en particulier. Thèse Médecine Paris.

RIOLAN, J. (1649) *Anthropographie.* Paris (cit. by Adachi. B. 1928).

ROSSI, G. and COVA, E. (1904) Studio morfologico delle arteria dello stomaco. *Arch. ital. Anat. Embriol.* **3**, 485.

RÖSCH, J. (1971) Die "superselektive" Arteriographie. *Röfo* **115**, 718.

RÖSCH, J. and BRET, J. (1963) Sleziná arteriografie. *Čs. Reatgenol.* **17**, 353.

RUBASCHEWA, A. (1930) Die Blutversorgung der Gallenblase. *Röfo* **41**, 957.

SABBAGH, A., ROBICSEK, F. and DAUGHERTY, H. K. (1970) Renal blood supply originating from the medial sacral vessels. *Vasc. Surg.* **4**, 19.

SCHMERBER, F. (1895) *Recherches anatomiques sur l'artère rénale.* Ass. Typographic, Lyon.

SCHMERBER, F. (1896) Les artères de la capsule graisseuse du rein. *Int. Mschr. Anat. Physiol.* **13**, 269.

SCHMIDT, H. and SCHIMANSKI, K. (1967) Die Stenose der Arteria coeliaca — ihre Diagnose und klinische Bedeutung. *Röfo* **106**, 1.

SCHORN, J., STENDER, H. ST. and VOEGT, H. (1957) Untersuchungen über die arterielle Strombahn der Leber, I – III. *Langenbecks Arch. Klin. Chir.* **286**, 187.

SELDINGER, S. I. (1953) Catheter replacement of needle in percutaneous arteriography; new technique. *Acta radiol. (Stockh.)* **39**, 368.

(SEROV, V. V.) CEPOV, B. B. (1959) Гиствонгиорентгелографические параллели при гломерулонефритах (Histoangiographic parallels in glomerulonephritis). *Urologiya* **24**, 15.

SOLANKE, T. F. (1968) The blood supply of the vermiform appendix in Nigerians. *J. Anat. (Lond.)* **102**, 353.

STEGER, C. and CRESTI, M. (1963) Über den Kollateralkreislauf bei chronischen Verschlüssen der Bauchaorta und der Beckenarterien. *Helv. chir. Acta* **3**, 322.

STEINBERG, I., FINBY, N. and EVANS, J. A. (1959) Safe and practical intravenous method for abdominal aortography, peripheral arteriography and cerebral angiography. *Amer. J. Roentgenol.* **82**, 758.

STEWARD, J. A. and RANKIN, F. W. (1933) Blood supply of the large intestine; its surgical considerations. *Arch. Surg.* **26**, 843.

STRÖM, B. G. and WINBERG, T. (1962) Percutaneous selective arteriography of the inferior mesenteric artery. *Acta radiol. (Stockh.)* **57**, 401.

SUHLER, A., PIETRI, J., KIENY, R. and FONTAINE, R. (1966) Le réseau artériel para-rénal et sa valeur comme circulation de suppléance dans les sténoses et oblitérations de l'artère rénale. *J. Chir. (Paris)* **92**, 613.

SUNDERGREN, R. (1970) Selective angiography of the left gastric artery. *Acta radiol. (Stockh)* Suppl. **299**.

SYKES, D. (1964) The correlation between renal vascularisation and lobulation of the kidney. *Brit. J. Urol.* **36**, 549.

TERNON, Y. (1959) *Chirurg* **78**, 517 (cit. by Mátyus, E. 1965).

TESTUT, L. (1902) *Trattato di anatomia umana II.* U.T.E.T., Torino.

THOMAS, D. P. (1966) Arteriographic localization of the placenta. *Aust. Radiol.* **10**, 127.

TILLE, D. (1961) *Die Aortographie des Abdomens aus klinischer Sicht.* Thieme, Leipzig.

TOMMASEO, T. (1958) Sul' una osservazione anatomica di dolicomegalia dell'arcuata arteriosa intermesenterica. *Riv. Anat. pat.* **13**, 719.

TONGIO, J., KIEMY, R., HAEHNEL, P. and WARTER, P. (1971) La circulation collatérale au cours des sténoses des artères rénales. Etude angiographique. *J. Radiol.Electrol.* **52**, 7.

VAN VOORTHUISEN, A. E. (1964) Selective angiografie van de lumbale arterien. *Ned. T. Geneesk.* **108**, 2461.

VOGLER, E. and HERBST, R. (1958) *Angiographie der Nieren.* Thieme, Stuttgart.

WITT, H. and KOURIK, W. (1969) Gemeinsame Versorgung des Gastrointestinaltraktes sowie der Leber und Milz durch erweiterte, schleifenförmig verlaufende A. mesenterica caudalis. *Röfo* **111**, 92.

ZWERINA, H. and POISEL, S. (1966) Über die Anastomose zwischen dem Tr. coeliacus, der Art. mes. sup. und Art. mes. inf. *Anat. Anz.* **119**, 427.

YAKUBI, K. (1920) Eck'sche Fistel etc. Chirurg. Anatomie des Stammes der V. portae und der umgebenden Organe. *Nippon Geka Gakki Zasshi* **21**, 12.

The inferior vena cava and its branches

AHLBERG, N. E., BARTLEY, O. and CHIDEKEL, N. (1968) Occurrence of valves in the main trunk of the renal vein. *Acta radiol. (Stockh.)* **7**, 431.

ANSON, B. J. and CAULDWELL, E. W. (1947) The blood supply of the kidney, suprarenal gland and associated structures. *Surg. Gynec. Obstet.* **84**, 313.

BANNER, R. L. and BRESFIELD, R. D. (1958) Surgical anatomy of the hepatic veins. *Cancer* **11**, 22.

BARTEL, J. and WIERNY, L. (1963) Zur Agenesie der Vena cava caudalis. *Röfo* **99**, 467.

BEUREN, A. J. (1966) *Die angiokardiographische Darstellung kongenitaler Herzfehler.* W. de Gruyter, Berlin.

BÖTTGER, E., SCHLICHT, I., BRANDS, W. and GRAJALES, R. (1972) Doppelung der Vena cava inferior — angiographischer Nachweis einer seltenen Anomalie. *Röfo* **117**, 521.

BÜCHELER, E., DÜX, A. and SOBBE, A. (1968) Die renolumbale Anastomose im direkten retroperitonealen Veno- und selektiven Azygogramm. *Röfo* **109**, 712.

BÜCHELER, E., DÜX, A. and THURN, P. (1966) Membranöser Verschluß und Agenesie der Vena cava inferior. *Röfo* **105**, 806.

BÜCHELER, E., DÜX, A. and THURN, P. (1967) Die Röntgendiagnostik der Nierenvenenthrombose. *Röfo* **106**, 800.

CARON, M. M. J. and RIBET, M. (1964) Phlébographie rénale sélective et anastomoses splénorénales. *Arch. Mal. Appar. dig.* **53**, 41.

CLEGG, E. J. (1970) The terminations of the left testicular and adrenal veins in man. *Fertil. and Steril.* **21**, 36.

COLBORN, G. L. (1964) A case of bilateral inferior vena cava joined only at the iliac anastomosis. *J. Urol.* **91**, 478.

DOEHNER, G. A. (1968) The hepatic venous system. *Radiology* **90**, 1119.

DOS SANTOS, R. (1935) Phlébographie d'une veine cave suturée. *J. Urol.* **39**, 585.

EDWARDS, E. A. (1951) Clinical anatomy of lesser variations of the inferior vena cava, and a proposal for classifying the anomalies of the vessel. *Angiology* **2**, 85.

ELIAS, H. (1963) Anatomy of the liver (in: *The Liver.* Ed. by Rouiler, Ch.). Academic Press, New York — London.

FUCHS, W. A. (1964) Vena cava inferior (in: *Handbuch der medizinischen Radiologie,* vol. 10/3. Ed. by Diethelm, L., Olsson, O., Strnad, F., Vieten, H. and Zuppinger, A.). Springer, Berlin — Göttingen — Heidelberg — New York.

GAGNON, R. (1956) The venous drainage of the human adrenal gland. *Rev. canad. Biol.* **14,** 350.

GANSAU, H. (1955) Retrograde Füllung der Beckenvenen durch perkutane Punction der Vena cava inferior. *Chirurg* **26,** 375.

GILLOT, C. and GALLEGOS, A. (1966) Anatomie topographique des veines rénales chez l'homme. *C. R. Ass. Anat.* **135,** 429.

GLADSTONE, R. J. (1929) Development of inferior vena cava in light of recent research. *J. Anat. (Lond.)* **64,** 70.

GŐSFAY, S. (1959) Untersuchungen der Vena spermatica interna durch retrograde Phlebographie bei Kranken mit Varikozele. *Z. Urol.* **52,** 105.

GRYSKA, P. R. and EARTHROWL, F. H. (1967) Left-sided inferior vena cava. *Arch. Surg.* **94,** 363.

HELANDER, C. G. and LINDBOM, A. (1959) Venography of the inferior vena cava. *Acta radiol. (Stockh.)* **52,** 257.

HIRSCH, D. M. and CHAN, K. F. (1963) Bilateral inferior vena cava. *J. Amer. med. Ass.* **185,** 729.

JACOBS, J. B. (1969) Selective gonadal venography. *Radiology* **92,** 885.

KNOPP, J. (1953) Ein Verfahren zur Abgrenzung der Stromgebiete großer intrahepatischer Gefäße. *Virchows Arch. path. Anat.* **323,** 563.

KOGUERMAN-LEPP, E. P. (1968) Hepatic veins and venous blood outflow from liver segments in man. *Arkh. Anat. Gistol. Embriol.* **55,** 105.

LEMAITRE, G., TOISON, G., DEFRANCE, G. and MAZEMAN, E. (1963) Deux observations d'uretère rétrocave. *J. Radiol. Électrol.* **44,** 332.

MERKLIN, R. J. and MICHELS, N. A. (1958) The variant renal and suprarenal blood supply with data on the inferior phrenic, ureteral and gonadal arteries. *J. int. Coll. Surg.* **29,** 41.

O'LOUGHLIN, B. J. *The inferior vena cava* (cit. by Abrams, H. L. 1961).

ORTMANN, R. (1968) Über Bedeutung, Häufigkeit und Variationsbild der linken retroaortalen Nierenvene. *Z. Anat. Entwickl.-Gesch.* **127,** 346.

PACOFSKY, K. B. and WOLFEL, D. A. (1971) Azygos continuation of the inferior vena cava. *Amer. J. Roentgenol.* **113,** 362.

PETERSEN, R. V. (1965) Intrahepatic interruption of the inferior vena cava with azygos continuation (Persistent right cardinal vein). *Radiology* **84,** 304.

RAPPAPORT, A. M. (1951) Hepatic venography. *Acta radiol. (Stockh.)* **36,** 165.

REUTER, S. R., BLAIR, A. J., SCHTEINGART, D. E. and BOOKSTEIN, J. J. (1967) Adrenal venography. *Radiology* **89,** 805.

RIGAUD, A., SENTENAE, J. and SENEGAS, J. (1962) Essai de systématisation de la circulation veineuse sus-hépatique extraparenchymateuse du foie en fonction de la forme et de l'orientation de ce viscère. *Bull. Ass. Anat. (Nancy)* **48,** 1161.

SCAVO, E. (1963) Sulla reale esistenza nell'uomo di sistemi sfinterici in corrispondenza dello sbocco delle vene epatiche. *Anat. e Chir.* **8,** 369.

STACKELBERG, B., LIND, J. and WEGELIUS, C. (1952) Absence of the inferior vena cava diagnosed by angiocardiography. *Cardiologia (Basel)* **21,** 583.

STARER, E. (1965) Percutaneous suprarenal venography. *Brit. J. Radiol.* **38,** 675.

STOLIC, E. and MRVALJEVIC, D. (1971) Les anastomoses intra-rénales des veines rénales chez l'homme. *C. R. Ass. Anal.* **146,** 632.

STUCKE, K. (1959) *Leberchirurgie.* Springer, Berlin — Göttingen — Heidelberg.

SURRINGTON, C. T. and JONAS, A. F., jr. (1952) Intraabdominal venography following inferior vena cava ligation. *Arch. Surg.* **65,** 605.

UNGVÁRY, GY. and FALLER, J. (1963) Vena-hepatica-Lappen in der Leber. *Zbl. Chir.* **88,** 1885.

System of the portal vein

ABEATICI, S. and CAMPI, L. (1951) La visualizzazione radiologica della porta per via splenica (Nota preventiva). *Minerva med.* **42,** 593.

BAYLY, J. H. and GONZALEZ, O. C. (1964) The umbilical vein in the adult: Diagnosis, treatment and research. *Amer. Surg.* **30,** 56.

BERGSTRAND, I. (1957) Roentgen anatomy of the intrahepatic portal rcmification. *Kgl. Fys. Sällsk. Lund Förh.* **27,** 85.

BERGSTRAND, I. (1964) Das Pfortadergebiet (in: *Handbuch der medizinischen Radiologie,* vol. 10/3. Ed. by Diethelm, L., Olsson, O., Strnad, F., Vieten, H. and Zuppinger, A.). Springer, Berlin — Göttingen — Heidelberg — NewYork.

BRAUS, H. and ELZE, C. (1956) *Anatomie des Menschen,* vol. 2. Springer, Berlin.

COUINAUD, C. (1957) *La foie.* Masson, Paris.

CRONQUIST, S. and RANNIGER, P. (1965) Spontaneous splenorenal shunts. *Acta radiol. (Stockh.)* **3,** 433.

DOEHNER, G. A., RUZICKA, F. F., HOFFMAN, G. and ROUSELOT, L. M. (1955) The portal venous system: Its roentgen-anatomy. *Radiology* **64,** 675.

DÜX, A., THURN, P. and SCHREIBER, H. W. (1962a) Der Kollateralkreislauf bei intra- und extrahepatischem Block im Serien-Splenoportogramm. *Röfo* **97,** 255.

DÜX, A., THURN, P., SCHREIBER, H. W. and BROICHER, H. (1962b) Die spontane splenorenale Anastomose im Splenoportogramm. *Röfo* **97,** 1.

EDWARDS, E. A. (1951a) Clinical anatomy of the lesser varieties of the inferior vena cava. *Angiology* **2,** 85.

EDWARDS, E. A. (1951b) Functional anatomy of the portasystematic communications. *Arch. intern. Med.* **88,** 137.

ELIAS, H. and PETTY, D. (1952) Gross anatomy of the blood vessels and ducts within the human liver. *Amer. J. Anat.* **90,** 52.

ENDER, L. A., OBMORNOV, L. E. and GOLUBKOVA, G. M. (1971) Certain normal variants and developmental anomalies of the splenoportal trunk. *Vestn. Rentg. Radiol.* **46,** 59.

GILLOT, C., HUREAU, J., AARON, C., MARTINI, R. and THALER, G. (1964) The superior mesenteric vein. *J. int. Coll. Surg.* **41,** 339.

GRÜNERT, R. D. (1960) *Chirurg* **31,** 534 (cit. by Düx, A., Thurn, P. and Schreiber, H. W. 1962a).

GUNTZ, M. and FARISSE, J. (1966) Les anastomoses intrahépatiques des branches de la veine porte. *Bull. Ass. Anat. (Nancy)* **51,** 471.

GVOZDANOVIĆ, V. and HAUPTMANN, E. (1955) Further experience with percutaneous lieno-portal venography. *Acta radiol. (Stockh.)* **43,** 177.

HABIGHORST, L. V., ALBERS, P. and ZEITLER, E. (1965) Die Gefäße der Gallenblase im postmortalen Angiogramm. *Röfo* **103,** 63.

HACH, W. (1971) Kollateralkreislauf beim Verschluss der V. cava inferior und der Beckenvenen. *Med. Klin.* **66**, 1574.

HEALEY, J. E. (1954) Clinical and anatomic aspects of radical hepatic surgery. *J. int. Coll. Surg.* **22**, 542.

HJORSTJÖ, C. H. (1948) Die Anatomie der intrahepatischen Gallengänge beim Menschen mittels Röntgen- und Injektionstechnik studiert. *Acta Univ. lund. N. S. II,* **44**, 3.

ILLARIONOVA, L. T. (1966) Veins of the human large intestine and their relation to the arteries. *Vop. Khir. Zheludochn. Kishechn. Trakta* **16**, [rep. Excerpta med. (Amst.), Sect. I 21 (1967) 277].

KIKKAWA, F. (1966) The segmental distribution of the trabecular veins in man. *Acta Anat. Nippon* **41**, 232.

KNIGHT, H. O. (1921) An anomalous portal vein with its surgical dangers. *Ann. Surg.* **74**, 697.

LEGER, L. (1955) *Splénoportographie.* Masson, Paris.

MAURER, H. J. (1964) Untersuchungen über Kollateralbahnen des lieno-portalen Systems. *Röntgen-Bl.* **17**, 509.

McINDOE, A. H. (1928) Vascular lesions of portal cirrhosis. *Arch. Path.* **5**, 23.

MYKING, A. O. and HALVORSEN, J. F. (1971) The cystic vein as a bypass in portal vein thrombosis. *Acta chir. scand.* **137**, 587.

PARCHWITZ, K. H. (1961) Das Röntgenbild der Magenvarizen. Diagnose und Differentialdiagnose. Thesis. Bonn.

PFUHL, W. (1932) (in: *Handbuch der mikroskopischen Anatomie des Menschen,* vol. V, pt 2. Ed. by Möllendorff, W.). Springer, Berlin.

PICCONE, V. A., LEVEEN, H. H., WHITE, J. J., SKINNER, G. B. and MACLEAN, L. D. (1967) Transumbical portal hepatography, a significant adjunct in the investigation of liver disease. *Surgery* **61**, 333.

PICK, L. (1909) Über totale hämangiomatöse Obliteration des Pfortaderstammes und über hepatopetale Kollateralbahnen. *Virchows Arch. path. Anat.* **197**, 490.

RÖSCH, J. (1962) Splenoportographie im Kindesalter. *Röfo* **96**, 61.

RÖSCH, J. (1964) Splenoportographie (in: *Ergebnisse der medizinischen Strahlenforschung,* vol. 1. Ed. by Schinz, H. R., Glauner, R. and Rüttmann, A.). Thieme, Stuttgart.

ROUSSELOT, L. M., RUZICKA, F. F. and DOEHNER, G. A. (1953) Portal venography via the portal and percutaneous splenic routes. *Surgery* **34**, 557.

SCHOENMACKERS, J. and VIETEN, H. (1953) Porto-cavale und porto-pulmonale Anastomosen im postmortalen Angiogramm. *Röfo* **79**, 488.

SCHOENMACKERS, J. and VIETEN, H. (1964) Postmortale Angiogramme des Pfortadergebietes (in: *Handbuch der medizinischen Radiologie,* vol. 10/1. Ed. by Diethelm, L., Olsson, O., Strnad, F., Vieten, H. and Zuppinger, A.). Springer, Berlin—Göttingen—Heidelberg—New York.

SHRYOCK, E. H., JANZEN, J. and BARNARD, M. C. (1942) Report of a newborn human presenting sympus dipus, anomalous umbilical vein transposition of the viscera and other anomalies. *Anat. Rec.* **82**, 347.

STAUBER, R. (1965) Ein seltener Fall von Doppelung der Pfortader. *Zbl. Chir.* **90**, 1896.

WALCKER, F. J. (1922) Beiträge zur kollateralen Blutzirkulation im Pfortadersystem. *Langenbecks Arch. Klin. Chir.* **120**, 819.

ZIELKE, K. (1962) Beitrag zur Frage von Verlauf und Mündungsgebiet der Gallenblasenvenen. *Acta hepatosplenol. (Stuttg.)* **9**, 33.

The common iliac artery and its branches

BELLMANN, G. and HERWIG, H. (1964) *Die Aortographie in der angiologischen Diagnostik.* Thieme, Leipzig.

BOIJSEN, E. and NILSSON, J. (1962) Angiography in the diagnosis of tumors of the urinary bladder. *Acta radiol. (Stockh.)* **57**, 241.

BRAEDEL, H. U. (1961) Arteriographischer Nachweis einer Gefäßanomalie des rechten Beines. *Röfo* **95**, 412.

BROOKS, V. (1924) Intra-arterial injection of sodium iodide. *J. Amer. med. Ass.* **82**, 1016.

BÜCHELER, E. and THURN, P. (1964) Zur Methodik der Blasenarteriographie. *Röfo* **101**, 238.

CARRIER, CH., MATTEAU, P. and JEAN, C. (1966) Aplasie d'une artère ombilicale. *J. Canad. med. Ass.* **94**, 1001.

DEHALLEUX, J. M., MULLER, G. and RITTER, J. (1966) Anomalie funiculaire: l'absence d'une artère ombilicale. *Recipe (Louvain)* **6**, 293.

DE LUCA, C. and DE SERIO, N. (1961): Studi di anatomia radiologica angiografica sul vivente. *Radiol. med. (Torino)* **47**, 1074.

DE LUCA, C. and DE SERIO, N. (1962a) Studi di anatomia radiologica angiografica sul vivente. *Radiol med. (Torino)* **48**, 222.

DE LUCA, C. and DE SERIO, N. (1962b) Studi di anatomia radiologica angiografica sul vivente. *Radiol. med. (Torino)* **48**, 886.

DIMTZA, A. and JÄGER, W. (1938) Zur Technik der Arteriographie der unteren Extremitäten. *Zbl. Chir.* **1**, 355.

DOS SANTOS, R., LAMAS, A. C. and CALDAS, J. P. (1929) L'artériographie des membres de l'aorte et de ses branches abdominales. *Bull. Soc. Chirurgie Paris* **55**, 587.

FERNSTRÖM, I. (1955) Arteriography of the uterine artery. *Acta radiol. (Stockh.) Suppl.* **122**.

FERRANTE, G., GIAMPAGLIA, F. and LEONE, F. (1967) Sulle anomalie di divisione delle arterie dell'arto inferiore. *Rif. Med.* **33**, 1.

FONTAINE, R. (1937) L'artériographie des membres. *J. int. Chir.* **2**, 559.

GARUSI, G. F. (1968) Étude artériographique du pied chez le sujet normal. *J. Rad. Électrol.* **49**, 15.

GESENIUS, H. (1949) Oscillographie und Arteriographie. *Dtsch. med. Wschr.* **74**, 1.

GOLLMANN, G. (1957) Eine Modifizierung der Seldingerschen Kathetermethode zur isolierten Kontrastfüllung der Aortenäste. *Röfo* **87**, 211.

GYURKÓ, GY. and SZABÓ, M. (1968) Adatok az emberi artériás rendszer nagyobb értörzseinek méreteire vonatkozóan (Data concerning the dimensions of the larger trunks of the human arterial system). *Magy. Sebész* **21**, 276.

HARSÁNYI, L. (1951) Az arteria és vena epigastrica inferior topográfiája a haspunkció szempontjából (Topography of the inferior epigastric artery and vein from the aspect of abdominal puncture). *Orv. Hetil.* **92**, 1303.

JASCHTSCHINSKI, S. N. (1891) Die typischen Verzweigungsformen der Arteria hypogastrica. *Int. Mschr. Anat. Physiol.* **8**, 111.

KELEMEN, J., KELENHEGYI, M. and HORVÁTH, GY. (1965) Retrograd arteriographia a hólyagdaganatok diagnosztikájában (Retrograde arteriography in the diagnostic of the tumours of the bladder). *Magy. Radiol.* **17**, 214.

KRASEMANN, P. H. (1972) Doppelte Arteria femoralis. *Röfo* **117**, 220.

LANZ, T. and WACHSMUTH, W. (1938) *Praktische Anatomie,* vol. 1/4. Springer, Berlin.

LÉRICHE, R. (1935) Sur la bénignité des artériographies au thorotrast. *Bull. Soc. Chirurgie Paris* **61**, 175.

LÉRICHE, R. (1940) De la résection du carrefour aortic-iliaque avec double sympathectomie lombaire pour thrombose artérique de l'aorte. *Presse méd.* **48**, 601.

LINDBOM, Å. (1952) Angiographie (in: *Lehrbuch der Röntgendiagnostik*, vol. 2. Ed. by Schinz, H. R., Baensch, W. E., Friedl, E. and Uehlinger, E.). Thieme, Stuttgart.

LOOSE, K. E. (1953) Die Bedeutung der Serienaortographie für die Gefäßdiagnostik des Beckens und der Nieren. *Radiol. clin. (Basel)* **23**, 325.

LOOSE, K. E. (1957) Aortographische Diagnostik. Indikation and Ergebnis. In: 74. *Tagung der Deutschen Gesellschaft für Chirurgie*, München.

MALCHIODI, L. and RUBERTI, U. (1957) Osservazioni anatomoradiologiche sulle anomalie congenite delle arterie dell'arto inferiore (dall'analisti di 650 arteriografie femorali). *Minerva Cardioangiol.* **5**, 297.

MANNERS-SMITH, T. (1912) The limb arteries of primates. *J. Anat. Physiol.* **46**, 95.

MARANTA, E., CAMPONOVO, F. and DEL BUONO, M. S. (1964) Die Beckenangiographie. *Röfo* **101**, 229.

MARTINEZ, L. O., JUDE, J. and BECKER, D. (1968) Bilateral persistent sciatic artery. A case report. *Angiology* **19**, 541.

MICHELS, N. A., SIDDHARTH, P., KORNBLITH, P. L. and PARKE, W. W. (1965) The variant blood supply to the descending colon, rectosigmoid and rectum based on 400 dissections. *Dis. Colon Rect.* **8**, 251.

MORRIS, G. C., BEALL, A. C., jr., BEARRY, W. B., FESTE, J. and DE BAKEY, M. E. (1960) *Surg. Forum* **10**, 498 (cit. by Pässler, H. W. and Pässler, H. H. 1963).

MÜLLER, J. H. A. (1967) Doppelung der Arteria femoralis. *Röfo* **106**, 152.

MÜSSBICHLER, H. (1971) Arteriographic investigations of the normal hip in adults. Evaluation of methods and vascular findings. *Acta radiol. (Stockh.)* **11**, 195.

ÖDMAN, P. (1956) Percutaneous selective angiography of the main branches of the aorta. *Acta radiol. (Stockh.)* **45**, 1.

OLOVSON, T. (1941) Beitrag zur Kenntnis der Verbindungen zwischen A. ilica interna und A. femoralis beim Menschen. *Acta chir. scand. Suppl.* **67**.

ORLANDI, G., PAVLICA, P., DAMELE, C. and TONELLI, B. (1968) Studio arteriografico dei circoli collaterali nelle obliterazioni dei iliaci e femorali. *Radiol. med. (Torino)* **54**, 1130.

PÄSSLER, H. W. (1952) *Die Angiographie zur Erkennung, Behandlung und Begutachtung peripherer Durchblutungsstörungen.* Thieme, Stuttgart.

PÄSSLER, H. W. (1957) Unsere Technik der automatischen Serienaortographie. *Röntgen-Bl.* **10**, 73.

PÄSSLER, H. W. (1958) *Begutachtung peripherer Durchblutungsstörungen.* Thieme, Stuttgart.

PÄSSLER, H. W. and PÄSSLER, H. H. (1963) Der Verlauf der Stammarterien im Bereich des Kniegelenkes und des Fußgelenkes. *Röntgen-Bl.* **16**, 177.

PERNKOPF, E. (1922) Über einen Fall von beiderseitiger Persistenz der Arteria ischiadica. *Anat. Anz.* **55**, 536.

PIRKER, E. and SCHMIDBERGER, H. (1972) Die Arteria ischiadica. Eine seltene Gefässvariante. *Röfo* **116**, 434.

RATSCHOW, M. (1937) Leistung und Bedeutung der Vasographie als Funktionsprüfung der peripheren Blutgefäße. *Röfo* **55**, 253.

RATSCHOW, M. (1959) *Angiologie.* Thieme, Stuttgart.

REICH, W. J. and NECHTOW, M. J. (1964) The iliac arteries. *J. int. Coll. Surg.* **41**, 53.

ROBERTS, W. H. and KRISHINGER, G. (1967) Comparative study of human internal iliac artery based on Adachi's classification. *Anat. Rec.* **158**, 191.

SGALITZER, M., DEMEL, R., KOLLERT, V. and RANZENHOFER, H. (1930) Darstellung und Behandlung der Erkrankungen peripherer Arterien. *Wien. klin. Wschr.* **2**, 833.

SHEHATA, R. (1964) The arterial supply of the urinary bladder. *J. Egypt. med. Ass.* **47**, 254.

VOELKER, F. and BOENINGHAUS, H. (1926) Anatomie und chirurgische Operationslehre der Blase (in: *Handbuch der Urologie.* Ed. by Lichtenberg, A., Voelker, F. and Wildbolz, H.). Springer, Berlin.

WELLAUER, J. (1957) Arteriographie der Extremitäten (in: *Lehrbuch der Röntgendiagnostik, Ergebnisse* 1952/56. Ed. by Schinz, H. R., Glauner, R. and Uehlinger, F. E.). Thieme, Stuttgart.

The common iliac vein and its branches

ABESHOUSE, B. S. and RUBEN, M. E. (1952) Prostatic and periprostatic phlebography. *J. Urol.* **68**, 640.

ALMÉN, T. and NYLANDER, G. (1962) Serial phlebography of the normal lower leg during muscular contraction and relaxation. *Acta radiol. (Stockh.)* **57**, 264.

ARNOLDI, C. C. (1961) A comparison between the phlebographic picture as seen in dynamic intraosseous phlebography and the clinical signs and symptoms of chronic venous insufficiency. *J. cardiovasc. Surg. (Torino)* **2**, 184.

BARBER, T. H. T. and ORLEY, A. (1932) Some X-ray observations in varicose disease of the leg. *Lancet.* **2**, 175.

BASMAJIAN, J. V. (1952) The distribution of valves in the femoral external iliac, and common iliac veins and their relationship to varicose veins. *Surg. Gynec. Obstet.* **95**, 537.

BERBERICH, J. and HIRSCH, S. (1923) Die röntgenologische Darstellung der Arterien und Venen am lebenden Menschen. *Klin. Wschr.* **2**, 2226.

BÉTOULIÈRES, P., CHAPTAL, G., THÉVENET, A., VIALLA, M. and BONNET, H. (1959) Un cas d'agénésie de la veine cave inférieure et des veines iliaques primitives. *J. Radiol. Électrol.* **40**, 810.

BRAUS, H. and ELZE, C. (1956) *Anatomie des Menschen.* Springer, Berlin.

CHARPY, A. and HOVELACQUE, A. (1920) Veines en particulier (in: *Traité d'anatomie humaine*, vol. 2/3. Ed. by Poirier, P. and Charpy, A.). Masson, Paris.

COCKETT, F. B. (1955) The pathology and treatment of venous ulcers of the leg. *Brit. J. Surg.* **179**, 260.

DE LA PENA, A. (1956) Flebografia de plexos y vasos pelvianos en el vivo. *Rev. esp. de Chirurg. Traum. Ortop.* **4**, 245.

DELORME, G., TAVERNIER, J., CAILLÉ, J. M., TESSIER, J. P. and LANGE, D. (1968) La phlébographie de l'utérus par la technique d'injection rétrograde de l'utéro-ovarienne gauche. *Ann. Radiol.* **11**, 11.

DOS SANTOS, I. G. (1938) Direct venography: conception, technic, first results. *J. Internat. Chir.* **3**, 625.

DRASNAR, V. (1946) Intraspongiöse Dauertropfinfusion. *Schweiz. med. Wschr.* **76**, 36.

FINE, I., FRANK, H. A. and STARR, A. (1942) Recent experiences with thrombophlebitis of the lower extremity and pulmonary embolism; value of venography as a diagnostic aid. *Ann. Surg.* **116**, 574.

GREITZ, T. (1955) Phlebography of the normal leg. *Acta radiol. (Stockh.)* **44**, 1.

GULLMO, A. (1957) Om flebografi. *Svenska Lök.-Tidn.* **54**, 3461.

GULLMO, A. (1959) Les localisations anatomiques de l'insuffisance veineuse des membres inférieurs. *Bull. Soc. franç. Phlébol.* **12**, 343.

GULLMO, A. (1964) Periphere Venen (in: *Handbuch der medizinischen Radiologie*, vol. 10/3. Ed. by Diethelm, L., Olsson, O., Strnad, F., Vieten, H. and Zuppinger, A.). Springer, Berlin – Göttingen – Heidelberg – New York.

KÜGELEN, A. (1951) Über den Wandbau der großen Venen. *Morph. Jb.* **91**, 447.

LEGER, L. and MASSE, P. (1951) La phlébographie transspongiocalcanéenne. *Presse méd.* **59**, 1560.

LIECHTI, A. (1948) *Die Röntgenuntersuchung der Wirbelsäule und ihre Grundlagen.* Springer, Wien.

LIMBORGH, J. (1963) La nomenclature des veines communicantes de l'extrémité inférieure. Rapport du Comité de Nomenclature de la Société Beneluxienne de Phlébologie (cit. by May, R. and Nissl, R. 1966).

LIMBORGH, J., BANGA, D. A., MEIJERINK, C. J. H. and LUIGIESI, H. H. (1962) De venae communicantes van het been. *Ned. T. Geneesk.* **106**, 415.

LINDBLOM, K. (1941) Phlebographische Untersuchungen des Unterschenkels bei Kontrastinjektion in eine subkutane Vene. *Acta radiol. (Stockh.)* **22**, 288.

LINTON, R. R. (1938) The communicating veins of the lower leg and the operative technique for their ligation. *Ann. Surg.* **107**, 582.

LUKE, J. C. (1951) The deep vein valves. *Surgery* **29**, 381.

LUZSA, GY. (1959/60) A venographia jelentősége a postthromboticus syndroma diagnosisában (Importance of venography in the diagnosis of postthrombotic syndrome). *Győr-Sopr. Megy. Tan. Kórh. Közl.* **2**, 251.

MARTINET, J. D. (1959) Die retrograde Phlebographie (in: *Die Phlebographie der unteren Extremität.* Ed. by May, R. and Nissl, R.). Thieme, Stuttgart.

MAVOR, G. E. and GALLOWAY, J. (1967) Collaterals of the deep venous circulation of the lower limb. *Surg. Gynec. Obstet.* **125**, 561.

MAY, R. and NISSL, R. (1959) *Die Phlebographie der unteren Extremität.* Thieme, Stuttgart.

MAY, R. and NISSL, R. (1966) Phlebographische Studien zur Anatomie der Beinvenen. *Röfo* **104**, 171.

MAY, R. and NISSL, R. (1968) Phlebographische Studien über die Venen der Kniekehle und der Wade. *Röfo* **109**, 614.

MAY, R. and NISSL, R. (1971) Aplasie der Vena femoralis communis ohne Begleitmissbildungen. *Röfo* **114**, 715.

MAY, R. and NISSL, R. (1973) Anormale Einmündung der Vena hypogastrica dextra. *Röfo* **118**, 224.

MOLNÁR, J. and HAJÓS, E. (1960) Kavernosogramme. *Z. Urol.* **53**, 441.

NETZER, C. O. (1958) Die normale und krankhaft veränderte Venenströmung in den unteren Gliedmaßen. Thesis. München.

OLIVIER, CL. (1957) *Maladies des veines.* Masson, Paris.

PETKOVIČ, S. (1953) Darstellung der Beckenvenen durch verschiedene Wege. *Röfo* **79**, 739.

PIRNER, R. (1956) Über die Bedeutung, Form und Art der Klappen in den Venae communicantes der unteren Extremitäten. *Anat. Anz.* **103**, 450.

RAIVIO, E. V. L. (1948) Untersuchungen über die Venen der unteren Extremitäten mit besonderer Berücksichtigung der gegenseitigen Venenverbindungen zwischen oberflächlichen und tiefen Venen. *Ann. Med. exp. Fenn.* *Suppl.* **4**, 26.

RATSCHOW, M. (1930) Uroselektan in der Vasographie unter spezieller Berücksichtigung der Varicographie. *Röfo* **42**, 37.

SCHLÜSSLER, R., HEINEN, G. and BETTE, L. (1966) Die röntgenkinematographische Darstellung der weiblichen Beckengefäße (in: *Angiographie.* Ed. by Loose, K. E and Fischer, A. W.). Thieme, Stuttgart.

SERVELLE, M. (1952) *Pathologie vasculaire.* Masson, Paris.

STAUBESAND, J. (1959) Funktionelle Morphologie der Arterien, Venen und arterio-venösen Anastomosen (in: *Angiologie.* Ed. by Ratschow, M.). Thieme, Stuttgart.

THOMAS, M. L., FLETSCHER, E. W. L., COCKETT, F. B. and NEGUS, D. (1967) Venous collaterals in external and common iliac vein obstruction. *Clin. Radiol.* **18**, 403.

TONITZA, P., TĂNASE, V., RUSU, M., BURDESCU, C., MOLDOVEANU, N. and FRUJINA, V. (1967) Agenezie de trunchiuri venoase profunde ale membrelor inferioare. *Viata med.* **14**, 1325.

VAS, GY. and KERPEL, M. (1954) Osteomedullaris phlebographia (Osteomedullary phlebography). *Magy. Sebész.* **4**, 280.

ZSEBŐK, Z., GERGELY, M. and CSILLAG, T. (1957) Intraspongiosus funkcionális venoscopia, venographia (Intraspongious functional venoscopy, venography). *Magy. Radiol.* **9**, 78.

Radiographic morphology of neonatal circulation

BAYLY, J. H. and GONZALEZ, O. C. (1964) The umbilical vein in the adult. *Amer. Surg.* **30**, 56.

DEHALLEUX, J. M., MULLER, G. and RITTER, J. (1966) Anomalie funiculaire: l'absence d'une artère ombilicale. *Recipe (Louvain)* **25**, 293.

EMMANOUILLIDES, G. C. and REIN, B. I. (1964) Abdominal aortography via the umbilical artery in newborn infant. *Radiology* **82**, 447.

HARANGHY, L. (1966) *A kórbonctan elemei* (Elements of pathological anatomy). Medicina Kiadó, Budapest.

HIRVONEN, L., PELTONEN, T. and RUOKA, M. (1961) Angiocardiography of the newborn with contrast injected into the umbilical vein. *Ann. Paediat. Fenn.* **7**, 124.

KAUFFMANN, H. J. and WEISSER, K. (1963) Die transumbilicale Aortographie und selective Arteriographie im Neugeborenenalter. *Röfo* **98**, 699.

AUTHOR INDEX

375

SUBJECT INDEX

383